Measures for Children with Developmental Disabilities

An ICF-CY Approach

Edited by

ANNETTE MAJNEMER
Director and Associate Dean, School of Physical and Occupational Therapy,
Faculty of Medicine, McGill University, Montreal, Quebec, Canada

2012

MAC KEITH PRESS

© 2012 Mac Keith Press
6 Market Road, London N7 9PW

Editor: Hilary M Hart
Managing Director: Ann-Marie Halligan
Production Manager: Udoka Ohuonu
Project Management: Prepress Projects Ltd

First published in this edition 2012

British Library Cataloguing-in-Publication data
A catalogue record for this book is available from the British Library

ISBN: 978-1-908316-45-5

Typeset by Prepress Projects Ltd, Perth, UK
Printed by Latimer Trend & Company, Plymouth, Devon, UK

Mac Keith Press is supported by Scope

CONTENTS

AUTHORS' APPOINTMENTS

Margareta Adolfsson   Affiliated researcher, CHILD, School of Education and Communication, Jonkoping University; the Swedish Institute for Disability Research, Jonkoping, Sweden

Sacha N. Bailey   Doctoral Candidate, School of Social Work, Centre for Research on Children and Families, McGill University, Montreal, Quebec, Canada

Gary Bedell   Associate Professor, Department of Occupational Therapy, Tufts University, Medford, MA, USA

Erna Imperatore Blanche   Associate Professor of Clinical Occupational Therapy, Division of Occupational Science and Occupational Therapy at the Ostrow School of Dentistry, University of Southern California, Los Angeles, CA, USA

Aline Bogossian   Doctoral Candidate, School of Social Work, Centre for Research for Children and Families, McGill University, Montreal, Quebec, Canada

Andrea R. Burch   Director of Special Academic Services at Alfred University, Alfred, NY, USA

Chantel C. Burkitt   Department of Educational Psychology, University of Minnesota, Minneapolis, USA

Patricia A. Burtner   Professor Emeritus, Occupational Therapy Graduate Program, University of New Mexico, Albuquerque, NM, USA

Katie Byford-Richardson   Research Assistant, School of Social Work, McGill University, Montreal, Quebec, Canada

Susana Castro   Faculty of Psychology and Educational Sciences, Porto University

Christine T. Chambers   Canada Research Chair in Pain and Child Health; Professor of Pediatrics and Psychology, Dalhousie University, Halifax, Nova Scotia, Canada

Emily B.J. Coffey   Montreal Neurological Institute, McGill University, Montreal, Quebec, Canada

Allan Colver   Professor of Community Child Health, Newcastle University, Newcastle, UK

Kim M. Cornish
Professor of Psychology, School of Psychology and Psychiatry, Monash University, Melbourne, Australia

Wendy J. Coster
Professor, Department of Occupational Therapy, Boston University, Boston, MA, USA

Martha Cousins
CanChild Centre for Childhood Disability Research, McMaster University, Hamilton, ON, Canada

Noemi Dahan-Oliel
Doctoral Student, School of Physical and Occupational Therapy, McGill University and McGill University Health Centre – Montreal Children's Hospital, Montreal, Quebec, Canada

Vasiliki Darsaklis
School of Physical & Occupational Therapy, McGill University, Montreal, Canada

Marina Dupasquier
PhD student, Department of Educational and Counselling Psychology, McGill University, Montreal, Canada

Kirsten M. Ellingsen
Postdoctoral Fellow in Pediatric Psychology, early childhood focus, Nemours, Alfred I duPont Hospital for Children, Wilmington, DE, USA

Nora Fayed
Department of Pediatrics, McMaster University, Hamilton, ON, Canada

Debbie Feldman
Professor, Université de Montréal, Faculty of Medicine, School of Rehabilitation; Researcher, Research Institute of Public Health of Université de Montréal and Centre for Interdisciplinary Research in Rehabilitation of Greater Montreal, Quebec, Canada

Frances Page Glascoe
Professor of Paediatrics, Vanderbilt University, Mertztown, Pennsylvania, USA

Reut Gruber
Department of Psychiatry, McGill University, Douglas Mental Health University Institute, Verdun, Quebec, Canada

Dennis C. Harper
Professor, Emeritus Lindquist Center, Department of Teaching and Learning, Center for Distabilities and Development, Colleges of Medicine, Education, Public Health, The University of Iowa, Iowa City, IA, USA

Diane Jacobs
Lecturer in Speech Pathology, La Trobe University, Melbourne, Australia

Celeste Johnston
Professor, School of Nursing, McGill University, Montreal, Canada

Mary A. Khetani
Assistant Professor, Department of Occupational Therapy, Colorado State University, Fort Collins, CO, USA

Sara King
Assistant Professor of Education (School Psychology), Mount Saint Vincent University, Halifax, Nova Scotia, Canada

Anne Klassen
Associate Professor, Department of Pediatrics, McMaster University, Hamilton, ON, Canada

Lucyna M. Lach
Associate Professor, School of Social Work, Centre for Research on Children and Families, McGill University, Montreal, Quebec, Canada

Mary Law
School of Rehabilitation Science, McMaster University, Hamilton, Canada

Andrea Lee	Psychologist, WakeMed Health and Hospitals, Raleigh, NC, USA; formerly doctoral student at University of North Carolina at Chapel Hill, NC, USA
Shannon Lewis	University of North Carolina at Chapel Hill
Catherine Limperopoulos	Director, MRI Research of the Developing Brain; Director, Advanced Pediatric Brain Imaging Research Laboratory, Diagnostic Imaging and Radiology/Fetal and Transitional Medicine, Children's National Medical Center; Associate Professor of Neurology, Radiology, and Pediatrics, George Washington University School of Medicine and Health Sciences, Washington, DC, USA
Elspeth McCartney	Speech and Language Therapy Division, University of Strathclyde, Glasgow, UK
Jane McCormack	Lecturer in Speech Pathology, Charles Stuart University, Albury, Australia
Sharynne McLeod	Professor in Speech and Language Acquisition, Charles Stuart University, Bathurst, Australia
Zoe Mailloux	Private practice, Redondo Beach, CA, USA
Annette Majnemer	Professor and Director, School of Physical and Occupational Therapy, McGill University, Montreal, Canada
Désirée B. Maltais	Assistant Professor, Department of Rehabilitation, Université Laval; Researcher, Centre for Interdisciplinary Research in Rehabilitation and Social Integration, Québec City, Canada
Kevin P. Marks	General Paediatrician and Clinical Assistant Professor, PeaceHealth Medical Group, Eugene, Oregon; Oregon Health & Science University School of Medicine, Department of Paediatrics, Division of General Paediatrics, Portland, Oregon
Barbara Mazer	Assistant Professor, School of Physical and Occupational Therapy, McGill University, Montreal; Research Associate, Centre for Interdisciplinary Research in Rehabilitation of Greater Montreal – Jewish Rehabilitation Hospital, Laval, Quebec, Canada
Kylee Miller	School of Education, University of North Carolina at Chapel Hill, NC, USA
Christopher Morris	Senior Research Fellow in Child Health, Peninsula Cerebra Research Unit, University of Exeter, Exeter, UK
Tim F. Oberlander	Professor, Paediatrics, University of British Columbia, Complex Pain Service, BC Children's Hospital, Centre for Community Child Health Research, Vancouver, Canada
Andy V. Pham	Assistant Professor, School of Psychology, Florida International University, Miami, FL, USA
Gustavo Reinoso	Director, Advance Therapy Systems, Dundalk, Ireland
Michael Saini	Assistant Professor, Factor-Inwentash Faculty of Social Work, University of Toronto, Toronto, Canada

Heidi Marie Sanders　Faculty, Occupational Therapy Graduate Program, University of New Mexico, Albuquerque, NM, USA

Veronica Schiariti　Department of Paediatrics, University of British Columbia, Vancouver, British Columbia, Canada

Irene Sebestyen　Research Associate, Jewish Rehabilitation Hospital, Laval, Quebec, Canada

Michael Shevell　Departments of Neurology and Neurosurgery and Pediatrics, Division of Pediatric Neurology, Montreal Children's Hospital, McGill University Health Center, Montreal, Canada

Mónica Silveira-Maia　Faculty of Psychology and Education Sciences, University of Porto, Portugal

Rune J. Simeonsson　Professor, School of Education, University of North Carolina at Chapel Hill; Adjunct Professor, School of Education and Communication, Jonkoping University, Sweden

Laurie M. Snider　Associate Professor, School of Physical & Occupational Therapy, McGill University; Research Associate, Montreal Children's Hospital; Research Associate, Centre for Interdisciplinary Research in Rehabilitation of Greater Montreal, Montreal, Canada

Michael J. Sornberger　PhD student, Department of Educational and Counselling Psychology, McGill University, Montreal, Canada

Myriam Srour　Departments of Neurology and Neurosurgery and Pediatrics, Division of Pediatric Neurology, Montreal Children's Hospital, McGill University Health Center, Montreal, Canada

Melanie Stelmazuk　Attention, Behavior and Sleep Lab, Douglas Mental Health University Institute, Verdun, Quebec, Canada

Bonnie Swaine　Professor, Université de Montréal, Faculty of Medicine, School of Rehabilitation; Scientific Director, Centre for Interdisciplinary Research in Rehabilitation of Greater Montreal, Quebec, Canada

Frank J. Symons　Associate Professor, Department of Educational Psychology, Center for Neurobehavioural Development, University of Minnesota, Minneapolis, USA

Karla Washington　Assistant Professor in Speech–Language Pathology, University of Cincinnati, Cincinnati, OH, USA

John Wilding　Emeritus Reader in Psychology, Royal Hollway, University of London, UK

Suzanne Woods-Grove　Assistant Professor, Special Education, Department of Teaching and Learning, The University of Iowa, Iowa City, IA, USA

F. Virginia Wright　Senior Scientist, Bloorview Research Institute; Associate Professor, Department of Physical Therapy, Faculty of Medicine, University of Toronto, Toronto, Canada

FOREWORD

Help! I am a new therapist trying to figure out which assessment tool I should use to evaluate a 3-year-old child with cerebral palsy whom I am seeing for the first time for a therapy needs assessment. I am a clinician researcher and want to choose outcomes across the International Classification of Functioning, Disability and Health (ICF) framework to ensure that I am assessing body structure/function, activities and participation and contextual factors such as the environment in my research. I am a health manager for a large paediatric rehabilitation hospital ambulatory service and want to develop an outcome-based framework to redesign our services. In particular, I want to focus on the promotion of participation for children with disabilities. In all these scenarios I am faced with the need to do hours of background searching and reading to identify the appropriate and best 'tools' or outcomes to use. Once I have made my decision, I will need to spend additional time trying to determine how to order the measure I want to use. I quickly realize that information on how to order the tool and the costs of the tool are hard to come by!

Now there is help! This beautifully crafted textbook, edited by Professor Annette Majnemer, with chapters written by measurement experts in the field, is going to establish itself as the 'go to' reference on assessment tools and outcome measures for children with neurodevelopmental disabilities. Health professionals, managers and researchers working with children who have a wide range of disabilities, such as cerebral palsy, spina bifida, autism and cognitive disabilities, can now easily identify relevant tools organized within the ICF-CY (Children and Youth) framework. In this volume, information is readily available on what a tool is assessing, its measurement properties, practical aspects of administration and where to find and order it. This book will make a significant difference in helping clinicians, researchers, managers and policy makers choose the best tool(s) for their purpose.

Importantly, it will also enhance the understanding and use of the ICF-CY framework, both in everyday practice and in our research. This can only help to bring about a better understanding of the multidimensional aspects of disability and foster a holistic approach towards childhood disability.

Following an excellent overview of outcome measures including determinants of health and an orientation to the ICF, the book is organized into sections on Body Functioning, Activities and Participation, and Contextual Factors (personal and environment) to provide an overview of the best measures in each area. Each chapter starts with an outline of the construct, general comments on measurement within the specific domain, and then a description of the best measures with an outline of their purpose, content and psychometric properties. Each chapter includes tables providing a capsule summary for easy reference. Measures of body structure are beyond the scope of the book, with two important exceptions: a chapter on brain imaging and a chapter on genetic assessment. These are excellent exceptions, given their important role in understanding childhood disability. In addition, recognizing the importance of global health and quality of life, this book builds on the ICF to include a final section devoted to health and quality of life measures.

Measures for Children with Developmental Disabilities: An ICF-CY Approach is a 'must have' for those individuals who wish to develop an outcome-based framework to their work. Outcome measure phobics fear no more, help is on the way!

Darcy L. Fehlings MD, MSc, FRCPC
Head of Division of Developmental Paediatrics,
Department of Paediatrics, University of Toronto;
Chair in Developmental Paediatrics, Bloorview
Children's Hospital, Toronto, Canada

PREFACE

This text was first conceptualized during a seemingly benign conversation with Hilary Hart, Book Editor, Mac Keith Press, at the annual meeting in 2005 of the American Academy of Cerebral Palsy and Developmental Medicine (AACPDM). Although the notion of putting together a textbook that described measures organized by the components of the International Classification of Functioning, Disability and Health (ICF) intrigued me, competing academic responsibilities and duties diverted my attention elsewhere. However, to Hilary's credit, she was quite persistent, and at each annual AACPDM meeting we would 'rediscuss'. Finally, several years later, I took on the challenge of editing this textbook.

The purpose of this text is to provide an overview of the measures that can be used with infants, children and young people who have a developmental disability. Chapter 1 guides the reader in the selection and use of measurement tools. A detailed description of the purpose and framework of this text appears in Chapter 2, and it would be helpful for readers to review this before using this textbook. The book is framed by the components within the ICF for Children and Youth (ICF-CY). A description of the measures used to evaluate the integrity of organs and systems within the body (i.e. body structures) was beyond the scope of this textbook. However, given the impressive advances in novel neuroimaging technologies that are highly relevant to the evaluation of brain structure and function in children with disabilities, a chapter on these measures was included. Furthermore, rapid advancement in genetic tools which are of relevance to our understanding of mechanisms that underlie the development and integrity of body structures and functions prompted the inclusion of a chapter on genetic testing. Chapters 5 to 16 cover body functions and describe a range of global and specific mental functions classified within the ICF as well as sensory, speech and neuromuscular functions. It was impossible to include all the components identified within each domain; however, every effort was made to emphasize the components that are most relevant to the field of childhood disability. Global measures of development (i.e. to assess developmental delays) do not readily fit within the categories of body functions or activities and participation; rather, they straddle both components and therefore appear as two chapters nestled in between these two sections. The nine domains within activities and participation each have their own chapters, with an introductory chapter describing global multidimensional measures of activities and participation (Chapters 19–28). Measures related to primary contextual factors appear in Chapters 29 to 32. Finally, the ICF-CY is meant to encapsulate an individual's health and functioning, taking into account the influence of intrinsic and extrinsic factors. Therefore, two final chapters on health status and quality of life measures were also added, although they are not technically domains within the ICF-CY.

Outlining this textbook was straightforward as the ICF-CY provided the headings to follow. However, it quickly become apparent that many of the domains within the components were diverse and complex, and finding appropriate measures suitable for the target population was often challenging. It was difficult to find content experts who were up to the challenge of synthesizing the measures that would be appropriate for a particular domain within the ICF-CY. Many of the contributors found that the constructs of the ICF-CY were not necessarily discrete. Furthermore, for the most part, measures were not developed to match a particular construct within the ICF-CY and therefore do not necessarily fit precisely within the domains of interest. However, the contributors were masterful and creative in finding the 'best fit' with respect to the measures that are currently available for use. Future research efforts linking items within standardized measures to the ICF-CY will be helpful in determining where particular measures best fit. For some areas, measures are still in the early development stage. For other areas, there are few, if any, tools available.

The chapters are meant to describe not every known measure but rather a sample of the best tools available within the domain of interest. For the most part, each chapter is organized with headings to include the construct, factors to consider when measuring this domain and an overview of recommended measures. Charts underlining the key attributes of selected measures are also included for quick reference. Some authors used a different format and the amount of information provided is variable. On occasion, a measure may be described in more than one chapter. Hopefully, readers will find it easy to navigate through this text and find the measures they are looking for.

The professional profile and expertise of the authors of these chapters reflect the multifaceted and specialized nature of the measures described. The authors represent a wide range of disciplines, from institutions and countries around the world. The knowledge and expertise of the authors is impressive, and I am extremely indebted to all the contributors for their significant efforts in conceptualizing and synthesizing their chapters. I recognize the difficulty of the task, and they should all be congratulated for their contributions. I also appreciate the encouragement that I received from contributors in putting this text together. Special thanks are due to Dr Rune Simeonsson for assembling teams to tackle some of the most complex domains.

I would like to thank my colleagues at the School of Physical and Occupational Therapy, McGill University, and especially the inquisitive graduate students I supervise. These individuals are a constant source of inspiration, reflection and encouragement. My wonderful, talented daughters, Meaghan and Allison, have always supported my career ambitions while simultaneously ensuring that I devote my energies to other vital elements of my life. Above all, I am so grateful to my husband Michael Shevell, who has been a valuable role model and my greatest supporter, both personally and professionally. I look forward to our adventures ahead as we continue to learn and enjoy life experiences together.

Disability is a multidimensional construct, and therefore clinicians and researchers need to consider all facets of functioning, disability and health, with reflection of the personal and environmental contextual factors that can influence disability status. As an occupational therapist, adopting this holistic view is intrinsic to my professional philosophy of practice, so that I can understand and appreciate the many factors that contribute to a child's adaptive capacity and capabilities. In searching for the most appropriate measures to evaluate all aspects of functioning, disability and health, it is difficult to find all the pieces to the puzzle. We are required to use what we have available to capture as complete a picture as possible so that we can identify strengths and address challenges.

Annette Majnemer
Montreal
May 2012

SECTION I OVERVIEW

1
SELECTION AND USE OF OUTCOME MEASURES

Annette Majnemer

What are outcome measures and their determinants?
An *outcome* is the consequence or end result of a process, which could be a treatment, programme or service or could simply be changes in the health condition over a phase or period of development.[1] The outcomes measured are linked to either the effects of a particular intervention or service delivery programme or the impact of the disease or health condition. *Outcome measures* are tools that may be used to assess a change in particular attributes that are deemed meaningful to a person's life over time.[2] They may be differentiated from enduring attributes such as personality traits, expectations or demographic characteristics. This last factor may include important determinants of outcomes, and therefore can also be measured for either clinical or research purposes, along with outcome measures. A *determinant* may be any factor that causes or influences the outcomes of interest.[3] The measurement of outcomes and their determinants is essential in informing decisions about treatment and targeting those who may benefit most. For example, the use of outcome measures as part of a randomized controlled trial may provide evidence that an injection of botulinum toxin for children with spastic cerebral palsy is effective in increasing range of motion, alleviating spasticity and improving movement quality and motor function.[4] However, evaluation of the determinants of responsiveness, that is the factors associated with greater improvements following Botulinum toxin treatments, reveals that age, number of previous treatments and contextual factors such as the child's mastery motivation and family stress levels can influence the degree of responsiveness to this expensive treatment modality.[5] Some variables may be confounders that are correlated with both the independent variable (determinants, exposures) and the dependent variable (outcome). These need to be accounted for in the analyses of relationships between determinants and outcomes.

Knowledge of determinants is therefore helpful in targeting those children who may benefit most from particular treatments or services, with the aim of enhancing the outcomes of interest. Similarly, a range of outcome measures may be used to characterize the development and functioning of a specified group of children with a developmental disability; however, measurement of particular determinants is also very helpful in differentiating factors that may positively or negatively influence disability level. Cassidy[6] presented a conceptual model that considered both medical factors (e.g. severity, comorbidities, aetiology) and demographic factors (e.g. age, sex, socioeconomic status) as important influences of outcomes. Similarly, the conceptual framework for the Canadian Health Measures Survey considers the dynamic interplay between non-modifiable and modifiable determinants together with health behaviours and characteristics as potential mediators (e.g. intermediary; intervenes between the exposure and the outcome) and moderators (e.g. alters the state or effect of a causal factor or variable) of health outcomes (Table 1.1). Whether in clinical practice or in the research setting, outcome assessment should involve consideration of factors that can potentially exert important influences on these outcomes. Therefore, appropriate tools need to be carefully selected to measure both outcomes and their determinants.

The measures used to assess outcomes and their determinants can be standardized, which implies that they are applied in a prescribed manner, as established by the developers of the instrument. Patient-centred outcomes are often measured using self-report questionnaires or interview formats to assess aspects of health and functioning from the individual's own perspective.[8] Often, clinical studies use surrogate end points (e.g. measurement of blood pressure and cholesterol) as a substitute for a more meaningful outcome (e.g. cardiovascular health/disease). Relationships are assumed and surrogates are used as they

TABLE 1.1

Conceptual framework for the Canadian Health Measures Survey[7]

Variables to consider	Examples of attributes
Non-modifiable determinants	Age, sex, ethnicity, genotype
Modifiable determinants	Family income, education, physical and social environment, healthcare system
Health behaviours	Physical activity, nutrition, substance abuse, stress exposures, medication use
Health characteristics	Functional status, body weight, cardiovascular fitness, reactivity to stress

TABLE 1.2

Utility of outcome measures for different stakeholders

Target group	Examples of benefits of use of outcome measures
Patients/clients and families	Identifies child's strengths and limitations
	Demonstrates changes over time
	Motivates the child and family to improve
	Outcomes research provides information on natural history of the population of interest
	Helpful in providing families with realistic goals and expectations
Service providers	Identifies areas of concern that may warrant treatment
	Enables surveillance of changes over time
	Encourages reflective practice approaches
	Promotes accountability
Administrators, clinical managers	Critical for programme evaluation
	Provides justification for new programmes or services
	Helpful in the evaluation of quality of services
Policy makers, health planners	Outcomes data can be used to guide decisions with respect to new policies and better services
	Useful in prioritizing resource needs
Researchers	Necessary to address a range of research questions, from the cell (causes, mechanisms, prevention) to the clinic (new tools, treatment effectiveness, service quality) and the community (epidemiological studies, systems of support, health promotion)

are more objectively and easily quantified. Whether in clinical practice or research, the measures used to describe the outcomes of interest should be valid, objective measures of the constructs of direct interest. There are several factors that need to be considered when selecting outcome measures, and these are outlined later in this chapter.

It should be emphasized that quantification of outcomes and their determinants using objective, standardized measurement tools is only one way of depicting and characterizing this important information. Qualitative methods or mixed methods can also be used as processes of inquiry to gather a more in-depth understanding of the constructs of interest.

Why are outcome measures important to use?

Outcome measurement has important benefits to consumers of services (patients/clients and their family members), service providers, clinical managers, policy makers and researchers (Table 1.2). For *patients* or *clients and their*

families, individualized application of outcome measures provides the family with objective, quantitative information regarding their child's relative strengths and weaknesses in the area(s) assessed, demonstrates changes in performance over time and serves to foster achievement and motivate children to improve their abilities in the areas measured by the assessment tool.[9,10] These measures would need to meet rigorous psychometric standards for use in individuals. Furthermore, outcomes data from research studies provide useful information regarding the natural history and developmental trajectories to be expected in particular childhood disability subgroups. Knowledge of these outcomes enables health service providers to more effectively counsel families regarding the outcomes to be expected for their child. It is important that parents and children have realistic expectations for the future and set personal goals that are attainable.

Measuring outcomes is important for health service providers as well. Outcome measures serve to identify areas of concern and to monitor changes over time. The use of outcome measures can promote a more reflective practice approach, thus providing clarity of purpose with respect to goal attainment.[10] Clinicians may carefully consider whether or not goals of intervention are being met, or whether new interventions or goals need to be pursued.[9,11] An outcomes-based framework for service delivery is an important cultural shift for clinicians. The focus is on achieving specified outcomes, with objective, measurable treatment goals and commitment to long-term changes.[10] Objective data encourage clinicians to be more accountable about the services they are providing, both to themselves and to others. Indeed, with increasing fiscal constraints, rehabilitation specialists are under greater scrutiny to provide high-quality care at the lowest cost, and outcome measurement can be an effective strategy to validate the usefulness of particular programmes or interventions.[9,12] For example, greater efforts at restructuring service delivery by using dyads (two children treated simultaneously by one health professional) or group treatment programmes, and by providing consultative services in addition to direct interventions, are cost-effective strategies that may need greater consideration in practice.

Clinical co-ordinators or managers and other *administrators of health services* value outcome measurement for a variety of reasons. First, interdisciplinary programmes are costly, and there is a need to demonstrate that the outcomes of the programme align well with the goals and objectives of the programme.[2,10] For example, if improving quality of life is the primary goal of a social support group or assistive technology service for children with developmental disabilities, it would be important to use an outcome measure at baseline and upon completion of the intervention to demonstrate such an effect. The use of outcome measures enables administrators and managers to better appreciate which goals are feasible and attainable for particular programmes or services. Outcomes research has highlighted new populations who are at risk of developmental disability. For example, outcomes data on infants with congenital heart defects who require open heart surgery clearly demonstrate that survival has improved dramatically; however, it is not known whether these neonates are at high risk for developmental and learning challenges as they grow and develop.[13] This emphasizes the need for new interdisciplinary health services for children with congenital heart defects that are directed at the periodic surveillance of developmental progress at key transition points as the child matures, as are routinely provided for infants who are born preterm. Therefore, new health service programmes can be justified by outcomes research on

new target populations that are at risk for developmental disabilities. As part of quality assurance, health administrators can use outcome measures to evaluate the quality of services to include the structure of the services, the process of care provided and the outcomes, and satisfaction with the services.[14–16] Performance measurement is a process whereby indicators and assessment tools are used to evaluate a programme's mission, goals and target outcomes.[10] This may include the evaluation of structural elements of a service such as access, frequency of treatments, and qualifications and expertise of the service provider. Furthermore, process elements may include attributes of the treatment such as respectful and supportive care and the appropriate selection of evidence-based treatment modalities. Finally, evaluation inevitably includes indicators and measures of the child's outcome in the domains in which improvements are expected. Satisfaction with services by family members should also be considered in programme evaluation and performance measurement.[15,17] This objective information not only sets performance standards but is essential in order for administrators and managers of health services to make decisions regarding resource allocation that will provide the best outcomes for children requiring these services.[10]

Public policy at the government level involves the development and adoption of principles, programmes and services in the health sector. Policy makers may take advantage of outcomes data as evidence to develop new policies or programmes for target populations in need of services.[18] Objective evidence provided by outcome measures can identify where the needs are greatest for services, resources and supports, which is required for effective and judicious resource allocation.

Researchers use outcome measures to answer a wide variety of questions related to childhood disability, including elucidation of mechanisms or causes of disability, understanding patterns of recovery and reorganization of the brain, validation of early identification tools, verification of treatment effectiveness, recognition of determinants of disability, evaluation of health promotion strategies, determination of quality of health services and effective knowledge translation efforts.[2] Invariably, outcome measures are needed to quantify objectively particular attributes or characteristics of the individual with or at risk for a disability, or aspects of their environment.

Clearly, the potential benefits of application of outcome measurement are broad and wide ranging. Therefore, consideration should be given to applying multiple measures to capture the spectrum of outcomes of interests, as well as possible indicators or determinants that may influence the outcomes.[16]

Factors to consider in the selection of outcome measures

Measures are widely used in clinical practice and research for a variety of purposes. Selection of the most appropriate outcome measures can raise a number of concerns and queries, for example:

- What are the best markers for success of your intervention?
- Which measures will enable you to specifically answer your research questions and test your hypotheses?
- Is the tool suitable for the population of interest (age, diagnosis, developmental level and abilities)?
- Will the findings on assessment provide useful clinical information?
- Will the evaluation tool accurately measure the 'right thing' (i.e. cohesive construct of interest) in your research or clinical hypotheses?
- Is the tool reliable, that is, is it consistent across multiple test administrations and raters?
- Is the measure affordable and easy to administer, and well tolerated by the participants being investigated or evaluated without the need for modification of the administration standards, which could jeopardize interpretability?
- Can you use only a portion of the measure without jeopardizing reliability and validity (do subscales stand alone)?

A number of criteria need to be considered in the selection of outcome measures, whether by clinicians or by researchers. Several authors[9,19–21] (see also www.hta. ac.uk/fullmono/mon214.pdf) have provided checklists of these criteria, and there is consensus that the key factors to consider in the selection of outcome measures include the following and are described further below:

- measures are specifically measuring the outcome(s) of interest;
- measures are relevant to the children being evaluated and to their families;
- administration is feasible and practical;
- measures were developed with a particular purpose, for a specific target population; and
- the instruments chosen are psychometrically sound.

MEASURES SELECTED ARE MEASURING THE OUTCOMES OF INTEREST

Clinicians need to be sure that the measures they select are relevant to the goals of treatment, and therefore goals of intervention should first be established before the selection of outcome measures.[9] What is the *intended purpose of the intervention* and what attributes of the child do you expect to change? If a treatment programme, for example, claims to improve developmental skills and enhance quality of life, then it is essential that the specific developmental domains targeted for improvement are measured using tools that are sensitive to change, and that quality of life is also measured. Therefore, clinicians need to carefully reflect on what outcomes are realistically likely to change in the time frame of the interventions being provided. Factors that might influence level of change (e.g. compliance with treatment) may need to be objectively quantified (measured) as well.[1,10] Table 1.3 provides an example of some of the issues and clinical questions that may be raised and considered in the selection of outcome measures for

TABLE 1.3

Example of factors to consider in the selection of measures for an early intervention programme[11]

Factors to consider	Clinical context
Relate outcome measures to the programme objectives	What areas of development do you hope to change? Does the family have specific goals that need to be considered and measured?
Seek the best available instruments	Are the changes quantitative (better scores) and/or qualitative (a change in quality of a particular behaviour or attribute)?
	Which tools will detect the degree or increment of change that you are hoping to accomplish?
Consider clinical significance and statistical significance of change	What level of change would be clinically meaningful for this child? To whom?
	Will criterion-referenced or norm-referenced tools be more appropriate in measuring clinically meaningful changes?
Apply a conceptual framework that will help guide the selection of measures	Which measures will best explain the effects of the intervention on the child and family?
	Which attributes or measures may help explain factors that are influencing level of improvement?

an early intervention programme or for a research study evaluating the effectiveness of such a programme on a target population.[11] Traditionally, many early intervention programmes have focused on measures of cognitive ability such as IQ; however, careful reflection a priori of the areas that should be measured will ensure that the effectiveness of such programmes is more broadly appreciated and understood.

Often, outcome measures are used for *clinical accountability*, so as to evaluate services and programmes. Outcomes are compared with baseline, and the proportion of patients or clients that meet or exceed treatment goals are determined. Increasingly, factors influencing 'treatment success' are considered, and may guide future service planning.[19] Programme evaluation could include family functioning, and child's self-concept and level of motivation, and programmes may therefore be interested in measuring these areas. In particular, these personal and environmental factors can potentially be modified by interdisciplinary teams, and therefore may be considered as part of the programme goals and interventions.[19]

Similarly, researchers need to carefully select the outcome measures that will specifically address their research questions, and can be used *to test the proposed hypotheses*.[22] It is often challenging to find an appropriate criterion standard measure of particular areas of behaviour and development, thus limiting the research questions that can be investigated. Indeed, often one of the first phases of research programmes involves the development of new measures that will then be utilized to pursue the research questions of investigators.

MEASURES ARE RELEVANT TO CHILDREN AND TO THEIR FAMILIES

The evaluation tools chosen for use must be acceptable to the children being assessed and to their families in terms of administration format and test requirements.[19] Furthermore, the areas selected for measurement should be of importance to the child and family, in line with health and developmental outcomes of relevance to them. *Family-centred care* involves a partnership between health service providers and families, whereby the parents and children are actively involved in the selection and prioritization of treatment goals, and the care provided must be respectful and supportive.[23] Family-centred approaches to care have been found to enhance developmental outcomes for the child, improve family adjustment and coping, and increase satisfaction with services.[24,25] Active involvement of families in the selection of pertinent outcomes will undoubtedly reinforce the positive attributes and benefits of family-centred service.

PRACTICALITY AND FEASIBILITY OF THE MEASURE

Measures should be 'user friendly', that is, easy to administer by the evaluator. The measure should have a clear (standardized) administration protocol. Indeed, some tools may require specific training or special qualifications to ensure standardized administration, scoring and interpretation. It is critical to follow the standardized administration and scoring procedures as outlined in the test manual rather than attempt to simplify the test administration, as deviation from the designated standardized approach can increase error and bias and jeopardize interpretation of the results.[20,22] Often, the time to complete the measure is a factor in its successful uptake as a clinical or research tool, with short administration times being an asset for children with disabilities.[8] Cost is another factor to consider, and investment in an expensive test kit is only likely to be necessary if there is broad applicability and utility. In summary, practical considerations in the selection of outcome measures include cost, time, ease of use, portability and availability of the instrument.[20] Often, clinicians will use what is already available in their department; however, consideration should be given to periodic investment in new outcome measures that may provide accurate new information that is not collected using existing measures.

THE PURPOSE OF THE MEASURE IS CONSIDERED

Tools are developed with a particular purpose. They may be discriminative tests, which provide information about children with disabilities compared with typically developing children (i.e. norm-referenced tests). Predictive measures and screening tools are used to identify children with or at risk of a particular attribute (now or in the future). Screening tests provide preliminary information, which is then followed up with a more detailed assessment in those who fail or obtain borderline results on the initial screen. Evaluative measures can detect changes over time. These tools are often criterion referenced (judged against a criterion standard, not compared with the 'norm') and thus are more likely to be sensitive to small changes in performance.[26,27] When selecting a particular measure, it is essential that evaluators verify the sample of children in whom the measure was standardized in order to be sure that it is representative and therefore appropriate for the children for whom it is intended. Thus, when selecting measures either for clinical practice or for research, it is important that the tools chosen are being used as intended. For example, if the intent is to demonstrate the effectiveness of a new aid or adaptation (e.g. built-up handles to facilitate grasp) in promoting independence in self-feeding, personal care and hygiene, then a measure such as the Pediatric Evaluation of Disability Inventory, which has been shown to reliably perceive small improvements (or deteriorations) in self-care activities, should be selected.[8] These tests must demonstrate that they are responsive tools that can be used to detect clinically important changes over time. Furthermore, the tool should be sensitive to change at various levels of performance. If the test is too difficult and scores tend to cluster at the lowest values (floor effect) or, conversely, if the test is too easy and scores cluster at the highest values (ceiling effect), then detecting small changes may not be possible.[20]

THE MEASURE IS PSYCHOMETRICALLY SOUND

Psychometric theory is the science of assessing the measurement properties of a tool. Collectively, this can include (1) data quality such as the impact of missing scores or non-response to items; (2) scaling assumptions and weighing of items to create scales; (3) acceptability of score distributions in representing the construct of interest; (4) reliability or consistency and reproducibility of the scores; (5) validity or the extent to which the tool is measuring the construct it claims to measure; and (6) responsiveness or the extent to which the measure can detect clinically important changes over time.[8]

Whether in clinical practice or in research, careful attention should be given to the psychometric properties of a measure to ensure that the measure selected was appropriately scaled and can accurately measure the construct of interest. Scoring the results must be done using the prescribed manner in which the tool was developed, including the interpretation of missing values and the ability to use only particular subscales. *Reliability* estimates the extent to which the scores produced are free from random error and are stable and accurate. Reliability can be estimated across time (test–retest), across raters (inter-rater) and within the measure (internal consistency).[21] Test–retest reliability verifies whether the score is consistent on repeated evaluation over a time frame in which you would not expect to observe any alteration in the results. For example, if too short a time interval is used, learning or practice effects may influence item execution. If the test is repeated right after completion of the first test, fatigue may influence performance. If too wide a time interval is used, there may be actual maturational or other (e.g. disease progression) changes in abilities. Inter-rater reliability ensures that any trained rater will achieve the same results when evaluating a group of individuals. Reliability decreases as a function of greater measurement error (i.e. the extent to which observed scores will vary from the true scores). Both the experience or training of the tester and the child's level of attention or compliance can contribute to measurement error. Indeed, the evaluator can introduce personal biases in the administration of the test and interpretation of the results, and therefore the

use of 'blind' evaluators in research, who are unaware of the study hypotheses or information about the research participants, is necessary to minimize evaluator bias. Reliability is typically represented statistically as a coefficient between 0 and 1.0, with 1.0 meaning no measurement error; the closer to 1.0, the more confident you can be about the stability of the scores produced. Correlations provide incomplete data, as they reflect only the degree of association and not the level of agreement. For example, one evaluator may consistently score children 10 points higher than another evaluator, and the resultant correlations between the two evaluators would be highly associated, but clearly with low agreement. The intraclass correlation coefficient (ICC) is a more appropriate analytical approach for continuous data to measure both association and level of agreement between multiple raters or scores obtained over repeated measurements. Kappa should be used for categorical data and weighted kappa should be used for ordinal data in order to determine the reliability between raters or tests. This provides the level of agreement as a ratio of observed agreement compared with the agreement expected by chance. Generally, ICC or kappa should be >0.70 or 0.75 (for group data; it should be higher for use with individuals), with scores of 0.5 to 0.75 considered moderate correlation. Confidence intervals (range of values of the actual reliability, as low as 'x' or as high as 'y') of these estimates of reliability are helpful to examine as well, as the narrower the confidence interval, the more precise the estimate of the true value.[20,27,28] When examining reliability estimates for a measure, it is critical to verify which group of participants (e.g. typically developing individuals or children with a particular diagnosis or health condition) were used in the reliability studies as the results cannot be generalized to other populations.

Validity refers to the extent to which a tool is measuring what it is designed to measure. First, in consultation with experts, the content of the tool is carefully evaluated to ensure that it includes all attributes of the phenomenon of interest and that it is logical and meaningful to the tester and the individuals being tested (face and content validity). The test can then be compared with a criterion standard measure which assesses the same characteristics or construct (concurrent validity). Another validation approach is to ascertain whether the measure correlates with scores obtained on a clinically relevant criterion standard in the future (predictive validity), thus verifying an association with behaviours in the future that you would expect it to predict. For these statistical comparisons, Spearman's or Pearson's correlation coefficient is generally used, and the closer the score is to 1.0, the stronger the association. Criterion standards often do not exist, and therefore the level of correlation is not perfect as the two measures being compared may be measuring similar but not identical attributes. Validity can also be estimated by demonstrating that the tool behaves as predicted in differentiating groups of individuals (discriminant validity) with high and low performance levels in known groups, for example, by using *t*-tests. Evidence that the tool relates to measures of a similar construct (convergent validity) and does not relate to measures of a different construct (divergent validity) can also be verified statistically, thus providing additional evidence for construct validity. In addition, the domains or subscales within the measure should aggregate well together to represent particular attributes of interest (internal consistency), and this can be verified using Cronbach's alpha. Factor analysis and principal components analysis are other statistical approaches that are used to verify that, conceptually,

several items or subscales collectively explain the variance in scores.[20,22,27,28]

As discussed above (i.e. the purpose of the measure), *responsiveness* of an instrument refers to its ability to detect clinically meaningful changes over time. This is particularly important to verify in the case of clinicians who want to use the tool to quantify the effectiveness of a treatment, or for researchers who are carrying out an intervention trial. A variety of statistical approaches may be used to evaluate the responsiveness of a tool, although often the effect size is reported, with an effect size >0.2 indicating a small effect, >0.5 a moderate effect and >0.8 a large effect.[20,27,28]

For a more detailed description of psychometric theory, Streiner and Norman[27] and Portnoy and Watkins[28] are excellent reference texts.

REFERENCES

1. Natsch S, Kullberg BJ, Hekster YA, van der Meer JWM (2003) Selecting outcome parameters in studies aimed at improving rational use of antibiotics: practical considerations. *J Clin Pharm Ther* 28: 475–478.
2. Majnemer A, Limperopoulos C (2002) Importance of outcome determination in pediatric rehabilitation. *Dev Med Child Neurol* 44: 773–777.
3. MSN Encarta Encyclopedia. *Definition of 'Determinants'.* Available at: http://encarta.msn.com/encnet/refpages/search. aspx?q=determinants (accessed 31 March 2008).
4. Tilton AH (2004) Management of spasticity in children with cerebral palsy. *Semin Pediatr Neurol* 11: 58–65.
5. Yap R, Majnemer A, Benaroch T, Cantin MA (2010) Determinants of responsiveness to botulinum toxin, casting, and bracing in the treatment of spastic equinus in children with cerebral palsy. *Dev Med Child Neurol* 52: 186–193.
6. Cassidy CA (1999) Panning for gold: Sifting through chart audit data for patient outcomes. *Outcomes Manag Nurs Pract* 3: 38–42.
7. Tremblay M, Wofson M, Gorber SC (2007) Canadian health measures survey: rationale, background and overview. *Suppl Health Reports* 18: 1–13.
8. Riazi A (2002) Patient-centred outcome measures. *Way Ahead* 5: 16–17. [Available at: www.mstrust.org.uk/publications/ wayahead/06022002_01.jsp]
9. Law M, King G, Russell D, MacKinnon E, Hurley P, Murphy C (1999) Measuring outcomes in children's rehabilitation: a decision protocol. *Arch Phys Med Rehabil* 80: 629–636.
10. Wells SJ, Johnson MA (2001) Selecting outcome measures for child welfare settings: lessons for use in performance management. *Child Youth Serv Rev* 23: 169–199.
11. Casto G, Lewis A (1986) Selecting outcome measures in early intervention. *J Div Early Child* 10: 118–123.
12. Kurtz LA (2002) Rehabilitation: physical therapy and occupational therapy. In: Batshaw ML, editor. *Children with Disabilities.* Baltimore: Paul H. Brookes Publishing, pp. 647–657.
13. Majnemer A, Limperopoulos C, Shevell MI, Rohlicek C, Rosenblatt B, Tchervenkov C (2009) A new look at outcomes of infants with congenital heart disease. *Pediatr Neurol* 40: 197–204.
14. Donabedian A (1988) The quality of care: how can it be assessed:? *J Am Med Assoc* 260: 1743–1748.
15. Mazer B, Majnemer A (2009) Service utilization and health promotion of children with neurodevelopmental disabilities. In: Shevell M, editor. *Neurodevelopmental Disabilities: Clinical and Scientific Foundations, International Review of Child Neurology Series.* London: Mac Keith Press, pp. 426–482.
16. Vivier PM, Bernier JA, Starfield B (1994) Current approaches to measuring health outcomes in pediatric research. *Curr Opin Pediatr* 6: 530–537.
17. Eldar R (2000) A conceptual proposal for the study of the quality of rehabilitation care. *Disabil Rehabil* 22: 163–169.
18. Lavis JN, Posada FB, Haines A, Osei E (2004) Use of research to inform public policymaking. *Lancet* 364: 1615–1621.
19. Graham K (1994) Guidelines for using standardized outcome measures following addictions treatment. *Eval Health Prof* 17: 43–59.
20. Jerosch-Herold C (2005) An evidence-based approach to choosing outcome measures: a checklist for the critical appraisal of validity, reliability and responsiveness studies. *Br J Occup Ther* 68: 347–353.
21. Teri L (1996) Selecting outcome measures for clinical trials of behavioral disturbances of dementia. *Int Psychogeriatr* 8: 347–349.
22. Kenny TJ, Holden EW, Santilli L (1991) The meaning of measures: pitfalls in behavioral and developmental research. *J Dev Behav Pediatr* 12: 355–360.
23. Rosenbaum P, King S, Law M, King G, Evans J (1998) Family-centred service: a conceptual framework and research review. *Phys Occup Ther Pediatr* 18: 1–20.
24. Hostler SL (1991) Family-centred care (review). *Pediatr Clin North Am* 38: 1545–1560.
25. Law M, Hanna S, King G, et al (2003) Factors affecting family-centred service delivery for children with disabilities. *Child Care Health Dev* 29: 357–366.
26. Rosenbaum P (1998) Screening tests and standardized assessments used to identify and characterize developmental delays. *Semin Pediatr Neurol* 5: 27–32.
27. Streiner DL, Norman GR (2003) *Health Measurement Scales: A Practical Guide to their Development and Use,* 3rd edition. Don Mills, Ontario: Oxford University Press.
28. Portnoy LG, Watkins MP (2000) *Foundations of Clinical Research: Applications to Practice,* 2nd edition. New Jersey: Prentice-Hall Health.

2
THE PURPOSE AND FRAMEWORK FOR THIS TEXT

Annette Majnemer

The purpose of this text

Disability status reflects a multidimensional experience, encapsulating both intrinsic attributes of the individual (e.g. physical, cognitive, behavioural, sensory) and extrinsic environmental factors that mediate disability. Descriptions of the developmental progress and outcomes of children and young people with developmental disabilities should be broadly framed to include all facets of the individual's physical and psychosocial functioning and health, with consideration of contextual factors that influence his or her capabilities and adaptive capacity.[1]

The primary aim of this text is to provide a representative sample of measures across a wide range of intrinsic and extrinsic attributes. The target readership for this text can be clinicians, educators or researchers who are looking for a particular measurement tool that can be used for children and young people with a developmental disability. *Developmental disability* is very broadly conceptualized as developmental delays or deficits in one or more developmental domains (e.g. gross/fine motor, cognitive, behavioural, speech) that have an impact on that person's ability to perform age-appropriate everyday activities and functions. Using the International Classification of Functioning, Disability and Health (ICF, described below) as a framework for organizing the various types of measures into sections and chapters, assessments across a wide range of domains are represented. The chapters are not meant to provide a description of every measure that exists within a particular domain or construct; rather, a representative sample of useful measures is depicted, with more detailed descriptions of those with the best properties and potential utility. Most chapters include tables with a capsule summary of the features of the best measures within the sphere of interest. The contributors to or authors of each chapter were selected for their expertise in the topic area. The contributors represent a broad range of disciplines from around the world, reflecting the multidimensional nature of the ICF.

Below is a description of the ICF, followed by a description of the organization of the content of the text and the chapters that follow. *It should be emphasized that biomedical investigations that evaluate the integrity of organs or systems, typically conducted by medical specialists, are not included in this text.* Rather, the focus of this text is to describe a broad range of assessments and questionnaires that might be used by health professionals who evaluate infants, children and young people with a developmental disability or by researchers investigating clinical research questions that relate to children with developmental disabilities.

The framework for this text

INTERNATIONAL CLASSIFICATION OF FUNCTIONING, DISABILITY AND HEALTH

The ICF was adopted in 2001 by the World Health Organization to replace the International Classification of Impairments, Disabilities and Handicaps.[2] The ICF is a scheme that is meant to comprehensively classify the functioning and health of individuals, and it complements the International Classification of Diseases (ICD) coding scheme.[3] The ICD explains what the health condition is (i.e. the diagnosis), and may reveal why it has occurred, and indirectly provides prognostic information, whereas the way in which the body systems and the individual are functioning in their environment and the extent to which the individual is participating in society are further elucidated by the ICF. An important advantage of the ICF is that it provides a common language that may be used across disciplines and sectors to describe human functioning[4–6] in individuals with or without disabilities. This conceptual framework of human functioning is cross-cutting and is therefore intended to be used by health professionals, policy makers, managers, educators, researchers and consumers of services.[5,7] Indeed, individuals from various health disciplines have mapped the ICF onto their discipline or programme so as to provide a holistic view of the clients or patients they are servicing.[3,8] There has been endorsement and gradual uptake by health professionals and researchers of the ICF as a model that guides the selection of measures, treatment goals and outcomes of interest,[9] and this ensures that intervention planning is family centred and collaborative.[10] In particular, reflection on the contextual factors that influence health and functioning has promoted a biopsychosocial view of disability, thus placing a greater emphasis on changing the environment (physical, social, attitudinal) rather than the child.[4,11,12]

The ICF for Children and Youth (ICF-CY) was published in 2007. It applies and modifies the categories, content and coding to the characteristics of children and young people (aged 0–18y). More specific detail was provided to the descriptions and new content was added where relevant. The criteria for inclusion and exclusion to the various categories were modified and qualifiers now consider developmental aspects.[5,7]

Part 1 of the ICF
Functioning and disability has two components:
(i)   body functions and structures
(ii)   activities and participation

Body structures refer to the anatomical parts of the body. These are classified by body systems, such as structures of the brain or the cardiovascular system or structures related to movement. Impairments of body structure are deviations from the population standard or norm and typically include a defect, injury or anomaly in the particular structure and are the anatomical manifestations of the underlying pathology. Body structures may be differentiated from the disease or health condition. Although impairments of body structure may relate to a health condition, the individual may not be 'ill' or unwell. Furthermore, body structures do not indicate or provide information on the aetiology of the impairment. *Body functions* refer to the physiological and psychological functions of the various body systems, and impairments describe alterations from the norm in the functioning of these systems. Physiological manifestations of particular body systems might include, for example, abnormal muscle tone or decreased visual acuity, whereas psychological

(behavioural) manifestations might include poor attention span or diminished fluency of speech. Impairments in body functions typically describe and refer to 'delayed, abnormal, decreased or poor' functioning of particular systems.

Activities and participation are classified together. *Activity* refers to the execution of a particular task or action, whereas these tasks can then be grouped within particular life situations or roles, referred to as *participation*. Activity limitations are the challenges or difficulties that an individual may experience in performing particular tasks. This could include discrete activities such as listening to a story, sitting on a chair or drinking from a cup. Participation restrictions refer to challenges in the ability to be involved or engaged in particular life roles, such as, learning and applying knowledge, mobility in different environments or interpersonal interactions and relationships. These activity limitations and participation restrictions are based on generally accepted standards of performance of typically developing infants, children and young people. Two qualifiers used to describe these components are capacity (i.e. the task[s] that an individual is able to execute in a standardized environment – 'can do') and performance (i.e. the task[s] that an individual typically carries out in his or her current environment – 'does do'). The gap between capacity and performance relates to the contextual factors below that exert powerful influences on functioning.

Part 2 of the ICF
Contextual factors has two components:
(i)   environmental factors
(ii)   personal factors

Contextual factors constitute the background within which an individual functions. *Environmental factors* include the physical, social and attitudinal environment that an individual lives in. These external factors can be viewed and subsequently coded as either facilitators or barriers, depending on their influence on an individual's functioning and health. There is the immediate 'individual' environment, including the home and work or school environments. The routine contacts made with others (e.g. family, peers, coworkers) and the physical attributes of these environments are considered. There is also the 'societal' environment, which includes services and organizations in the community and government (e.g. laws, transportation services, social networks) that can affect the physical, social and attitudinal environment.

Features of the individual that are not part of their health condition or health status would constitute their *personal factors*. These include, for example, demographic characteristics such as age, sex and ethnic origin, but also lifestyle preferences and habits, upbringing, education, coping style, motivation and other personality traits. It should be noted that personal factors are not classified in the ICF. However, their important contribution is recognized and is part of the framework.

Organizational structure of this text

SECTIONS AND CHAPTERS OF THE TEXT: ICF FRAMEWORK

The ICF was used as a framework for creating various sections and chapters to group different types of measurement tools. It should be noted at the outset that these various measures, for the most part, were not specifically developed to capture a particular construct or group of constructs within the ICF framework. The authors of this text have done their best to identify the best available measures that capture attributes within the domains of the ICF classification. This is a challenging task and the fit within the codes listed for each domain is not always exact. Nonetheless, the key conceptual attributes across the spectrum of human functioning and health are included.

Section I provides an overview on the selection and use of outcome measures and outlines the organizational structure of the text. Section II focuses on two particular biomedical tools related to body structure and function that have advanced considerably owing to novel technological capabilities. Section II then elaborates on measures of domains within body function. Section III provides an overview of global measures of developmental impairments (delays) across a range of body function domains. Activities and participation measures appear in Section IV, and tools that may be used to assess contextual factors are in Section V. Finally, Section VI has been added to provide insights into measuring a child holistically, in terms of both health and well-being.

Body structure measures would include those that evaluate the structural integrity of each of the organs and systems within the body. These biomedical instruments were beyond the scope of this text and were not included. Nonetheless, given the important advances in *novel neuroimaging technologies* such as magnetic resonance spectroscopy, diffusion tensor imaging and volumetric studies of brain microstructure, a chapter was included to update the reader on neuroimaging tools as a measure of brain structure and function. Furthermore, a chapter on *genetic testing* was also included. It should be noted that the gene integrity within the body conceptually is not part of the ICF; rather it considers the mechanisms that underlie the integrity (whether intact or impaired) of the structures and functions of the organs and systems. The rapid evolution and advancement of genetic testing is resulting in rapid expansion of new knowledge of the genetic determinants of developmental disabilities or of the enhanced risk for early brain injury or maldevelopment, which are ultimately associated with disability. Therefore, the chapter on genetic testing provides an overview of these new tests that are increasingly being used in clinical practice and research to elucidate causal pathways of developmental disability.

Component: Body structures and functions
Chapter 3 Brain structure and function: novel neuroimaging tools
Chapter 4 Body structure and function: genetic testing

Body functions within the ICF cover a wide range of system functions and are listed in Table 2.1. The measures available for particular ICF domains that were felt to be most relevant to the clinicians who provide services to children and young people with developmental disabilities and to researchers who investigate clinical research questions pertaining to the field of childhood disability are included in this text. Therefore, chapters describing measures of the functions of the digestive, metabolic and endocrine systems, genitourinary and reproductive systems, or skin and related structures were not included. Similarly, several of the sensory functions (seeing, hearing) involve medical tests and are not described in this text. An effort was made to include chapters related to all global mental functions and specific mental functions; however, some particular mental functions are unfortunately excluded from this edition. For global mental functions, there is no chapter that specifically describes measures of dispositions and intrapersonal functions (b125; although this is acknowledged by ICF-CY coding as related to temperament and personality functions) or energy and drive functions (b130). For specific mental functions, chapters describing measures of psychomotor functions (b147), thought functions (b160), basic cognitive functions (b163), calculation functions (b172) or mental function of sequencing complex movements (b176) also are not included.

There are numerous measures available that evaluate a child's *global developmental abilities* and thus cover many of the domains of body functions (e.g. sensory, motor, perceptual, speech, behavioural). These may be in

TABLE 2.1
Component: Body functions

ICF domain	Chapters included	
Mental functions		
(a) Global mental functions (b110–b139)	Chapter 5	Consciousness (b110), orientation (b114), sleep (b134)
	Chapter 6	Intellectual (b117)
	Chapter 7	Psychosocial (b122)
	Chapter 8	Temperament and personality (b126)
(b) Specific mental functions (b140–b189)	Chapter 9	Attention (b140), memory (b144), higher-order cognitive (b164)
	Chapter 10	Emotional (b152), experience of self/time (b180)
	Chapter 11	Perceptual (b156)
	Chapter 12	Mental functions of language (b167)
Sensory functions and pain	Chapter 13	General sensory functions (b210–b270)
	Chapter 14	Pain (b280–b289)
Voice and speech functions	Chapter 15	Voice and speech functions (b310–b340)
Functions of the digestive, metabolic and endocrine systems	Not included	
Genitourinary and reproductive functions	Not included	
Neuromusculoskeletal and movement-related functions	Chapter 16	Neuromuscular and movement-related functions (b710–b789)
Functions of the skin and related structures	Not included	

TABLE 2.2
Component: Activities and participation

ICF domain	Chapters included
	Chapter 19 Overview
Learning and applying knowledge	Chapter 20
General tasks and demands	Chapter 21
Communication	Chapter 22
Mobility	Chapter 23
Self-care	Chapter 24
Domestic life	Chapter 25
Interpersonal interactions and relationships	Chapter 26
Major life areas	Chapter 27
Community, social and civic life	Chapter 28

the form of screening tools (Chapter 17) or standardized instruments (Chapter 18). It is challenging to classify these measures to fit within either body functions or activities and participation, and indeed this remains a point of controversy. In my view, the purpose of these measures, for the most part, is to determine whether or not a child exhibits delays or abnormalities in one or more developmental domains. They do not necessarily demonstrate or illustrate whether or not these delays have an impact on everyday activities and participation in age-appropriate life roles. Therefore, these global developmental measures appear to be a better fit with body functions, but nevertheless they appear in their own section (Section III), between body functions and activities and participation.

For *activities and participation measures* (Table 2.2), there is a chapter that provides an overview of the terminology and challenges with measurement of this multifaceted component. Six measures that cross several of the domains within activities and participation are described in detail in this overview. For the specific domains, each chapter describes the construct and summarizes the fundamental attributes of some of the best measures available

TABLE 2.3
Component: Environmental factors

ICF domain	Chapters included
Products and technology	
Natural environment and human-made changes to environment	Chapter 30 Physical, social and attitudinal environment
Support and relationships	Chapter 31 Health services and systems
Attitudes	Chapter 32 Family functioning
Services, systems and policies	

in the domain of interest. Some of the chapters have few measures available that fully capture the particular ICF domain, whereas others have many measures available that evaluate parts of the domain of interest.

For *contextual factors*, although personal factors are not classified within the ICF, this particular area is described in Chapter 29, and measures that may be helpful for evaluating some relevant personal attributes are suggested. Finally, elements of the environment that are most pertinent to children and young people with a disability are conceptualized in three separate chapters (see Table 2.3). The chapters that cover particular environmental factors do not easily separate out within the five ICF domains within this component, as there are overlapping concepts.

Finally, in an effort to acknowledge the importance of a holistic view of *health and well-being*, two additional chapters were added. Chapter 33 provides an overview of measures of health status whereas Chapter 34 focuses on quality of life measures. From my perspective, health and well-being encapsulate all elements of the ICF, with all components (Part 1, 'Functioning and disability', and Part 2, 'Contextual factors') interacting to influence these global spheres. Considerable controversy exists with respect to defining and delineating the unique attributes of health and quality of life, as these concepts and their measures continue to be further developed and refined.

Format for each chapter

A suggested format was provided to each of the contributors of this book, and in most but not all cases the chapters adhere to this format. The first section of each chapter is entitled 'What is the construct?' and is meant to clarify what specific aspects or attributes within the ICF framework are the focus of the measures described within the chapter. In some cases, there may be several constructs or characteristics within an ICF component that are grouped together and collectively defined within this section. It

should be re-emphasized that most measures were not developed with a particular ICF construct in mind, and therefore measures often do not match or adhere precisely to particular elements of the ICF. Nonetheless, the information gathered by using the recommended measures in each chapter should be helpful in informing the ICF coding of the particular attributes of interest. Minimum data sets and structured interviews are some of the methods currently being explored to facilitate specific coding strategies for the ICF-CY.[13,14] Coding is described in detail in the text by the World Health Organization on the ICF-CY 2007.[7]

For most chapters, the second section is entitled 'General factors to consider when measuring this domain'. The authors put forth a variety of issues that are important to consider when measuring the particular area of interest. These could include, for example, methods of measurement, factors related to type of disability, the effect of age, feasibility issues and limitations in the use of measures in children with developmental disabilities. A common issue raised is the need for proxy reporters for some of the measures and the inherent biases that can accompany their perspectives of what the child would report. Another concern frequently raised is the challenge of assessing a domain against a backdrop of ongoing growth and development, implying that children (with a permanent lifelong condition) are maturing and evolving continuously, and therefore age and stage of development must be considered as part of the interpretation of assessment results.[1]

Each chapter provides an overview of recommended measures, which describes the various tools and their purpose and content, as well as their psychometric properties. In most chapters, a tabular format of the best measures is also included with headings such as purpose, population, description of domains, administration and test format, psychometric properties, how to order and key references. These tables are meant to provide a capsule summary of the measure for easy reference.

REFERENCES

1. Lollar DJ, Simeonsson RJ, Nanda U (2000) Measures of outcomes for children and youth. *Arch Phys Med Rehabil* 81(Suppl 2): S46–S52.
2. World Health Organization (2010) *International Classification of Functioning, Disability and Health (ICF)*. Available at: www3.who.int/icf/icftemplate.cfm (accessed 1 August 2011).
3. Simeonsson RJ, Scarborough AA, Hebbeler KM (2006) ICF and ICD codes provide a standard language of disability in young children. *J Clin Epidemiol* 59: 365–373.
4. Colver A (2005) A shared framework and language for childhood disability. *Dev Med Child Neurol* 47: 780–784.
5. Lollar DJ, Simeonsson RJ (2005) Diagnosis to function: classification for children and youths. *J Dev Behav Pediatr* 26: 323–330.
6. Mandich M (2007) International classification of functioning, disability and health. Editorial. *Phys Occup Ther Pediatr* 27: 1–4.
7. World Health Organization (2007) *International Classification of Functioning, Disability and Health – Children and Youth*. Geneva: World Health Organization.
8. McCormack J, Worrall LE (2008) The ICF body functions and structures related to speech–language pathology. *Int J Speech-Lang Pathol* 10: 9–17.
9. Majnemer A (2006) Assessment tools for cerebral palsy: new directions. *Future Neurol* 1: 755–763.
10. McDougall J, Wright V (2009) The ICF-CY and goal attainment scaling: benefits of their combined use for pediatric practice. *Disabil Rehabil* 31: 1362–1372.
11. Majnemer A, Darrah J (2009) New concepts in the rehabilitation of children with developmental disabilities: occupational therapy and physical therapy perspectives. In: Shevell M, editor. *Neurodevelopmental Disabilities: Clinical and Scientific Foundations. International Review of Child Neurology Series*. London: Mac Keith Press, pp. 394–409.
12. Manns PJ, Darrah J (2006) Linking research and clinical practice in physical therapy: strategies for integration. *Physiotherapy* 92: 88–94.
13. Kronk RA, Ogonowski JA, Rice CN, Feldman HM (2005) Reliability in assigning ICF codes to children with special health care needs using a developmentally structured interview. *Disabil Rehabil* 27: 977–983.
14. Simeonsson RJ, Leonardi M, Lollar D, Bjorck-Akesson E, Hollenweger J, Martinuzzi A (2003) Applying the international classification of functioning, disability and health (ICF) to measure childhood disability. *Disabil Rehabil* 25: 602–610.

SECTION II BODY STRUCTURES AND FUNCTIONS

3
NOVEL NEUROIMAGING TOOLS

Catherine Limperopoulos

What is the construct?

Magnetic resonance imaging (MRI) uses a strong magnetic field to align the nuclear magnetization of hydrogen protons in water in organ systems (e.g. the brain). Application of a radiofrequency pulse then alters the alignment of this magnetization, causing the hydrogen nuclei to produce a rotating magnetic field, which is detectable by the scanner.[1] A magnetic resonance image is then produced because the protons in different tissues return to their baseline (equilibrium state) at different rates. When the radiofrequency wave is turned off, the net magnetization is realigned through a process of T1 or T2 recovery or relaxation properties. The T1- or T2-weighted image is mainly determined by the repetition time of the pulse sequence. Different tissues have different T1 or T2 recovery. For example, T1-weighted images have a larger longitudinal and transverse magnetization; fat has a higher signal and will appear bright on a T1-weighted image, whereas water (e.g. cerebrospinal fluid) will appear dark on T1-weighted images. Similarly, cerebral grey matter will appear darker and white matter will appear brighter on T1-weighted images. Conversely, on T2-weighted images, water- and fluid-containing tissues will appear bright and fat will appear dark, while cerebral grey matter will appear brighter than white matter.

One of the advantages of MRI as a clinical and research tool is that it is non-invasive and does not use ionizing radiation, which is potentially harmful. This built-in safety feature makes MRI an ideal tool for imaging healthy children or children with developmental disabilities. Additionally, MRI of the brain increasingly plays an important role in (1) understanding the progression of normal brain development, (2) defining the nature, location and extent of cerebral injury or maldevelopment in children with developmental disabilities, (3) assisting with prognostication by identifying imaging biomarkers that predict adverse neurodevelopmental outcome and

(4) guiding the implementation of targeted medical (e.g. pharmacological and rehabilitation) therapies aimed at restoring function or monitoring interventions aimed at circumventing brain injury.

CONVENTIONAL MRI IN CHILDREN WITH DEVELOPMENTAL DISABILITIES

Conventional MRI has the potential to identify normal and pathological brain morphology and provide objective information about the structure of the developing brain in children with developmental disabilities. The identification of congenital malformations of the brain can assist with determining causation, prognosis and the need for genetic counselling.[2] To date, the neuroradiological work-up of children with developmental disabilities has demonstrated an important role for MRI. Although earlier neuroimaging studies generally reported brains to be structurally normal in appearance in this population irrespective of the type and severity of the delay, recent studies have reported a high incidence of MRI brain abnormalities that are generally minor or subtle in severity (e.g. asymmetrical lateral ventricles, megacisterna magna, diffuse increase in white matter signal, abnormal corpus callosum, cerebellar abnormalities).[3–9] Children with idiopathic developmental delay have been shown to have a high prevalence of abnormalities in the ventricles and corpus callosum.[5] MRI abnormalities have been strongly correlated with the presence of neurological signs, but not with isolated abnormal head circumference.[3,4]

More recently, proton magnetic resonance spectroscopy (^{1}H-MRS) has been combined with conventional MRI as part of the neuroimaging evaluation of children with developmental disabilities. MRS non-invasively evaluates the metabolic status of brain tissue in vivo. Owing to the simplicity and robustness of their detection, peaks of *N*-acetylaspartate (NAA, neuronal marker), choline (Cho, marker of myelination), creatine (Cr, marker of cellular metabolism) and lactate (marker of anaerobic metabolism) are investigated in most studies. Several studies have reported ^{1}H-MRS abnormalities in children with developmental disabilities, including a decreased NAA/Cr ratio and an elevated Cho/Cr ratio as well as higher choline in the white matter,[3,4,10,11] suggesting delayed myelination. From a clinical perspective, these data suggest that performing conventional MRI studies together with MRS has diagnostic value and may contribute to the diagnostic yield in children with developmental disabilities.

Factors to consider when measuring this domain
The human brain is not fully developed at birth. In fact, brain development comprises a continuum that unfolds through the lifespan, albeit most strikingly and dynamically during the fetal and early postnatal periods.[12] During these critical periods, the fundamental neural architecture is laid down and subsequent fine-tuning of neuronal networks takes place.[13] This protracted time course of human brain maturation extends beyond the first decade of life. For example, although it has been suggested that the most rapid pace of maturation of white matter occurs during the first 2 years of life, studies have shown that the process of white matter myelination continues through adolescence and well into adulthood.[14,15] Therefore, an understanding of *normal or typical* brain development and *variability* in developmental milestones of brain maturity is essential in order to understand the timing, extent and progression of aberrant development in children with developmental disabilities.

Another important consideration when imaging a child with a developmental disability for an aetiological determination is the presence of *acquired* injury to the developing brain or *developmental* abnormalities. Adverse events during the first and second trimesters affect the brain during critical periods of neuronal proliferation, migration and cortical organization, resulting in brain malformations. Conversely, injury in the third trimester typically results in acquired injury that may be in the form of glottic or cystic lesions of the brain, primarily affecting the white matter.[16] Late third-trimester injury (after 36 weeks of gestation) predominantly affects the cortical and subcortical grey matter. It is important to note that this grey–white matter classification is now believed to be less distinct, and that there is overlap between lesion types and timing periods.

Reorganization or plasticity after early brain injury also needs to be considered when interpreting MRI studies. Importantly, it is often unclear whether compensation occurs as an alteration of an already existing network (i.e. reorganization) or whether the lesion alters the normal developmental trajectory, leading to a primary abnormal organization.[16]

Lastly, every morphometric MRI measure by which the brain may be characterized is dependent upon the developmental stage. Moreover, the developing brain undergoes massive transformation from conception to adult life. Accordingly, keeping in mind that the developmental trajectory of the normal brain is a 'moving' target, there are unique challenges in interpreting paediatric MRI studies.

Overview of recommended measures
The recent successful application of advanced MRI techniques in young children is providing an unprecedented window to better understand the developing brain in vivo. Over the last decade, there has been rapid advancement in magnetic resonance image acquisition and in the development of dedicated image analysis tools for the quantification of brain development in children. A number of novel MRI measures/tools are now available to evaluate brain structure and function in children with developmental disabilities. These tools, summarized below, are revolutionizing our understanding of how the developing human brain unfolds throughout childhood, and of its functional correlates.

VOLUMETRIC MEASUREMENTS: THREE-DIMENSIONAL MRI
Three-dimensional volumetric MRI techniques and postacquisition image analysis are used to quantify brain growth and characterize brain tissue development. Volumetric MRI analysis is achieved by segmentation of the brain volume into tissue types depending on their difference in signal intensity, followed by three-dimensional renderings. This analysis includes global (e.g. total brain volume) and tissue-specific volumes (e.g. cortical grey matter, white matter, subcortical grey matter, cerebrospinal fluid) to characterize impaired growth in specific tissue subtypes that yield local information about neuronal and axonal development (Fig. 3.1). Additionally, regional brain volumetric measures (e.g. premotor region, dorsolateral prefrontal region) can be performed (Fig. 3.2). Surface-based measures can also be obtained. For example, surface representation of the cerebral cortex can be made by measuring cortical thickness, which provides information about the columnar dimension of cortical organization.[14,17] MRI-based cortical thickness quantification follows cortical folding patterns and captures the distance between white matter surface and pial grey matter surface, producing scalar measures throughout the cerebrum[18–20] (Fig. 3.3).

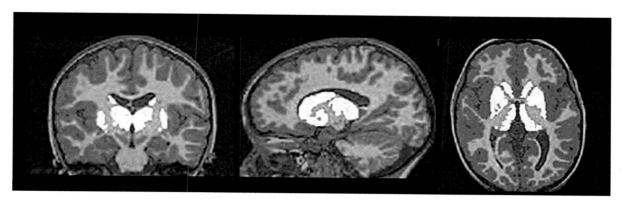

Figure 3.1 Three-dimensional volumetric segmentation of the brain in coronal (left), sagittal (middle) and axial (right) planes. Dark grey, cortical grey matter; light grey, white matter; white, subcortical grey matter.

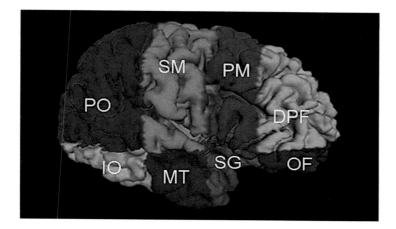

Figure 3.2 Parcellation of the brain into eight regions. DPF, dorsolateral prefrontal region; IO, inferior occipital region; MT, midtemporal region; OF, orbitofrontal region; PM, premotor region; PO, parieto-occipital region; SG, subgenual region; SM, sensorimotor region.

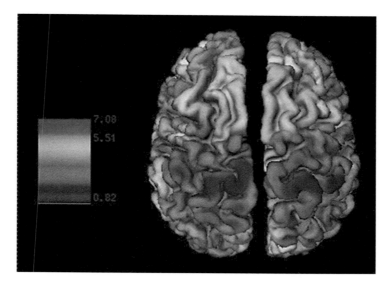

Figure 3.3 Cortical thickness measurements with corresponding scalar values measured in millimetres.

Voxel-based Morphometry

Voxel-based morphometry is a relatively new image-processing technique used to examine regional differences in tissue density throughout the brain.[21] This automated technique characterizes morphometric differences between children using a voxel-by-voxel examination of regional brain tissue concentration and volume from high-resolution structural MRI. Voxel-based morphometry can be used to study normal development with increasing age, as well as pathological conditions such as seizures and malformations of cortical development.[22]

Microstructural Measurements: Diffusion Tensor Imaging

Diffusion tensor imaging (DTI) techniques allow us to probe even deeper into white matter development in children with developmental disabilities. This MRI technique assesses the diffusion of water across the axes of white matter bundles and provides important information at a microarchitectural level about maturational processes and the impact of cerebral injury or maldevelopment on the developing brain.[23–25] Specifically, the motion (or diffusion) of water molecules in biological tissues can be measured by the apparent diffusion coefficient (ADC). Diffusion of water is influenced by many factors. For example, water diffusion is impeded by white matter bundles that themselves delineate functional connectivity. Fractional anisotropy is used to measure fibre tract organization and connectivity in specific regions of interest (e.g. the posterior limb of the internal capsule) and can provide important prognostic information on disturbances in axonal microstructure in children with developmental disabilities. Using DTI, a progressive decrease in white matter ADC together with an increase in fractional anisotropy has been demonstrated between 28 and 40 weeks in preterm infants, reflecting increased white matter fibre organization.[26] More recently, DTI fibre-tracking methods have been developed and applied to young children. These tractography techniques delineate and measure different fibre tracts within the brain through diffusion methods[25] (Fig. 3.4) and can help elucidate the mechanisms governing altered microcircuitry of specific white matter tracts in the developing brain.

Functional Measurements: Functional MRI

Functional MRI (fMRI) is a powerful MRI modality that uses the different magnetic properties of oxygenated and deoxygenated blood in response to neuronal activity.[27] Neuronal activation results in an increase in tissue oxygenation that occurs on top of the increase in oxygen demand. It is precisely this haemodynamic activity, referred to as blood oxygenation level dependent (BOLD), that enables the assessment of neural processing in response to cerebral tasks. fMRI is one of the most important methods for in vivo non-invasive investigation of cognitive development in children. However, an important challenge in performing fMRI in young children is compliance. Moreover, fMRI paradigms are not feasible

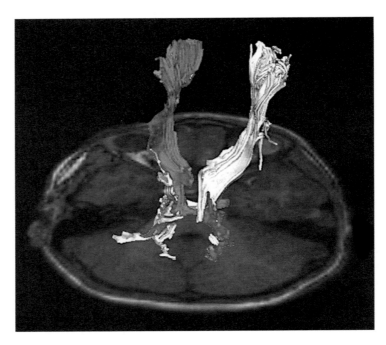

Figure 3.4 Example of diffusion tensor tractography images depicting the cerebro-ponto-cerebellar tracts.

in young infants. The very recent successful application of resting-state functional connectivity MRI to study young infants promises to be an exciting method to assess the earliest forms of cerebral connectivity and to characterize its early development in the human brain.[28–31] This modified fMRI technique measures spontaneous fluctuations in the BOLD signal during the resting state, fluctuations which represent neural networks.

MEASUREMENT CHALLENGES OF ADVANCED MRI MEASUREMENTS: RELIABILITY

Advanced MRI techniques offer a powerful tool for the non-invasive assessment of brain development in children; however, they also present unique challenges to those who perform the studies and those who interpret them. *Reliability* is a cornerstone of clinical research measurement. The accurate and reliable measurement of brain structure from MRI data is not a trivial task. For example, reliability can differ depending on the MRI tool being used and what is being measured (i.e. structure, function, metabolism).[32] Hence, it is important to establish the reliability of quantitative MRI measurements in children and to take into account factors that can influence the reliability of these measures (e.g. developmental age, brain injury, compliance). Defining the psychometric properties of these novel MRI measures is important in order to reliably detect differences in global and regional cortical development in children with developmental disabilities. Despite the critical importance of measurement accuracy in neuroimaging research, MRI reliability and validation studies have received relatively little systematic investigation, particularly in children. These data are summarized below.

BRAIN STRUCTURE AND MICROSTRUCTURE

Diffusion tensor imaging techniques have been used by several groups to investigate white matter development in infants and young children;[23,33–35] however, very few studies have examined the reproducibility of these imaging tools in children. One study reported highly reproducible (intrarater coefficients of variation <2.8% and inter-rater coefficients of variation <4.9%) measures of ADC and fractional anisotropy using region of interest-based methods. Test–retest reliability was also found to be high (coefficients of variation <9.6%).[36] More recently, the reliability of fibre-tracking measurements in DTI studies has been examined in adult populations, and results demonstrate high intrarater intraclass correlation coefficients (>0.92) and moderate to high inter-rater (>0.76) correlation coefficients for geometric alignment and diffusion property measurements, respectively.[37]

Available data suggest moderate to high intra- and inter-rater reliability, with correlation coefficients ranging between 0.73 and 0.99 for manually derived measurements of tissue-specific types (e.g. cortical grey matter, myelinated and unmyelinated white matter, thalami and basal ganglia)[38] and cerebral structures (e.g. cerebellum, hippocampus, amygdala, corpus callosum)[38–42] in newborn infants and young children using manual or semi-automated tools. Similarly, intrarater reliability coefficient values for regional cerebral measurements (e.g. premotor region, midtemporal region) have also been reported to be above 0.77 (range 0.77–0.98).[38,42,43] Manual measurements of the brain are difficult and labour intensive. For example, it can take a trained anatomist several days to manually label a single set of high-resolution structural brain magnetic resonance images.[44] Therefore, manual labelling is not feasible when dealing with large MRI data sets. Moreover, manual measurements performed by a skilled operator are susceptible to operator bias.

Advanced automated postprocessing MRI tools (described earlier) have been developed to facilitate efficient, operator-independent brain structure quantification. These include atlas-based methods,[45,46] voxel-based morphometry[21] and tensor-based morphometry,[47] to name a few. Several studies have compared automated MRI measurements (e.g. cortical thickness, brain segmentation) with regional manual measurements derived from both in vivo and post-mortem brain MRI studies,[44,48] primarily in adults. Overall, the results suggest high accuracy and reliability when comparing cortical thickness within-patient and cross-patient differences, as well as test–retest reliability.[44,49] Similarly, whole-brain segmentation tools have also been shown to perform well in the presence of anatomical variability and to be comparable in accuracy to manual labelling methods.[48,50] The contrast-to-noise ratio (e.g. grey/white matter contrast) and the fidelity of the underlying magnetic resonance data have been reported to be important determinants of the overall precision of MRI measurements. These factors are particularly vital in paediatric MRI studies, which are often affected by poor image quality secondary to motion, especially in young children, and by the well-known challenges of reliably segmenting the immature brain secondary to its decreased tissue contrast/image quality. Nevertheless, a surge of research activities are focused on the application of these automated MRI measurements of cerebral structure, microstructure and function in young infants.[28,51–57] Studies on the accuracy of these techniques are currently under way, and preliminary reports are promising.

Brain function

Several approaches have been used to measure the reliability of estimated activity using fMRI. Some studies have estimated the reliability of fMRI data to be highly accurate for some tasks and brain regions.[58–60] Others have reported low reliability.[61,62] In a recent survey of fMRI test–retest reliability, the average intraclass correlation coefficient value was 0.50. Notably, most studies have been carried out in adolescents or adults. Reliability has been shown to vary by cognitive task and experimental design. In general, simple motor and sensory tasks have greater reliability than tasks involving higher cognition.[31] The test–retest interval also plays a role; overall, an increase in time between the initial scan and the retest scan decreases reliability. Another important consideration is that MRI measures differ between healthy individuals and individuals with brain disorders; such disorders can be progressive in nature or may result in functional recovery, either of which can impact the results of fMRI.[31] Finally, reliability in fMRI studies can also be affected by the degree of stability of the patterns of activation within an individual (test–retest reliability), especially given that the cognitive state of an individual is variable over time (i.e. because of differences in arousal, attention, etc.).

Factors that influence the reproducibility of MRI-driven measures

The potential influence of magnetic resonance image acquisition and data analysis parameters on the reliability of the MRI-derived measures is an important consideration. The reliability of MRI-driven automated measures can be influenced by a number of factors, including (1) individual-related factors (e.g. hydration status, age, cognitive level, compliance),[48,49] (2) instrument-related factors (e.g. field strength, thermal noise, scanner manufacturer, imaging magnet gradients,[50] pulse sequence) and (3) data postprocessing-related factors (e.g. software package and version, parameters selected for analyses).[49,63] Although some degree of standardization exists in the preprocessing and postprocessing of MRI data, the increasingly broad range of available computational pipelines increases the variability between results. All of these factors may affect the ability to detect structural and functional differences between groups, not only in studies using cross-sectional designs but in longitudinal studies as well. Prospective studies describing normal development or studies characterizing the progression of neurological disorders face additional challenges from individual-related factors (described above) as well as instrument-related factors (i.e. major scanner upgrades, across-session system instabilities). Moreover, multisite studies can be particularly flawed in study design and interpretation because of instrument-related differences between sites, such as scanner manufacturer, field strength and other hardware components.

More recently, studies have begun to investigate the effects of field strength, scanner upgrade and manufacture on the reliability of MRI measurements. Available evidence suggests that, although within-scanner measurements are very reliable across MRI sessions even after upgrades, the use of different MRI scanners and MRI acquisitions (e.g. the use of different pulse sequences), as well as different parameters in postprocessing, negatively affects the reliability of MRI measurements. Therefore, combining data across platforms and across field strength (e.g. 1.5T vs 3.0T) introduces bias.[49,50] These factors are important to consider and to control for when designing multisite or longitudinal studies in order to optimize measurement accuracy and minimize systematic error. Similar studies are needed in paediatric populations.

Summary

Recent advances in the rapidly evolving field of paediatric MRI-driven research are revolutionizing our ability to study in vivo brain development to an unprecedented level of detail. The successful application of advanced MRI acquisition techniques and sophisticated computational pipelines, including diffusion tractography, functional brain connectivity maps and advanced brain morphometric studies, will undoubtedly provide new insights into the complex and intricate relationships between normal development, maldevelopment or acquired injury, and brain plasticity. These newer neuroimaging techniques offer higher sensitivity to more subtle structural and functional alterations detected by conventional MRI, and have the potential to better elucidate the anatomical substrates that underlie impaired motor, cognitive and sociobehavioural development in children with developmental disabilities. However, important work lies ahead in carefully assessing the psychometric properties of these novel MRI-based quantification methodologies in order to optimize their measurement sensitivity and specificity and to minimize measurement error. Large-scale collaborative multicentre studies are needed to effectively understand the influence of reliability and reproducibility of MRI-driven measurements across the lifespan.

REFERENCES

1. Bitar R, Leung G, Perng R, et al (2006) MR pulse sequences: what every radiologist wants to know but is afraid to ask. *Radiographics* 26: 513–537.

2. Battaglia A (2003) Neuroimaging studies in the evaluation of developmental delay/mental retardation. *Am J Med Genet C Semin Med Genet* 117C: 25–30.

3. Verbruggen KT, Maurits NM, Meiners LC, Brouwer OF, van Spronsen FJ, Sijens PE (2009) Quantitative multivoxel proton spectroscopy of the brain in developmental delay. *J Magn Reson Imaging* 30: 716–721.

4. Verbruggen KT, Meiners LC, Sijens PE, Lunsing RJ, van Spronsen FJ, Brouwer OF (2009) Magnetic resonance imaging and proton magnetic resonance spectroscopy of the brain in the diagnostic evaluation of developmental delay. *Eur J Paediatr Neurol* 13: 181–190.

5. Widjaja E, Nilsson D, Blaser S, Raybaud C (2008) White matter abnormalities in children with idiopathic developmental delay. *Acta Radiol* 49: 589–595.

6. Soto-Ares G, Joyes B, Lemaitre MP, Vallee L, Pruvo JP (2003) MRI in children with mental retardation. *Pediatr Radiol* 33: 334–345.

7. Bouhadiba Z, Dacher J, Monroc M, Vanhulle C, Menard JF, Kalifa G (2000) [MRI of the brain in the evaluation of children with developmental delay]. *J Radiol* 81: 870–873.

8. Trauner D, Wulfeck B, Tallal P, Hesselink J (2000) Neurological and MRI profiles of children with developmental language impairment. *Dev Med Child Neurol* 42: 470–475.

9. Webster RI, Erdos C, Evans K, et al (2008) Neurological and magnetic resonance imaging findings in children with developmental language impairment. *J Child Neurol* 23: 870–877.

10. Filippi CG, Ulug AM, Deck MD, Zimmerman RD, Heier LA (2002) Developmental delay in children: assessment with proton MR spectroscopy. *AJNR Am J Neuroradiol* 23: 882–888.

11. Fayed N, Morales H, Modrego PJ, Munoz-Mingarro J (2006) White matter proton MR spectroscopy in children with isolated developmental delay: does it mean delayed myelination? *Acad Radiol* 13: 229–235.

12. Limperopoulos C (2010) Advanced neuroimaging techniques: their role in the development of future fetal and neonatal neuroprotection. *Semin Perinatol* 34: 93–101.

13. Toga AW, Thompson PM, Sowell ER (2006) Mapping brain maturation. *Trends Neurosci* 29: 148–159.

14. Caviness VS, Jr., Kennedy DN, Richelme C, Rademacher J, Filipek PA (1996) The human brain age 7–11 years: a volumetric analysis based on magnetic resonance images. *Cereb Cortex* 6: 726–736.

15. Rajapakse JC, DeCarli C, McLaughlin A, et al (1996) Cerebral magnetic resonance image segmentation using data fusion. *J Comput Assist Tomogr* 20: 206–218.

16. Staudt M (2010) Brain plasticity following early life brain injury: insights from neuroimaging. *Semin Perinatol* 34: 87–92.

17. Caviness VS Jr, Lange NT, Makris N, Herbert MR, Kennedy DN (1999) MRI-based brain volumetrics: emergence of a developmental brain science. *Brain Dev* 21: 289–295.

18. Lerch JP, Evans AC (2005) Cortical thickness analysis examined through power analysis and a population simulation. *NeuroImage* 24: 163–173.

19. Kim JS, Singh V, Lee JK, et al (2005) Automated 3-D extraction and evaluation of the inner and outer cortical surfaces using a Laplacian map and partial volume effect classification. *NeuroImage* 27: 210–221.

20. Karama S, Ad-Dab'bagh Y, Haier RJ, et al (2009) Positive association between cognitive ability and cortical thickness in a representative US sample of healthy 6 to 18 year-olds. *Intelligence* 37: 145–155.

21. Ashburner J, Friston KJ (2000) Voxel-based morphometry – the methods. *NeuroImage* 11: 805–821.

22. Bonilha L, Montenegro MA, Rorden C, et al (2006) Voxel-based morphometry reveals excess gray matter concentration in patients with focal cortical dysplasia. *Epilepsia* 47: 908–915.

23. Mukherjee P, Miller JH, Shimony JS, et al (2001) Normal brain maturation during childhood: developmental trends characterized with diffusion-tensor MR imaging. *Radiology* 221: 349–358.

24. Miller JH, McKinstry RC, Philip JV, Mukherjee P, Neil JJ (2003) Diffusion-tensor MR imaging of normal brain maturation: a guide to structural development and myelination. *AJR Am J Roentgenol* 180: 851–859.

25. Neil JJ (2008) Diffusion imaging concepts for clinicians. *J Magn Reson Imaging* 27: 1–7.

26. Huppi PS, Maier SE, Peled S, et al (1998) Microstructural development of human newborn cerebral white matter assessed in vivo by diffusion tensor magnetic resonance imaging. *Pediatr Res* 44: 584–590.

27. Ment LR, Constable RT (2007) Injury and recovery in the developing brain: evidence from functional MRI studies of prematurely born children. *Nat Clin Pract Neurol* 3: 558–571.

28. Smyser CD, Inder TE, Shimony JS, et al (2010) Longitudinal analysis of neural network development in preterm infants. *Cereb Cortex* 20: 2852–2862.

29. Lin W, Zhu Q, Gao W, et al (2008) Functional connectivity MR imaging reveals cortical functional connectivity in the developing brain. *AJNR Am J Neuroradiol* 29: 1883–1889.

30. Fair DA, Cohen AL, Dosenbach NU, et al (2008) The maturing architecture of the brain's default network. *Proc Natl Acad Sci U S A* 105: 4028–4032.

31. Fransson P, Skiold B, Horsch S, et al (2007) Resting-state networks in the infant brain. *Proc Natl Acad Sci U S A* 104: 15531–15536.

32. Bennett CM, Miller MB (2010) How reliable are the results from functional magnetic resonance imaging? *Ann N Y Acad Sci* 1191: 133–155.

33. Hermoye L, Saint-Martin C, Cosnard G, et al (2006) Pediatric diffusion tensor imaging: normal database and observation of the white matter maturation in early childhood. *NeuroImage* 29: 493–504.

34. Jones RA, Palasis S, Grattan-Smith JD (2003) The evolution of the apparent diffusion coefficient in the pediatric brain at low and high diffusion weightings. *J Magn Reson Imaging* 18: 665–674.

35. McKinstry RC, Mathur A, Miller JH, et al (2002) Radial organization of developing preterm human cerebral cortex revealed by non-invasive water diffusion anisotropy MRI. *Cereb Cortex* 12: 1237–1243.

36. Bonekamp D, Nagae LM, Degaonkar M, et al (2007) Diffusion tensor imaging in children and adolescents: reproducibility, hemispheric, and age-related differences. *NeuroImage* 34: 733–742.

37. Danielian LE, Iwata NK, Thomasson DM, Floeter MK (2010) Reliability of fiber tracking measurements in diffusion tensor imaging for longitudinal study. *NeuroImage* 49: 1572–1580.

38. Thompson DK, Warfield SK, Carlin JB, et al (2007) Perinatal risk factors altering regional brain structure in the preterm infant. *Brain* 130: 667–677.

39. Limperopoulos C, Soul JS, Gauvreau K, et al (2005) Late gestation cerebellar growth is rapid and impeded by premature birth. *Pediatrics* 115: 688–695.

40. Thompson DK, Wood SJ, Doyle LW, et al (2008) Neonate hippocampal volumes: prematurity, perinatal predictors, and 2-year outcome. *Ann Neurol* 63: 642–651.

41. Allin M, Matsumoto H, Santhouse AM, et al (2001) Cognitive and motor function and the size of the cerebellum in adolescents born very pre-term. *Brain* 124: 60–66.

42. Peterson BS, Vohr B, Staib LH, et al (2000) Regional brain volume abnormalities and long-term cognitive outcome in preterm infants. *JAMA* 284: 1939–1947.

43. Limperopoulos C, Tworetzky W, McElhinney D, et al (2010) Brain volume and metabolism in fetuses with congenital heart disease: evaluation with quantitative magnetic resonance imaging and spectroscopy. *Circulation* 121: 26–33.

44. Fischl B, Dale AM (2000) Measuring the thickness of the human cerebral cortex from magnetic resonance images. *Proc Natl Acad Sci U S A* 97: 11050–11055.

45. Collins DL, Zijdenbos AP, Kollokian V, et al (1998) Design and construction of a realistic digital brain phantom. *IEEE Trans Med Imaging* 17: 463–468.

46. Fischl B, Salat DH, van der Kouwe AJ, et al (2004) Sequence-independent segmentation of magnetic resonance images. *NeuroImage* 23(Suppl 1): S69–84.

47. Leow A, Huang SC, Geng A, et al (2005) Inverse consistent mapping in 3D deformable image registration: its construction and statistical properties. *Inf Process Med Imaging* 19: 493–503.

48. Fischl B, Salat DH, Busa E, et al (2002) Whole brain segmentation: automated labeling of neuroanatomical structures in the human brain. *Neuron* 33: 341–355.

49. Han X, Jovicich J, Salat D, et al (2006) Reliability of MRI-derived measurements of human cerebral cortical thickness: the effects of field strength, scanner upgrade and manufacturer. *NeuroImage* 32: 180–194.

50. Jovicich J, Czanner S, Han X, et al (2009) MRI-derived measurements of human subcortical, ventricular and intracranial brain volumes: reliability effects of scan sessions, acquisition sequences, data analyses, scanner upgrade, scanner vendors and field strengths. *NeuroImage* 46: 177–192.

51. Hill J, Dierker D, Neil J, et al (2010) A surface-based analysis of hemispheric asymmetries and folding of cerebral cortex in term-born human infants. *J Neurosci* 30: 2268–2276.

52. Shi F, Fan Y, Tang S, Gilmore JH, Lin W, Shen D (2010) Neonatal brain image segmentation in longitudinal MRI studies. *NeuroImage* 49: 391–400.

53. Weisenfeld NI, Warfield SK (2009) Automatic segmentation of newborn brain MRI. *NeuroImage* 47: 564–572.

54. Murgasova M, Dyet L, Edwards D, Rutherford M, Hajnal J, Rueckert D (2007) Segmentation of brain MRI in young children. *Acad Radiol* 14: 1350–1366.

55. Seghier ML, Huppi PS (2010) The role of functional magnetic resonance imaging in the study of brain development, injury, and recovery in the newborn. *Semin Perinatol* 34: 79–86.

56. Bassi L, Ricci D, Volzone A, et al (2008) Probabilistic diffusion tractography of the optic radiations and visual function in preterm infants at term equivalent age. *Brain* 131: 573–582.

57. Adams E, Chau V, Poskitt KJ, Grunau RE, Synnes A, Miller SP (2010) Tractography-based quantitation of corticospinal tract development in premature newborns. *J Pediatr* 156: 882–888.

58. Aron AR, Gluck MA, Poldrack RA (2006) Long-term test–retest reliability of functional MRI in a classification learning task. *NeuroImage* 29: 1000–1006.

59. Maldjian JA, Laurienti PJ, Driskill L, Burdette JH (2002) Multiple reproducibility indices for evaluation of cognitive functional MR imaging paradigms. *AJNR Am J Neuroradiol* 23: 1030–1037.

60. Raemaekers M, Vink M, Zandbelt B, van Wezel RJ, Kahn RS, Ramsey NF (2007) Test–retest reliability of fMRI activation during prosaccades and antisaccades. *NeuroImage* 36: 532–542.

61. Duncan KJ, Pattamadilok C, Knierim I, Devlin JT (2009) Consistency and variability in functional localisers. *NeuroImage* 46: 1018–1026.

62. Rau S, Fesl G, Bruhns P, et al (2007) Reproducibility of activations in Broca area with two language tasks: a functional MR imaging study. *AJNR Am J Neuroradiol* 28: 1346–1353.

63. Senjem ML, Gunter JL, Shiung MM, Petersen RC, Jack CR Jr (2005) Comparison of different methodological implementations of voxel-based morphometry in neurodegenerative disease. *NeuroImage* 26: 600–608.

4
GENETIC TESTING

Myriam Srour and Michael I. Shevell

Introduction

This chapter is not intended as a comprehensive guide to genetic testing and diagnostic work-up. Technology in this field is advancing at an extremely fast rate, quickly rendering information out of date. Thus, this chapter is intended as an overview of the basic genetic concepts, approaches and currently available techniques in genetic testing.

What is the construct?

Genetic testing refers to a medical test performed to identify changes in DNA, chromosomes, proteins and certain metabolites.[1] Over the past decade, our knowledge of human genetics has exploded owing to substantial advances in molecular technologies and the completion of the human genome project in 2003. The human genome comprises 3 billion base-pairs and 20 000 to 25 000 genes, of which approximately half exert an effect within the central nervous system.[2] Sequence information is stored in widely accessible public databases such as the UCSC genome browser (http://genome.ucsc.edu) or the Ensembl genome browser (http://uswest.ensembl.org). Briefly, a gene comprises (1) exonic sequences which encode a specific protein product; (2) intronic sequences between the exons that are not translated into protein; and (3) transcribed (mRNA-produced) but non-translated (i.e. not incorporated into protein) sequences that have a regulatory role in protein synthesis. A gene can have alternative splice isoforms by skipping or incorporating different exons depending on differential spatial (e.g. different organs) and/or temporal (e.g. different stages of brain development) expression.

The aim of clinical genetic testing is to answer questions associated with the health of the individual and includes (1) diagnostic, (2) presymptomatic, (3) carrier and (4) predispositional tests. Predispositional tests mostly remain in the research domain and refer to establishing risk estimation of developing a disease which is usually complex and multifactorial, such as type 2 diabetes or arthritis.

Identifying the specific genetic aetiology of a condition allows for the (1) possible implementation of specific treatment, (2) introduction of preventative measures for complications associated with the disease, (3) avoidance of unnecessary costly and burdensome further testing, (4) refined prognostication and (5) estimation for inheritance and possible risk of recurrence in family members.

General factors to consider when measuring this domain

Genetic tests can be performed in several clinical situations. They can be performed in a *symptomatic* individual for confirmation or exclusion of a genetic condition, or in an *asymptomatic* individual who has a positive family history and is at risk of inheriting a genetic mutation. The latter includes *carrier testing* and *presymptomatic testing*. In this situation, testing may be performed to identify whether the individual is a carrier of the mutation (i.e. is not at risk of developing the disease but can transmit the mutation to his or her offspring, as in autosomal recessive or X-linked disorders). Alternatively, genetic testing could identify a presymptomatic individual (i.e. someone who is at high risk of developing the disease, such as someone with X-linked adrenoleukodystrophy or Huntington disease). In general, presymptomatic testing is usually performed for diseases for which treatment is available (e.g. metabolic disease) or preventative or screening measures can be instituted (e.g. von Hippel–Lindau syndrome). Genetic testing should be performed only when its benefits clearly outweigh its disadvantages. Genetic counselling is strongly recommended before and after genetic testing, but especially presymptomatic and carrier testing. This involves informing the individual of the inheritance, natural history and management of the disease, the rationale for the test, its potential benefits, and disadvantages and possible consequences on future reproductive, health, employment and insurance prospects. Genetic counselling is also important to address the psychosocial, emotional and familial implications.

It is always important to consider the possibility of a genetic aetiology when assessing a child with a developmental disability. A family history of a similar condition should always be sought. It is important to keep in mind that the lack of a positive family history of disease does not exclude a genetic aetiology, for several reasons. First, the mutation may have arisen de novo in the child. Second, the condition may be autosomal recessive, and so there may not be other affected family members. Third, one should keep in mind the sensitive issue of non-paternity, especially in autosomal dominant conditions. Fourth, many disorders have variable penetrance or expression; thus, a parent carrying the same mutation may have very mild or absent symptoms (e.g. Charcot–Marie–Tooth disease, hereditary spastic paraparesis, myotonic muscular dystrophy). Other important questions to ask when taking a family history include consanguinity, a history of multiple miscarriages, ethnicity and place of origin. Some geographic regions and ethnic minorities have an increased incidence of genetic disease owing to recognized founder effects (e.g. French-Canadians for myotonic dystrophy, individuals of Ashkenazi Jewish ancestry for Tay–Sachs disease).

Overview of recommended measures

Types of genetic testing include cytogenetic, molecular and biochemical/analyte analysis. Cytogenetic testing surveys the chromosomes for aneuploidy (i.e. additional or missing chromosomes), deletions, duplications and structural rearrangements such as translocations, inversions and marker chromosomes. The main cytogenetic techniques include karyotype analysis, fluorescence in situ hybridization (FISH) and the more novel chromosomal microarray (CMA). Cytogenetic testing is most often used as a first-tier diagnostic test for children with global developmental delay, intellectual disability and/or autism spectrum disorders in the absence of features suggestive of a specific genetic disorder. When clinical features are suggestive of a known Mendelian disorder(s), specific genes can be tested for mutations using different molecular techniques such as targeted mutation analysis, deletion/duplication analysis and sequence analysis of an entire coding region. For inborn errors of metabolism, testing usually begins with biochemical analysis of enzymes or analytes in blood, urine, cerebrospinal fluid or other body tissues. If a biochemical diagnosis is reached, molecular testing of the causative gene can be performed to identify the specific genetic defect (mutation).

CYTOGENETIC ANALYSIS

Cytogenetic analysis refers to the study of chromosomes and aims to detect chromosomal aberrations such as deletions, duplications, translocations, or supernumerary or marker chromosomes. Karyotype analysis, FISH and CMA will be discussed. Although each technique has its advantages and disadvantages, the main difference lies in the size of the aberration that can be detected. CMA has become the technique of first choice.

Karyotype analysis

Karyotype analysis is the classic method of visualizing chromosomes in cells that have been arrested during cell division using special stains (such as Giemsa) to allow for the recognition of structural or numerical rearrangements. The chromosomes take on a striped appearance under the microscope. The chromosomes are examined for irregularities in banding patterns that correspond to deletions, duplications or translocations. Marker or supernumerary chromosomes can be detected. The resolution is typically at the level of approximately 550 bands, which enables detection of deletions in the range of 5 to 10 million base-pairs.[3] Even high-resolution karyotypes are unreliable for detecting deletions in the range of 3 to 5 million base-pairs in size (which contain, on average, 50 genes). The poor sensitivity and resolution of the karyotype are its main limiting factors. As a comparison, CMA can detect deletions smaller than 50 000 base-pairs to 1 million base-pairs.[4–6] Other disadvantages of karyotype analysis include cost, time and labour requirements. In addition, mosaicism (chromosomal aberration present only in a fraction of cells or tissue types) may be missed – its detection is dependent on the tissue sampled.

A karyotype analysis may be ordered to confirm a specific diagnosis that is apparent on clinical grounds such as Down syndrome or cri du chat syndrome. However, a karyotype is often used to interrogate the genome for a chromosomal aberration to explain a non-specific presentation, such as children with global developmental delay, mental retardation[a]/intellectual disabilities and multiple congenital abnormalities. Until it was supplanted by CMA, a karyotype was recommended as part of the work-up of all children with an intellectual disability or global developmental delay (GDD) regardless of the presence of dysmorphic features, small stature, congenital abnormalities or unusual behaviours. The reported yield from a standard karyotype in children with GDD is between 3% and 11%, with a mean of 3.7%.[7] Yields are more elevated with high-resolution karyotyping (>550 bands). The yield is similar between sexes and across the severity of delay.

---

[a]UK usage: learning disability

It also may be increased in the presence of clinically recognized dysmorphisms.[8]

Fluorescence in situ hybridization and subtelomere studies

Fluorescence in situ hybridization (FISH) is the annealing of fluorescently labelled locus-specific probes to their complementary sequences in the genome. As the fluorescent probes can bind to short, specific sequences, small deletions that are not otherwise detected by classic karyotype analysis can be uncovered. Thus, FISH studies carry a higher resolution than karyotype studies, being able to detect deletions smaller than 1 million base-pairs.

FISH can be locus specific and target a specific region in the genome where a deletion results in a known clinical syndrome. For example, a FISH probe targeting 15q11 can look for a deletion causing Angelman or Prader–Willi syndrome. In addition, FISH can simultaneously assess multiple loci, such as the subtelomeric regions, which are responsible for half of all structural chromosomal abnormalities.[9]

The utility of a complete set of subtelomeric probes has been demonstrated in several studies with a yield of approximately 2.5% in the presence of a normal karyotype.[7,10–12] The yield is higher in moderate to severe intellectual disability (0.5% yield in mild intellectual

KARYOTYPE ANALYSIS	
Purpose	To visualize chromosomes within a cell using special stains (such as Giemsa) to enable recognition of structural or numerical rearrangements
Indications	Detection of supernumerary (additional) chromosomes, deleted or duplicated chromosomal segments, balanced translocations and marker chromosomes
	Evaluation of any child with unexplained global developmental delay
	Evaluation of a child with dysmorphisms or multiple congenital malformations
Limitations	Cannot reliably detect deletions or rearrangements of segments smaller than 3–5 million base-pairs
	May not identify subtle rearrangements of the subtelomeric regions
	Determination of the chromosomal origin of a small supernumerary marker chromosomes may be difficult if size is insufficient to provide a recognizable characteristic banding pattern
	Mosaicism may be missed
	Elevated labour, time and cost requirements

FLUORESCENCE IN SITU HYBRIDIZATION	
Purpose	To detect the presence or absence of specific chromosomes or chromosomal regions through annealing (attachment) of fluorescence-labelled DNA probes to a patient's DNA. Presence of a tested chromosomal region is confirmed by detection of the hybridized fluorescent signal, while deletion of a region is detected by the absence of the expected fluorescent signal
Indications	Testing specific loci for recognized microdeletion or duplication syndromes
	Evaluating subtelomeric regions for rearrangements in unexplained intellectual disability
	Defining chromosomal origin in segmental rearrangements or marker chromosomes
Limitations	Dependent on the karyotype
	Usually hypothesis driven (patient must have features consistent with a recognizable syndrome)
	Does not detect abnormalities distinct from the genomic segments for which probes have been designed and used
	Duplications, triplications, etc. are problematic to characterize as an increase in signal is difficult to quantify
	Largely replaced by chromosomal microarray

disability).[12] The yield is higher in the presence of a positive family history.[8]

It is important to note that FISH remains dependent on the karyotype because the fluorescent probe anneals to the chromosomes in a karyotype preparation. A major limitation of this technique is its dependence on a pretesting hypothesis. The presence of specific recognizable features is a requisite to choosing a specific set of probes. Furthermore, when assessing multiple loci, as in the setting of subtelomeres, this technique does not give additional information on the remainder of the genome (i.e. FISH analyses do not detect abnormalities distinct from the genomic segments for which probes have been designed and used). For these reasons, the use of FISH has been largely supplanted by CMA. FISH is now mostly used as a confirmatory tool to validate deletions detected by CMA.

Chromosomal microarray

Chromosomal microarray (CMA) is a molecular technique with cytogenetic applications. The term CMA includes all types of array-based genomic copy number analyses (i.e. array-based comparative genomic hybridization [aCGH] and single nucleotide polymorphism [SNP] arrays). Since its development a decade ago and its rapid technological refinement, CMA has quickly replaced the methods of karyotype analysis and FISH to become a first-line cytogenetic technique. There are a number of different types of arrays that are available depending on the substrate which is immobilized to the glass slide: bacterial artificial chromosome (BAC), complementary DNAs, oligonucleotides, and SNPs. The principle of aCGH relies on the comparison of two differentially fluorescent-labelled DNA samples: one from the patient and one from a control reference. The labelled DNA is hybridized to DNA fragment targets immobilized on glass slides (array). The arrays are scanned and the data are analysed by software that computes the log2 ratios for a variety of copy number differences, or copy number variations (CNVs), between the patient and reference sample. Thus, it can detect CNVs (i.e. a ratio between a patient and control not equal to 1). For SNP arrays, only a single test DNA is labelled and hybridized to the array for comparison with previously run controls. BAC arrays have largely disappeared from use. Oligonucleotide-based arrays have the greatest resolution and genome coverage, and thus other types of arrays have been mostly phased out. In addition, the arrays vary based on the choice of oligomers on the slide: (1) targeted arrays contain oligomers that target specific regions of the genome, such as the subtelomeres and those responsible for known microdeletion or microduplication syndromes, whereas (2) whole-genome or tiling path arrays offer full genome coverage, with spacing between probes of 50 000 to 1 million base-pairs, and often additional coverage in the subtelomeres and known microdeletion/duplication syndrome regions. Whole-genome arrays should be used in the postnatal setting. The resolution of CMA is determined by the size of the oligomer targets and the density and distribution of the targets throughout the genome. Thus, the smaller the size of the oligo probes and the tighter the spacing, the higher the resolution. The latest microarrays achieve kilobase-level resolution.[13] In addition to its increased resolution, another advantage of CMA over FISH is the array's ability to detect duplications and amplifications and evaluate multiple loci simultaneously without previous targeting. SNP arrays have the advantage of also detecting long stretches of homozygosity, suggesting either consanguinity or uniparental disomy (when both copies of a chromosome or part of a chromosome are inherited from the same parent). Abnormalities on CMA are validated by FISH (especially to detect deletions) or quantitative polymerase chain reaction (qPCR, for duplication).

The most important challenge of CMA is the interpretation of an abnormal result, and the determination of whether a CNV is pathogenic (i.e. responsible for the clinical phenotype) or alternatively represents a normal variation. Guidelines for the interpretation of CNVs are detailed in Kearney et al.[14] Many CNVs described in the literature are present in phenotypically normal individuals. Thus, an initial step in the evaluation of the significance of a CNV is establishing whether it is inherited from a phenotypically normal parent (i.e. thus it is likely to be non-pathogenic) or is de novo (i.e. more likely to be pathogenic). Discrimination between common and rare CNVs is also important in establishing the clinical significance of a CNV. CNVs identified in healthy controls are documented in publicly available online databases such as the Database of Genomic Variants (http://projects.tcag.ca/variation/). The DECIPHER database (https://decipher.sanger.ac.uk/), for example, catalogues chromosomal imbalances and lists the associated phenotypes with appropriate references. Another limitation of CMA is the inability to detect balanced rearrangements. However, several reports have demonstrated that 40% of the balanced translocations as assessed by karyotype are in fact unbalanced.[15] In addition, balanced rearrangements are relatively common in the typical population, with one study estimating the incidence of de novo reciprocal translocation in the typical population at 1 in 2000.[16]

Chromosomal microarray is currently recommended as a first-tier clinical diagnostic test for individuals with developmental disabilities or congenital anomalies.[17] Overall, the yield from CMA in patients with

CHROMOSOMAL MICROARRAY	
Purpose	To detect copy number variations (deletions/duplications) across the genome by comparing hybridization of labelled patient and reference DNA to immobilized DNA fragments. Arrays can be targeted (i.e. contain immobilized fragments of specific regions of the genome known to be responsible for microdeletion syndromes) or can offer whole-genome coverage
Indication	Evaluation for copy number variations (deletions/duplications) in children with unexplained developmental delay, dysmorphisms or multiple congenital malformations
Limitations	Will not detect completely balanced translocations
	May detect variants of unclear clinical significance or deletions/duplications unrelated to the patient's phenotype

developmental delay and intellectual disabilities ranges from 15% to 20% depending on the patient selection and the type of array used.[17] Shoumans et al[18] showed a yield of 9.8% in 41 patients with idiopathic intellectual disability and dysmorphic features using a BAC CMA.[18] In a study by DeVries et al,[19] whole-genome CMA detected pathogenic abnormalities in 10 of 100 patients with intellectual disabilities.[19] Shevell et al[20] performed BAC CMA in 94 patients with non-syndromic global developmental delay and previously normal studies (including karyotyping) and obtained a 6.4% yield. In a large series of 1500 cases submitted to a single laboratory for BAC CMA testing, clinically relevant abnormalities were detected in 5.6% of cases.[21] Engels et al[22] reported on a series of 60 patients with intellectual disability using genome-wide oligo CGH and found a 10% yield of pathogenic CNVs. A number of microdeletion syndromes have been identified as a result of CMA testing. Examples include the microdeletion 17q21.31 syndrome (which is associated with intellectual disability, a characteristic facial appearance and white matter periventricular changes[23,24]) and the 16p11.2 microdeletion syndrome, which is now estimated to occur in 1% of children with autism.[25,26]

In recent years, CMA has become a routine first-line investigation and is replacing conventional karyotyping in the genetic diagnosis of patients with intellectual and developmental disabilities. The interpretation, however, is complicated by the presence of a high variability in large segments of the human genome.

MOLECULAR GENETIC TESTING

Molecular genetic analysis refers to testing for disease-causing changes (i.e. mutations) in specific genes. Targeted mutation screening involves testing either for nucleotide repeat expansion or for one or more specific mutations at specific locations in a gene that are known to be the most frequent in the general or specific population at risk for the disorder (e.g. Glu6Val for sickle cell anaemia). Molecular sequence analysis involves the sequencing and analysis of a gene, and can include either only the exons or both introns and exons and other regions. This enables the detection of nucleotide changes or frameshifts throughout the gene. Sequencing will not be able to detect larger deletions, and therefore other methods such as qPCR or multiplex ligation-dependent probe amplification may need to be used.

Choosing which genetic test to order can be a challenging and daunting task. Knowledge about the disease, the types of genetic tests available and their sensitivity and specificity must be taken into account. The clinician is usually faced with three main clinical situations. First, there may be suspicion of a disorder that is genetically and molecularly homogeneous: the clinical phenotype is associated with a very limited number of mutations in only one gene. Examples of such disorders include myotonic muscular dystrophy, which results from a triplet repeat CTG expansion in *DMPK,* found in 100% of patients, and spinal muscular atrophy type 1, which results from a homozygous deletion of exons 7 and 8 of the *SMN1* gene, found in 95% to 98% of patients.[27] Here, genetic testing usually consists of looking for only the specific mutations and the techniques are usually standardized in regional laboratories with high sensitivity. In the second type of clinical situation, the physician may be facing a disorder that is genetically homogeneous but molecularly heterogeneous: the phenotype is associated with a wide range of mutations in only one gene. Such an example is Duchenne muscular dystrophy, in which all patients have mutations in the dystrophin gene. However, these mutations can be distributed throughout the gene and include point mutations, small insertions or deletions, larger deletions or multiplications of one or several exons, or involve large genomic rearrangements. Thus, targeted mutation analysis is not a good option, and multiple steps and techniques are required such as deletion and duplication analysis, mutation sequence analysis and others.

MOLECULAR GENETIC TESTING	
Purpose	Testing for disease-causing changes (i.e. mutations) in specific genes
	There are multiple methods available: (1) targeted mutation analysis – testing for either a nucleotide repeat expansion or one or more specific mutations in a given gene; (2) sequence analysis of entire coding region – nucleotide sequence is determined for the entire coding region of a gene; and (3) deletion/duplication analysis – testing that identifies deletions/duplications of an entire exon, multiple exons or a whole gene that are not readily detectable by sequence analysis
Indications	Testing for mutations in specific causative genes in patients with a suggestive phenotype
Limitations	False negatives: mutations may be located in regions of the gene that are not tested. With targeted mutation analysis, mutations occurring outside the specific locations that are examined will not be detected
	Mutations in regulatory regions or introns will not be detected with sequence analysis of the entire coding region. Deletions/duplications of entire exon(s) or whole gene are usually not detected on sequencing – specific deletion/duplication analysis needs to be carried out in such cases
	Interpretation of pathogenicity of missense mutations
	Cost can be high

Sensitivity in testing in these conditions varies depending on what level of diagnostic testing is offered by the regional laboratory. Sensitivity is usually lower than in conditions that are genetically and molecularly homogeneous. In the third clinical situation, the physician is faced with a disorder that is genetically and molecularly heterogeneous, whereby the phenotype is associated with multiple mutations in different genes. Disorders that are genetically and molecularly heterogeneous are common. These include, among others, non-syndromic intellectual disability, congenital myasthenic syndromes, Joubert syndrome, Charcot–Marie–Tooth type 1 disease and hereditary spastic paraplegias. There are at least 12 genes known to be mutated in congenital myasthenic syndrome, and as a group they account at present for only 60% of clinically diagnosed cases. Testing for mutations in all the associated genes can sometimes be cost-inefficient; however, with the advances in sequencing technology, many laboratories are now offering sequencing panels for a number of different disorders at relatively affordable prices.

The interpretation of an abnormal test result rests on determining whether the detected abnormality is pathogenic and responsible for the individual's phenotype or, alternatively, represents a non-causal variant. Guidelines to the interpretation of abnormal genetic tests are detailed in the 2007 American College of Medical Genetics and Genomics Recommendations for Standards for Interpretation and Reporting of Sequence Variations.[28] Some mutations are clearly pathogenic. Mutations that have been previously described to cause a given disease,

especially in genetically and molecularly homogeneous disorders, are definitely pathogenic. Nonsense (i.e. resulting in a 'stop' codon) and frameshift (i.e. insertion or deletion of a number of nucleotides that is a multiple of three, thus resulting in the disruption of the triplet reading frame and in a different translation of the sequence) mutations are usually always pathogenic as they result in either a truncated or an absent protein product. Interpretation of a missense mutation is more complicated. One must attempt to predict the functional impact of the mutation on the resulting protein. Is the missense mutation silent (i.e. the coded amino acid remains the same)? Does it result in an amino acid change? Is it present in an important functional domain of the protein? Is this particular nucleotide highly conserved across species? Many laboratories will include an interpretation of the abnormal result. Sometimes, the abnormality will remain of unclear significance. Another important clue to determining whether a mutation is pathogenic is to verify whether the variant is observed in an asymptomatic relative and (when there are multiple affected family members) whether the mutation segregates with the phenotype. A mutation found in an asymptomatic parent renders it less likely to be pathogenic, although caution must be taken as some disorders have incomplete penetrance and significant intrafamilial phenotypic variability.

A negative result, or the absence of the identification of a mutation, must also be carefully interpreted. It must always be considered in light of what exactly was looked for and which technique was used. Thus, a normal result of targeted mutation analysis will only eliminate the possibility of mutations in the specific sites tested. In a molecularly homogeneous disorder, one can be more confident that the disease specifically tested for is excluded. However, in cases of molecular heterogeneity, one cannot exclude the possibility of a mutation at another site. Furthermore, one must be aware that sequencing of a gene will miss deletions, and additional techniques must be utilized to eliminate deletions or more complex intragenic rearrangements. Thus, a negative result must always be interpreted in light of the sensitivity of the test (its ability to detect certain mutations) and the allelic heterogeneity of the disorder at both a genotypic and a phenotypic level.

SINGLE NUCLEOTIDE POLYMORPHISMS AND GENOME-WIDE ASSOCIATION STUDIES

The sequencing of the human genome reveals many types of variations. The most common type of variation is at the level of a single nucleotide and is referred to as a single nucleotide polymorphism (SNP). More than 9 million SNPs have been reported. These are distributed every few hundred bases and are more frequent in non-coding (intronic) regions of the genome. The great majority are binary, which means that at a given position there are two possible alleles (C or G, for example). The development of microarray and bead technology has made it possible to easily sample and genotype (i.e. test for) over 1 million SNPs per individual in a cost-effective way. This has allowed the use of SNPs as molecular markers in many studies of monogenetic or complex diseases. Genome-wide association studies (GWASs) look for associations between common SNPs and a particular clinical phenotype. More recently, GWASs have been extended to also include CNVs. Significant differences in allele frequency between controls and clinically affected individuals would imply that the corresponding region of the genome contains functional DNA sequence variants that

influence the disease trait in question. GWASs are used primarily in complex diseases, such as diabetes, where a large number of genetic susceptibility variants are thought to be involved. To date, these studies have identified risk and protective factors for asthma,[29] cancer,[30] diabetes,[31,32] heart disease,[33,34] schizophrenia and bipolar disorder.[35] SNP association studies can also be performed by testing only a restricted number of SNPs (located for example in or surrounding a candidate gene, such as genes involved in the dopaminergic pathway in attention-deficit–hyperactivity disorder).

Although GWASs are increasingly utilized, the approach has important limitations. The first is that despite the observation that many susceptibility loci have been identified, very few have been replicated. Associations that have been identified from a single genome-wide association data set rarely have definite statistical support. A *p*-value of approximately 10^{-7} is required for significance and corresponds to a significance of $p=0.05$ in traditional, classical epidemiological studies. Very large sample sizes are required for adequate power. Adequate matching of the control population is extremely important and should include matching for ethnic origin as SNP frequencies vary significantly from one ethnic population to the next. Unrecognized subpopulations in a cohort may produce false-positive or false-negative results. A major limitation of GWASs lies in the assumption that the risk allele is common and is directly being tested. Thus, an association with rare alleles will be missed as they are not tested or because the signal is lost. Furthermore, certain conditions are genetically heterogeneous, making the search for allele associations unlikely to be fruitful. Intellectual disability is a good example of a genetically heterogeneous condition that is already associated with mutations in over 300 genes,[36] and thus is not suited to be studied by a GWAS approach. Finally, although the GWAS approach has led to the identification of a small number of causative

GENOME-WIDE ASSOCIATION STUDIES	
Purpose	To determine associations between single nucleotide polymorphisms or copy number variations and a particular clinical phenotype
	Used primarily to look for susceptibility loci in complex diseases
Indications	Still only used at the research level to identify susceptibility loci and identify genes implicated in disease pathogenicity
Limitations	Requirement of very large sample sizes
	Biases due to inappropriate selection of cases and controls
	Insensitivity to rare and structural variants
	Unsuitable for the study of heterogeneous disorders

genes and susceptibility loci (such as *CARD15*, *IL23R* and *ATG16L1* in Crohn disease, implicating autophagy in disease pathogenesis[37]), most identified susceptibility loci are of little or no diagnostic relevance.[38] Most of these factors account only for a small proportion of the total genetic risk, and their presence or absence will rarely increase risk for a disorder by over twofold.

WHOLE-EXOME SEQUENCING

The recent introduction of what is termed 'next-generation sequencing' has revolutionized the methods of large-scale sequencing, bringing in a high level of efficiency and significantly reducing associated time, labour and financial costs. Because most recognized disease-causing mutations (>80%) affect either the protein-coding or splice sites,[39] sequencing all the exons of the genome – that is, whole-exome sequencing (WES) – represents a cost-effective strategy. Indeed, the protein-coding regions of the human genome are estimated to represent approximately 1% of the entire genome. The costs of WES are diminishing very rapidly, and at the end of 2011 the US$1000 exome became a reality. WES first requires the targeting and amplification of exonic fragments (i.e. 'exome capture'), which is followed by parallel sequencing. The generated sequences are then aligned onto a reference sequence, and variants are annotated.

Of course, there are important challenges associated with WES. The generated data are incomplete, the coverage of the exomes is not uniform and some regions can be completely missed. This may be due to biases in capture, sequencing and alignment. Sequence alignment can be difficult with highly homogeneous sequences, or in regions of repeated sequences. There can be sequencing errors resulting in false variant calls. Interpretation is a large challenge because WES generates a huge number of data: millions of bases and over 10 000 variants per individual. Interpretation of novel variants is a difficult task that will be facilitated by databases and catalogues of variants found in healthy individuals compared with those known to be associated with disease. Complex ethical issues also arise as extensive data are generated that are not related to the disorder being tested. Information related to risk for other disease or carrier status for another disease may be uncovered. This raises ethical concerns over which information should be returned to the patient. Currently, a targeted analysis approach is often used, in which a full exome sequence is generated, but the analysis is limited to genes already known to play a role in the presenting symptom.

Summary

Genetic testing in children and young people with developmental disabilities can offer numerous benefits to the patient and family, such as possible implementation of specific treatment, introduction of preventative measures, improved prognostication, estimation of recurrence risk in family members and avoidance of additional testing. Detailed and careful clinical history, family history and neurological examination remain the cornerstones of the genetic evaluation of a child with a developmental disability. In the presence of a specific suspected diagnosis, testing for mutations in specific genes may be performed using targeted mutation analysis, gene sequencing or deletion/duplication analysis. Screening tests include CMA, karyotype analysis and FISH, although CMA is becoming the preferred choice. GWASs remain in the research domain and the evaluation of risk-conferring variation is not yet performed in a clinical setting. Genetic counselling is an integral part of the process of genetic testing. Results should be interpreted with careful consideration

WHOLE-EXOME SEQUENCING	
Purpose	To sequence all the protein-coding regions of the genome
Indications	Still mainly used on a research basis. Few laboratories offer whole-exome sequencing on a clinical basis. Used to search for mutations in genes known to be associated with a particular disorder and for the discovery of disease-causing genes
Limitations	Many exonic regions missed
	Capture and sequencing bias
	Sequencing and alignment errors
	Interpretation of large number of variants very challenging
	Significant ethical issues regarding generation of information not related to disorder being tested

of (1) the heterogeneity of the disease, (2) the ability of the given test to identify causative mutations and (3) the normal human genetic variation.

Technological advances continue to refine and improve available techniques. The recent introduction of next-generation sequencing has made the affordable sequencing of the 'personal genome' a reality. Technical challenges are being replaced by the challenge of correct contextual interpretation of the massive amounts of generated data. The systematic clinical phenotyping of patients together with the classification of variants in databases as well as the functional validation of results will be of critical importance for distinguishing between disease-causing and normal variants.

REFERENCES

1. Holtzman NA, Watson MS (1999) Promoting safe and effective genetic testing in the United States. Final report of the Task Force on Genetic Testing. *J Child Fam Nurs* 2: 388–390.
2. Luo Z, Geschwind DH (2001) Microarray applications in neuroscience. *Neurobiol Dis* 8: 183–193.
3. Yunis JJ (1976) High resolution of human chromosomes. *Science* 191: 1268–1270.
4. Baldwin EL, Lee JY, Blake DM, et al (2008) Enhanced detection of clinically relevant genomic imbalances using a targeted plus whole genome oligonucleotide microarray. *Genet Med* 10: 415–429.
5. Toruner GA, Streck DL, Schwalb MN, Dermody JJ (2007) An oligonucleotide based array-CGH system for detection of genome wide copy number changes including subtelomeric regions for genetic evaluation of mental retardation. *Am J Med Genet A* 143A: 824–829.
6. Veltman JA, de Vries BB (2006) Diagnostic genome profiling: unbiased whole genome or targeted analysis? *J Mol Diagn* 8: 534–537.
7. Shevell M, Ashwal S, Donley D, et al (2003) Practice parameter: evaluation of the child with global developmental delay: report of the Quality Standards Subcommittee of the American Academy of Neurology and The Practice Committee of the Child Neurology Society. *Neurology* 60: 367–380.
8. Ravnan JB, Tepperberg JH, Papenhausen P, et al (2006) Subtelomere FISH analysis of 11 688 cases: an evaluation of the frequency and pattern of subtelomere rearrangements in individuals with developmental disabilities. *J Med Genet* 43: 478–489.
9. Biesecker LG (2002) The end of the beginning of chromosome ends. *Am J Med Genet* 107: 263–266.
10. Ballif BC, Sulpizio SG, Lloyd RM, Minier SL, Theisen A, Bejjani BA, Shaffer LG (2007) The clinical utility of enhanced subtelomeric coverage in array CGH. *Am J Med Genet A* 143A: 1850–1857.
11. Borgaonkar DS (1997) *Chromosomal Variation in Man: A Catalog of Chromosomal Variants and Anomalies.* New York: Wiley–Liss.
12. Knight SJ, Regan R, Nicod A, et al (1999) Subtle chromosomal rearrangements in children with unexplained mental retardation. *Lancet* 354: 1676–1681.
13. Koolen DA, Pfundt R, de Leeuw N, et al (2009) Genomic microarrays in mental retardation: a practical workflow for diagnostic applications. *Hum Mutat* 30: 283–292.
14. Kearney HM, Thorland EC, Brown KK, Quintero-Rivera F, South ST (2011) A Working Group of the American College of Medical Genetics (ACMG) Laboratory Quality Assurance Committee. American College of Medical Genetics Standards and Guidelines for Interpretation and Reporting of Postnatal Constitutional Copy Number Variants. *Genet Med* 13: 680–685.
15. De Gregori M, Ciccone R, Magini P, et al (2007) Cryptic deletions are a common finding in 'balanced' reciprocal and complex chromosome rearrangements: a study of 59 patients. *J Med Genet* 44: 750–762.
16. Warburton D (1991) De novo balanced chromosome rearrangements and extra marker chromosomes identified at prenatal diagnosis: clinical significance and distribution of breakpoints. *Am J Hum Genet* 49: 995–1013.
17. Miller DT, Adam MP, Aradhya S, et al (2010) Consensus statement: Chromosomal microarray is a first-tier clinical diagnostic test for individuals with developmental disabilities or congenital anomalies. *Am J Hum Genet.* 86: 749–764.
18. Schoumans J, Ruivenkamp C, Holmberg E, Kyllerman M, Anderlid BM, Nordenskjold M (2005) Detection of chromosomal imbalances in children with idiopathic mental retardation by array based comparative genomic hybridisation (array-CGH). *J Med Genet* 42: 699–705.
19. de Vries BB, Pfundt R, Leisink M, et al (2005) Diagnostic genome profiling in mental retardation. *Am J Hum Genet* 77: 606–616.
20. Shevell MI, Bejjani BA, Srour M, Rorem EA, Hall N, Shaffer LG (2008) Array comparative genomic hybridization in global developmental delay. *Am J Med Genet B Neuropsychiatr Genet* 147B: 1101–1108.
21. Shaffer LG, Kashork CD, Saleki R, et al (2006) Targeted genomic microarray analysis for identification of chromosome abnormalities in 1500 consecutive clinical cases. *J Pediatr* 149: 98–102.
22. Engels H, Brockschmidt A, Hoischen A, et al (2007) DNA microarray analysis identifies candidate regions and genes in unexplained mental retardation. *Neurology* 68: 743–50.
23. Koolen DA, Vissers LE, Pfundt R, et al (2006) A new chromosome 17q21.31 microdeletion syndrome associated with a common inversion polymorphism. *Nat Genet* 38: 999–1001.
24. Sharp AJ, Hansen S, Selzer RR, et al (2006) Discovery of previously unidentified genomic disorders from the duplication architecture of the human genome. *Nat Genet* 38: 1038–1042.
25. Weiss LA, Shen Y, Korn JM, et al (2008) Association between microdeletion and microduplication at 16p11.2 and autism. *N Engl J Med* 358: 667–675.
26. Kumar RA, Karamohamed S, Sudi J, et al (2008) Recurrent 16p11.2 microdeletions in autism. *Hum Mol Genet* 17: 628–638.
27. Ogino S, Wilson RB (2002) Genetic testing and risk assessment for spinal muscular atrophy (SMA). *Hum Genet* 111: 477–500.
28. Richards CS, Bale S, Bellissimo DB, Das S, Grody WW, Hegde MR, Lyon E, Ward BE; Molecular Subcommittee of the ACMG Laboratory Quality Assurance Committee (2008) ACMG Recommendations for Standards for Interpretation and Reporting of Sequence Variations: Revisions 2007. *Genet Med* 10: 294–300.
29. Weidinger S, Gieger C, Rodriguez E, et al (2008) Genome-wide scan on total serum IgE levels identifies FCER1A as novel susceptibility locus. *PLoS Genet* 4: e1000166.
30. Haiman CA, Patterson N, Freedman ML, et al (2007) Multiple regions within 8q24 independently affect risk for prostate cancer. *Nat Genet* 39: 638–644.

31. Grant SF, Thorleifsson G, Reynisdottir I, et al (2006) Variant of transcription factor 7-like 2 (TCF7L2) gene confers risk of type 2 diabetes. *Nat Genet* 38: 320–323.

32. Helgason A, Palsson S, Thorleifsson G, et al (2007) Refining the impact of TCF7L2 gene variants on type 2 diabetes and adaptive evolution. *Nat Genet* 39: 218–225.

33. Helgadottir A, Thorleifsson G, Manolescu A, et al (2007) A common variant on chromosome 9p21 affects the risk of myocardial infarction. *Science* 316: 1491–1493.

34. McPherson R, Pertsemlidis A, Kavaslar N, et al (2007) A common allele on chromosome 9 associated with coronary heart disease. *Science* 316: 1488–1491.

35. Moskvina V, Craddock N, Holmans P, et al (2009) Gene-wide analyses of genome-wide association data sets: evidence for multiple common risk alleles for schizophrenia and bipolar disorder and for overlap in genetic risk. *Mol Psychiatry* 14: 252–260.

36. Inlow JK, Restifo LL (2004) Molecular and comparative genetics of mental retardation. *Genetics* 166: 835–881.

37. Rioux JD, Xavier RJ, Taylor KD, et al (2007) Genome-wide association study identifies new susceptibility loci for Crohn disease and implicates autophagy in disease pathogenesis. *Nat Genet* 39: 596–604.

38. Ropers HH (2007) New perspectives for the elucidation of genetic disorders. *Am J Hum Genet* 81: 199–207.

39. Stenson PD, Ball EV, Mort M, et al (2003) Human Gene Mutation Database (HGMD): 2003 update. *Hum Mutat* 21: 577–581.

40. Topper S, Ober C, Das S (2011) Exome sequencing and the genetics of intellectual disability. *Clin Genet* 80: 117–126.

41. Ng SB, Bigham AW, Buckingham KJ, et al (2010) Exome sequencing identifies MLL2 mutations as a cause of Kabuki syndrome. *Nat Genet* 42: 790–793.

42. Hoischen A, van Bon BW, Gilissen C, et al (2010) *De novo* mutations of SETBP1 cause Schinzel–Giedion syndrome. *Nat Genet* 42: 483–485.

5
GLOBAL MENTAL FUNCTIONS: WAKEFULNESS AND SLEEP (B110, B134)

Reut Gruber, Emily B.J. Coffey and Melanie Stelmazuk

What is the construct?

Approximately one-third of otherwise healthy, typically developing children and a similar proportion of adolescents have impaired or insufficient sleep.[1,2] The most common complaints include bedtime problems, difficulties falling asleep, frequent and/or prolonged night wakings or excessive daytime sleepiness.[1,2] Poor sleep appears to interfere with prefrontal cortical function, which particularly affects executive functions such as working memory, emotional regulation and behavioural inhibition.[2] This may manifest itself in daytime impairments such as decreased memory and learning and behavioural problems.[2]

Sleep problems occur at even greater rates in children with disabilities, medical illnesses and common psychiatric disorders such as attention-deficit–hyperactivity disorder, autism and mood/anxiety disorders.[1–3] In the case of some psychiatric illnesses presenting in childhood, sleep complaints are included in the diagnostic criteria.[3,4] The relationship between primary and secondary causes of similar symptoms is not always clear, such as in the case of an illness causing anxiety or discomfort at night interfering with sleep, or conversely when a primary sleep disorder leads to poor social and academic functioning. Nevertheless, treating sleep problems can lead to improvements in the cognitive, social and emotional functioning of children and adolescents, and a reduction in symptoms of other problems,[1,2] and may even prevent the development of psychiatric illnesses such as major depressive disorder.[4]

The causes, diagnoses and treatments of sleep disorders in children and adolescents vary depending on the nature of existing illnesses and disorders and the age of the individual, as well as a host of social, environmental and psychological factors.[1,2] Accurate detection and classification of sleep disorders depends on a detailed examination of sleep, medical, developmental and family histories, past diagnosis, treatment and response, along with a physical and psychological examination.[1,2] Insights into relationships within the family and the health and well-being of the caregivers are particularly important because of their potential causal or maintenance role in sleep problems, and because parents' perception of the child's sleep may be influenced by an inaccurate understanding of typical development.[1,2] When considered within the appropriate contexts, results from the tests and tools described below may be useful for understanding a child or adolescent's sleep-related problem, to compare results before and after an intervention or to address research questions.

WHAT DOES THIS DOMAIN ENCOMPASS AND WHAT ASPECTS ARE MEASURED?

Sleep is a reversible global state which is generally characterized by a decrease in bodily movement and responsiveness to external stimuli. Sleep and wakefulness form the highest level of a hierarchical structure of attentive behaviours.[5] Each can be subdivided into finer levels of description, which can be placed on a continuum of attentive or alertness states. At one extreme lies states of hyperalertness, such as when a life-threatening situation arises, and at the other lies deep sleep stages known as slow-wave sleep in which low or non-existent levels of wakefulness are experienced.

During sleep, the brain undergoes characteristic activities which can be measured physiologically, most commonly by electroencephalography (EEG), in which small voltage differences associated with neural activity are measured between electrodes placed on the scalp. Sleep is divided into rapid eye movement (REM) sleep, which is a form of sleep associated with muscular atonia and dreaming, and four stages of non-REM sleep of increasing depth. Healthy individuals experience cycles of different sleep stages approximately every 90 minutes, with periods of REM sleep increasing in duration towards the end of the night. Sleep patterns change over development, indicating a possible role of sleep in brain maturation. For example, most healthy adults sleep between 7 and 8 hours each night, with about 20% to 25% of total sleep being REM sleep. Infants, in contrast, spend 16 or more hours per day sleeping, nearly half of that in REM sleep. At all ages, there is considerable variation among individuals in the amount and composition of sleep required.

Although the functions of sleep are not completely understood, it is clear that inadequate sleep negatively impacts waking states, resulting in unpleasant subjective feelings of fatigue, daytime sleepiness, altered mood and behavioural patterns, and reduced alertness, and interfering with attentive and learning mechanisms. These may significantly affect the health, development, education, well-being and even safety of individuals.

For these reasons, the measurement of factors influencing sleep, the quality of sleep itself and the effects of sleep are all of interest for clinical and experimental work. Factors that influence sleep may include aspects of the patient's social and family life, the sleeping environment, stressors, diet, medication, exercise, and habits and routines associated with going to sleep. The quality of sleep may be monitored to assess duration, depth, fragmentation and phase and to detect physiological irregularities in breathing and muscular activity during sleep. The effects of variations in sleep can be assessed objectively by performance measures addressing cognitive functioning as well as by measures of daytime sleepiness, mood or behaviour.

General factors to consider when measuring this domain

METHODS OF MEASUREMENT

Sleep-related measures can be roughly divided into subjective and objective measures. Subjective measures generally take the form of questionnaires filled out either by the patient or by proxy (i.e. by the parent, caregiver, bedmate, etc.), and may require some degree of judgement of the patient's behaviour, symptoms and condition. Objective measures directly record and evaluate physiological, activity or performance aspects according to well-defined standards or guidelines, often using special equipment and administered by trained specialists. Common objective measures used in the study of sleep and wakefulness focus on brain activity, including such methods as EEG or functional magnetic resonance imaging, muscle movement during the night or patterns of physical activity over a period of several days (actigraphy), breathing or performance on cognitive tasks.

Subjective and objective measures each have advantages and disadvantages. Subjective data are inexpensive and easy to collect, can offer a great deal of insight into the patient's situation including behaviours and habits that may contribute to problems and can provide information about patterns over time which is impossible to obtain from a one-time physiological evaluation. However, the integrity of subjective data is dependent upon accurate and honest reporting. The retrospective nature of most questionnaires introduces errors as the most recent events may be overgeneralized and results may be biased towards socially desirable answers. Respondants may also have difficulty accurately recalling nocturnal events, for example night wakings, and may be unable to estimate sleep and wake times accurately.

While objective measures often provide more consistent, reliable and quantifiable measurements, they are generally much more expensive and time-consuming to administer and are limited in their scope. For example, measuring the physical activity of a teenager over the course of several days might be useful for identifying whether that patient is sleepy during morning classes because he or she does not fall asleep until very late at night. However, this objective measurement would not tell the examiner if the adolescent frequently smoked cigarettes, drank highly caffeinated beverages and played exciting video games late in the evening – thus possibly missing the opportunity for a relatively easy solution.

Another consideration when selecting a measure is the relative burden to the patient. Filling in a short paper-and-pen questionnaire or keeping a sleep log can provide a surprising amount of information in a short amount of execution time, and asks little of the patient. Overnight sleep recordings or repeated clinical visits instead involve disturbance to the lives and schedules of patients and their caregivers. For families already dealing with a disability or disorder, this may be an additional burden.

Regardless of the measure used, sleep quality, alertness and cognitive performance are sensitive to the effects of prescription medication, the ingestion of substances such as caffeine, habits such as smoking and the use of non-prescription and illicit drugs. The voluntary use of substances is particularly problematic in the adolescent age range, but younger children may also ingest significant quantities of caffeinated beverages. Before carrying out tests which look at sleep quality, patients should (if possible) be asked to discontinue any medication known to affect sleep for some days or weeks such that a pure measure of the underlying problem may be taken. If this is not possible, knowledge of the individual's habitual and recent consumption of these substances is necessary to interpret the results of any sleep-related measure correctly.

FACTORS RELATING TO TYPE/LEVEL OF DISABILITY: GENERIC VERSUS DISEASE SPECIFIC

Developmental conditions or disabilities which coexist with sleep problems may diminish the level of co-operation to be expected, therefore making lengthy examinations such as polysomnography (PSG; see below) difficult and less effective. Subjective measures which rely on self-reporting require a minimum level of literacy and understanding which may not be present in children with certain developmental disabilities. Simple measures that are easy to administer by a third party (parent or clinician) or are not intrusive (e.g. actigraphy) can generally be used regardless of the level and type of disability.

AGE OF THE CHILD

Infants, children, adolescents and adults differ in the causes and manifestations of sleep-related problems; the duration, structure and timing of normal sleep; and the symptoms and effects of inadequate sleep. Hence, measures should be age sensitive and modified for use with children. The main difference in testing adults and children is that young, preliterate children may not be able to complete questionnaires themselves. Subjective measures for young children can be completed by the child's caregiver, for example to collect information about the child's bedtime routine and sleep–wake cycle. Self-report questionnaires may be used with literate school-aged children provided that the language used is simple and clear and that straightforward, factual questions are asked. Like adults, adolescents are generally able to understand more conceptual test items, for example asking them to assess their overall level of alertness during the day on a scale of one to five. However, to obtain useful information, questionnaires for this age range must be sensitive to the fact that the stressors, priorities and issues related to this period of life are different from those of adults. In addition, children may not be able to comply with instructions for objective tests. Many problems administering objective tests can be resolved by using the simplest, least intrusive measures, and, when more extensive tests are required, a good bedside manner and enlisting the assistance of the caregiver to help to explain the procedures and reassure the child. It is critical that the results obtained by these measures are interpreted in relation to normative data collected for the age group of the test individual.

CLINICAL AND RESEARCH APPLICATIONS

For the reasons discussed above, there is no simple answer as to which measures are the best to use. Most research studies benefit from the use of a combination of subjective and objective measures, taking into consideration the desired information and relative costs and benefits of each measure for the individual or group in question.

In the following section, an assortment of useful measures which cover the age range of infancy to adolescence are described. Where possible, measures that are available free of charge from the authors have been included. To assist the user in identifying appropriate measures, key characteristics of these tools are summarized in Table 5.1. These characteristics include the age range, whether the measure is subjective or objective, the time required to administer the measure, the type of information obtainable from the measure, any cautions or conditions which preclude the measure's use and the relative expense and burden to the patient.

Overview of recommended measures

SLEEP LOG

Description of purpose

A sleep log or diary is a brief daily record of a number of sleep- and waking-related parameters kept by a patient or, if this is not possible, by his or her caregiver. Sleep logs may be used as a starting point to better understand a complaint (particularly relating to sleep phase), may be used in conjunction with other measures such as actigraphy (see below) or may be helpful on their own to allow a patient to recognize habits and behaviours that are contributing to sleeping problems. A sleep log can provide a baseline at the beginning of a treatment to help assess the outcome. Although sleep log data are not as objective as other measures, they can unobtrusively and inexpensively provide a valuable insight into the patient's condition over time, which is not easy to obtain using other methods. Sleep logs also address the patient's perception of a problem, which may differ significantly from objectively recorded data. For example, healthy individuals often overestimate and insomniacs tend to underestimate their ability to sleep.[6]

Population

Literate children, adolescents and adults may use sleep logs. Sleep logs using simplified words and scales are available for young school-age children. Very young children and infants may have a sleep log kept for them by a caregiver based on their observations and questions asked verbally to the child.

Administration/test format

Sleep logs can be self-reported or administered by a caregiver. Two types are available: a simple hourly grid to record sleep and wake times graphically in order to assess

TABLE 5.1

Summary of sleep measures

Measure	Description	Ages (y)	Subjective/ objective	Type of objective data	Time to administer	Suitable for examining				Relative expense	Relative burden to patients/ caregivers
						Behaviour and habits	Sleep quality and related disorders	Daytime function/ sleepiness	Circadian rhythm/ sleep duration		
Sleep log	Self-report measure completed daily	All	Subjective	Not applicable	10min/day for 2–3 wk	Y	Y	Y	Y	Low	Low
Children's Sleep Habits Questionnaire	Questionnaire completed by caregiver which indicates need for further diagnosis	4–12	Subjective	Not applicable	15min	Y	Y	Y	Y	Low	Low
Epworth Sleepiness Scale (Modified)	Short questionnaire completed by caregiver (or child >6y)	5–12	Subjective	Not applicable	10min			Y		Low	Low
Sleep Habits Survey (Adolescent)	Comprehensive self-rated questionnaire	13–19	Subjective	Not applicable	45min	Y	Y	Y	Y	Low	Low
Pittsburg Sleep Quality Index	Short self-rated questionnaire	>13	Subjective	Not applicable	10min		Y	Y	Y	Low	Low
PSG	Multiple physiological measures taken during an overnight sleep recording	All	Objective	EEG, EMG, ECG, etc.	~12h		Y			High	High
Actigraphy	A watch-like instrument worn on the wrist or ankle records information about movement; may be used during PSG or independently for a longer period	All	Objective	Movement	~2 wk		Y		Y	Medium	Low
Multiple Sleep Latency Test	A daytime study involving multiple short naps and multiple measures; often used after PSG	All	Objective	EEG	~8h			Y		High	High
Cognitive Function and Performance Testing	Various tests used to assess the effects of poor sleep on daytime functioning and cognitive functions	>6	Objective	RT, accuracy, errors	Varies			Y	Y	Medium	Medium

PSG, polysomnography; RT;, yes; EEG, electroencephalogram; EMG, electromyogram; ECG, electrocardiogram; RT, reaction time.

sleep phase, and a more involved version which consists of a log sheet, usually one per week, with a small space allotted per question per day for a brief answer or rating. The information collected usually includes the time the person tried to fall asleep, the estimated time of sleep onset, the length of any awakenings, any sleep disturbances, the intended and actual awake times, feelings of drowsiness and mood during the day, the timing of daytime naps and meals and any drinks or activities preceding bedtime. Other information can be added to customize the measure to the patient's needs, and editable spreadsheets are available.

Psychometric properties
Psychometric data are scarce, as much of the information included is highly subjective in nature. Comparisons can be made between sleeping and waking times reported by the patient and PSG or actigraphy (see below), which generally demonstrate a wide range of accuracies across individuals and sleep settings.[6,7] However, patients' reported sleep times can be valuable as approximations, and the discrepancy between a sleep log and other measures can also be helpful to understand the patient's perception of a sleep problem.

Cost/how to order
Sleep log sheets are available for download free of charge on the internet from a number of sources, in basic printable and/or computer spreadsheet form, which can be customized.

Key references
IsHak DWW, Burt T, Sederer LI, editors (2002) *Outcome Measurement in Psychiatry: A Critical Review.* Washington, DC: American Psychiatric Publishing, Inc.
Means MK, Edinger JD, Glennc M, Fins AI (2003) Accuracy of sleep perceptions among insomnia sufferers and normal sleepers. *Sleep Med* 4: 285–296.

CHILDREN'S SLEEP HABITS QUESTIONNAIRE

Description of purpose
The Children's Sleep Habits Questionnaire (CSHQ) is a sleep questionnaire for preschool and school-aged children developed by clinical researchers at Brown University to screen for both behaviourally and medically based sleep disorders most common to this age group, including dyssomnias (difficulty getting to sleep or staying asleep), parasomnias (e.g. sleepwalking or sleeptalking, night terrors, bedwetting, restless leg syndrome) and sleep-disordered breathing. The CSHQ is intended to be used to identify the need and direction for possible

further evaluation rather than to diagnose sleep problems. It yields both a total score and eight subscale scores on bedtime resistance, sleep onset delay, sleep duration, sleep anxiety, night wakings, parasomnias, sleep-disordered breathing and daytime sleepiness.

Population
The CSHQ is designed for children aged 4 to 12 years.

Administration/test format
The measure is completed by the child's caregiver regarding the child's sleep and wake activities over the past week (or another reference week if the last week was unusual for some reason). Each item is rated on a three-point scale (i.e. 'usually', 'sometimes', 'rarely'), as well as a binary indication of whether the sleep habit is a problem.

The full version of the CSHQ contains items which are used in the scoring of the scale, as well as additional items which are not used for scoring but may nonetheless yield clinically relevant information. An abbreviated version of the scale exists which contains only those items that are included in scoring the survey; these are the 35 individual items which constitute the CSHQ subscales. Scoring is accomplished by summing the numbers associated with responses (some items are reverse scored). A higher score is indicative of more sleep problems, and a total score of 41 or higher on the abbreviated CSHQ is considered by the test's authors to be an indicator for referral to a sleep specialist.

Psychometric properties
Reliability and validity data have been collected on a sample of 495 elementary school children and on a clinical sample from a paediatric sleep clinic. The test showed adequate internal consistency and test–retest reliability (0.68 for community sample and 0.78 for clinical sample) of 0.62 to 0.79, and was able to consistently differentiate a sleep-disordered group from a healthy group of individuals.[8] As there are no established norms for the total and subscale scores, the authors suggest that it is most useful in comparing samples or in assessing sleep pre and post intervention.

Cost/how to order
The CSHQ and scoring instructions are freely available from the author. http://research.brown.edu/research/profile.php?id=1100924889

Key references
Owens J, Nobile C, McGuinn M, Spirito A (2000) The Children's Sleep Habits Questionnaire: Construction and

validation of a sleep survey for school-aged children. *Sleep* 23: 1043–1051.

Owens J, Spirito A, McGuinn M, Nobile C (2000) Sleep habits and sleep disturbance in school-aged children. *J Dev Behav Paediatr* 21: 27–36.

Spruyt K, Gozal D (2011) Pediatric sleep questionnaires as diagnostic or epidemiological tools: a review of currently available instruments. *Sleep Med Rev* 15: 19–32.

Spruyt K, Gozal D (2011) Development of pediatric sleep questionnaires as diagnostic or epidemiological tools: a brief review of do's and don'ts. *Sleep Med Rev* 15: 7–17.

EPWORTH SLEEPINESS SCALE (MODIFIED)

Description of purpose

Excessive daytime sleepiness is a common and under-recognized symptom in children which may accompany a variety of intrinsic and extrinsic sleep disorders.[9] In children, daytime sleepiness may not be suspected by the caregiver, as fatigued children tend to exhibit hyperactivity. The Epworth Sleepiness Scale (ESS) was designed to assess an adult's general level of daytime sleepiness. The propensity of the individual to fall asleep during eight common situations, such as sitting and reading, watching television or driving, is reported on a four-point scale. The ESS was modified slightly by Melendres et al[10] to be applicable to children by removing a reference to alcohol consumption and changing a question about driving a car to being a passenger in a car.

Population

Melendres et al[10] found the modified ESS to be useful for children aged 5 to 12 years. The daytime sleepiness of children younger than 5 years of age may be mitigated by daytime napping, which is common in this age range, leading to decreased sensitivity of the measure.

Administration/test format

The modified ESS for children is usually completed by a child's caregiver. Melendres et al[10] also compared answers from caregivers and children older than 6 years and found a strong correlation between scores.[10] The questionnaire contains eight items, which are rated on a scale of 0 to 3 (no, slight, moderate or high chance of dozing while engaging in the activity). The responses are summed to obtain an overall score. In adults, an ESS score of >10 is taken to indicate increased daytime sleepiness. Children's scores are generally less than those of adults and so the cut-off score should not be used, but nonetheless scores of patient populations for children with suspected sleep-disordered breathing had scores significantly higher than those of a comparison population.[10]

Psychometric properties

Comprehensive normative data are not available for use of the modified ESS with children. Similarly, there is a lack of psychometric data. Scores in adults tend to be stable over time, yet do not correlate precisely with objective measures of sleep quality such as PSG, suggesting that different aspects are being measured.

Cost/how to order

The ESS is publicly available online and printed in Johns,[11] among other scientific publications. The modified scale is published in Melendres et al.[10]

Key references

Hoban TF, Chervin RD (2001) Assessment of sleepiness in children. *Semin Pediatr Neurobiol* 8: 216–228.

Melendres CS, Lutz JM, Rubin ED, Marcus CL (2004) Daytime sleepiness and hyperactivity in children with suspected sleep-disordered breathing. *Pediatrics* 114: 768–775.

Johns MW (1991) A new method for measuring daytime sleepiness: the Epsworth Sleepiness Scale. *Sleep* 14: 540–545.

Johns MW (1992) Reliability and factor analysis of the Epworth Sleepiness Scale. *Sleep* 15: 376–381.

SLEEP HABITS SURVEY FOR ADOLESCENTS

Description of purpose

The Sleep Habits Survey for Adolescents is a self-report questionnaire developed to address sleep-related factors and habits of particular concern for the period of adolescence, including school, social and work activities, as well as aspects of well-being that may be influenced by inadequate sleep such as school performance and mood. The Sleep Habits Survey for Adolescents can be used to examine potentially problematic sleep-related behaviours and habits, to identify a need and direction for possible further evaluation and to compare populations and experimental groups.

Population

Normative data are available for adolescents aged 13 to 19 years.

Administration/test format

The survey is completed by self-report if possible, with reference to the previous 2-week period. The measure contains approximately 60 items, which are presented in various formats to include short-answer, fill in the blank, multiple choice and graphic scale questions. There are slightly different versions for males and females owing to questions regarding physical development. The Sleep Habits Survey does not have an associated scoring system, but the information taken as a whole can be helpful to understand the patient's case, and results on individual items of interest can be compared with normative data or between study conditions or groups.

Psychometric properties
Normative data are available from a large sample (>3000) of high school students in Rhode Island (USA), the results of which are reported in Wolfson and Carskadon.[12] Wolfson et al[13] found that adolescents' self-reports of sleep-related activity correlated well with results from a sleep diary and as estimated by actigraphy, although results from the weekends were less accurate than weekdays.

Cost/how to order
The survey is published and publicly available from: http://research.brown.edu/research/profile. php?id=1100924889

Key references
Wolfson R, Carskadon MA (1998) Sleep schedules and daytime functioning in adolescents. *Child Dev* 69: 875–887.
Wolfson AR, Carskadon MA, Acebo C, et al (2003) Evidence for the validity of a Sleep Habits Survey for Adolescents. *Sleep* 26: 213–216.

PITTSBURG SLEEP QUALITY INDEX

Description of purpose
The Pittsburgh Sleep Quality Index (PSQI) is a short, retrospective self-rated questionnaire that looks at sleep quality and disturbances over a 1-month period. The results of the test are not sufficient to diagnose sleep disorders, but can be useful to roughly categorize sleep quality of patients, and to observe patterns and identify directions for further analysis. The results are divided into seven subscales: subjective sleep quality, sleep latency, sleep duration, habitual sleep efficiency, sleep disturbances, use of sleeping medication and daytime dysfunction.

Population
The PSQI is designed for use with adults but can also be used with adolescents, as all items are brief and easy to understand.

Administration/test format
The test is usually self-rated, although items have also been adapted so that they can be administered by a

clinician or assistant. It takes most patients 5 to 10 minutes to complete. No training is needed to administer or score the test. The PSQI is composed of 19 self-rated questions and five questions rated by a bed partner or room-mate if applicable. The first four items collect information about the approximate start, end and duration of sleep periods. Several questions ask specific questions about the causes of sleep problems and daytime mood and sleepiness on a four-point scale that ranges from 'not during the last month' to 'three or more times per week'. The final question asks for a general rating of subjective sleep quality on a four-point scale. Only self-rated questions are used in the scoring, which produces a score from 0 (no difficulty) to 3 (severe difficulty) for each component listed above, and a global score. Global scores >5 are suggestive of clinically significant sleep disturbance, whereas relative scores on the component scales help clinicians to understand the nature of the disturbance.

Psychometric properties
As the test has been in use for more than 20 years, normative data are available for a variety of healthy and patient populations. Adequate internal consistency and reliability (0.83) has been demonstrated in healthy comparison groups, patients with sleep disorders and depressed patients. Global scores are significantly higher in psychiatric and sleep-disordered populations than in healthy comparison individuals. Component scales significantly differentiate between diagnostic groups. PSG measures of sleep latency for the whole sample (r=0.33) and for the depressive subgroup (r=0.37), sleep duration in the comparison group (r=0.34) and the number of arousals in depressives (r=0.47) were correlated to scores from the PSQI results, although PSQI component scale scores were not all significantly correlated with corresponding PSG measures.

Cost/how to order
The PSQI is copyrighted, but there is no charge for its use. The scale and scoring instructions are available in the original publication.[14]

Key references
Buysse DJ, Reynolds CF III, Monk TH, Berman SR, Kupfer DJ (1989) Pittsburgh Sleep Quality Index: a new instrument for psychiatric practice and research. *Psychiatry Res* 28: 193–213.
Buysse DJ, Reynolds CF III, Monk TH, Berman SR, Kupfer DJ, editors (2000) *Handbook of Psychiatric Measures*. Washington, DC: American Psychological Association.

POLYSOMNOGRAPHY

Description of purpose

Polysomnography is a multicomponent recording of the biophysiological changes that occur during sleep, including brain activity (EEG), skeletal muscle activation (electromyography [EMG]), heart rhythm (ECG), respiratory functions and peripheral pulse oximetry. Additional procedures that provide further information may be used depending on the nature of the problem or research question, for example the measurements of limb movements by actigraphy or video recording nocturnal events.[1,2] If performed in a sleep laboratory, technicians will make behavioural observations which are useful to understand the resulting polysomnogram. PSG can also be used in combination with questionnaires such as those mentioned in this chapter in order to provide a broad picture of the patient's or participant's situation. A sleep diary kept over a period of several weeks can provide a sufficient account of sleep problems in many cases; however, PSG is essential for the diagnosis of sleep apnoea, narcolepsy and some parasomnias or sleep-related seizure disorders that do not respond to conventional therapy, or where periodic limb movement sleep disorder is suspected.[1,2,15] PSG is not suitable for examining aspects or disorders of the circadian rhythm, but can help in ruling out other sleep problems.

Population

Paediatric PSG has evolved from adult PSG. As sleep disorders in children are different to those in adults in many ways,[1,2] paediatric PSG has become a specialized area of study.[16] PSG can be performed on children of any age with minor modifications to equipment and procedures. The resulting data are evaluated in a similar manner to those of adults, although special classification systems for sleep-related disorders are used which consider age-related differences.[1,2] The age and medical or psychological condition of the patient may compromise the ability to collect quality information. For example, young children may be frightened by the equipment or may intentionally or unintentionally remove sensors. Many problems can be reduced by an experienced paediatric polysomnographic technologist who can establish a good relationship with the child or young person and can enlist the parents' assistance for reassurance so as to maximize co-operation. It may also be helpful to review aspects of the procedure with the parent and, if appropriate, the child, before the PSG.[9] Home PSG is a relatively new alternative to traditional laboratory PSG, in which a technician connects sensors either in the home or in the laboratory, and patients sleep in their own bed. Home PSG is especially appropriate for use in children, for whom the new setting

of the sleep laboratory is likely to cause sleep disturbances known as first-night effects. For example, studies show that children sleep longer and have more pronounced slow-wave sleep with a reduction in stage 2 non-REM sleep at home compared with sleep in a clinic.[17]

Administration/test format

Polysomnography generally requires an overnight stay in a sleep laboratory, with provision for adult accompaniment, preceded by several additional hours for children in the laboratory to allow sensor hook-up, to become accustomed to their environment and to go through their normal bedtime routine. If PSG is used to diagnose a sleep disorder, it is also necessary to take a detailed sleep history and comprehensive developmental, medical and family histories, and to perform physical and psychological examinations.[1,2] Home PSG generally requires that a technician visit the patient's home with portable measuring equipment, which is connected before the normal sleep time. A technician may monitor the system remotely, or more commonly will collect the equipment for data analysis the following day. Scoring of the polysomnogram is generally performed by hand by a trained technician, who makes a subjective decision based on each 30-second 'epoch' of sleep or wake units during the observation period, based on accepted standards.[18] This analysis may take 2 to 3 hours for an experienced technologist.[18] Automatic and computer-aided scoring are also available; however, to date they have shown limited accuracy without significant input and verification from a technician.[18,19] Fully automated systems are not yet in widespread use. If possible, medications which may disrupt night-time sleep such as stimulants and antidepressants should be discontinued 2 weeks before the study.[9]

Psychometric properties

Polysomnography is considered the 'criterion standard' for evaluation of sleep and sleep-related breathing against which other methods such as actigraphy are compared.[15,16] As the number of sensors is increased, the diagnostic accuracy improves. The accuracy of scoring of the PSG is dependent on the training and experience of the technologist. Cronbach's α and intraclass correlation coefficients (ICCs) may be calculated to assess inter-rater reliability, which in most studies is between 80% and 90%. For example, in a study by Montgomery-Downs et al,[20] the combined reliability for all polysomnographic measures was α=0.996 ($p<0.001$). As PSG has been used for more than 40 years, normative data are available for a wide range of populations including children and adolescents (e.g. see Montgomery-Downs et al[20] and Stores et al[21]). Home PSG is a newer development and thus has a shorter history, yet appears to provide data comparable to those obtained in the laboratory.[22] Normative data have also been published for several populations including healthy preschool and early school-aged children.[17] It has been suggested that sleep would be more disrupted by extraneous factors in the home environment than in the controlled and standardized laboratory environment, but various reports suggest that this is not the case and that sleep is of better quality and is more consolidated at home.[21] Diagnosis of some sleep-related disorders such as obstructive sleep apnoea syndrome may be less accurate using home PSG.[23]

Cost/how to order
Polysomnography is inherently expensive because of the time required for set-up, monitoring and data analysis by a trained technician.[18] The costs involved of course depend heavily on the location and country. Chervin et al[23] estimated the cost of one night's PSG at between US$1000 and US$1400, whereas a home study was approximately US$500.

Key references
Chervin RD, Murman DL, Malow BA, Totten V (1999) Cost–utility of three approaches to the diagnosis of sleep apnea: polysomnography, home testing, and empirical therapy. *Ann Intern Med* 130: 496–505.
Feinsilver SH (1998) How sleep labs can survive managed care [guest editorial]. Available at: www.rtmagazine.com/issues/articles/1998–04_11.asp.
Goodwin JL, Enright PL, Kaemingk KL, et al (2001) Feasibility of using unattended polysomnography in children for research – Report of the Tucson Children's Assessment of Sleep Apnea Study (TuCASA). *Sleep* 24: 937–1044.
Kushida CA, Littner MR, Morgenthaler T, et al (2005) Practice parameters for the indications for polysomnography and related procedures: an update for 2005. *Sleep* 28: 499–519.
Montgomery-Downs HE, O'Brian LM, Gulliver TE, Gozal D (2006) Polysomnographic characteristics in normal preschool and early school-aged children. *Pediatrics* 117: 741–753.
Penzel T, Kesper K, Gross V, Becker HF, Vogelmeier C, editors (2003) Problems in automatic sleep scoring applied to sleep apnea. Engineering in Medicine and Biology Society 2003. Proceedings of the 25th Annual International Conference of the IEEE, Piscataway, NJ: IEEE.
Stores G (1999) Children's sleep disorders: Modern approaches, developmental effects, and children at special risk. *Dev Med Child Neurol* 41: 568–573. Piscataway, NJ: IEEE.

Stores G, Crawford C (2000) Arousal norms for children age 5–16 years based on home polysomnography. *Technol Health Care* 8: 285–290.
Stores G, Crawford C, Selman J, Wiggs L (1998) Home polysomnography norms for children. *Technol Health Care* 6: 231–236.

ACTIGRAPHY

Description of purpose
Actigraphy is a method used to study sleep–wake patterns and circadian rhythms by assessing movement.[24] This is achieved using a small device that is usually attached to the wrist of the non-dominant hand or an ankle, which records data from accelerometers several times per second. Actigraphy cannot provide sleep staging information and is not used for routine diagnosis or management of sleep disorders, but may be useful to evaluate insomnia, circadian rhythm sleep disorders, excessive sleepiness and restless legs syndrome, and to assess the effectiveness of treatments.[24] It may be used in addition to PSG to provide complementary information, or may replace full PSG if the nature of the suspected problem is related predominantly to arousal and movement or when PSG is not possible. Actigraphy may also be useful to assess daytime sleepiness in situations in which standard techniques such as the Multiple Sleep Latency Test are not practical.[24]

Population
Actigraphy can be used for the analysis of circadian rhythm patterns and arousal disturbances for people of all ages. It may be preferable to PSG for children and people with certain physical or psychiatric conditions which make recording good-quality PSG data problematic. Actigraphy is less valuable for use with individuals who have long motionless periods of wakefulness or who have disorders that involve altered patterns of motility.[25]

Administration/test format
If actigraphy is used as part of PSG, the device is attached for the duration of the study and the data are recorded and scored in combination with the other PSG measures. If actigraphy is performed by itself, the individual under study is usually asked to wear the device continuously for about a week. During the period of observation, a sleep diary is commonly kept to assist in determining lights on and off times.[24] The data are then uploaded to a computer and processed, providing information such as average activity during different periods, estimated wake and sleep periods based on predefined cut-off

values, circadian rhythm patterns and average time of peak activity.

Psychometric properties

The accuracy of actigraphy sleep–wake estimates is usually determined by comparing the actigraphy results with simultaneously recorded full PSG results and tends to be fairly high in healthy populations (for examples see Jean-Louis et al[26]). For example, correlations for total sleep time for PSG data and actigraphy have been reported as being 0.97, with high inter-rater agreement of 94.8 between actigraphy and PSG. Normative data on sleep–wake patterns across development are available, from adults to newborns.[25,27] Multiple studies have documented the ability of actigraphy to distinguish between rest and wakefulness, and to differentiate between clinical groups and identify certain sleep-related disorders.[25] However, differences in the validity of specific devices and scoring algorithms have not been established for all equipment and for all clinical groups. Certain conditions such as motor disorders or high motility during sleep may preclude the accurate use of actigraphy.[25]

Cost/how to order

Actigraphy assessments vary in cost by location and company. Advertised prices per assessment are around US$250. Available at: http://learnactiware.com/documentation/clinicalimplementationguide.pdf and http://ribn.respironics.com

Key references

Jean-Louis G, Kripke DF, Mason WJ, Elliott JA, Youngstedt SD (2001) Sleep estimation from wrist movement quantified by different actigraphic modalities. *J Neurosci Methods* 105: 185–191.
Littner M, Kushida CA, McDowell Anderson W, et al (2003) Practice parameters for the role of actigraphy in the study of sleep and circadian rhythms: an update for 2002. *Sleep* 26: 337–341.
Sahed A, Acebo C (2002) The role of actigraphy in sleep medicine. *Sleep Med Rev* 6: 113–124.

MULTIPLE SLEEP LATENCY TEST

Description of purpose

The Multiple Sleep Latency Test (MSLT) is an objective measure of daytime sleepiness commonly performed after an overnight sleep study. The patient or participant is left lying in a darkened room for short periods of time repeatedly throughout the day, while measurements such as EEG, muscle activity and eye movements are recorded to determine when the participant falls asleep. Additional information may be optionally obtained from oximetry, airflow detection, respiratory effort and limb EMG. Scores on the MSLT are taken to represent a measure of physiological sleep tendency.[28] The test is commonly performed after an overnight sleep study. It is particularly useful to evaluate excessive daytime sleepiness and narcolepsy, and to assess the effectiveness of treatments for sleep-related problems or interventions.

Population

Children may be tested in the same manner as adults, with the recommendation that the standard nap period used for adults (20min) is lengthened to 30 minutes to allow for longer sleep onset times found in children.[29]

Administration/test format

The standard MSLT nap periods are 20 minutes, repeated five times at about 2-hour intervals, making the total test duration approximately 8 hours. The results are then analysed, in a similar manner to PSG, by a technician trained in PSG and sleep staging to determine sleep latency and REM onset scores. The nap is discontinued after a preset elapsed time (20 or 30min) or after 15 minutes from the onset of sleep.

Psychometric properties

The MSLT has been used widely since the 1970s, therefore considerable normative data for various populations are available. It has also been shown to be sensitive to the effects of sleep deprivation and pharmacological manipulations of alertness.[28] The clinical MSLT displays excellent inter-rater and intrarater reliability estimates for both sleep latency (0.9 and 0.87, respectively) and REM onset scores (0.88 and 0.81, respectively) in both healthy individuals and individuals with sleep disorders.[28]

Cost/how to order

Most sleep laboratories routinely performing overnight polysomnograms have the resources in place to perform MSLT procedures, even if they do not regularly do so. As with the PSG, the MSLT is relatively costly owing to the need for a technician to monitor and score the data. The cost of the analysis varies according to location, facilities and optional equipment used, but based on currently available estimates is in the range of US$1000. Available at: http://bit.ly/HCD4LT.

Key references

Drake CL, Rice MF, Roehrs TA, Rosenthal L, Guido P, Roth T (2000) Scoring reliability of the Multiple Sleep Latency Test in a clinical population. *Sleep* 23: 1–3.

Golan N, Shahar E, Ravid S, Pillar G (2004) Sleep disorders and daytime sleepiness in children with attention-deficit/hyperactivity disorder. *Sleep* 27: 261–266.

COGNITIVE FUNCTION AND PERFORMANCE TESTING

Description of purpose
Computerized tests can be used to assess the behavioural effects of sleepiness and effects of changes in sleep quality on various performance measures. Parameters of interest include reaction time, sustained attention, vigilance, inhibition and executive function, all of which are sensitive to sleep loss. Test scores for a single session are not very informative in understanding individual cases because of normal interindividual differences, but may be valuable for comparing differences between conditions or the outcome of interventions over repeated sessions. Many of these tests have been used extensively in testing cognitive functions for research purposes, as stand-alone measures and in combination with various neuroimaging techniques. The Psychomotor Vigilance Test (PVT) has been found to be highly sensitive to sleep restriction, and is reliable and not subject to practice effects,[30,31] therefore we report it here as an example. Other well-studied tests include the 'go/no-go task', which focuses on inhibitory functions; the 'attention network task', which involves the measurement of orientation, alertness and executive attention; and the Posner paradigm, which looks at spatial cueing and attention. The PVT has been used extensively in sleep research to objectively measure aspects of alertness and sustained attention.[31] The paradigm consists of a visual stimulus or stimuli presented for very short periods of time at random intervals on a computer or hand-held device. The individual must press a button whenever the image appears on the screen, from which various measures of reaction time and accuracy are calculated.

Population
The PVT can be used with both adults and children who are old enough to understand the instructions (as young as age 6y has been reported in the literature[31]). Existing physical or psychological conditions which impair perception or attention may preclude the use of the PVT to expose sleep-related vigilance changes.

Administration/test format
Neurocognitive assessments such as the PVT can be administered by trained technicians under professional supervision as appropriate. The test lasts for approximately 10 minutes, during which time the stimuli are presented about 100 times with interstimulus intervals varying from about 2 to 10 seconds.[31,32] A shorter portable

version of the test has also been validated for use in field studies with adults.[33] Commercially available software can then be used to analyse the results and produce summary statistics for the test taker's performance, including reaction time, standard deviation of reaction time, the number of lapses (missed stimuli) and total number of errors (wrong keys and false starts).

Psychometric properties
Normative data are available for a number of adult populations (for an example, see Sforza et al[32]), and for children aged 6–11 years.[31] ICCs have been reported in the 'almost perfect' range for the number of PVT lapses (0.89) as well as for median response times (0.83).[34] Age and sex significantly affect PVT scores in children.[31]

Cost/how to order
In principle, the PVT can be implemented by computer application capable of submillisecond resolution for recording responses and analysed in any spreadsheet or statistical application. Ready-made PVTs with comfortable user interfaces and automatic processing of results are also commercially available.

Key references
Kushida CA (2008) *Handbook of Sleep Disorders*, 2nd edition. New York: Informa Healthcare.
Lamond N, Dawson D, Roach GD (2005) Fatigue assessment in the field: Validation of a hand-held electronic psychomotor vigilance task. *Aviation Space Environ Med* 76: 486–489.
Sforza E, Haba-Rubio J, De Bilbao F, Rochat T, Ibanez V (2004) Performance vigilance task and sleepiness in patients with sleep-disordered breathing. *Eur Respir J* 24: 279–285.
Venker CC, Goodwin JL, Roe DJ, Kaemingk KL, Mulvaney S, Quan SF (2007) Normative Psychomotor Vigilance Task performance in children aged 6 to 11 – the Tucson Children's Assessment of Sleep Apnea (TuCASA). *Sleep Breath* 11: 217–224.

Summary
Sleep-related difficulties negatively impact the health, well-being and development of a high proportion of otherwise healthy children and adolescents, and exacerbate existing problems in an even higher proportion among those with disabilities, medical illnesses and common psychiatric disorders. Sleep problems are complex and may involve two-way interactions with many aspects of waking life. Since no single scale or technique can provide an adequate measure of all sleep-related problems, a measurement tool must be carefully selected for

a given target population and purpose. The first sections of this chapter introduced factors to be considered when selecting appropriate measures, such as the compromises necessary between the goals of obtaining useful data and limiting the burden on the patient, and the relative benefits of objective and subjective data.

The measures summarized in Table 5.1 and described in more detail in the chapter provide a range of starting points to better understand relevant aspects of individual cases and to assess the progress of their treatment. These measures can also be used for basic and clinical research, perhaps leading us closer to understanding what sleep is for and why it is of such critical importance during the first years of our lives.

REFERENCES

1. Stores G (2001) *A Clinical Guide to Sleep Disorders in Children and Adolescents*. Cambridge: Cambridge University Press.
2. Mindell JA, Owens JA (2010) *A Clinical Guide to Pediatric Sleep, Diagnosis and Management of Sleep Problems*, 2nd edition. Philadelphia: Wolters Kluwer.
3. Stores G (2001) Sleep–wake function in children with neuro-developmental and psychiatric disorders. *Semin Pediatr Neurol* 8: 188–197.
4. Richardson MA, Friedman NR, editors (2007) *Clinician's Guide to Pediatric Sleep Disorders*. New York: Informa Healthcare.
5. Gazzaniga MS, Ivry RB, Mangun GR, editors (2002) *Cognitive Neuroscience: The Biology of the Mind*, 2nd edition. New York: W. W. Norton & Company.
6. IsHak DWW, Burt T, Sederer LI, editors (2002) *Outcome Measurement in Psychiatry: A Critical Review*. Washington, DC: American Psychiatric Publishing, Inc.
7. Means MK, Edinger JD, Glennc M, Fins AI (2003) Accuracy of sleep perceptions among insomnia sufferers and normal sleepers. *Sleep Med* 4: 285–296.
8. Owens J, Nobile C, McGuinn M, Spirito A (2000) The Children's Sleep Habits Questionnaire: construction and validation of a sleep survey for school-aged children. *Sleep* 23: 1043–1051.
9. Hoban TF, Chervin RD (2001) Assessment of sleepiness in children. *Semin Pediatr Neurobiol* 8: 216–228.
10. Melendres CS, Lutz JM, Ruben DE, Marcus CL (2004) Daytime sleepiness and hyperactivity in children with suspected sleep-disordered breathing. *Pediatrics* 114: 768–775.
11. Johns MW (1991) A new method for measuring daytime sleepiness: the Epsworth Sleepiness Scale. *Sleep* 14: 540–545.
12. Wolfson R, Carskadon MA (1998) Sleep schedules and daytime functioning in adolescents. *Child Dev* 69: 875–887.
13. Wolfson AR, Carskadon MA, Acebo C, et al (2003) Evidence for the validity of a sleep habits survey for adolescents. *Sleep* 26: 213–216.
14. Buysse DJ, Reynolds III CF, Monk TH, Berman SR, Kupfer DJ (1989) Pittsburgh Sleep Quality Index: a new instrument for psychiatric practice and research. *Psychiatry Res* 28: 193–213.
15. Kushida CA, Littner MR, Morgenthaler T, et al (2005) Practice parameters for the indications for polysomnography and related procedures: an update for 2005. *Sleep* 28: 499–519.
16. Wong TK (2007) Polysomnography in children: 2006 update. *HK J Paediatr* 12: 42–46.
17. Stores G, Crawford C, Selman J, Wiggs L (1998) Home polysomnography norms for children. *Technol Health Care* 6: 231–236.
18. Feinsilver SH (1998) *How Sleep Labs can Survive Managed Care* [guest editorial]. Available at: www.rtmagazine.com/issues/articles/1998-04_11.asp.
19. Penzel T, Kesper K, Gross V, Becker HF, Vogelmeier C, editors (2003) Problems in automatic sleep scoring applied to sleep apnea. Engineering in Medicine and Biology Society 2003 Proceedings of the 25th Annual International Conference of the IEEE. Piscataway, NJ: IEEE.
20. Montgomery-Downs HE, O'Brian LM, Gulliver TE, Gozal D (2006) Polysomnographic characteristics in normal preschool and early school-aged children. *Pediatrics* 117: 741–753.
21. Stores G, Crawford C (2000) Arousal norms for children age 5–16 years based on home polysomnography. *Technol Health Care* 8: 285–290.
22. Goodwin JL, Enright PL, Kaemingk KL, et al (2001) Feasibility of using unattended polysomnography in children for research – Report of the Tucson Children's Assessment of Sleep Apnea Study (TuCASA). *Sleep* 24: 937–1044.
23. Chervin RD, Murman DL, Malow BA, Totten V (1999) Cost–utility of three approaches to the diagnosis of sleep apnea: polysomnography, home testing, and empirical therapy. *Ann Intern Med* 130: 496–505.
24. Littner M, Kushida CA, McDowell Anderson W, et al (2003) Practice parameters for the role of actigraphy in the study of sleep and circadian rhythms: and update for 2002. *Sleep* 26: 337–341.
25. Sadeh A, Acebo C (2002) The role of actigraphy in sleep medicine. *Sleep Med Rev* 6: 113–124.
26. Jean-Louis G, Kripke DF, Mason WJ, Elliott JA, Youngstedt SD (2001) Sleep estimation from wrist movement quantified by different actigraphic modalities. *J Neurosci Methods* 105: 185–191.
27. So K, Buckley P, Adamson TM, Horne RC (2005) Actigraphy correctly predicts sleep behavior in infants who are younger than six months, when compared with polysomnography. *Pediatr Res* 58: 761–765.
28. Drake CL, Rice MF, Roehrs TA, Rosenthal L, Guido P, Roth T (2000) Scoring reliability of the multiple sleep latency test in a clinical population. *Sleep* 23: 1–3.
29. Golan N, Shahar E, Ravid S, Pillar G (2004) Sleep disorders and daytime sleepiness in children with attention-deficit/hyperactive disorder. *Sleep* 27: 261–266.
30. Kushida CA (2008) *Handbook of Sleep Disorders*, 2nd edition. New York: Informa Healthcare.
31. Venker CC, Goodwin JL, Roe DJ, Kaemingk KL, Mulvaney S, Quan SF (2007) Normative Psychomotor Vigilance Task Performance in Children Aged 6 to 11 – the Tucson Children's Assessment of Sleep Apnea (TuCASA). *Sleep Breath* 11: 217–224.
32. Sforza E, Haba-Rubio J, De Bilbao F, Rochat T, Ibanez V (2004) Performance vigilance task and sleepiness in patients with sleep-disordered breathing. *Eur Respir J* 24: 279–285.
33. Lamond N, Dawson D, Roach GD (2005) Fatigue assessment in the field: validation of a hand-held electronic psychomotor vigilance task. *Aviation Space Environ Med* 76: 486–489.
34. Dorrian J, Rogers NL, Dinges DF (2005) Psychomotor vigilance performance: a neurocognitive assay sensitive to sleep loss. In: Kushida CA, editor. *Sleep Deprivation*. New York: Marcel Dekker, Inc., pp. 39–70.

6
GLOBAL MENTAL FUNCTIONS: INTELLECTUAL (B117)

Kim M. Cornish, Michael J. Sornberger, Marina Dupasquier and John Wilding

What is the construct?

The concept of 'intelligence' is one that seems, at first glance, to lend itself to an almost instinctive understanding. However, after decades of intensive study there still remains a lack of consensus as to what exactly intelligence comprises. Is it a single, unified construct or can it be divided into varying subdomains that constitute proficiencies in various types of skill and ability? The latter is the most widely accepted model and most current intelligence quotient (IQ) batteries incorporate measures that cluster within two broadly defined cognitive domains – verbal and non-verbal (performance) functions. Another important distinction is that between fluid and crystallized intelligence; the former is demonstrated in the ability to adapt knowledge to solve novel problems and the latter in the possession of knowledge gained during experience.

Later in the chapter we highlight four of the most widely employed batteries designed to tap intellectual functioning: the Wechsler Intelligence Scale for Children (WISC), the Stanford–Binet Intelligence Scales (SB5), the Kaufman Assessment Battery for Children (K-ABC) and the Leiter International Performance Scale.

Scores from the different subtests in these batteries are combined to produce an estimate of IQ, indicating where the individual falls on the distribution of scores from the typical population; in the case of children, the comparison is made with children of the same age group. The average child in each age group has an IQ of 100, and 68% of the normal population will fall between scores of 85 and 115 (1 standard deviation from the mean). Another measure that can be used is mental age, indicating the average age at which the obtained score is attained.

The questions that guide this chapter are twofold. First, can IQ measures that are standardized on typically developing individuals be of value in elucidating profiles of intellectual function and dysfunction in atypical populations? In essence, are the measures themselves appropriately designed to tap the range and profiles of abilities that fall outside of the typical range? Should the focus be on the overall full-scale standard 'score' (a combination of the standardized subscale scores) or on individual subtest raw scores that might indicate profiles of strengths and weaknesses across different subtests and domains? We will argue strongly that the latter approach is the only feasible way to capture some aspects of intellectual functioning in atypical populations as defined by IQ measures. Second, can traditional measures of intellectual functioning capture developmental changes or do they mask more subtle trajectories of change? We attempt to address these questions in three genetically determined disorders in order to discuss the critical importance of aetiology and disorder-specific 'signatures' in the context of intellectual functions. We conclude with a plea for research and practice to embrace a more experimental approach to understanding the often subtle disorder-specific profiles of strengths and weaknesses – profiles that might be masked using more traditional, standardized IQ measures.

Overview of recommended measures

In brief, intellectual functioning is typically assessed in most standardized batteries using a number of subtests that combine to create an IQ score, which is perceived as being a standardized measure of intelligence. In any given battery, a variety of scores can be derived and there are slight variations in domain structures across batteries. For example, the WISC domains are described as *verbal* versus *performance*, whereas in the K-ABC, domains are described as *sequential* versus *simultaneous*. Each battery will allow for a comparison of raw scores within and across domains as well as providing standard scores that fall within a normal distribution. It is impossible here to describe in detail all current IQ batteries that are used in clinical and educational practice. Instead we highlight four core batteries that have played a pivotal role in research that has focused on intellectual functioning in typical and atypical populations.

The most common measures for assessing intellectual functioning across childhood are the WISC-IV[1] and the SB5.[2] However, there are a number of alternative batteries that use slightly different scales and subtests but have been used extensively in atypical populations. We describe two here: the K-ABC II[3] (see also K-ABC[4]) and the Leiter International Performance Scale – Revised (Leiter-R).[5]

WECHSLER INTELLIGENCE SCALE FOR CHILDREN, FOURTH EDITION

Overview and purpose
The WISC-IV is the most widely used assessment tool for measuring intelligence in children.[6,7] The original goal in developing the Wechsler scales was to provide a set of tools that could clinically assess intelligence in children.

Administration and scoring
The WISC-IV is made up of 10 core subtests (similarities, vocabulary, comprehension, block design, picture concepts, matrix reasoning, digit span, coding, letter–number sequencing and symbol search). The test also includes five supplementary subtests (information, word reasoning, picture completion, arithmetic and cancellation); these subtests are optional and may be used in place of or in addition to core subtests, at the administrator's discretion. These subtests vary in nature; they can involve the child giving oral or written responses to questions, as well as object manipulation.

To score the test, the administrator uses normative data to transform the raw scores into standardized scores. Each domain receives its own score, which is calculated as a combination of its subtests; similarly, the WISC-IV full-scale IQ is a combination of the scores of all the subtests.

STANFORD–BINET INTELLIGENCE SCALES, FIFTH EDITION

Overview and purpose
Alongside the WISC-IV, the SB5 is likely to be the most commonly used intelligence assessment instrument. It stands out for its use of both verbal and non-verbal domains of intellectual functioning.

Administration and scoring
The administration of the SB5 is divided into 10 subtests: five are verbal and five are non-verbal. The test begins with the administration of a non-verbal subtest (object series/matrices) followed by a verbal subtest (vocabulary). The child's score on these tests is used to determine level of functionality and will inform the administrator as to the ability levels for the remaining subtests. The administrator then proceeds to the remaining eight subtests, some of which are divided into multiple smaller activities, or 'testlets.'

The non-verbal subtests are performed first. These subtests include the following testlets: procedural knowledge, picture absurdities, non-verbal quantitative reasoning, form board, form patterns, delayed response and block span. Next, the administrator presents the verbal subtests, which include these testlets: early reasoning, verbal absurdities, verbal analogies, verbal quantitative reasoning, position and direction, memory for sentences and last word.

As mentioned earlier, scoring begins after the first two subtests are complete in order to determine the functional ability for the remainder of the test. Once the entire test is complete, the administrator uses standardized data to convert the raw scores into normative scores. Scores are provided for non-verbal IQ, verbal IQ and a full-scale IQ; each is measured on a mean of 100, with a standard deviation of 15.

KAUFMAN ASSESSMENT BATTERY FOR CHILDREN, SECOND EDITION

Overview and purpose
The KABC-II was developed to provide more flexibility in terms of interpretative freedom when working with final scores and also in the range of subtests that can be used or omitted, depending on the child.[8]

One benefit of the KABC-II is that the construction of the test allows administrators to decide between two theoretical models: the Cattell–Horn–Carroll (CHC) model and the Luria model. The more psychometrically based CHC model is influenced by fluid and crystallized abilities as the basis of intelligence; the more neuropsychological Luria model focuses instead on cognitive processing abilities. Before using the KABC-II, an administrator can decide which theoretical model to apply. The authors recommend CHC interpretation for children with disabilities in reading, written expression or mathematics, children with learning disabilities and children with emotional, behavioural or attentional disorders. For children with autism or language disorders, the authors instead recommend the Luria model. The theoretical model will influence the administration of subtests; different subtests are deemed 'core' or 'supplementary' depending on the model chosen, and the scoring of scales is also different between the CHC and Luria models.

WECHSLER INTELLIGENCE SCALE FOR CHILDREN, FOURTH EDITION (WISC-IV)	
Purpose	To provide a clinical assessment and measure of intelligence The most widely used measure of intelligence Revisions from older versions have updated this test to reduce the incidence of zero or maximum (floor or ceiling) scores, to be engaging to children and to improve clinical utility
Population	Age 6–16y
Description of domains (subscales)	One global score made up of four indices: verbal comprehension, perceptual reasoning, working memory and processing speed
Administration and test format	Time to complete 60–90 min Testing format: 10 core and five supplementary subtests items; direct assessment of child using activities and stimuli Scoring: objective scoring – for subtests that require verbal answers, the WISC-IV manual provides detailed descriptions of acceptable answers and their respective score values. This keeps administrators from having to make subjective decisions about scoring, which could affect reliability Time bonuses for some subtests Training: a training CD is available to order from the publisher
Psychometric properties	Normative sample: 2200 children selected to match US census data *Reliability* Internal consistency *r*-values range from 0.72 to 0.94; test–retest reliability *r*-values range from 0.86 to 0.93 *Validity* Research suggests that a five-factor structure based on Cattell–Horn–Carroll theory may be more valid than the current four-factor structure; correlates with earlier versions of the WISC, as well as with other Wechsler measures, including (1) WISC-III at *r*=0.89; (2) Wechsler Preschool and Primary Scale of Intelligence at *r*=0.89; (3) Wechsler Adult Intelligence Scale at *r*=0.89; and (4) Wechsler Abbreviated Scale of Intelligence at *r*=0.86 Standardization included studies of special groups, including children with autistic disorder, Asperger syndrome, language disorders, attention-deficit–hyperactivity disorder, learning disability, brain injury and motor impairment. However, research suggests that these studies used small groups, and so should not be used for differential diagnosis
How to order	The full WISC-IV can be ordered from http://pearsonassess.ca. The complete WISC-IV kit (Canadian edition) costs between US$1595 and 2215, depending on packaging options
Key references	Hebben N (2004) Review of special group studies and utility of the process approach with the WISC-IV. In: Flanagan DP, Kaufman AS, editors. *Essentials of WISC-IV Assessment*. New York: John Wiley, pp. 183–199. Kaufman AS, Flanagan DP, Alfonso VC, Mascolo JT (2006) Test review: Wechsler Intelligence Scale for Children, 4th edition (WISC-IV). *J Psychoed Assess* 24: 278–295. Ryan JJ, Glass LA, Brown CN (2007) Administration time estimates for Wechsler Intelligence Scale for Children-IV subtests, composites, and short forms. *J Clin Psychol* 63: 309–318.

The subtests include word order, number recall, hand movements, triangles, face recognition, conceptual thinking, rover, block counting, gestalt closure, pattern reasoning, story completion, atlantis, rebus, delayed recall, riddles, expressive vocabulary and verbal knowledge. Whether or not these subtests are core or supplementary depends on the age of the child being assessed and the theoretical model being used.

Stanford–Binet Intelligence Scales, fifth edition (SB5)

Purpose	To assess intelligence and cognitive abilities
	Adaptive test wherein test item difficulty adapts to examinee's responses, reducing frustration, increasing reliability and economizing administration time
	Used as part of a diagnostic battery of tests to determine presence of cognitive delays in young children, learning disabilities and intellectual giftedness
	Used in research on cognitive abilities, as well as in psychoeducational, clinical and neuropsychological assessments
	Provides information for interventions, career assessment
Population	2y to 85+y
Description of domains (subscales)	Two domains (non-verbal, verbal), each made up of five factors (knowledge, fluid reasoning, visuospatial reasoning, quantitative reasoning, working memory). These domains and factors combine for a total of 10 unique subtests
Administration and test format	Time to complete: 45–90min to administer full-scale IQ
	Testing format: A verbal and a non-verbal routing task determine in which level to begin within each domain, and age determines start points within each level. Questions administered with visual aid from stimulus books (easel format) and/or with blocks, chips, shapes, toys
	Scoring: norm-referenced; mean=100, SD 15, for composite scores; mean=10, SD 3, for subtests, allowing for easy comparison with other tests; can be scored manually or by computer
	Training: psychologists, psychiatrists or psychometricians can use this instrument
Psychometric properties	Normative sample: 4800 participants aged 2y to 85+y who were representative of the US 2001 census data
	Reliability Split-half reliability: r-values ranged from 0.84 to 0.89 across subtests; reliability coefficients between non-verbal IQ, verbal IQ and full-scale IQ for all age groups range from r-values of 0.95 to r-values of 0.98
	FSIQ: standard error of measurement averaged 2.30. Test–retest correlations for all age groups range from 0.93 to 0.95. Inter-rater reliability averaged 0.89
	Validity Concurrent validity: correlates with (1) Woodcock–Johnson Test of General Intellectual Ability at 0.79; (2) Wechsler Adult Intelligence Scale at 0.81; (3) Wechsler Intelligence Scales for Children at 0.69; differentiates between children with and without disabilities; validity for special populations is extensive; children/adults with autism, speech disorders, learning disabilities, developmental delay, emotional disturbance, English as second language, motor impairments and attention-deficit–hyperactivity disorder tested and results found to match other comparative tests
How to order	The full SB5 can be ordered from www.assess.nelson.com/test-ind/stan-b5. The complete kit costs C\$1545, or C\$1826 with scoring software
Key references	Bain SK, Allin JD (2005). Book Review: Stanford–Binet Intelligence Scales, 5th edition. *J Psychoedu Assess* 23: 87–95.
	Becker KA (2003) *History of the Stanford–Binet Intelligence Scales: Content and Psychometrics. (Stanford–Binet Intelligence Scales, Fifth Edition Assessment Service Bulletin No. 1)*. Itasca, IL: Riverside Publishing.
	Thorndike RL, Hagen EP, Sattler JM (1986) *Technical Manual, Stanford–Binet Intelligence Scale*, 4th edition. Chicago: Riverside.

KAUFMAN ASSESSMENT BATTERY FOR CHILDREN, SECOND EDITION (KABC-II)	
Purpose	Uses two theoretical models – Luria's Model of Mental Processing and the Cattell–Horn–Carroll (CHC) hierarchically organized model – to evaluate simultaneous and sequential processing in children and adolescents
	Two theoretical models allow for two separate methods of interpretation
	CHC interpretation is recommended for children with disabilities in reading, written expression or mathematics, children with learning disabilities and children with emotional, behavioural or attentional disorders
	Luria interpretation is recommended for children with autism or language disorder
Population	3–18y
Description of domains (subscales)	CHC interpretation: one global score, Fluid-crystallized Index (FCI), made up of five scales: long-term storage and retrieval, (Glr), short-term memory (Gsm), visual processing (Gv), fluid reasoning (Gf) and crystallized ability (Gc)
	Luria interpretation: one global score, Mental Processing Index (MPI), made up of four scales: learning ability, sequential processing, simultaneous processing and planning ability. A fifth scale, knowledge, is not included in the global score
	Note that the scales from the two interpretations are divided the same way, and therefore parallel one another. These parallels are learning ability/Glr, sequential processing/Gsm, simultaneous processing/Gv, planning ability/Gf and knowledge/Gc
Administration and test format	Time to complete:
	30–55min to administer core Luria model
	40–70min to administer core CHC model
	60–100min to administer entire battery
	Testing format:16 subtests; direct assessment of child using activities and stimuli
	Scoring: objective; standardized software available for scoring; focus is on global and scale scores rather than individual tasks
	Training: training video available to order from publisher
Psychometric properties	Normative sample: >3000 children and adolescents
	Reliability Test–retest reliability of subtests established (range: r=0.50–0.86 for ages 3–5y; r=0.53–0.88 for ages 7–12y; r=0.60–0.92 for ages 13–18y)
	Validity Confirmatory factor analyses support construct validity; Comparative Fit Index scores support theory-based scale structure for KABC-II
How to order	The KABC-II can be ordered from Pearson Assessments at www.pearsonassessments.com/kabcassess.aspx
	A complete price list is available on this website
Key references	Bain SK Grey R (2008) Test reviews. In: Kaufman AS, Kaufman NL (eds) Kaufman Assessment Battery for Children, 2nd edition. Circle Pines, MN: AGS. Also in *J Psychoedu Assess* 26: 92–101.
	Kaufman JC, Kaufman AS, Kaufman-Singer J, Kaufman NL (2005) The Kaufman Assessment Battery for Children – second edition; and the Kaufman Adolescent and Adult Intelligence Test. In: Flanagan DP, Harrison PL, editors. *Contemporary Intellectual Assessment*. New York: Guildford Press, pp. 344–370.
	Reynolds MR, Keith TZ, Goldenring Fine J, Fisher ME, Low J (2007) Confirmatory factor structure of the Kaufman Assessment Battery for Children – Second Edition: Consistency with Cattell–Horn–Carroll theory. *School Psychol Quart* 22: 511–539.

Administration and scoring

Before administration of the KABC-II, it is crucial for the administrator to know which theoretical model is being applied. In terms of the actual scores, Lichtenberger and Kaufman[9] note that the first and most important scale is the global score, and that subscale scores should be analysed to determine relative strengths and weaknesses.

LEITER INTERNATIONAL PERFORMANCE SCALE – REVISED

Overview and purpose

The Leiter-R is a completely non-verbal test designed to evaluate an individual's intellectual ability, memory and attention. A main strength of this scale is its usefulness in assessing children with severe communication

LEITER INTERNATIONAL PERFORMANCE SCALE, REVISED (LEITER-R)	
Purpose	To evaluate an individual's intellectual ability, memory and attention using non-verbal tasks
	May be used with children who cannot be tested using conventional testing owing to such circumstances as cognitive delay or English as a second language
	May be used as an outcome measure of medical and rehabilitation interventions – can measure small increments of improvement
Population	Ages 2y 0mo to 20y 11mo
Description of domains (subscales)	Four domains (reasoning, visualization, attention, memory and memory span), divided into two batteries (visualization and reasoning, VR; and attention and memory, AM), comprising 20 subtest items
Administration and test format	Time to complete: 90min; a shorter version called the brief IQ is also available
	Testing format: individually administered using response easels and stimulus cards
	Scoring: mean=100, SD 15, for composite scores; mean=10, SD 3, for subtests, allowing for easy comparison with other tests
	Can be scored manually or by computer
	Training: video available for purchase from website
Psychometric properties	Normative sample: VR battery: 1719 individuals; AM battery: subset of VR battery sample totalling 763 individuals. Samples were representative of 1993 US census data
	Reliability Test–retest reliability: VR battery r-values ranged within 0.80 across age groups (less reliable at younger ages); AM battery r-values ranged from 0.55 to 0.85 with a median estimate of 0.62 (too low to be used for diagnostic purposes); internal consistency as measured by Cronbach's alpha: VR battery ranged from 0.75 to 0.90; AM battery ranged from 0.69 to 0.87; several subtests and composite scores showed practice effects
	Validity 174 examiners rated the tests on content validity in piloting stages. Only subtests that received high ratings were included; correlates with (1) WISC-III (0.85–0.86), (2) the original Leiter (0.85–0.93); validity for special populations: test was found to identify children/adults with speech disorders, cognitive delay, learning disabilities, attention-deficit–hyperactivity disorder and giftedness
How to order	The full Leiter-R can be ordered from https://www.stoeltingco.com. The complete kit costs US$925, or US$1060 with scoring software
Key references	Roid GH, Miller LJ (1997) *Leiter International Performance Scale – Revised: Examiner's Manual*. Wood Dale, IL: Stoelting Co.
	Stinnet TA (2001) Review of the Leiter International Performance Scale – Revised. In: Plake BS, Impara JC, editors, Murphy LL, managing editor. *The Fourteenth Mental Measurements Yearbook* Lincoln, NB: Buros Institute of Mental Measurements of the University of Nebraska-Lincoln, pp. 687–692.

impairments who have little or no expressive language capability. The Leiter-R is also useful in cases where the child being assessed has difficulties with motor coordination.[10] It therefore allows an assessment of intellectual functioning in children who would otherwise be excluded from measures that include significant verbal components such as the WISC, SB5 and K-ABC. The Leiter-R focuses on four domains of intellectual functioning: reasoning, visualization, attention, and memory and memory span.

In developing normative data for the Leiter-R, the authors used special criterion groups, including children identified as gifted and children with specific developmental disorders including attention-deficit–hyperactivity disorder, and learning disabilities.

Administration and scoring
The Leiter-R is made up of two batteries: visualization and reasoning, and attention and memory. Responses are given by inserting cards into appropriate slots, manipulating foam shapes or pointing to stimuli. Scoring is compared with either normative data or special criterion data, scored on a scale with a mean of 100 and a standard deviation of 15.

General factors to consider when measuring this domain

ATYPICAL DEVELOPMENT AND INTELLECTUAL FUNCTIONING
As discussed above, scores tend to cluster around a mean of 100 with a standard deviation of 15. However, in those individuals with delay, there will be a graded skew to the lower end of the distribution, depending on the severity of the intellectual delay. Until recently, intellectual impairment was, in many cases, categorized solely on the basis of the child's IQ score as profound (score 0–19), severe (20–34), moderate (score 35–49) or mild (score 50–69).[11] In these cases, the underlying assumption was that impairment in intellectual functioning, as measured by an IQ test, implied a 'global' delay with differences lying on a continuum of severity, irrespective of the aetiology of the intellectual delay, that is whether arising from trisomy 21 (Down syndrome) or from a single gene being switched off on the X chromosome (fragile X syndrome). However, this assumption has been challenged by a decade of exciting research discoveries that have clearly identified that aetiology does matter and that the intellectual functioning of children with different disorders will vary to some significant degree because of their different aetiologies. See Cornish et al[12] and Visootsak and Sherman[13] for examples related to fragile X syndrome and Down syndrome. Most recently, research has also begun to acknowledge the

critical role of gene and environmental interactions in shaping cognitive outcomes in individuals with developmental disorders.[14] The impact of development itself in shaping cognitive profiles across different developmental disorders has also come to the forefront of recent research endeavours and findings clearly demonstrate that performance does not remain static with age but instead has a dynamic trajectory from infancy onwards.[14–16]

Taken together, these findings emphasize the importance of aetiology and age as important factors in the assessment of children with developmental delays. In the following section, we will highlight three developmental disorders that have received considerable attention in recent years: fragile X syndrome, Down syndrome and Williams syndrome. All three disorders cause significant intellectual delay and at first glance they seem to result in a comparable level of functioning. However, when recent investigations have looked at the profiles of individual subtest scores rather than at global IQ scores, findings have revealed important syndrome-specific *signatures*. Having said that, we do offer the reader a note of caution because, on the one hand, these new findings suggest that IQ batteries can play a role in identifying strengths as well as challenges in intellectual functioning across different disorders, and on the other hand they will have limited validity and reliability in terms of comparing performance with that of typically developing children using the standardized norms.

FRAGILE X SYNDROME
Fragile X syndrome is a well-recognized cause of hereditary developmental delay in males and to lesser extent in females. It is one of the most widely studied genetic disorders worldwide, affecting an estimated 1 in 2500 males and females.[17] Several imaging studies reveal a vulnerability in fragile X in specific brain regions that are involved in intellectual functioning, visuospatial ability and executive function.[18,19]

Intellectual functioning
Intellectual disability and behavioural difficulties characterize many children and adolescents with fragile X syndrome. Almost all males, with fragile X syndrome present with IQ scores that fall within the moderate–severe range of impairment, with profiles emerging from as young as 3 years of age.[20] Some females with this disorder only show learning disabilities that do not qualify as 'clinical';[21] on the other hand, approximately 50% display more moderate–severe intellectual impairments.[12] The reason for this sex difference is that females with fragile X have only one inactive X chromosome. The second unaffected chromosome will therefore serve as 'buffer' to the full effect of

the disorder, resulting in the broader range of intellectual functioning and cognitive deficits that we associate with females compared with fragile X males.

When studies have teased apart performance to look specifically at discrepancies across IQ domains and subtests, some important findings have emerged: (1) at the *domain* level, some of the earliest research studies demonstrated higher verbal IQ than performance IQ (e.g. WISC),[22] with a similar discrepancy observed between simultaneous and sequential processing, with the former a relative strength (K-ABC);[23,24] (2) other studies have focused on the *subdomain* level, specifically comparing individual subtests within and across domains. With this methodology, detailed profiles have emerged that indicate relative strengths on subtests that involve vocabulary, gestalt processing and visuospatial construction[25–28] with specific weaknesses on subtests that involve arithmetic, visual motor skills and sequential processing.[28–30] Taken together, these findings indicate that skills that make heavy demands on sequential processing, such as those required for planning, cognitive flexibility and working memory, are especially vulnerable in fragile X, but other skills, such as those that require simultaneous and verbal processing, are relative strengths. It is important though to note that we refer only to *relative* strengths, not absolute strengths, which would indicate a sparing of impairment.

Does IQ decline with age in fragile X?

In terms of age-related changes in intellectual functioning, a recent longitudinal study using the Leiter performance scales has found IQ to decline significantly at around 8 years of age with continued decline in the twelfth year.[20] Other studies have also found a similar profile of decline in intellectual functions as measured by standardized IQ batteries,[31,32] especially on measures of non-verbal functioning such as the Leiter scales. However, we suggest caution in how these scores are used to infer decline and argue that development would be expected to be slower and so the gap between a child with developmental delay and a typically developing child will increase with age, impacting on IQ score. There may be no actual deterioration, only a slower development, and so we strongly recommend that future studies track developmental changes very carefully using more experimentally driven measures that tap specific intellectual strengths as well as weaknesses.

DOWN SYNDROME

Down syndrome is the most common genetic cause of developmental delay (96% of cases) and results from an extra copy of chromosome 21, known as *trisomy 21*. The syndrome has an estimated frequency of 1 in 730 people[33]

and has a distinct clinical phenotype that includes a number of unique facial feature characteristics.

Intellectual functioning

Down syndrome is always associated with intellectual impairment, which can range from mild to severe with an IQ range of 30–70.[34] Research suggests a less definitive profile of domain strengths and weaknesses than reported in other syndrome groups (see fragile X above) but, nonetheless, some specific strengths do emerge. For example, Hodapp et al[23] identified slightly better performance on the simultaneous processing domain than on the sequential processing domain using the K-ABC, but in a comparison of subtests a specific strength was observed on a task that required imitating a series of hand movements in a sequence. This relative strength was not observed in fragile X syndrome.

Does IQ decline with age in Down syndrome?

Although intellectual decline associated with Alzheimer dementia is well documented in mid to late adulthood in Down syndrome,[35] few studies have assessed intellectual decline in the childhood years. An interesting early study by Gibson et al[36] suggested that performance on the WISC remained relatively stable with increasing age but with a specific and pervasive decline on the block design subtests that requires visuospatial processing. The authors speculate that this particular test can potentially serve as a useful early marker of later intellectual decline in individuals with Down syndrome. In a 7-year longitudinal study, Kittler et al[37] sought to determine whether sex differences in cognitive functioning are present in individuals with Down syndrome, whether there are changes in cognitive functioning over time and whether there is an interaction between sex and cognitive functioning over time. The authors found that females scored higher on the coding subtest of the WISC, but found a general decline in the overall performance of adults with Down syndrome, particularly on the verbal subscale subtests of the WISC (i.e. information, similarities, vocabulary and comprehension), which each tap different nuances of verbal ability. Conversely, Burt et al's[38] longitudinal study spanning over 4 years did not find an age-related decline in the cognitive functioning of adults with Down syndrome apart from the previously mentioned deterioration associated with Alzheimer disease. In this study, the authors chose to assess cognitive functioning with the Leiter scales, a measure of non-verbal intelligence. Perhaps the discrepancies in the findings of these studies are indicative of a subtler and more specific decline in cognitive functioning that is more easily detected by the subtests of the WISC, but we suggest that more comprehensive research is required to make any definitive conclusions on the presence of age-related cognitive decline in people with Down syndrome.

WILLIAMS SYNDROME

Williams syndrome is a relatively rare disorder that results from a microdeletion on one copy of chromosome 7. Until quite recently, it was assumed to be a quite rare disorder – 1 in 15 000 to 20 000 – but one recent study estimates the frequency at 1 in 7500.[39]

Intellectual functioning

Almost all children with Williams syndrome will have some degree of intellectual impairment, with some children showing mild impairment and others being more severely affected. At a more fine-tuned level, one recent study found a discrepancy in a verbal performance, with verbal processing skills greater than non-verbal processing skills.[40,41] Few studies have focused on comparing subtests but those that have, especially in relation to the Stanford–Binet measure, have found comparable performance across all subtests.[42] One subtest that appears to be especially weak, with little change, is the object assembly subtest from the Weschler Preschool and Primary Scale of Intelligence and WISC, which requires spatial manipulation and construction to make a meaningful design (e.g. a ball).[43] However, the paucity of evidence does contrast with many other experimental studies that have used similar but non-standardized measures of verbal and performance abilities and report significant discrepancies between components of visuospatial abilities and verbal abilities.[44–46]

Does IQ decline with age in Williams syndrome?

There is still some debate regarding age-related changes in IQ in children and adults with Williams syndrome. For example, in a series of cross-sectional and longitudinal studies, Fisch et al[47] found a decline in IQ (e.g. Stanford–Binet) from late childhood (around age 8y) that accelerated with age such that, by 15 years, many individuals performed at floor level.[47] In contrast, an earlier study by Udwin et al[48] reported an increase in IQ from the mid-teens to early adulthood.

Interpreting IQ assessment outcomes in atypical populations: issues of complexity

Studies using IQ measures to assess intellectual functioning in children with developmental disorders are instantly confronted with a number of issues that need careful consideration. A core issue relates to how one interprets actual IQ scores in a population that has intellectual delay and their relevance to clinical and academic practice. Is it most appropriate to view IQ scores as definitive outcome measures that guide practice, or should these measures be viewed as a 'filter' or signpost to explore specific areas of proficiencies and deficiencies in more detail using experimental paradigms that can tap subtle signatures? From our brief review of current studies focused on three different developmental disorders, it is clear that cognitive delay does not imply global delay across all cognitive domains. We question here the feasibility of using IQ measures as an indicator of cognitive function and dysfunction in developmental disorders.

The global score derived from an IQ battery comprises the sum of scores on a range of different tasks. In the general population, performance on these tasks tends to be correlated. An individual who does well on one task will also generally do well on the others, implying that some common process is involved in all such tasks; some theorists have suggested that speed of neural functioning is the relevant process.

Use of the global score to estimate the potential of an individual with a developmental disability assumes that this is also the case in atypical populations and that impairment of this single underlying function will produce a similar reduction in efficiency across the board. However, as we have stressed, evidence is accumulating that such an assumption is unjustified and that different developmental disorders involve different areas of the brain and hence different cognitive functions (e.g. memory, inhibition of distraction, spatial abilities). Thus, a reduced global score will tell us little more than that some aspects of cognitive function are impaired (which was probably known before testing!). Obviously we would not accept that two people with the same overall score on a range of physical activities were really equivalent if one failed on all tests requiring use of the left hand owing to some muscular problem while the other performed poorly on tasks requiring eye–hand coordination. Equally, the profile of IQ test scores must be examined to decide whether a pervasive reduction is apparent or there is a weakness in a specific area of testing. For example, in a child with a developmental disability, cognitive age will commonly be below chronological age, and equivalent to that of a younger typically developing child; however, the difference will often lie principally in weak fluid intelligence (ability to cope with novel tasks rather than crystallized intelligence [knowledge of the world]), which should have benefited from their greater age.[49]

The subcomponents identified in most of the four batteries that we have discussed (e.g. verbal ability, speed, visuospatial reasoning) do provide a better guide to specific weaknesses, but even these are relatively coarse measures of performance that invite further questions about the precise problem in the relevant domain. There is a huge range of tasks claiming to test specific functions, but evaluation of these is beyond the scope of this chapter. However, standardized versions of such tasks are as yet not well developed, particularly for children, and often a task must be purpose built to test a specific hypothesis. It is likely that, with increasingly sophisticated identification of key functions and the use of brain imaging to aid in this process, more and better-standardized tasks of this type will be developed.

We therefore see IQ batteries as initial 'coarse filters' that can suggest areas of weakness to be pursued using finer-grain testing within specific cognitive functions, but users should be aware of the temptation to conclude that equivalent overall scores on such batteries imply equivalence in intellectual functioning.

Summary

We began this chapter by asking two important questions. The first was whether IQ batteries standardized on typically developing individuals would be of value in elucidating profiles of intellectual function and dysfunction in atypical populations. We have argued that as a global measure of intellectual functioning, they have limited value other than to describe levels of impairment across broad cognitive domains. When domains are teased apart to examine subtest performance, then much more useful information emerges that highlights putative strengths and weaknesses that are disorder specific. But this information

can also be of limited value if not combined with experimentally based cognitive measures that can provide more accurate and more fine-tuned assessments of differing aspects of intellectual functioning.

Our second question focused on whether IQ changes with age and the value of that assessment. We would argue that such studies provide minimal information of value for practice and instead we urge readers to consider the critical need for longitudinal assessments that focus on core cognitive weaknesses and strengths that are syndrome specific. The seminal work of Karmiloff-Smith and colleagues[14–16] and Cornish and Wilding[50] attests to the importance of tracing trajectories of cognitive function from infancy onwards and not making the a priori assumption that decline follows a linear trajectory with increasing age, producing exponentially poorer performance. It is highly likely that some cognitive abilities change with age in the expected direction, but others may follow a typical trajectory and timeline. The key is to utilize measures that are appropriately designed to assess the wide range of intellectual functioning in children with atypical development. Relying on standardized measures may mask important but subtle strengths as well as difficulties.

In summary, assessment of intellectual functioning through traditional batteries has some value but perhaps should be viewed as a starting point in understanding disorder-specific profiles of, and trajectories over age of, proficiencies and deficiencies.

REFERENCES

1. Wechsler D (2004) *The Wechsler Intelligence Scale for Children*, 4th edition. London: Pearson Assessment.
2. Roid GH (2003) *Stanford–Binet Intelligence Scales*, 5th edition. Itasca, IL: Riverside.
3. Kaufman AS, Kaufman NL (2004) *Kaufman Assessment Battery for Children – 2*. Circle Pines, MN: American Guidance Service.
4. Kaufman AS, Kaufman NL (1983) *Kaufman Assessment Battery for Children: Interpretive Manual*. Circle Pines, MN: American Guidance Service.
5. Roid GH, Miller LJ (1997) *Leiter International Performance Scale-Revised: Examiner's Manual*. Wood Dale, IL: Stoelting Co.
6. Flanagan DP, Kaufman AS (2004) *Essentials of WISC-IV Assessment*. New York: Wiley.
7. Kaufman AS, Flanagan DP, Alfonso VC, Mascolo T (2006) Test review: Wechsler Intelligence Scale for Children, fourth edition (WISC-IV). *J Psychoeduc Assess* 9: 278–295.
8. Bain SK, Grey R (2008) Test reviews: Kaufman AS, Kaufman NL (eds) Kaufman Assessment Battery for Children, second edition. Circle Pines, MN: AGS. Also in *J Psychoeduc Assess* 26: 92.
9. Lichtenberger EO, Kaufman AS (2006) *Essentials of WAIS-IV Assessment*. New York: John Wiley.
10. Sandler AG, Hatt CV (2004) Mental retardation. In: Hersen M, editor. *Psychological Assessment in Clinical Practice: A Pragmatic Guide*. New York: Brunner-Routledge, pp. 321–345.
11. Huberman R, Cahill L (2000) Childhood mental disorders and child psychiatry. In: Goldman HH, editor. *Review of General Psychiatry*, 5th edition. New York: Lange Medical Books/McGraw-Hill, pp. 399–422.
12. Cornish KM, Turk J, Hagerman R (2008) The fragile X continuum: new advances and perspectives. *J Intellect Disabil Res* 52: 469–482.
13. Visootsak J, Sherman S (2007) Neuropsychiatric and behavioral aspects of trisomy 21. *Curr Psychiatry Rep* 9: 135–140.
14. Karmiloff-Smith A (2009) Nativism versus neuroconstructivism: rethinking the study of developmental disorders. *Dev Psychol* 45: 56–63.
15. Cornish K, Scerif G, Karmiloff-Smith A (2007) Tracing syndrome-specific trajectories of attention across the lifespan. *Cortex* 43: 672–85.
16. Karmiloff-Smith A (1998) Development itself is the key to understanding developmental disorders. *Trends Cogn Sci* 2: 389–298.
17. Hagerman PJ (2008) The fragile X prevalence paradox. *J Med Genet* 45: 498–499.
18. Schaer M, Eliez S (2007) From genes to brain: understanding brain development in neurogenetic disorders using neuroimaging techniques. *Child Adolesc Psychiatric Clin N Am* 16: 557–579.
19. Walter E, Mazaika PK, Reiss AL (2009) Insights into brain development from neurogenetic syndromes: evidence from

fragile X syndrome, Williams syndrome, Turner syndrome, and velocardiofacial syndrome. *Neuroscience* 164: 257–271.

20. Skinner M, Hooper S, Hatton DD, et al (2005) Mapping non-verbal IQ in young boys with fragile X syndrome. *Am J Med Genet A* 132: 25–32.

21. Bennetto L, Pennington BF (2002) Neuropsychology. In: Hagerman RJ, Hagerman PJ, editors. *Fragile X Syndrome: Diagnosis, Treatment, and Research*, 3rd edition. Baltimore: Johns Hopkins University Press, pp. 206–248.

22. Veenema H, Veenema T, Geraedts JPM (1987) The fragile X syndrome in a large family: two psychological investigations. *J Med Genet* 24: 32–38.

23. Hodapp RM, Leckman JF, Dykens EM, Sparrow SS, Zelinsky DG, Ort SI (1992) K-ABC profiles of children with fragile X syndrome, Down syndrome and non-specific mental retardation. *Am J Ment Retard* 97: 39–46.

24. Kemper MB, Hagerman RJ, Altshul-Stark D (1988) Cognitive profiles of boys with the fragile X syndrome. *Am J Med Genet* 30: 191–200.

25. Backes M, Genc B, Schreck J, Doerfler W, Lehmkuhl G, von Gontard A (2000) Cognitive and behavioral profile of fragile X boys: correlations to molecular data. *Am J Med Genet* 95: 150–156

26. Cornish KM, Munir F, Cross G (1998) The nature of the spatial deficit in young females with fragile X syndrome: a neuropsychological and molecular perspective. *Neuropsychologia* 36: 1239–1246.

27. Cornish KM, Munir F, Cross G (1999) Spatial cognition in males with fragile X syndrome: evidence for a neuropsychological phenotype. *Cortex* 35: 263–271.

28. Jäkälä P, Hanninen T, Ryynanen M, et al (1997) Fragile-X: neuropsychological test performance, CGG triplet repeat lengths, and hippocampal volumes. *J Clin Invest* 100: 331–338.

29. Cornish K, Turk J, Wilding J, Sudhalter V, Kooy F, Hagerman R (2004) Deconstructing the attention deficit in fragile X syndrome: a developmental neuropsychological approach. *J Child Psychol Psychiatr* 45: 1042–1053.

30. Freund LS, Reiss AL (1991) Cognitive profiles associated with the fra(X) syndrome in males and females. *Am J Med Genet* 38: 542–547.

31. Fisch GS, Simensen RJ, Schroer RJ (2002) Longitudinal changes in cognitive and adaptive behavior scores in children and adolescents with the fragile X mutation or autism. *J Autism Dev Disord* 32: 107–114.

32. Hall SS, Burns DD, Lightbody AA, Reiss AL (2008) Longitudinal changes in intellectual development in children with fragile X syndrome. *J Abnorm Child Psychol* 36: 927–939.

33. Canfield MA, Honein MA, Yuskiv N, et al (2006) National estimates and race/ethnic-specific variation of selected birth defects in the United States, 1999–2001. *Birth Defects Res A Clin Mol Teratol* 76: 747–756.

34. Chapman RS, Hesketh LJ (2001) Language, cognition, and short-term memory in individuals with Down syndrome. *Downs Syndr Res Pract* 7: 1–7.

35. Nieuwenhuis-Mark RE (2009) Diagnosing Alzheimer's dementia in Down syndrome: problems and possible solutions. *Res Dev Disabil* 30: 827–838.

36. Gibson D, Groeneweg G, Jerry P, Harris A (1988) Age and pattern of intellectual decline among Down syndrome and other mentally retarded adults. *Int J Rehabil Res* 11: 47–55.

37. Kittler P, Krinsky-McHale SJ, Devenny DA (2004) Sex differences in performance over 7 years on the Wechsler Intelligence Scale for Children – Revised among adults with intellectual disability. *J Intell Disabil Res* 48: 114–122.

38. Burt DB, Loveland KA, Chen Y-W, Chuang A, Lewis KR, Cherry L (1995) Aging in adults with Down syndrome: report from a longitudinal study. *Am J Ment Retard* 100: 262–270.

39. Stromme P, Bjornstad PG, Ramstad K. (2002) Prevalence estimation of Williams syndrome. *J Child Neurol* 17: 269–271.

40. Campbell LE, Stevens A, Daly E, et al (2009) A comparative study of cognition and brain anatomy between two neurodevelopmental disorders: 22q11.2 deletion syndrome and Williams syndrome. *Neuropsychologia* 47: 1034–1044.

41. Levy Y, Bechar T (2003) Cognitive, lexical, and morpho-syntactic profiles of Israeli children with Williams syndrome. *Cortex* 29: 255–271.

42. Greer MK, Brown FR, Pai GS, Choudry SH, Klein AJ (1997) Cognitive, adaptive, and behavioral characteristics of Williams syndrome. *Am J Med Genet* 74: 521–525.

43. Atkinson J, Anker S, Braddick O, Nokes L, Mason A, Braddick F (2001) Visual and visuospatial development in young children with Williams syndrome. *Dev Med Child Neurol* 43: 330–337.

44. Ansari D, Donlan C, Karmiloff-Smith A (2007) Atypical and typical development of visual estimation abilities. *Cortex* 43: 758–768.

45. Brock J, Jarrold C, Farran EK, Laws G, Riby D (2007) Do children with Williams syndrome have really good vocabulary knowledge? Methods for comparing cognitive and linguistic abilities in developmental disorders. *Clin Linguist Phon* 21: 673–688.

46. Farran EK, Jarrold C, Gathercole SE (2001) Block design performance in the Williams syndrome phenotype: a problem with mental imagery? *J Child Psychol Psychiatr* 42: 719–728.

47. Fisch GS, Carpenter N, Howard-Peebles PN, et al (2007) Studies of age-correlated features of cognitive-behavioral development in children and adolescents with genetic disorders. *Am J Med Genet* 143: 2478–2489.

48. Udwin O, Davies M, Howlin P (1996) A longitudinal study of cognitive abilities and educational attainment in Williams syndrome. *Dev Med Child Neurol* 38: 1020–1029.

49. Anderson M (1992) *Intelligence and Development: a Cognitive Theory*. Oxford: Blackwell Publishing.

50. Cornish KM, Wilding J (2009) *Attention, Genes and Developmental Disorders*. New York: Oxford University Press.

7
GLOBAL MENTAL FUNCTIONS: PSYCHOSOCIAL (B122)

Sara King and Christine T. Chambers

What is the construct?

Global psychosocial functions, as defined by the International Classification of Functioning, Disability and Health for Children and Youth (ICF-CY), refer to those developmental functions involved with '[understanding] and constructively [integrating] the mental functions that lead to the formation of the personal and interpersonal skills needed to establish reciprocal social interactions, in terms of both meaning and purpose'. Psychosocial functions are constantly developing to meet the child's needs with respect to his or her environment; for example, infants begin to develop psychosocial skills as they learn to regulate their emotions and affect in relation to their environment, whereas toddlers must develop skills that allow them to interact with their peers. As the child matures, these skills are constantly evolving to make it possible for the child or adolescent to adapt to the environment. Parents, therefore, play an important role in guiding the child through each stage of psychosocial development, certainly when the child is very young. Assessment of psychosocial functions must consider the developmental stage of the child, as well as factors leading to difficulty in self–other relationships and factors leading to difficulties in establishing an attachment to a caregiver. Commonly assessed aspects of psychosocial functioning include internalizing symptoms (e.g. anxiety, depression), externalizing symptoms (e.g. hyperactivity), social competence (i.e. social skills and social adjustment), school competence, autonomy development and self-concept/self-esteem. Recent advances in medical treatment (e.g. drug development, surgical procedures) have resulted in a dramatic increase in the prevalence of children with chronic conditions and disabilities that may have previously led to preterm death but can now be effectively treated and managed.[1] As such, children with chronic conditions and developmental disabilities are now able to participate in many typical activities of childhood (e.g. regular school, extracurricular and social activities). However, with increased survival rates and integration

with typically developing children comes new challenges for children and families affected by disability. One such challenge is the assessment of psychosocial functioning.

Psychosocial functioning is an especially important component of typical development, as the emergence of the skills noted above ensures that the individual is able to function competently in social situations and develop meaningful social relationships with other individuals in his or her environment. Indeed, the development of psychosocial functioning has lasting effects for the individual, as competent social functioning and the development of social relationships in childhood has been shown to be predictive of better social, academic and occupational outcomes later in life.[2–5]

Several authors have suggested that children with chronic illness and physical disabilities often show increased rates of internalizing and externalizing disorders and lower self-esteem when compared with normative data and with typically developing children.[6,7] Despite such suggestions, examinations of psychosocial functioning in this population are somewhat rare;[1] that is, a clear clinical picture of psychosocial functioning in children with disabilities is lacking. The assessment of psychosocial functioning in children with disabilities has perhaps been overlooked because caregivers and clinicians involved with this population are often concerned with ensuring that the child is medically stable and placed in an appropriate educational environment. However, the importance of assessing psychosocial functioning in children with disabilities cannot be understated given that this population has been shown to be at risk for development of social and peer difficulties.[8] Assessment of psychosocial functioning in children must, therefore, be emphasized, as potential risk factors in this domain of functioning can be identified and remediated.

Psychosocial functioning encompasses a large range of functions. Many of the measures of this construct focus on psychological symptoms such as anxiety, depression and withdrawal, as well as functions such as leadership ability, social skills, self-esteem, sports participation and school functioning. Another area that has received a great deal of attention in recent years is quality of life. Quality of life can be defined as 'the combination of objectively and subjectively indicated well-being in multiple domains of life considered salient in one's culture and time, while adhering to universal standards of human rights.'[9] Quality of life can be assessed from the perspective of the disease/condition (i.e. health-related quality of life, often using disease-specific quality of life tools)[10] and in a more generic fashion. As noted by Wallander et al,[9] it is important to assess both types of quality of life in children with chronic conditions, as it is imperative to view this group as whole people and not just as children with a disability. An overview of quality of life measures is provided in Chapter 34.

Aside from quality of life, it is important to assess self-esteem. Children with disabilities may be unable to participate in the same activities as typically developing children, thereby preventing interactions with their social environment that normally contribute to the child's growth, development and self-esteem. School functioning is another important facet of psychosocial functioning that should be assessed in children with disabilities. Attending school provides the child with the opportunity to experience successes and failures, which assist the development of self-esteem and relationships with peers, as well as the ability to learn effective coping skills. School absences, then, could lead to decreased opportunities to interact with other children and establish relationships, and therefore the child may end up feeling neglected by the school community. Children with disabilities often miss school for extended periods of time and may therefore be at risk for school functioning difficulties. For this reason, it is essential to consider measures that capture psychosocial elements of school functioning when assessing psychosocial functioning more globally in this group.

General factors to consider when measuring this domain

Measurement of psychosocial functioning in children with disabilities is challenging for a number of reasons, one of the most salient being the lack of empirical research on evidence-based measures of psychosocial functioning in this population. Indeed, Holmbeck and colleagues[11] noted that there has traditionally been greater focus on evidence-based practice in the intervention literature, but less so in the assessment literature. Using evidence-based measures for assessment assures that we have reliable and valid tools with which to assess functioning.

A second issue with respect to measurement of psychosocial functioning is the traditional focus on

psychopathology when assessing the construct. Many measures of psychosocial functioning focus on psychopathology and *Diagnostic and Statistical Manual of Mental Disorders*, 4th edition (DSM-IV),[12] criteria; however, diagnosing psychological disorders is not necessarily the main focus of psychosocial assessment in children with disabilities. Rather, the main focus is to determine whether these children differ from typically developing children with respect to psychosocial functioning. It has been suggested that many of the scales or instruments, such as the Child Behavior Checklist (CBCL),[13] become overly inflated when used to assess psychosocial functioning in children with chronic illness or disability.[14] It should be noted, however, that these suggestions have not always been supported by research, as shown in a study examining behavioural difficulties in children with diabetes.[15]

There is debate as to whether psychosocial functioning should be assessed from a categorical (i.e. diagnosis-specific) or non-categorical (i.e. general) perspective.[6,7] Given that the psychosocial implications of many chronic conditions are very similar, it has been suggested that psychosocial functioning be assessed using a non-categorical approach.[16] Specifically, these authors suggest that chronic physical conditions can be placed on various common dimensions, with each dimension having a different impact on psychosocial functioning. According to Pless and Pinkerton,[16] dimensions include the nature of onset and course, the life-threat potential, the intrusiveness of pain treatment, visibility and social stigma, stability versus crises, and secondary functional and cognitive disability. Although this work is based on chronic conditions, it is probably appropriate to consider disability in the same manner; therefore, the following discussion of measurement will be based on the non-categorical approach to assessment. Finally, it is worth mentioning that it is difficult to assess psychosocial functioning in the context of the ICF, as many of the measures currently used to assess the construct are not designed with the ICF in mind (i.e. whereas most measures assess capability in psychosocial functioning, the ICF often emphasizes loss of or impairment in this area).

There is no preferred method of assessing psychosocial functioning in typically developing children or in children with chronic illness or disability.[1] Paper and pencil questionnaire measures are often administered to assess psychosocial functioning, with the CBCL[13] being the most widely used measure.[1] Depending on the disability or illness and the age of the child being assessed, parents and teachers are often the most commonly used informants; however, if at all possible, it is essential to include self-report measures of psychosocial functioning in order to gain perspective on the child's perceptions of his or her experiences and level of functioning. Indeed, research in the area of chronic illness[1,15,17,18] suggests that a multidimensional approach to assessment of psychosocial functioning is best, as different measures show varying degrees of sensitivity to psychosocial functioning and varied informants allow for assessment of functioning across settings. These findings can probably be applied to children with disabilities, as many disabilities share commonalities that allow for a non-categorical approach to assessment.

A recent review of evidence-based assessment of psychosocial functioning in paediatric populations provides an excellent resource for measures that can be used in paediatric populations with chronic illness.[11] As members of the Psychosocial Adjustment and Psychopathology Workgroup of Division 54 (Pediatric Psychology) of the American Psychological Association (APA), Holmbeck and colleagues[11] generated a list of 28 possible measures of psychosocial adjustment and psychopathology in children. This master list was then distributed to members of APA Division 54 and respondents were asked to identify measures they had used or would consider using in either research or clinical settings. Measures with the highest endorsement rates were chosen for inclusion in the final review and suggestions for additional measures were taken into consideration. Overall, Holmbeck and colleagues[11] identified a group of 37 measures of psychosocial adjustment and psychopathology suitable for use in paediatric populations, with 34 of these measures being classified as 'well established' according to evidence-based assessment criteria. When preparing the current review, we examined the measures suggested by Holmbeck and colleagues[11] in their comprehensive review and selected those that have the most potential to be useful when assessing psychosocial functioning in children with developmental disabilities. For a full list of measures identified by Holmbeck and colleagues,[11] we direct the reader to the comprehensive review article published in the *Journal of Pediatric Psychology*.[11]

Although primarily validated for use in typically developing populations and those with chronic illness, the majority of measures selected for inclusion in this chapter can be used in many different populations, including children with disabilities. The key issue with self-report measures, though, is whether or not the child will be able to provide a self-report. If the child has a physical disability that precludes him or her from providing a self-report, it may be possible to pose questions orally and have the clinician or researcher record the child's responses. However, if the child has a cognitive disability, it may be more difficult to obtain self-report ratings of psychosocial functioning. If the child is unable to respond using a self-report measure, then it is important

to obtain reports from as many sources as possible (e.g. parents, teachers, other caregivers). It is also important to note that some subscales on the measures identified in this chapter may be falsely inflated for children with chronic illness or disability, as some scales probe for symptoms of physical illness (e.g. Behavior Assessment System for Children, second edition (BASC-2), somatization subscale). Care should be taken when interpreting these scales in children with disabilities, especially if these children have comorbid medical conditions, as symptoms common to the illness or disability may be falsely interpreted as somatization. However, as noted above, some evidence suggests that, even when illness-related factors are accounted for, children with type I diabetes still show elevated behavioural profiles on the CBCL, suggesting that important information can be gleaned from such questionnaires despite the apparent confound of a physical disorder or chronic condition.[14]

Overview of recommended measures
Diagnostic interviews will not be discussed in this chapter as they are often used for the purpose of diagnosing psychopathology, which is not the purpose of assessing psychosocial functioning in children with disabilities.[11] If, in the course of assessing psychosocial functioning in a child with a disability, the examiner determines that a more thorough investigation of psychopathology is warranted, then he or she is encouraged to use a more structured diagnostic interview. The following measures were selected by consulting the Holmbeck et al[11] review and selecting those measures that, based on clinical experience, are most applicable for children with disabilities.

ADAPTIVE BEHAVIOR ASSESSMENT SYSTEM, SECOND EDITION

Description
The Adaptive Behavior Assessment System, second edition (ABAS-II), is a norm-referenced tool designed to assess global adaptive functioning across the lifespan (i.e. from birth to age 89y). It is possible to calculate scores across three domains of functioning: conceptual, social and practical. These domain scores can be useful for diagnosing mental retardation[a] according to current diagnostic criteria from the DSM-IV and the American Association on Mental Retardation. The ABAS-II is currently the only measure that assesses all 10 adaptive behaviour skills listed in the DSM-IV diagnostic criteria for learning disabilities. With respect to psychosocial functioning, probably the most helpful scale on the ABAS-II is the social

---

[a]UK usage: learning disability.

scale, although use of this measure provides a good estimate of functioning in many areas. Despite the fact that the ABAS is often used as a diagnostic tool for learning disabilities, it has good clinical utility in other populations with chronic illness/disabilities as it provides information about the child's current level of functioning across several domains, meaning that treatment can be targeted to specific areas if needed.

ADAPTIVE BEHAVIOR ASSESSMENT SYSTEM, SECOND EDITION (ABAS-II)	
Purpose	To evaluate adaptive skills and activities of daily living. May also be used as part of a diagnosis of learning disability
	Provides a complete assessment of adaptive skills, with social domain most relevant to psychosocial functioning
	Provides an indication of severity of impairment in multiple areas of functioning
	Incorporates the American Association on Mental Retardation (AAMR) guidelines by providing norms in conceptual, social and practical domains of functioning
	Can be used with other populations (e.g. attention-deficit–hyperactivity disorder, learning disabilities, other speech, hearing, neurological disorders)
Population	Children and adults from birth to age 89y
Description of domains (subscales)	Three domains: conceptual, social, practical
	Nine subscales: communication, functional academics, self-direction, leisure, social, community use, home living, health and safety, self-care, work (if appropriate)
Administration and test format	Time to complete: 15–20min to administer
	Testing format: parent report form (age 0–5y or age 5–21y); teacher report form (age 0–5y or 5–21y); adult form (age 16–89y)
	Scoring: uses between 193 and 241 items to calculate General Adaptive Composite (GAC) four-point Likert scale ('is not able' to 'always when needed'): is not able (0), never when needed (1), sometimes when needed (2), always when needed (3)
	Training: level B (assessor is required to have Master's-level training in psychology, education or a related field with specific training in assessment)
Psychometric properties	Normative sample: >3200 individuals spanning 31 age groups – stratified by sex, race/ethnicity and level of education; sample also included individuals in 20 clinical groups including autism, attention-deficit–hyperactivity disorder and visual impairment
	Reliability Average internal consistency coefficient for standardization sample's GAC ranges from 0.97 to 0.99; moderate correlations among skill levels (0.40–0.70s) – suggests related but independent skills; test–retest reliability correlations for the GAC near or above 0.90
	Validity Theory and constructs from AAMR and DSM-IV used to provide framework for ABAS-II content; factor analytical support for GAC and individual scales; construct validity supported by intercorrelational data among skill areas, domains and GAC ranges from moderate to high; concurrent validity with Vineland Adaptive Behaviour Scale (0.70–0.84) Behavioural Assessment System for Children (0.80); correlations in the 0.40–0.50s range with various measures of intelligence (WPPSI-III, WAIS-III, WISC-IV); differentiates between children with and without disabilities (construct validity)
How to order	Online ordering through Pearson Assessment. Cost depends on type of kit ordered. The complete kit with scoring software costs US$365
Key references	Harrison PL, Oakland T (2003) *Adaptive Behavior Assessment System*, 2nd edition. San Antonio, TX: Harcourt Assessment.
	Rust JO, Wallace MA (2004) Book review: Adaptive Behavior Assessment System, 2nd edition. *J Psychoedu Assess* 22: 367–373.

BEHAVIOUR ASSESSMENT SYSTEM FOR CHILDREN, SECOND EDITION

Description

The BASC-2 provides the clinician or researcher with a multi-informant, integrated assessment of the child or adolescent's functioning across a wide range of psychosocial functioning. The BASC-2 can be completed by parents and teachers or as a self-report (for children and adolescents over age 8y). Additionally, the BASC-2 can be used for behavioural observation using the Student Observation System. Items on the parent and teacher forms yield scores for four composite indices (externalizing problems, internalizing problems, behavioural symptoms and adaptive skills); the teacher report also consists of a 'school problems' composite index. Items on the self-report form also yield composite scores across four domains (school problems, internalizing problems, emotional symptoms and personal adjustment). The BASC-2 is a broad-based measure of behaviour; however, the composite scores provide the clinician with important information with respect to psychosocial functioning. Of particular relevance to clinicians and researchers who are interested in psychosocial functioning are the internalizing problems, emotional symptoms and personal adjustment indices. Although based on a normative sample, the BASC-2 has clinical utility in children with disabilities and chronic illness and is widely used when assessing and treating this population.[19,20] With this in mind, care should be taken when interpreting scores on scales and composites for two reasons. First, children with disabilities may indicate more physical complaints, thereby obtaining clinically significant scores on the Somatization subscale.[20] The clinician should use clinical judgement to determine whether these physical complaints are significantly increased in relation to the child's disability. Second, the BASC-2 is focused on identifying DSM-IV disorders; therefore, children with disabilities may not reach clinical significance on any of the subscales or composites; however, the clinician should again use clinical judgement to determine whether the child shows increased rates of symptomatology in relation to his or her disability.

CHILD BEHAVIOR CHECKLIST

Description

The CBCL is the most commonly used broad-based measure of psychological and behavioural functioning in children.[1] The CBCL is completed by the parent (or other primary caregiver) and, as with the BASC-2, this measure provides the clinician or researcher with an assessment of the child or adolescent's functioning across a wide range

of behavioural and adaptive functioning domains. Items on the CBCL yield scores on eight scales of co-occurring difficulties: anxious/depressed, withdrawn/depressed, somatic complaints, rule-breaking behaviour, aggressive behaviour, social problems, thought problems and attention problems. Along with the parent questionnaire, there are teacher (teacher report form; TRF) and self-report (youth self-report; YSR) versions of the CBCL, allowing for a multi-informant, integrated approach. Again, as discussed above, when using this measure with children with disabilities, the clinician or researcher should use clinical judgement when determining whether the child exhibits elevated symptoms relative to what would be expected given the disability.

CHILDREN'S GLOBAL ASSESSMENT SCALE

Description

The Children's Global Assessment Scale (CGAS) is a modified version of the Global Assessment Scale and is a clinician-rated measure of social and psychological functioning in children aged 4–16 years. This is a global scale on which the child's functioning is rated on a scale from 1 (most functionally impaired) to 100 (healthiest), with any score above 70 indicating typical functioning. This type of scale is a useful way for the clinician to synthesize knowledge about the individual's specific social and psychological functioning and integrate this information into a single, clinically meaningful index of overall functioning. The authors also note that global ratings of functioning may be more sensitive to treatment than single ratings of psychological symptomatology. The CGAS may be especially helpful when assessing children with disabilities, as it provides the rater with guidelines with which to score functioning, allowing for a good general picture of psychosocial functioning.

FUNCTIONAL EMOTIONAL ASSESSMENT SCALE

Description

The Functional Emotional Assessment Scale (FEAS) is an observational play-based assessment tool designed to measure the very young child's social and emotional competence in the context of the relationship with the caregiver. In addition, the tool measures the caregiver's ability to support the child's development. The FEAS is not intended for use as a formal diagnostic tool, rather the purpose is to allow the clinician to screen areas of social and emotional development that may need further inquiry. The FEAS can also be used descriptively to profile the child's development across social, emotional and related developmental domains. An additional

BEHAVIOUR ASSESSMENT SYSTEM FOR CHILDREN, SECOND EDITION (BASC-2)	
Purpose	To evaluate behaviour and self-perceptions of children and young adults
	Multimethod: parent, teacher, self-report, scales; structured developmental history form; observed classroom behaviour form
	Multidimensional: assesses multiple aspects of behaviour and personality, including positive (i.e. adaptive) and negative (i.e. clinical) dimensions
	Can be used for clinical diagnosis, educational classification, manifestation determination, programme evaluation, forensic evaluation and research
	Can be used with individuals with sensory impairments
Population	Children and adults aged 2–25y
Description of domains (subscales)	Parent form: four composites (externalizing problems, internalizing problems, behavioural symptoms index, adaptive skills); 14 scales (hyperactivity, aggression, conduct problems, anxiety, depression, somatization, attention problems, atypicality, withdrawal, adaptability, social skills, leadership, activities of daily living, functional communication)
	Teacher form: five composites (externalizing problems, internalizing problems, school problems, behavioural symptoms index, adaptive skills); 15 scales (hyperactivity, aggression, conduct problems, anxiety, depression, somatization, attention problems, learning problems, atypicality, withdrawal, adaptability, social skills, leadership, study skills, functional communication)
	Self-report form: four composites (school problems, internalizing problems, inattention/hyperactivity, personal adjustment); 14 scales (attitude to school, attitude to teachers, atypicality, locus of control, social stress, anxiety, depression, sense of inadequacy, attention problems, hyperactivity, relations with parents, interpersonal relations, self-esteem, self-reliance)
Administration and test format	Time to complete: 15–30min to administer (depending on type of form)
	Testing format: parent report form (ages 2–5, 6–11 or 12–21y); teacher report form (ages 2–5, 6–11 or 12–21y); self-report form (ages 8–11 or 12–21y); observed classroom behaviour form; structured developmental history form
	Scoring: between 100 and 176 items (depending on form); four-point Likert scale (0, never; 1, sometimes; 2, often; 3, always)
	Training: level C
Psychometric properties	Normative sample: >13 000 between the ages of 2 and 18y; overall sample came from over 375 sites in 257 cities and 40 states; equal numbers of males and females in each age group
	Reliability Teacher form: average internal consistency coefficient for standardization sample ranges from high 0.80s (internalizing problems) to high 0.90s (adaptive skills)
	Teacher form: test–retest reliability correlations for composite scales in mid-0.80s to low 0.90s
	Parent form: reliabilities slightly lower than teacher form; median values range from 0.80 to 0.87; scales with highest reliability: hyperactivity, attention problems, social skills and functional communication
	Parent form: test–retest reliability correlations for composite scales range from low 0.80s to low 0.90s, except for internalizing problems (0.78)
	Validity Factor analytical support for BASC-2 composites and scales. Moderate to high concurrent validity with Achenbach System of Empirically Based Assessment (ASEBA) CBCL (0.64–0.85). Moderate to high concurrent validity with Conners' scales (0.26–0.85). Moderate to high concurrent validity with Behaviour Rating Inventory of Executive Functioning (BRIEF; parent form) (0.58–0.86)

How to order	Online ordering through Pearson Assessment. Cost depends on type of kit ordered. The complete starter kit with scoring software costs US$628.50
Key references	Reynolds CR, Kamphaus RW (2004) *Behaviour Assessment System for Children*, 2nd edition. San Antonio, TX: NCS Pearson, Inc.
	Rescorla LA (2009) Rating scale systems for assessing psychopathology: The Achenbach System of Empirically Based Assessment (ASEBA) and the Behaviour Assessment System for Children-2 (BASC-2). In: Matson JL, Andrasik F, Matson ML, editors. *Assessing Childhood Psychopathology and Developmental Disabilities*. New York: Springer.
	Holmbeck GN, Thill AW, Bachanas P, et al (2007) Evidence-based practice in paediatric psychology: measures of psychosocial adjustment and psychopathology. *J Paediatr Psychol* 33: 958–980.

ACHENBACH SYSTEM OF EMPIRICALLY BASED ASSESSMENT (ASEBA) – CHILD BEHAVIOR CHECKLIST (CBL), TEACHER REPORT FORM (TRF), YOUTH SELF-REPORT (YSR)

Purpose	Measure of competences, adaptive functioning, and behavioural, emotional and social problems
	Utilizes quantitative scores and individualized descriptors (i.e. respondents can include narrative descriptions of the child)
	Includes scales evaluating DSM-IV diagnostic categories
Population	Children and adults aged 1.5–90+y
Description of domains (subscales)	School-age form (parent, TFR, YSR): competence and adaptive (activities, social, school); empirically based (anxious/depressed, withdrawn/depressed, somatic complaints, social problems, thought problems, attention problems, rule-breaking behaviour, aggressive behaviour); DSM-orientated (affective problems, anxiety problems, somatic problems, attention-deficit–hyperactivity disorder, oppositional defiant problems, conduct problems)
Administration and test format	Time to complete: 15–30min to administer (depending on type of form)
	Testing format: CBCL (ages 1.5–5 and 6–18y); TRF (ages 1.5–5 and 6–18y); YSR (ages 11–18y)
	Scoring: 113 items; three-point Likert scale [not true (0), somewhat or sometimes true (1), very true or often true (2)]; seven additional items assessing social and academic involvement; five open-ended questions assessing disabilities, additional concerns, descriptions
	Training: graduate training – at least a Master's degree
Psychometric properties	Normative sample: CBCL (6–18y): 3600 children between the ages of 6 and 18y; standardization sample came from 100 sites in 40 states; included children from several ethnic backgrounds and socioeconomic groups; clinical and non-clinical populations; sex-specific norms
	Reliability (for school-age forms)
	CBCL: test–retest reliability coefficients ranged from 0.63 to 0.97; cross-informant agreement coefficients ranged from 0.69 to 0.76
	TRF: test–retest reliability coefficients ranged from 0.55 to 0.95; cross-informant agreement coefficients ranged from 0.49 to 0.60
	YSR: test–retest reliability coefficients ranged from 0.72 to 0.97
	Validity
	Factor analytical support for ASEBA forms; moderate to high concurrent validity with BASC-2 (0.64–0.85); differentiates between referred and non-referred samples

How to order	Online ordering through ASEBA (www.aseba.org). Cost depends on type of kit ordered. CBCL 6–18 module costs US$295
Key references	Achenbach TM, Edelbrock CS (1983) *Manual for the Child Behavior Checklist and Revised Child Behaviour Profile*. Burlington, VT: University Associates in Psychiatry.
	Holmbeck GN, Thill AW, Bachanas P, et al (2008) Evidence-based practice in pediatric psychology: measures of psychosocial adjustment and psychopathology. *J Pediatr Psychol* 33: 958–980.
	Rescorla LA (2009) Rating scale systems for assessing psychopathology: the Achenbach System of Empirically Based Assessment (ASEBA) and the Behaviour Assessment System for Children-2 (BASC-2). In Matson JL, Andrasik F, Matson ML, editors. *Assessing Childhood Psychopathology and Developmental Disabilities*. New York: Springer.

CHILDREN'S GLOBAL ASSESSMENT SCALE (CGAS)

Purpose	Unidimensional global measure of disturbance and adequacy of social functioning
	Allows clinician to synthesize knowledge of many aspects of the individual's functioning into a single, clinically meaningful index of severity
Population	Children aged 4–16y
Description of domains (subscales)	Rater is asked to consider the individual's lowest level of functioning over the past month and is given the following guidelines:
	100–91: doing very well
	90–81: doing well
	80–71: doing all right – minor impairment
	70–61: some problems – in one area only
	60–51: some noticeable problems – in more than one area
	50–41: obvious problems – moderate impairment in most areas or severe in one area
	40–31: serious problems – major impairment in several areas and unable to function in one area
	30–21: severe problems – unable to function in almost all situations
	20–11: very severely impaired – considerable supervision is required for safety
	10–1: extremely impaired – constant supervision is required for safety
Administration and test format	Time to complete: the actual rating takes very little time; however, the clinician will probably spend a significant amount of time interviewing the individual and gathering collateral information on which to base the CGAS rating
	Training: graduate/medical training in interviewing
Psychometric properties	Normative sample: 19 case histories evaluated by second-year child psychiatry fellows to determine reliability and validity
	Reliability High inter-rater reliability (0.84); high test–retest reliability (0.85)
	Validity Discriminant validity: differentiates between inpatients and outpatients with respect to level of severity
	Concurrent validity: moderate correlation with Conners' Abbreviated Parent Index (−0.25)
How to order	Available online and from author

Key references	Shaffer D, Gould MS, Brasic J, et al (1983) A children's global assessment scale. *Arch Gen Psychiatry* 40: 1228–1231.
	Holmbeck GN, Thill AW, Bachanas P, et al (2008) Evidence-based practice in pediatric psychology: measures of psychosocial adjustment and psychopathology. *J Pediatr Psychol* 33: 958–980.

FUNCTIONAL EMOTIONAL ASSESSMENT SCALE (FEAS)

Purpose	To evaluate emotional functioning in children with constitutional- and maturation-based difficulties (i.e. regulatory disorders), children with interactional difficulties and children with pervasive developmental disorders
	Systematic assessment of the child and caregiver's functional emotional capacities
	Observational (play-based)
	Intended for use in infants and young children
	Distinguishes between children with high-risk profiles of emotional functioning and those without
Population	Infants and children 7mo–4y
Description of domains (subscales)	The infant or child is assessed on six levels of social and emotional development: regulation and interest in the world, forming relationships (attachment), intentional two-way communications, development of a complex sense of self, representational capacity and elaboration of symbolic thinking, emotional thinking or development, and expression of thematic play
Administration and test format	Time to complete: 15–20min to administer
	Testing format: observational/play-based: caregiver asked to interact with child and then examiner facilitates interaction to elicit behaviours not observed previously
	Scoring: scored on a three-point Likert scale for most items (0, not at all or very brief; 1, present some of the time/observed several times; 2, consistently present). Ratings can be summed to obtain category and subtest scores for caregiver and child, as well as combined total scores for caregiver and child
	Training: training required (watching at least 10 videotapes and achieving 80% reliability is recommended)
Psychometric properties	Normative sample: four non-nationally representative samples of children between 7mo and 48mo used to validate the FEAS: (1) 197 typically developing children; (2) 190 children with regulatory disorder; (3) 41 children with pervasive developmental disorder (aged 19–48mo); (4) 40 children with multiple difficulties
	Reliability Inter-rater reliability (Cronbach's alpha) ranges from 0.90 to 0.92 for caregiver scale and from 0.90 to 0.98 for the child scale
	Validity Very few data on construct or concurrent validity; scores obtained by typically developing and clinical samples compared using discrimination analysis, *t*-tests and analysis of variance – the authors consider this information to reflect construct validity; intercorrelations between FEAS scores and two other measures developed by the authors were not significant – authors interpret this finding to mean that the FEAS provides unique information

How to order	Online ordering through the Interdisciplinary Council on Developmental and Learning Disorders (www.icdl.com). Test book: US$40 for ICDL members/US$47 for non-members. Additional protocol booklets: US$8
Key references	Greenspan SI, DeGangi GA, Wieder S (2001) *The Functional Emotional Assessment Scale (FEAS) for Infancy and Early Childhood: Clinical and Research Applications*. Bethesda: Interdisciplinary Council on Developmental and Learning Disorders.

benefit of the FEAS is that it was specifically designed to detect difficulties across a range of disorders, such as regulatory disorders and pervasive developmental disorders.

PEDIATRIC QUALITY OF LIFE INVENTORY

Description
The Pediatric Quality of Life Inventory (PedsQL) is a generic, standardized instrument designed to assess parent and child perceptions of health-related quality of life in paediatric populations. This measure has been used to assess health-related quality of life in individuals with disabilities and has been shown to be an effective measure of quality of life in this population.[21] Several of the subscales capture psychosocial functioning of the child and therefore this measure is included in this chapter. The PedsQL consists of three core scales: physical functioning (i.e. functional status in activities of daily living), psychological functioning (i.e. emotional distress) and social functioning (i.e. interpersonal functioning/ peer relations). In addition to the three core scales, the PedsQL consists of eight other modules assessing specific symptoms and health-related concerns: pain, nausea, procedural anxiety, treatment anxiety, worry, cognitive problems, perceived physical appearance and physician/ nurse communication.

SELF-PERCEPTION PROFILE FOR ADOLESCENTS

Description
The Self-perception Profile for Adolescents (SPPA) is a self-report measure that assesses self-concept from a multidimensional perspective in young people aged 13–20 years. The 45 items on this measure load on to five subscales: scholastic competence, social acceptance, athletic competence, physical appearance and behavioural conduct. Also included is a global self-worth scale. This measure may be particularly useful in adolescents with disabilities, as it assesses many areas of functioning that contribute to psychosocial adjustment (i.e. school functioning, athletic competence, self-worth).

SELF-PERCEPTION PROFILE FOR CHILDREN

Description
The Self-perception Profile for Children (SPPC) is a 36-item self-report measure designed to assess self-concept in children aged 8 to 15 years. Items on this measure load onto five subscales: scholastic competence, social acceptance, athletic competence, physical appearance and behavioural conduct. Like the SPPA, the SPPC includes a global self-worth scale. As noted above, this measure may be particularly useful in adolescents with disabilities, as it assesses many areas of functioning that contribute to psychosocial adjustment (i.e. school functioning, athletic competence, self-worth).

SOCIAL SKILLS RATING SYSTEM

Description
The Social Skills Rating System (SSRS) has been described in the literature as a comprehensive instrument with a multisource approach that can be linked to interventions. This measure can be used with preschool, elementary school and secondary school children and consists of self-report, parent and teacher forms. Items on the SSRS load onto three primary scales: social skills, problem behaviours and academic competence. Three subscales make up all versions of the SSRS: co-operation, assertion and self-control. Additionally, the parent version includes a responsibility subscale, whereas the self-report version includes an empathy subscale.

SOCIAL ADJUSTMENT INVENTORY FOR CHILDREN AND ADOLESCENTS

Description
The Social Adjustment Inventory for Children and Adolescents (SAICA) is a semi-structured interview that can be administered to either the child or the child's parent(s) to assess social and psychological functioning. This measure has been included because, although it is designed to be completed in an interview setting, it specifically targets social functioning; this measure can also

PEDIATRIC QUALITY OF LIFE INVENTORY (PEDSQL)

Purpose	Brief, standardized assessment instrument designed to measure parents' and patients' perceptions of health-related quality of life in paediatric populations with chronic illness. Designed to measure the core dimensions of health, as defined by the World Health Organization, along with school functioning
Population	Children aged 2–18y
Description of domains (subscales)	Four multidimensional scales: physical functioning, emotional functioning, social functioning, school functioning
	Eight modules: pain, nausea, procedural anxiety, treatment anxiety, worry, cognitive problems, perceived physical appearance, physician/nurse communication
	Three summary scores: total scale score, physical health summary score, psychosocial health summary score
Administration and test format	Time to complete: <4min
	Testing format: child self-report form (ages 8–12y), adolescent self-report form (ages 13–18y), parent proxy forms (child and adolescent)
	Scoring: 45 items; responses on a four-point Likert scale (0, never a problem; 1, sometimes a problem; 2, often a problem; 3, always a problem)
	Training: training in administration of standardized questionnaires (i.e. graduate training)
Psychometric properties	Normative sample: 291 English-speaking individuals with cancer (aged 8–18y) and their parents; measure has also been validated for use in several other paediatric populations
	Reliability
	Child report: good internal consistency – alphas range from 0.67 to 0.83; parent proxy report: good internal consistency – alphas range from 0.59 to 0.89
	Validity
	Factor analytic support for the scales; discriminant validity – differentiates between healthy children and children with acute or chronic health conditions; distinguishes disease severity within a chronic health condition; concurrent validity – correlated with other standardized measures of psychosocial functioning (CDI, State-Trait Anxiety Inventory for Children, Social Support Scale for Children, Self-perception Profile for Children, Self-perception Profile for Adolescents, CBCL)
How to order	Available online at www.pedsql.org and from author
Key references	Holmbeck GN, Thill AW, Bachanas P, et al (2008) Evidence-based practice in paediatric psychology: measures of psychosocial adjustment and psychopathology. *J Paediatr Psychol* 33: 958–980.
	Varni JW, Seid M, Rode CA (1999) The PedsQL: measurement model for the paediatric quality of life inventory. *Med Care* 37: 126–139.

SELF-PERCEPTION PROFILE FOR ADOLESCENTS (SPPA)

Purpose	Adaptation of the Self-perception Profile for Children. Assesses the adolescent's domain-specific perceptions of competence, as well as global perception of worth/esteem as a person – domains designed to be more specific to adolescents
Population	Adolescents aged 13–20y

Description of domains (subscales)	Eight specific domains: scholastic competence, social acceptance, athletic competence, physical appearance, job competence, close friendship, romantic appeal and behavioural conduct Global self-worth subscale
Administration and test format	Time to complete: 20–30min depending on age of adolescent Testing format: questionnaire Scoring: 45 items; responses on a four-point Likert scale, from low perceived competence (1) to high perceived competence (4); adolescents asked to choose between two choices and indicate whether their choice is 'really true for me' or 'sort of true for me' (reduces social desirability bias) Training: training in administration of standardized questionnaires (i.e. graduate training)
Psychometric properties	Normative sample: 1543 Colorado school children – predominantly middle class and 90% white. Measure has since been normed in other, more diverse, samples of children *Reliability* No data on test–retest reliability; moderate internal consistency – coefficients range from 0.74 to 0.92 *Validity* Mixed findings for factor structure; no data provided for construct validity in original manual
How to order	Available from author: Dr S Harter, Department of Psychology, University of Denver, Denver, CO, USA
Key references	Harter S (1988) *Manual for the Self Perception Scale for Children. Revision of the Perceived Competence Scale for Children.* University of Denver: unpublished manuscript. Holmbeck GN, Thill AW, Bachanas P, et al (2008) Evidence-based practice in pediatric psychology: measures of psychosocial adjustment and psychopathology. *J Pediatr Psychol* 33: 958–980. Wichstrom L (1995) Harter's self perception profile for adolescents: reliability, validity, and evaluation of the question format. *J Personality Assess* 65: 100–116.

SELF-PERCEPTION PROFILE FOR CHILDREN (SPPC)

Purpose	Assesses the child's domain-specific perceptions of competence, as well as global perception of worth/esteem as a person
Population	Children aged 8–15y
Description of domains (subscales)	Five specific domains: scholastic competence, social acceptance, athletic competence, physical appearance and behavioural conduct Global self-worth subscale
Administration and test format	Time to complete: 20–30min depending on age of child Testing format: questionnaire Scoring: 36 items; responses on four-point Likert scale – low perceived competence (1) to high perceived competence (4); children asked to choose between two choices and indicate whether their choice is 'really true for me' or 'sort of true for me' (reduces social desirability bias) Training: training in administration of standardized questionnaires (i.e. graduate training)

Psychometric properties	Normative sample: 1543 Colorado school children – predominantly middle class and 90% white. Measure has since been normed in other, more diverse, samples of children *Reliability* No data on test–retest reliability; moderate internal consistency – coefficients range from 0.71 to 0.86 *Validity* Factor analytic support for the scales; no data provided for criterion validity
How to order	Available from author: Dr S Harter, Department of Psychology, University of Denver, Denver, CO, USA
Key references	Harter S (1985) *Manual for the Self Perception Scale for Children. Revision of the Perceived Competence Scale for Children*. University of Denver: unpublished manuscript. Holmbeck GN, Thill AW, Bachanas P, et al (2008) Evidence-based practice in pediatric psychology: measures of psychosocial adjustment and psychopathology. *J Pediatr Psychol* 33: 958–980. Naar-King S, Ellis DA, Frey MA (2004) *Assessing Children's Well-being: A Handbook of Measures*. Mahwah, NJ: Erlbaum.

Social Skills Rating System (SSRS)

Purpose	To obtain a complete picture of social behaviours based on parent, teacher and student ratings. Allows for evaluation of a wide range of behaviours that affect relationships, peer acceptance and academic performance. Can be useful in intervention planning
Population	Children and adolescents aged 3–18y
Description of domains (subscales)	Three scales: social skills (co-operation, empathy, assertion, self-control, responsibility), problem behaviours (externalizing, internalizing, hyperactivity), academic competence (teachers rate academic performance in the areas of reading, maths, general cognitive functioning and parental support)
Administration and test format	Time to complete: 10–25min, depending on the rater Testing format: questionnaire Scoring: 34–57 items, depending on form used; responses on three-point Likert scale (0, never; 1, sometimes; 2, very often) Training: level B
Psychometric properties	Normative sample: 4170 American children (self-rated); 1027 parents; 259 teachers; samples consisted of children from a wide range of educational classifications (i.e. 'learning disabled', 'behaviour disordered' and 'mentally handicapped') *Reliability* Good internal consistency – coefficients ranged from 0.84 to 0.95 for scales; adequate test–retest reliability – coefficients ranged from 0.65 to 0.93 *Validity* Adequate construct/convergent validity – SSRS validated against several other tools (e.g. Social Behaviour Assessment, CBCL-TRF, CBCL, CBCL-YSR) – coefficients ranged from 0.20s to 0.70s, suggesting that the tool is measuring a valid construct
How to order	Online ordering through Pearson Assessment. Cost depends on type of kit ordered. Elementary starter kit with scoring software costs US$386. Secondary starter kit with scoring software costs US$365

Key references	Diperna JC, Volpe RJ (2005) Self-report on the Social Skills Rating System: analysis of reliability for an elementary sample. *Psychol Schools* 42: 345–354.
	Gresham FM, Elliot SN (1990) *Social Skills Rating System Manual*. Circle Pines, MN: American Guidance Service.

SOCIAL ADJUSTMENT INVENTORY FOR CHILDREN AND ADOLESCENTS (SAICA)

Purpose	Semi-structured interview designed to assess social functioning in clinical and epidemiological settings
Population	Children and adolescents aged 6–18y
Description of domains (subscales)	Functioning is assessed in four areas: school functioning, spare-time activities, peer relationships and home adjustment
Administration and test format	Time to complete: approximately 30min Testing format: semi-structured interview Scoring: 77 items (35 competence items, 42 problem behaviour items); responses on four-point Likert scale Competence items: very competent(1) to not at all competent(4) Problem behaviour items: not at all a problem(1) to severe problem(4) Training: Master's, PhD or MD training with knowledge of child development
Psychometric properties	Normative sample: 124 children aged 6–18y of 38 depressed and 28 comparison parents *Reliability* High internal consistency for subscale scores within a given role area – coefficients range from 0.11 to 1.00; adequate inter-rater reliability – coefficients range from 0.14 to 0.84; test–retest reliability not reported *Validity* Factor analytic support for scales Convergent validity with IQ scores – coefficients range from –0.11 to 0.41 Convergent validity with CBCL – coefficients range from –0.71 to –0.02 (negative correlations result from opposite scoring of SAICA and CBCL) Differentiates between those with a history of psychiatric disorders and those without
How to order	Available from: Myrna Weissman, Columbia University, New York State Psychiatric Institute, New York, USA
Key references	Holmbeck GN, Thill AW, Bachanas P, et al. (2007) Evidence-based practice in pediatric psychology: measures of psychosocial adjustment and psychopathology. *J Pediatr Psychol* 33: 958–980. John K, Gammon G, Prusoff B, Warner V (1987) The Social Adjustment Scale for Children and Adolescents (SAICA): testing of a new semi-structured interview. *J Am Acad Child Adolesc Psychiatry* 26: 898–911.

be used in both clinical and epidemiological settings. The SAICA can be an important supplement in diagnostic assessments. Four areas are assessed: school functioning, spare-time activities, peer relationships and home adjustment.

Conclusion

This review, coupled with the comprehensive review conducted by Holmbeck and colleagues,[11] identifies several measures that may provide insight into dimensions of psychosocial functioning of children with physical and/

or cognitive disabilities. It should be noted, however, that the measures outlined above, while useful, have not been adequately tested and validated in populations with chronic illness/disability. Therefore, it is evident that more research on evidence-based assessment must be conducted to establish a set of universally accepted psychosocial measures for use with children presenting with a unique set of challenges. By establishing a set of standards for assessment, it will be possible to ensure the best possible outcomes for children with disabilities and their families.

REFERENCES

1. Wallander JL, Thompson RJ, Alriksson-Schmidt A (2003) Psychosocial adjustment of children with chronic physical conditions. In: Roberts MC, editor. *Handbook of Pediatric Psychology*, 3rd edition. New York: Guilford Press, pp. 141–158.

2. Crick NR, Dodge KA (1994) A review and reformulation of social information-processing mechanisms in children's social adjustment. *Psychol Bull* 115: 74–101.

3. Dodge KA, Murphy RR, Buchsbaum K (1984) The assessment of intention-cue detection skills in children: implications for developmental psychopathology. *Child Dev* 55: 163–173.

4. Dodge KA, Pettit GS, McClaskey CL, Brown MM (1986) Social competence in children. *Monographs Soc Res Child Dev* 51: 1–85.

5. Woodward LJ, Fergusson DM (2000) Childhood peer relationship problems and later risks of educational under-achievement and unemployment. *J Child Psychol Psychiatry* 41: 191–201.

6. Holmbeck GN, Westhoven VC, Shapera Phillips W, et al (2003) A multimethod, multi-informant, and multidimensional perspective on psychosocial adjustment in preadolescents with spina bifida. *J Consulting Clin Psychol* 71: 782–796.

7. Lavigne JV, Faier-Routman J (1992) Psychological adjustment to pediatric physical disorders: a metaanalytic review. *J Pediatr Psychol* 17: 133–157.

8. Cadman DT, Boyle M, Szatmari P, Offord DR (1987) Chronic illness, disability, and mental and social well-being: findings of the Ontario Child Health Study. *Pediatrics* 79: 805–813.

9. Wallander JL (2001) Theoretical and developmental issues in quality of life for children and adolescents. In: Koot HM, Wallander JL, editors. *Quality of Life in Child and Adolescent Illness: Concepts, Methods, and Findings*. Hove, East Sussex: Brunner-Routledge, pp. 23–48.

10. Varni JW, Seid M, Rode CA (1999) The PedsQL: Measurement model for the pediatric quality of life inventory. *Med Care* 37: 126–139.

11. Holmbeck GN, Thill AW, Bachanas P, et al (2007) Evidence-based practice in pediatric psychology: measures of psychosocial adjustment and psychopathology. *J Pediatr Psychol* 33: 958–980.

12. American Psychiatric Association (2000) *Diagnostic and Statisical Manual of Mental Disordes* (4th edn). Washington, DC: American Psychiatric Association.

13. Achenbach TM (2002) *Manual for the ASEBA School-Age Forms and Profiles*. Burlington, VT: Research Centre for Children, Youth, and Families.

14. Perrin EC, Stein REK, Drotar D (1991) Cautions in using the child behavior checklist: observations based on research about children with a chronic illness. *J Pediatr Psychol* 16: 411–421.

15. Holmes CS, Respess D, Greer T, Frentz J (1998) Behavior problems in children with diabetes: Disentangling possible scoring confounds on the child behavior checklist. *J Pediatr Psychol* 23: 179–185.

16. Pless IB, Pinkerton P (1975) *Chronic Childhood Disorder: Promoting Patterns of Adjustment*. Chicago: Year Book Medical Publishers.

17. Radcliffe J, Bennett D, Kazak A, Foley B, Phillips PC (1996) Adjustment in childhood brain tumor survival: child, mother, and teacher report. *J Pediatr Psychol* 21: 529–539.

18. Klinnert MD, McQuaid EL, McCormick D, Adinoff AD, Bryant NE (2000) A multimethod assessment of behavioral and emotional adjustment in children with asthma. *J Pediatr Psychol* 25: 35–46.

19. Robins PM, Schoff KM, Glutting JJ, Abelkop AS (2003) Discriminative validity of the behavior assessment system for children-parent rating scales in children with recurrent abdominal pain and matched controls. *Psychol Schools* 40: 145–154.

20. Titus JB, Kanive R, Sanders SJ, Blackburn LB (2008) Behavioural profiles of children with epilepsy: parent and teacher reports of emotional, behavioural, and educational concerns on the BASC-2. *Psychol Schools* 45: 893–904.

21. Varni JW, Burwinkle TM, Sherman SA, et al (2005) Health-related quality of life of children and adolescents with cerebral palsy: hearing the voices of the children. *Dev Med Child Neurol* 47: 592–597.

8
GLOBAL MENTAL FUNCTIONS: TEMPERAMENT AND PERSONALITY (B126)

Suzanne Woods-Groves and Dennis C. Harper

What is the construct?

Temperament and *personality* are included under mental functions and global mental functions and are described as 'general mental functions of constitutional disposition of the individual to react in a particular way to situations, including the set of mental characteristics that makes the individual distinct from others'.[1] As further noted in the International Classification of Functioning, Disability and Health (ICF) text on classification, the codes on temperament and personality functions can be related to codes on expression and intrapersonal functions (b12s). Either or both dimensions may be used. The specific properties of these codes and their relationship await development according to the authors. These descriptions (codes) in temperament and personality include extraversion, introversion, agreeableness, conscientiousness, psychic and emotional stability, openness to experience, optimism, novelty, confidence and trustworthiness. Exclusions are noted as intellectual functions, energy and drive functions, psychomotor functions and emotional functions. As is evident from this foregoing information, this construct of temperament and personality is very broad, quite descriptive and not currently well defined or related to the other existing codes and strategies within the ICF system.

A contemporary definition of temperament and personality from the existing literature reveals a long, detailed and very comprehensive measurement history. Temperament is noted by Allport[2] to be 'the characteristic phenomena of an individual's emotional nature including his susceptibilities to emotional stimulation, his customary strength and speedy response, the quality of his prevailing mood, these phenomena's being regarded as dependent upon constitutional make up' (p.34). Although more contemporary definitions exist, they are fundamentally the same and emphasize biological/hereditary or constitutional factors as underlying and enduring. Personality is defined by Allport[3] as 'the dynamic organization within

the individual of those psychophysical systems that determine his unique adjustment to his environment' (p.4). Contemporary emphasis focuses on taxometric definition of traits.[4] Both of these historical definitions are fundamentally consistent with the 'constitutional disposition' emphasis present in the current ICF descriptions. These are enduring characteristics that define individuals' uniqueness in relating to their environment and others. The forms of the current ICF taxonomic codes (each area, e.g. extroversion, confidence) are not easily represented in currently available temperament and/or personality tests or measures, especially for children. Some of the codes (descriptors) exist, but many do not specifically exist as tests or measures in the personality assessment literature and even less so for young people with developmental disabilities. This chapter will offer options for measurement, suggestions for alternatives and recommendations for development of measures where possible.

General factors to consider when measuring this domain

The methods and purpose for assessment in these areas are related to several key application issues. The purpose of measurement focuses on screening to determine estimates of prevalence/incidence of selected descriptions, identifying characteristics or functional outcomes of the individual as well. This may include, for example, assessment of depressive symptoms or motivational behaviours. Furthermore, personality assessment should be completed from and within an ecological/environmental contextual perspective.[5] Again, this perspective is entirely consistent with the ICF evaluation and methodology. Measurement should be multimethod, multisource and multisetting focused, emphasizing that identification and analysis is more accurate when the assessment involves multiple techniques and multiple informants who have had contact with the child/young person in a variety of settings.[5] This assessment emphasis increases the reliability and validity of the selected evaluations and tests and is a general tenet of valid and reliable psychometric measurement.

Assessment of temperament and personality can be completed by self-report, observation or by proxy (observer, teacher and/or parent), to note the more common strategies. The validity and reliability of measures selected need to be referenced as they apply to the child/adolescent age group and their accessibility to the individual with special needs. However, the majority of instruments available are designed on and for individuals with 'average' physical and cognitive skill levels. As an example, many instruments include questions, items or rankings based on normative skills and assumed common experiences. In some instances, limitations due to a particular disability may result in an inappropriate deficit outcome reflective only of the inability of the individual to complete the item or respond to the item reflective of physical, cognitive or experiential limitations. This outcome is often common in tests that do not include children with particular disabilities in the original development and norming of outcomes. Although this deficit may be valid, it may also reflect test access limitations. Deficits for children/adolescents on such measures may give a faulty interpretation and document only that the test is not a suitable measure for the particular construct with this particular disability or individual's limitations. Children and young people with neurodevelopmental disabilities display complicated variations in growth, and in some instances idiosyncratic rates of growth in all skill and developmental areas. In some situations skill growth is hampered by a lag or a delay and may emerge at a later time and in varying and often uneven degrees or patterns. In other instances, the rates of growth reach a level and subsequently reflect a deficit in a particular area. Fundamental caution is needed in understanding and interpreting test outcome measures. The young people under study need to be understood in a test's basic characteristics for assessment to be meaningful and useful in treatment.

Generally few personality instruments have been developed on and for children/adolescents with developmental disabilities. Consequently, interpretation of results should be approached with caution. The child's age, developmental levels and ability to complete the measures are all key issues in this process. As noted previously, multiple methods and multiple sources are always recommended in using methods of this domain. Where possible, proxy measures should be evaluated within their context and in reference to the particular respondent and potential bias, or at least perspective. If possible, direct contact with the individual through some type of interview (usually structured) is a helpful aid to validating findings and understanding the outcome. Knowledge of the specific limitations of the child/adolescent with a disability is always useful in understanding their particular impact on measurement results. One noteworthy area that affects a subgroup of individuals with neurodevelopmental disabilities and assessment of temperamental and personalities is referred to as *behavioural phenotypes*. These behavioural phenotypes refer to a characteristic pattern of motor, cognitive, linguistic and/or social abnormalities which are consistently associated with a biological disorder, for example autism – stereotypies; Down syndrome – facial characteristics; fragile X – self-mutilation. There is increasing evidence that certain neurodevelopmental disorders may be associated with particular behaviour patterns, for example tempos and temperaments.[6] These characteristics can affect a wide range of measurement outcomes. The impact on the measure may not reflect what the test authors intended, and such behaviours are often very difficult to accommodate or remediate. Aetiologies of these behavioural phenotypes are often linked genetically in these neurodevelopmental disorders.[7] Such behavioural patterns are found in those with Down syndrome, autism and Williams syndrome, to mention those that are better known. Knowledge of these behavioural phenotypes is important in understanding the results of any measurement or evaluation of those with developmental disabilities.

Overview of recommended measures

We recommend several key online resources for locating and reviewing tests. By far the best-known site is the Buros Institute Mental Measurements. This institute produces a comprehensive review of all known tests on a regular basis, reviewed by professionals in the field. It has a website (www.unl.edu/buros/) and produces an extensive text every few years. The American Psychological Association has a site that may assist as well, APAPsycNet (http://psycnet.apa.org/); this lists numerous resources and journals. Another useful text that reviews many psychological measures is the *Handbook of Psychiatric Measures*.[8] Finally, the Cochrane Library is a resource for evidence for healthcare decision-making (www.cochrane.org/reviews/) and may be helpful as well.

Research development in personality and emotional assessment for children with developmental disabilities has not been a high priority, nor has it focused on dispositional characteristics defined by the ICF schema. However, there is a need for research on assessment strategies and measures that include descriptive features, motivational intentions and positive behaviours for children and young people with selected disabilities similar to the five scales of the Five Factor Personality Inventory – Children,[9] i.e., agreeableness, extraversion, openness to experience, conscientiousness and emotional regulation. This type of instrument often has a broad theoretical orientation and seeks to provide personality descriptions that are applicable across a wide range of individuals and experiences. Investigations that sample larger and representative groups, which should include those with some disabilities, is often mandatory to ensure applicability and utility across groups. Inclusion of special normative groups is desirable and can be useful, primarily for comparisons. Importantly, the interpretation of outcomes in these 'special groups' must be done with a cautious awareness of their differences as they may affect the test's validity. Test limitations that occur are often related to cognitive deficits affecting the understanding of test items and the validity of the test. Applicability of new measures is often related to how many samples have been included in the test's development and their relevance to the specific child under consideration. All measures must be placed in context and be part of a broader overall approach.

Finally, we selected measures that gave focus to the intent of the ICF in this area – a dispositional description of individuals as well as functional status, which includes a more direct clinicopathological assessment. Measures included are different types of assessment, for example structured, behavioural, ratings of others, self-report, objective and projective. We are aware of the controversies that surround these instruments, which reflect both philosophical bias and psychometric requirements. Nevertheless, we offer some variety across these measures for children.

TEMPERAMENT AND PERSONALITY MEASURES
We considered the following criteria when selecting instruments to review: (1) commercial availability of the instrument; (2) psychometric properties of the instrument; and (3) the purpose of the instrument, that is, whether the instrument was designed to assess temperament and personality. It is essential that instruments used for screening and diagnostic purposes are reliable and valid and as such should meet certain criteria. Reliability coefficients of 0.90 or above are acceptable for diagnostic decisions, while instruments with reliability coefficients of 0.80 can be used in screening decisions.[10] Nunnally[11] noted that reliability coefficients of 0.90 are acceptable for diagnostic decisions, while coefficients of 0.95 are the goal. An examiner should consult the test manual for relevant information regarding specific types of reliability for each group the test will be used with.

TEMPERAMENT AND ATYPICAL BEHAVIOR SCALE: EARLY CHILDHOOD INDICATORS OF DEVELOPMENTAL DYSFUNCTION

Overview and purpose
The Temperament and Atypical Behavior Scale (TABS)[12] is designed to detect self-regulation behaviours and dispositions that may be symptomatic of children who are at risk of or who have atypical development. Atypical aberrant behaviour can interfere with an individual's ability to adapt to his or her environment and can result in socioemotional difficulties. The TABS provides a norm-referenced assessment that can be used as a screener and diagnostic tool for children aged 11 to 71 months. This assessment can aid in the early identification of behaviour problems and should be used in conjunction with a comprehensive evaluation that includes other psychometric measures such as performance assessments, adaptive behaviour rating scales, interviews and naturalistic observations.

Administration and scoring
The TABS assessment consists of the TABS Screener and the TABS Assessment Tool, both of which are completed by a parent or caregiver. The TABS Screener has 15 items, drawn from the TABS Assessment Tool, that are designed to quickly identify individuals who require further evaluation and can be completed in 5 minutes. If this assessment indicates a need, then the rater completes the TABS Assessment Tool, a 55-item rating scale that can be completed in 15 minutes. For each item, raters indicate 'yes' or 'no'. Raters select 'yes' if the item describes a current problem behaviour and then select 'need help' if they would like assistance with this problem. Raters select 'no' for each item that is not currently considered a problem behaviour. The rater completes all the items.

The TABS Assessment Tool consists of the following four subtests designed to measure atypical temperament and self-regulatory behaviours: detached, hypersensitive–active, under-reactive and dysregulated.[12] The 'detached' subtest addresses behaviours that are indicative of being disconnected from one's environment. The 'hypersensitive–active' subtest addresses behaviours that may be construed as being over-reactive to one's environment. The 'under-reactive' subtest addresses unresponsive behaviours, while the 'dysregulated' subtest describes behaviours that indicate problems in self-regulating. The TABS Assessment yields four subtest T-scores with a mean of 50 and a standard deviation of 10 and the Temperament Regulatory Index (TRI) total score with a mean of 100 and a standard deviation of 15. The examiner is encouraged to use the TRI score in screening and diagnostic decisions.[12]

The manual reports cut-off scores, centiles and normalized standard scores. The authors indicated that the TABS assessment was written at a third-grade reading level and designed to be relatively easy for parents to complete.[12]

Psychometric properties

The TABS norms were developed through a national sample of 833 children aged 11 to 71 months. The manual reported that agencies from 33 states and three provinces in Canada participated. The demographic characteristics of the sample indicated that 212 children in the normative sample were labelled as disabled, with 621 students identified as non-disabled. The authors indicated they did not consider socioeconomic status, ethnicity and geographical region to be factors in atypical development.[12] They determined there was no effect for sex or age and did not report separate norms for those variables. The manual provided a description of individuals with disabilities who were included in the sample. Disabilities ranged from mild to severe. The internal consistency of the TABS Assessment was examined. Split-half reliability coefficients for the TRI total score were 0.88 for children not at risk, 0.95 for children with disabilities and 0.95 for the pooled sample.[12] Across the four subtests, split-half reliabilities ranged from 0.66 to 0.77 for those without disabilities, from 0.81 to 0.92 for children with disabilities and from 0.79 to 91 for the pooled sample. The stability of the TABS Assessment was investigated. The assessment was administered then re-administered after a 2- to 3-week period. The sample consisted of 157 children, 97 without disabilities and 60 with disabilities. Test–retest reliability coefficients for the TRI score across the three samples ranged from $r=0.91$ to $r=0.94$. For the three samples across the four subtests, test–retest reliability coefficients ranged from $r=0.73$ to $r=0.92$. The internal consistency of the TABS Screener yielded a coefficient alpha of 0.83, indicating its utility as a screening device.

As evidence of content validity, the items of the TABS Assessment were constructed by examining reviews of literature and previous research concerning temperament and self-regulatory maladaptive behaviours.[12] The items were submitted to factor analysis and ultimately resulted in the identification of four factors: detached, hypersensitive–active, under-reactive and dysregulated. This factor structure is similar to the Diagnostic Classification 0–3.[13] As evidence of construct validity, the authors asserted that the subtest and total test scores should not reflect differences with regard to age for the pooled sample. The data supported this assertion. Subtest and total mean scores exhibited statistically significant differences when individuals with disabilities scores were compared with individuals without disabilities scores.[12] According to the

manual, the TABS Screener correctly identified 72% of the children who were screened as being at risk for or having a disability.[12]

CAREY TEMPERAMENT SCALES

Overview and purpose

The Carey Temperament Scales (CTS)[14] refer to a collection of five questionnaires designed to assess nine dimensions of temperament: activity, rhythmicity, approach–withdrawal, adaptability, intensity, mood, persistence, distractibility and sensitivity. The CTS are designed for individuals who range in age from 1 month to 12 years. The scales are recommended for use in clinical settings and for research. The CTS can be employed in conjunction with developmental assessments, adaptive behaviour scales, systematic observations and ecological assessments to provide a comprehensive evaluation.

Administration and scoring

The CTS encompass the following five questionnaires: (1) the Early Infancy Temperament Scales, for ages 1 to 4 months; (2) the Revised Infant Temperament Questionnaire, for ages 4 to 11 months; (3) the Toddler Temperament Scales, for ages 1 to 2 years; (4) the Behavioral Style Questionnaire, for ages 3 to 7 years; and (5) the Middle Childhood Temperament Questionnaire, for ages 8 to 12 years. The questionnaires are to be completed by a parent or caregiver. The approximate completion time for a questionnaire is 20 minutes. Each questionnaire addresses the following dimensions: activity, rhythmicity, approach–withdrawal, adaptability, intensity, mood, persistence, distractibility and sensitivity. Items depict typical childhood behaviours, which are rated on a scale from 1 (almost never) to 6 (almost always) according to their occurrence. A category score is derived for each temperament dimension. With regard to administration, the manual recommends that examiners are licensed or certified professionals in the field of child development and psychology.

Psychometric properties

Newman[15] noted that the CTS represent 30 years of research. The scales were normed with 200 to 500 children, who were mainly white and middle class and ranged in age from 1 month to 12 years.[15] This limits the use of the CTS in individuals of other ethnicities and socioeconomic status. Langlois[16] reported that the test–retest reliability coefficients for the CTS ranged from $r=0.64$ to $r=94$ for an administration interval that spanned 20 to 75 days. Internal consistency investigations yielded alpha coefficients that ranged from 0.43 to 0.76 with a median of

TEMPERAMENT AND ATYPICAL BEHAVIOR SCALE (TABS): EARLY CHILDHOOD INDICATORS OF DEVELOPMENTAL DYSFUNCTION	
Purpose	To detect self-regulation behaviours and dispositions that may be symptomatic of children who are at risk for or who have atypical development
	Can be used as part of a comprehensive evaluation for determining eligibility for special education services
	Can be used for planning individualized education programmes
Population	11–71mo
Description of domains (subscales)	The TABS assessment contains 55 items designed to assess four dimensions: detached, hypersensitive–active, under-reactive and dysregulated
Administration and test format	Time to complete: The TABS Screener can be completed in 5min; the TABS Assessment can be completed in 15min
	Testing format: TABS Screener 15 items – primary caregiver completes; TABS Assessment 55 items – primary caregiver completes
	Scoring: yes or no response, norm-referenced; TABS Assessment yields four subtest T-scores, a Temperment and Regularity Index total score with a mean of 100 and a standard deviation of 15, cut-off scores, centiles and normalized standard scores
	Training: the TABS can be administered by someone familiar with the administration procedures. An individual trained in psychometric assessment should interpret the results
Psychometric properties	Normative sample: 621 children without disabilities; 212 children with disabilities
	Reliability
	Split-half reliabilities with a Spearman–Brown correction for the TRI total score were 0.88 for children not at risk, 0.95 for children with disabilities and 0.95 for the pooled sample. Across the four subtests, split-half reliabilities ranged from 0.66 to 0.77 for the sample without disabilities, from 0.81 to 0.92 for the children with disabilities and from 0.79 to 91 for the pooled sample
	Test–retest reliability coefficients for the TRI score across the three samples ranged from 0.91 to 0.94. Across the four subtests, test–retest reliability coefficients were 0.73 to 0.92 for the sample without disabilities, 0.78 to 0.91 for children with disabilities and 0.81 to 0.92 for the pooled sample; the TABS Screener yielded an alpha coefficient of 0.83
	Validity
	As evidence of content validity, items were developed through a review of pertinent literature and research; content validity was also supported by an overlap of the four factors of the TABS and the Diagnostic Classification 0–3.[13] As evidence of construct validity, subtest and total test scores differentiate between children with and without disabilities; the TABS Screener correctly identified 72% of the children who were screened as being at risk for or having a disability 0.[12]
How to order	The TABS is published by Paul H. Brookes Publishing Co., Inc. Total cost for the manual, a pad of screeners and a packet of assessment tools is US$95
Key references	Neisworth JT, Bagnato SJ, Salvia J, Hunt FM (1999) *TABS Manual for the Temperament and Atypical Behaviour Scale: Early Childhood Indicators of Developmental Dysfunction*. Baltimore: Paul H. Brooks Publishing Co.
	Zero to Three (1994). Diagnostic classification: 0–3. Washington, DC: National Center for Infants, Toddlers, and Families. Available at: www.zerotothree.org.

0.62 for the Early Infancy Temperament Scales and from 0.49 to 0.71 with a median of 0.57 for the Revised Infant Temperament Questionnaire. The Toddler Temperament Scale's alpha coefficients ranged from 0.53 to 0.86 with a median of 0.70. The Behavioral Style Questionnaire yielded alpha coefficients that ranged from 0.47 to 0.80 with a median of 0.70.[17] The Middle Childhood Temperament Questionnaire's alpha coefficients ranged from 0.71 to 0.83 with a median of 0.82.

With regard to content validity, the items of the CTS were developed based on a New York longitudinal study[18] that identified nine dimensions of temperament. Researchers familiar with temperament literature evaluated questionnaire items. Pilot testing of the instruments facilitated item analysis and further revision.[15] Construct validity was addressed by Carey and McDevitt, who provided a comprehensive review of the nine purported dimensions of temperament and the efficacy of the CTS in their book *Coping with Children's Temperament*.[19,20] As noted earlier, 30 years of research into the CTS has contributed to the evolving study of temperament and child development.

PERSONALITY INVENTORY FOR CHILDREN, SECOND EDITION

Overview and purpose

The Personality Inventory for Children, second edition (PIC-2),[21] is designed to assess an individual's cognitive, emotional, interpersonal and behavioural functioning.[21] The authors purported that the PIC-2 can be used to identify areas of adjustment that are problematic for an individual and that may warrant further psychometric investigation. It is designed for use with individuals ranging in age from 5 to 19 years.[21] The authors recommended using the PIC-2 along with the child self-report Personality Inventory for Youth[22] and the teacher-report Student Behavior Survey[23] in order to provide a 'multidimensional assessment' that consists of parent, child and teacher reports.[21] Results from the PIC-2 can be assimilated with other diagnostic assessments such as child and teacher interviews, behavioural observations, achievement and intellectual assessments for a comprehensive evaluation.

Administration and scoring

The PIC-2 is a questionnaire that consists of 275 true or false items that can be completed by parents or caregivers within 40 minutes. The standard form includes three response validity scales, nine adjustment scales, 21 adjustment subscales and a critical item response set.[21] The response validity scales consist of three dimensions that address an examinee's defensiveness, problem minimization or denial; dissimulation, problem exaggeration or malingering; and inconsistency and inadequate attention to or comprehension of the PIC-2 statements.[21] The nine adjustment scales measure cognitive impairment, impulsivity and distractibility, delinquency, family dysfunction, reality distortion, somatic concern, psychological discomfort, social withdrawal and social skills deficits. Each adjustment scale consists of two or three adjustment subscales. The PIC-2 Behavioral Summary is a screener that can be completed by parents or caregivers within 15 minutes. It incorporates the first 96 items of the PIC-2 and consists of eight short adjustment scales and three composite scales: externalization, internalization and social adjustment.

The authors asserted that all items are written below a fourth-grade level.[21] For both assessments, the parent or caregiver is provided with an answer sheet and the administration booklet. He or she is asked to complete the demographic information listed on the answer sheet and is then instructed to read the directions for completing the questionnaire.[21] The assessments can also be completed through computerized administration.

Thirteen scoring templates are employed to hand score the PIC-2 Standard Form. Computerized scoring is also available. A critical items summary is provided. For both assessments, raw scores are used to derive T-scores for each of the scales and subscales. Composite scales and a total score are available for the Behavioral Summary. The administration of the assessments is relatively easy and can be conducted by someone familiar with the administration procedures; however, a person trained in psychometric assessment should interpret the results.

Psychometric properties

The manual reports that the PIC-2 and the Behavioral Summary were standardized with 2306 parents of individuals without disabilities and involved 23 different schools in 12 US states. The sample consisted of 47.6% males and 52.4% females, who ranged in age from 5 to 19 years. Each age group comprised an average, more than 100 individuals, except for the age 18 and above group, which consisted of 67 individuals. The following demographic variables of the sample were reflective of the 1998 US Bureau of the Census[24] statistics: sex, ethnic background, geographic region, parents' educational level and guardianship status. Separate normative tables were provided for males and females.

The authors also employed a referred sample that consisted of 1551 protocols from parents of children and adolescents referred for evaluation and included 39 sites in 17 US states that represented four geographical regions.

PERSONALITY INVENTORY FOR CHILDREN, SECOND EDITION (PIC-2)	
Purpose	To assess an individual's cognitive, emotional, interpersonal and behavioural functioning
	Can be used in conjunction with other assessments as part of an eligibility process for special education services
	Can be used to examine changes in behaviour after intervention strategies have been implemented
Population	5–19y
Description of domains (subscales)	The PIC-2 consists of the following scales: three response validity scales, nine adjustment scales and 21 adjustment subscales
	The Behavior Summary yields eight short adjustment scales and three composite scales
Administration and test format	Time to complete: the PIC-2 can be completed in 40min; the Behavior Summary can be completed in 15min
	Testing format: The PIC-2 has 275 items – the parent completes; the Behavior Summary contains the first 96 items of the PIC-2 – the parent completes
	Scoring: true or false response, norm-referenced; the PIC-2 yields T-scores with a mean of 50 and a standard deviation of 10 for each of its adjustment scales and subscales. The Behavioral Summary yields T-scores for three composite scales and a total composite score
	Training: the administration of the assessments is relatively easy and can be conducted by someone familiar with the administration procedures. However, the results should be interpreted by a person trained in psychometric assessment
Psychometric properties	Normative sample: the standardization sample consisted of 2306 protocols from parents of individuals without disabilities; the referred sample consisted of 1551 protocols from parents of children and adolescents referred for evaluation.
	Reliability
	Alpha coefficients across the adjustment scales ranged from 0.81 to 0.95 with a median of 0.89 for the referred sample and from 0.75 to 0.91 with a median of 0.84 for the standardization sample. The test–retest reliabilities for the adjustment scales after a 1-week interval ranged from 0.88 to 0.94 with a median of 0.90 for the referred sample and 0.66–0.90 with a median of 0.82 for the standardization sample. For the referred sample, mother and father inter-rater agreement yielded coefficients that ranged from 0.67 to 0.88 with a median of 0.73. The Behavioral Summary's total score had high alpha coefficients of 0.95 for the referred sample and 0.93 for the standardization sample
	Validity
	With regard to content validity, previous versions of the PIC were examined. A combination of item analysis, factor analysis and clinical judgement were used to create the adjustment scales and subscales. Concurrent validity was supported by the moderate to high correlation of the PIC-2 items with a clinical rating scale, the PIY 21, a self-report scale, and the SBS 22, a teacher report scale. The authors examined PIC-2 results for 11 clinical groups. The data indicated statistically significant differences between the means for each group.[21] As evidence of construct validity, the PIC-2 items and Behavioral Summary were submitted to factor analysis. The PIC-2 items formed the following five factors: externalizing symptoms, internalizing symptoms, cognitive status, social adjustment and family dysfunction. The Behavioral Summary items resulted in two factors: externalizing and internalizing
How to order	The PIC-2 is published by Western Psychological Services. The total cost for the computer scoring kit is US$203.50. This includes the manual, two reusable administration booklets, 50 answer sheets and PIC-2/PIY/SBS scoring CD (25 uses)

Key references	Lachar D, Gruber CP (1995) *Personality Inventory for Youth (PIY) Manual: Administration and Interpretation Guide; Technical Guide*. Los Angeles: Western Psychological Services.
	Lachar D, Gruber CP (2001) *Personality Inventory for Children: Standard Form and Behavioral Summary Manual*. Los Angeles: Western Psychological Services.
	Lachar D, Wingenfeld SA, Kline RB, Gruber CP (2000) *Student Behavior Survey Manual*. Los Angeles: Western Psychological Services.

This sample included 68% males and 32% females, who ranged in age from 5 to 18 years. With regard to ethnicity, the sample included 1.1% Asian American, 15.9% African American, 11% Hispanic, 70.9% white and 1.2% other. The referral sources included 17.1% school based, 73.1% clinic based and 9.8% juvenile justice.[21]

The internal consistency of the PIC-2 was examined for the referred and standardization samples. Alpha coefficients across the adjustment scales ranged from 0.81 to 0.95 with a median of 0.89 for the referred sample and from 0.75 to 0.91 with a median of 0.84 for the standardization sample. The test–retest reliabilities for the adjustment scales after a 1-week interval ranged from $r=0.88$ to $r=0.94$ with a median of $r=90$ for the referred sample and from $r=0.66$ to $r=0.90$ with a median of $r=0.82$ for the standardization sample. For the referred sample, mother and father inter-rater agreement yielded coefficients that ranged from $r=0.67$ to $r=0.88$ with a median of $r=0.73$.[21] The results lent support to the overall stability and consistency of the PIC-2 adjustment scales. The Behavioral Summary's total score yielded high alpha coefficients of 0.95 for the referred sample and 0.93 for the standardization sample.

With regard to content validity, the previous versions of the PIC were examined. Existing items were retained, revised or eliminated and new items were created. The authors indicated that they used a combination of item analysis, factor analysis and clinical judgement to create the adjustment scales and subscales.[21] Evidence of concurrent validity included examining the relationship of the PIC-2 items with the following assessments: a clinical rating scale, the Personality Inventory for Youth,[22] a self-report scale, and the Student Behavior Survey,[23] a teacher report scale. The results indicated that the PIC-2 items have a moderate to high relationship with the instruments employed.

The authors examined PIC-2 results for 11 clinical groups. The data indicated statistically significant differences between the means for each group.[21] As evidence of construct validity, the PIC-2 items and Behavioral Summary were submitted to factor analysis. The PIC-2 items formed the following five factors: externalizing

symptoms, internalizing symptoms, cognitive status, social adjustment and family dysfunction. The Behavioral Summary items resulted in two factors: externalizing and internalizing. The manual provided extensive evidence of the reliability and validity of the PIC-2 and the Behavioral Summary.

MINNESOTA MULTIPHASIC PERSONALITY INVENTORY – ADOLESCENT

Overview and purpose
The Minnesota Multiphasic Personality Inventory – Adolescent (MMPI-A)[25] is a self-report inventory that is designed to appraise personal, social and behavioural functioning. Information from the MMPI-A can reveal areas of dysfunction that need to be further investigated. The MMPI-A is recommended for adolescents between the ages of 14 and 18 years. School, clinical and counselling psychologists can incorporate results from the MMPI-A along with other psychometric assessments such as behavioural observations, interviews and intellectual and achievement performance measures to provide a comprehensive evaluation.

Administration and scoring
The MMPI-A is a 478-item self-report that can be completed within 45 to 60 minutes according to the manual. Examinees are instructed to read each item and respond by marking true or false. The authors report that the items are written at the sixth-grade reading level. The examinee can read the items or use an audiocassette/compact disc. The items can be completed using paper and pencil or a computer.

The MMPI-A consists of the following scales: six validity scales, 10 clinical scales, 31 clinical subscales, 15 content scales, 31 content component subscales, 11 supplementary scales and a number of supplemental indices. The six validity scales are cannot say, lie, infrequency, defensiveness, variable response inconsistency and true-response consistency. These scales are useful in determining the response profile of the examinee. Delman et al[26] acknowledged that the validity scales were 'suitable for use when an assessment of the accuracy of the person's self-report is questionable and/or considered an important component of the evaluation'. The 10 clinical scales are hypochondriasis, depression, hysteria, psychopathic deviate, masculinity–femininity, paranoia, psychasthenia, schizophrenia, mania and social introversion or extroversion. The supplemental indices include the MacAndrew Alcoholism Scale – Revised, alcohol/drug problem acknowledgment, alcohol/drug problem proneness, immaturity, anxiety, repression and the Personality Psychopathology Five scales.

An extended score report and basic service report are available. Scoring options include hand scoring, a mail-in scoring service, software scoring and optical scan scoring. Raw scores are used to derive T-scores with a mean of 50 and a standard deviation of 10 for the clinical and validity scales. Butcher and Williams[27] authored *The Minnesota Report Adolescent Interpretive System*, second edition, a guide that incorporates qualitative statements, supplementary indices and scale scores to aid examiners in the interpretation of the MMPI-A. Individuals with a background in psychometrics can administer this assessment; however, psychologists or individuals with comparable training should interpret the results.

Psychometric properties
The manual reports that the MMPI-A was standardized with 1620 individuals without disabilities and involved junior high and high schools in eight states within the USA. Overall, the MMPI-A normative sample provides a fair representation of the US adolescent population. The sample consisted of 805 males and 815 females, who ranged in age from 14 to 18 years. Demographic variables (i.e. age, sex, ethnic background and urban–rural residency) were adequately represented in the sample. With regard to parental education and occupation, the majority of the sample consisted of parents who completed high school, graduated from college or graduate school and held upper-level jobs, such as managerial and professional positions.[25] The authors also employed a clinical sample of 713 individuals aged 14 to 18 years. There were 420 males and 293 females, who were solicited from treatment facilities in the Minneapolis area. The sample included individuals from inpatient alcohol and drug treatment facilities, inpatient mental health facilities, day treatment programmes and a special school programme.

With regard to the internal consistency of the clinical scales, the manual reported the following alpha coefficients: 0.40 to 0.89 for the normative sample and 0.35 to 0.91 for the clinical sample for males and females across the 10 scales. The test–retest reliability of the clinical scales involved 154 individuals who completed the

MMPI-A twice, with a 1-week interval between administrations. Test–retest reliability coefficients ranging from $r=0.65$ to $r=0.84$ for the normative sample across the 10 scales were reported. The authors noted that the standard error of measurement should be taken into account when interpreting the MMPI-A scales. The typical standard error of measurement for the basic scales was reported to be four to six T-score points.[25]

With regard to content validity, the MMPI-A was constructed by omitting, revising or retaining items from the MMPI.[25] The manual reported that the validity and clinical scales were submitted to factor analysis. The following four factors were revealed: general maladjustment, overcontrol, social introversion and masculinity–femininity.[25] These results lent support for the construct validity of the scales. There is an extensive record of research concerning the validity and clinical utility of the MMPI-A. Delman et al[26] noted that the MMPI and MMPI-2 have more than 10 000 references that support their validity. The authors acknowledged 'Findings from studies of the MMPI-2[28] and MMPI-A have mostly been consistent with those from studies of the original MMPI'.[26] The MMPI-A has a history of use with adolescents and allows the clinician to have many options for interpretation and application.

FIVE-FACTOR PERSONALITY INVENTORY – CHILDREN

Overview and purpose
The Five-factor Personality Inventory – Children (FFPI-C)[9] is a self-report inventory designed to assess personality dispositions in children and adolescents that may place individuals at risk for or result in social or emotional adjustment problems. It is designed for individuals aged from 9 years to 18 years 11 months and is recommended for use in school and community cognitive health settings. The authors employed Allport and Odbert's[29] five-factor personality theory in the construction of the FFPI-C.[9] This theory purported that the construct of personality encompasses the following five factors: agreeableness, extroversion, openness to experience, conscientiousness and neuroticism.[29] The FFPI-C can be used in conjunction with intelligence and achievement performance assessments, parent and teacher reports, and systematic observations to provide a comprehensive evaluation.

Administration and scoring
The FFPI-C is a 75-item inventory that can be completed by the examinee within 15 to 40 minutes. The manual states that the FFPI-C can be self-administered, individually administered or group administered.[9] The protocol requires a third-grade reading level for self-administration. Each item is presented as two opposing statements.

Five empty bubbles are positioned between the two statements. The examinee is asked to read each statement and mark how much he or she agrees with it. The protocol states 'If you agree with a sentence, colour in the circle closest to that sentence. If you somewhat agree with a sentence, colour in the second closest circle to that sentence'.[9] If the examinee has trouble choosing between statements, he or she is instructed to choose the middle circle.

The five scales of the FFPI-C are agreeableness, extraversion, openness to experience, conscientiousness and emotional regulation.[9] The agreeableness scale addresses aspects of trust, straightforwardness, altruism, compliance, modesty and tender-mindedness. Extraversion addresses warmth, gregariousness, assertiveness, activity, excitement seeking and positive emotions. Openness to experience addresses fantasy, aesthetics, feelings, actions, ideas and values. Conscientiousness addresses competence, order, dutifulness, achievement striving, self-discipline and deliberation. The emotional regulation scale addresses anxiety, angry hostility, depression, self-consciousness, impulsiveness and vulnerability.[9]

The FFPI-C employs raw scores to derive T-scores with a mean of 50 and a standard deviation of 10 for each of the five scales. The manual reports the standard error of measurement, centile rank and a descriptive rating for each scale. The authors provide a table for converting T-scores into other standardized scores and centile ranks. The manual recommends examiners have formal training in psychometric measurement and personality theory and assessment.[9]

FIVE-FACTOR PERSONALITY INVENTORY – CHILDREN (FFPI-C)	
Purpose	To assess personality dispositions in children and adolescents that may place individuals at risk for or result in social or emotional adjustment problems
	Can be used in conjunction with other assessments as part of a comprehensive evaluation process
	Can be used as a screening instrument to determine if further social and emotional assessment is warranted
Population	9y–18y 11mo
Description of domains (subscales)	The FFPI-C consists of five scales: agreeableness, extraversion, openness to experience, conscientiousness and emotional regulation
Administration and test format	Time to complete: the FFPI-C can be completed within 15–40min
	Testing format: the FFPI-C has 75 items; the child/adolescent completes
	Scoring: each item is presented as two opposing statements. Five empty bubbles are positioned between the two statements. The examinee is asked to read each statement and mark how much he or she agrees with them. Norm-referenced. The FFPI-C yields T-scores with a mean of 50 and a standard deviation of 10
	Training: the manual recommends that examiners have formal training in psychometric measurement and personality theory and assessment
Psychometric properties	Normative sample: 1284 individuals aged 9–18y. With regard to individuals with disabilities, the sample included 81% no exceptionality, 3% learning disorder, <1% articulation disorder, 6% emotional disturbance, <1% blind/partially sighted, <1% physical impairment, <1% autistic, 1% language disorder, 3% attention-deficit–hyperactivity disorder, 3% gifted and talented, 4% other disabilities
	Reliability The manual also reported alpha coefficients for age, ethnicity and sex. Alpha coefficients across the five scales ranged from 0.74 to 0.86 for the total sample, from 0.85 to 0.96 for individuals with ADHD, from 0.73 to 0.84 for individuals with emotional disorders and from 0.85 to 0.91 for individuals with learning disorders. Test–retest reliability was examined with 192 children and adolescents who were aged 9–18y. The examinees completed the FFPI-C and after a 2-week interval completed the assessment again. Test–retest reliabilities ranged from 0.84 to 0.88 across the five scales

Psychometric properties	*Validity*
	As evidence of content validity, the construction of the FFPI-C involved a review of research, a panel of experts in the field and item analyses. The authors addressed criterion-related validity through multiple studies in which the FFPI-C was administered in conjunction with comparable instruments. The results indicated that the majority of items had a moderate to high relationship with the instruments employed and thus lent support for the concurrent validity of the FFPI-C. With regard to construct validity, the FFPI-C mean T-scores for the normative sample were compared for the following groups: individuals with emotional disorders, learning disabilities and ADHD. The authors reported that the majority of the scores for the disability groups were significantly lower than for the normative sample.[9] A discriminant analysis employed the normative sample for the following comparisons: individuals with emotional disorders but no disability and individuals with learning disabilities but no other disability. The data revealed that the FFPI-C scales significantly differentiated between the individuals with emotional disorders and learning disabilities when they were compared with individuals without disabilities. The FFPI-C scales correctly identified 72.8% of individuals with emotional disorders and no disability, and 70.8% of individuals with learning disabilities and no disabilities.[9] As further evidence of construct validity, each of the five FFPI-C scales was submitted to a confirmatory factor analysis. The manual reported that three of the four model fit indices employed supported the proposed structure of the scale in question. The intercorrelation of the FFPI-C scales was examined. As hypothesized, correlations revealed a small to moderate relationship between the scales, thus indicating that, although related, the scales retained a degree of specificity
How to order	The FFPI-C is published by Pro-Ed. The total cost for the computer scoring kit is US$150.00 This includes the examiner's manual and 25 administration and scoring forms
Key references	McGhee RL, Ehrler DJ, Buckhalt JA (2007) *FFPI-C Five-Factor Personality Inventory-Children Examiner's Manual*. Austin, TX: Pro-Ed.

Psychometric properties

The manual states that the FFPI-C was standardized with 1284 individuals across 18 US states. The sample consisted of 49% males and 51% females, who ranged in age from 9 to 18 years. For each age group there was an average of more than 100 individuals, except for the 18-year-old group, which consisted of 99 individuals. Sex, geographic region and ethnicities within the sample were reflective of the 2002 Statistical Abstract of the USA,[30] with the exception of individuals who were of Hispanic descent, who constituted 8% of the normative sample compared with 13% reported by the US census date. With regard to individuals with disabilities, the sample included 81% no exceptionality, 3% learning disorder, <1% articulation disorder, 6% emotional disturbance, <1% blind/partially sighted, <1% physical impairment, <1% autistic, 1% language disorder, 3% attention-deficit–hyperactivity disorder (ADHD), 3% gifted and talented and 4% other disabilities. Separate normative tables were provided for males and females.

The internal consistency of the FFPI-C was examined for the normative sample. Alpha coefficients across the five scales ranged from 0.74 to 0.86 for the total sample, from 0.85 to 0.96 for individuals with ADHD, from 0.73

to 0.84 for individuals with emotional disorders and from 0.85 to 0.91 for individuals with learning disorders. The manual also reported alpha coefficients for age, ethnicity and sex. Test–retest reliability was examined with 192 children and adolescents who were 9 to 18 years of age. The examinees completed the FFPI-C and after a 2-week interval completed the assessment again. Test–retest reliabilities ranged from $r=0.84$ to $r=0.88$ across the five scales. The standard error of measurements for each scale for the 68%, 90% and 99% confidence intervals were reported in the manual for males and females. The results lent support to the overall stability and consistency of the FFPI-C scales.

As evidence of content validity, the construction of the FFPI-C involved the review of previous personality research and existing assessments that employed the five-factor model of personality.[9] A team of experts in the area of child development, personality and psychology examined a pool of 100 items. The final 75 items were examined. The discriminating power of each item exceeded the recommended 0.35 value for all the FFPI-C scales.[9] A differential item functioning analysis was conducted. A logistic regression procedure compared the scores for African Americans and non-African Americans, and Hispanic Americans and non-Hispanic Americans, and revealed that the 75 items were ultimately not biased across ethnicity and race.

The authors addressed criterion-related validity through multiple studies in which the FFPI-C was administered with one or more of the following assessments: the NEO Five-factor Inventory,[31] the Junior Eysenck Personality Questionnaire,[32] the Behavioral and Emotional Rating Scale, second edition,[33] the Behavior Dimensions Rating Scale[34] and the Hammill Multiability Intelligence Test.[35] The results indicated that the majority of items had a moderate to high relationship with the instruments employed and thus lent support for the concurrent validity of the FFPI-C. With regard to construct validity, the authors compared the FFPI-C mean T-scores for the normative sample and the following groups: individuals with emotional disorders, with specific learning disabilities and with ADHD. The data revealed that the emotional disorders group achieved a low score on the emotional regulation scale. The group with learning disabilities scored within the low average range on the conscientiousness scale, while the group with ADHD achieved a low score on the conscientiousness scale and a score within the low average range for the openness to experience and emotional regulation scales. The authors reported that the majority of scores for the groups with disabilities were significantly lower than those of the normative sample.[9]

A discriminant analysis employed the normative sample for the following comparisons: individuals with emotional disorders but no disability and individuals with learning disabilities but no other disability. The data revealed that the FFPI-C scales significantly differentiated between the individuals with emotional disorders and learning disabilities when they were compared with individuals without disabilities. The classification accuracy of the FFPI-C scales correctly identified 72.8% of individuals with emotional disorders and no disability and 70.8% of individuals with learning disabilities but no other disabilities.[9] As further evidence of construct validity, each of the FFPI-C scales was submitted to a confirmatory factor analysis. The manual reports that three of the four model fit indices employed supported the proposed structure of the scale in question. The intercorrelation of the FFPI-C scales was examined. As hypothesized, correlations revealed a small to moderate relationship between the scales, thus indicating that, although related, the scales retained a degree of specificity. The authors provided extensive data to support the reliability and validity of the FFPI-C. The authors welcomed the use of the FFPI-C in future research studies.

DRAW A PERSON: SCREENING PROCEDURE FOR EMOTIONAL DISTURBANCE

OVERVIEW AND PURPOSE

The Draw a Person: Screening Procedure for Emotional Disturbance (DAP:SPED)[36] is a standardized procedure for scoring examinees' drawings in order to screen children and adolescents for emotional problems.[36] It is designed for use with individuals who range in age from 6 to 17 years. The DAP projective technique is steeped in controversy, with proponents and opponents on each side of the aisle.[37,38] Laak et al[38] acknowledged that historically two general approaches to the DAP test have been utilized: (1) the thinking approach – the use of norms and quantification methods; and (2) the global approach – the assessment of specific attributes of the content and quality of drawings and the use of a judgement approach. These two approaches have been employed in the use of the DAP as a tool to investigate cognitive and developmental levels and as a tool to investigate personality and emotional disturbance.[38] It is strongly advised that the DAP:SPED be used as a screener and in conjunction with intellectual and achievement assessments, parent, teacher and child interviews, and systematic observations in order to provide a comprehensive assessment.

Administration and scoring

The DAP:SPED can be administered in a group format and individually, with a total administration time of approximately 15 to 20 minutes. The examinee is directed to draw three separate pictures: of a man, of a woman and of themselves. The manual reported that a maximum of 5 minutes should be allowed for the examinee to complete each drawing. The manual provided a comprehensive scoring system for the examiner that categorized 55 criteria for scoring into two groups: those that pertained to figure dimension and those that rated the content of the drawing for attributes such as shading, frowning mouth, etc.[36] Ten templates are provided to facilitate scoring the DAP:SPED. The raw scores for the man, woman and self drawings are summed and used to derive a total score, which is reported as a T-score with a mean of 50 and a standard deviation of 10. Centile ranks are also provided along with confidence intervals. With regard to administration, the authors recommended that the DAP:SPED be administered and interpreted by trained professionals such as school counsellors, school psychologists and evaluation specialists.[36]

Psychometric properties

The DAP:SPED normative data were obtained in 2260 individuals who were also used to standardize the DAP:A

Quantitative Scoring System.[39] The sample comprised 50.1% males and 49.9% females, who ranged in age from 6 to 17 years. The demographic variables of sex, ethnicity, geographic region, age, socioeconomic status and parental occupation were examined and deemed to adequately represent the 1980 US Bureau of the Census population data.[40] Norms were reported for males and females for the following age groups: 6 to 8 years (*n*=530), 9 to 12 years (*n*=818) and 13 to 17 years (*n*=912).

The internal consistency, inter-rater, intrarater and test–retest reliability of the DAP:SPED were examined. Alpha coefficients were calculated for males and females for each age group and employed the summed raw scores for the three drawings. Alpha coefficients ranged from 0.67 to 0.78. for males and females across the three age groups. The authors provided standard errors of measurements for males and females for each age group. The inter-rater and intrarater reliability of the DAP:SPED was examined for 54 cases that were scored by two different raters and the same rater twice during a 1-month interval.[36] The inter-rater reliability was *r*=0.84 while the intrarater reliability was *r*=0.83. Test–retest reliability was investigated by administering the DAP:SPED to 67 individuals twice with a 1-week interval between administrations. The examinees attended a school for individuals with disabilities, which served individuals with learning disabilities, emotional/behaviour problems and brain injuries, ranging in age from 5 to 17 years.[36] The correlation between administrations was *r*=0.67.

With regard to validity, the authors examined the utility of the DAP:SPED and its ability to differentiate between individuals with and without disabilities through four separate studies. Each of the studies indicated that the DAP:SPED successfully differentiated groups of individuals described as having emotional/behavioural disorders from groups of individuals without disabilities. The relationship of the DAP:SPED and the Matrix Analogies Test – Short Form,[41] an intelligence test, was examined. As hypothesized, there was a low, non-significant, correlation between the measure of intelligence and the DAP:SPED. Although the DAP:SPED may be surrounded by controversy, it still remains a very popular instrument that is used by psychologists worldwide.[37,38] Naglieri et al[36] provided a comprehensive approach that standardized and quantified the application of the DAP assessment for use as a screener for individuals with emotional/behaviour problems.

REFERENCES

1. World Health Organization (2007) *International Classification of Functioning, Disability and Health Version for Children and Youth ICF-CY*. Geneva: World Health Organization.
2. Allport GW (1961) *Pattern and Growth in Personality*. New York: Holt.
3. Allport GW (1937) *Personality: A Psychological Interpretation*. New York: Holt.
4. Wiggins JS, Pincus AL (1992) Personality: structure and assessment. *Annu Rev Psychol* 43: 473–504.
5. Knoff HM (1990) Best practices in personality assessment. *Preventing School Failure* 34: 25–30.
6. Harris JC (2002) Behavioral phenotypes of neurodevelopmental disorders: Portals into the developing brain. In: Davis KL, Charney D, Coyle JT, Nemeroff C, editors. *Neuropsycholopharmacology: The Fifth Generation of Progress*. New York: Lippincott Williams & Wilkins, pp. 625–638.
7. Tome SA, Williamson N, Pauli R (1990) Temperament in Williams syndrome. *J Med Genet* 36: 345–352.
8. Rush AJ, First MB, Blacker D, editor (2008) *Handbook of Psychiatric Measures*, 2nd edition. Washington, DC: American Psychiatric Publishing, Inc.
9. McGhee RL, Ehrler DJ, Buckhalt JA (2007) *FFPI-C Five-Factor Personality Inventory–Children Examiner's Manual*. Austin, TX: Pro-Ed.
10. Salvia J, Ysseldyke JE, Bolt S (2007) *Assessment: In Special and Inclusive Education*, 10th edition. New York: Houghton Mifflin Company.
11. Nunnally J (1978) *Psychometric Theory*. New York: McGraw Hill, Inc.
12. Neisworth JT, Bagnato SJ, Salvia J, Hunt FM (1999) *TABS Manual for the Temperament and Atypical Behavior Scale: Early Childhood Indicators of Developmental Dysfunction*. Baltimore: Paul H. Brookes Publishing Co.
13. Zero to Three (1994) National Center for Infants, Toddlers, and Families. Diagnostic classification: 0–3. Available at: www.zerotothree.org/child-development/early-childhood-mental-health/diagnostic-classification-of-mental-health-and-developmental-disorders-of-infancy-and-early-childhood-revised.html.
14. Carey WB (2000) *The Carey Temperament Scales Test Manual*. Scottsdale, AZ: Behavioral-Developmental Initiatives.
15. Newman J (2001) Test review of the Carey Temperament Scales. In: Plake BS, Impara JC, editors. *The Fourteenth Mental Measurements Yearbook* (accessed April 20 2009). Available at: www.unl.edu/buros
16. Langlois A. Test review of the Carey Temperament Scales. In: Plake BS, Impara JC, editors. *The Fourteenth Mental Measurements Yearbook*. Available from www.unl.edu/buros (accessed 20 April 2010).
17. McDevitt SC, Carey WB (1996) *Manual for the Behavioral Style Questionnaire*. Scottsdale, AZ: Behavioral-Developmental Initiatives.
18. Thomas A, Chess S, Birch HG, Hertzig ME, Korn S (1963) *Behavioral Individuality in Early Childhood*. New York: New York University Press.
19. Carey WB, McDevitt SC (1995) *The Carey Temperament Scales*. Scottsdale, AZ: Behavioral-Development Initiatives.
20. Carey WB, McDevitt SC (1995) *Coping with Children's Temperament: A Guide for Professionals*. New York: Basic Books.
21. Lachar D, Gruber CP (2001) *Personality Inventory for Children: Standard Form and Behavioral Summary Manual*. Los Angeles: Western Psychological Services.
22. Lachar D, Gruber CP (1995) Personality Inventory for Youth (PIY) *Manual: Administration and Interpretation Guide; Technical Guide*. Los Angeles: Western Psychological Services.

23. Lachar D, Wingenfeld SA, Kline R B, Gruber CP (2000) *Student Behavior Survey Manual*. Los Angeles: Western Psychological Services.

24. US Bureau of the Census (1998) *Statistical Abstract of the United States: 1998*, 117th edition. Washington, DC: US Bureau of the Census.

25. Butcher JN, Williams CL, Graham JR, et al (1992) *Minnesota Multiphasic Personality Inventory–Adolescent: Manual for Administration, Scoring, and Interpretation*. Minneapolis, MN: University of Minnesota Press.

26. Delman HM, Robinson DG, Kimmelblatt CA, McCormack J (2008) General psychiatric symptoms measures. In: Rush AJ, First MB, Blacker D, editors. *Handbook of Psychiatric Measures*, 2nd edition. Washington, DC: American Psychiatric Publishing, Inc., pp. 61–82.

27. Butcher JN, Williams CL (2007) *The Minnesota Report Adolescent Interpretive System*. 2nd edition, Minneapolis, MN: University of Minnesota Press.

28. Butcher JN, Graham JR, Ben-Porath YS, et al (2001) *Minnesota Multiphasic Personality Inventory-2 (MMPI-2): Manual for Administration and Scoring*, revised edition. Minneapolis: University of Minnesota Press.

29. Allport GW, Odbert HS (1936) Trait names: A psycho-lexical study. *Psychol Monogr* 47: 211.

30. US Bureau of the Census (2002) *Statistical Abstract of the United States: 2002*, 122nd edition. Washington, DC: US Bureau of the Census.

31. Costa PT Jr, McCrae RR (1991) *NEO Five Factor Inventory*. Odessa, FL: Psychological Assessment Resources.

32. Wysenck HJ, Eysenck SBG (1975) *Junior Eysenck Personality Questionnaire*. San Diego: Educational and Industrial Testing Service.

33. Epstein MH (2004) *Behavioral and Emotional Rating Scale*, 2nd edition. Austin, TX: Pro-Ed.

34. Bullock LM, Wilson MJ (1989) *Behavior Dimensions Rating Scale*. Allen: DLM Teaching Resources.

35. Hammill DD, Bryant BR, Pearson NA (2001) *Hammill Multiability Intelligence Test*. Austin, TX: Pro-Ed.

36. Naglieri JA, McNeish TJ, Bardos AN (1991) *DAP: SPED: Draw a Person: Screening Procedure for Emotional Disturbance: Examiner's Manual*. Austin, TX: Pro-Ed.

37. Williams TO Jr, Fall A, Eaves RC, Woods-Groves S (2006) The reliability of scores for the Draw-A-Person Intellectual Ability Test for Children, Adolescents, and Adults. *J Psychoedu Assess* 24: 137–144.

38. Laak JT, Goede MD, Aleva A, Rijswijk PV (2005) The Draw-A-Person Test: An indicator of children's cognitive and socio-emotional adaptation? *J Genet Psychol* 166: 77–93.

39. Naglieri JA (1988) *Draw A Person: A Quantitative Scoring System*. San Antonio, TX: Psychological Corporation.

40. U. S. Bureau of the Census (1980) *Statistical Abstract of the United States*: 1980, 101st edition. Washington, DC: US Bureau of the Census.

41. Naglieri JA (1985) *Matrix Analogies Test – Short Form*. San Antonio, TX: Psychological Corporation.

9

SPECIFIC MENTAL FUNCTIONS: ATTENTION AND EXECUTIVE FUNCTIONS (B140, B144, B164)

John Wilding and Kim M. Cornish

What is the construct?

The past decade has witnessed an explosion of research focused on identifying different components of *attention*. This research has been driven in part by the increase in awareness of specific disorders of attention, in particular attention-deficit–hyperactivity disorder (ADHD), and a growing awareness that attention is not a single unitary construct but rather a complex, multidimensional concept. In a classroom setting, inattentive behaviours are often observed as difficulties in concentration and focus, distractibility, impulsivity and disorganization. This constellation of behaviours is included in clinical diagnostic assessments of inattention, for example the *Diagnostic and Statistical Manual of Mental Disorders*, fourth edition (DSM-IV; American Psychiatric Association, 1994), and in parent/teacher-based assessments such as the Conners Rating Scales.[1,2] Commonly, three subtypes of attention-deficit disorder are defined – inattention only, hyperactivity only and combined inattention and hyperactivity (ADHD). The severity and impact of these behaviours vary across development such that, in some cases, early problems dissipate as the child matures and is able to focus more effectively. However, other children remain inattentive throughout their childhood, making them vulnerable to the development of more serious clinical disorders such as ADHD.

Alongside the behavioural symptoms of inattention, it has become widely recognized that cognitive impairments in attention need to be recognized and identified early in development. Although behavioural ratings can play an important role in demonstrating overt manifestations of inattention and can identify children at risk of more serious developmental disorders of attention, they do not pinpoint the precise underlying causes of the behaviour. In order to identify such causes, many tasks have been devised in an attempt to define the specific processes that may be impaired. Although opinions differ about the various cognitive processes involved in attention, there is general consensus of a division between *selective attention* (the ability to selectively attend to specific information while ignoring distractions – this is a pivotal component of attention and undergoes a rapid development in the preschool and childhood years), *sustained attention* (the ability to focus for prolonged periods in an otherwise unchanging situation and to ignore irrelevant distractions – this is a critical component for successful performance across many cognitive skills, for example decision-making and learning) and *control processes* (such as the ability to inhibit prepotent responses, switch attention from one focus to another and to complete a planned sequence of actions – these complex skills undergo significant developmental changes across childhood and are essential for efficient selection and maintenance of information).

In addition, *divided attention*, required when performing more than one task at a time, and *alertness* (or arousal) are often added, the latter being important for the maintenance of attention on prolonged and, in particular, boring tasks. Hence, attention can be viewed as a complex of interconnected functions, with control processes co-ordinating more basic operations in order to achieve selection, maintenance of attention and detailed sequences of behaviour. These control processes are commonly regarded as equivalent to *executive function* as identified by neuropsychologists, which depends principally on the functioning of the frontal lobes of the brain and which co-ordinates a wide range of control processes such as planning, inhibition of interference and unnecessary motor activity, attention switching, maintenance of attentional focus and updating working memory. The areas of the brain that underpin these processes are the last to mature during development. See Cornish and Wilding[3] for a comprehensive review of attention and executive function.

It should be noted that several findings demonstrate that attentional ability is relatively independent of intelligence quotient (IQ). Scores on the Test of Everyday Attention for Children (TEA-Ch) battery, described below, were not significantly related to IQ if a correction for multiple correlations was applied (see Table 4 in Manly et al[4]), and the studies carried out by the present authors (summarised in Cornish and Wilding[3]) have shown that relations between attention and performance differ from those between IQ and performance.

We first describe a selection of behavioural and cognitive measures commonly used by researchers and clinicians to examine attention and executive function. Given the space limitations, it is impossible to include all the measures that are currently available, and the choice of an instrument in a specific situation will invariably depend upon the clinical population under investigation. Secondly, we will describe examples of atypical attention and executive function in individuals diagnosed with developmental disorders of attention but whose genetic aetiologies are different: ADHD, fragile X syndrome and Down syndrome. We ask to what extent similar behavioural symptomatology implies commonalities in cognitive mechanisms and therefore necessitates similar treatment approaches. We will be arguing that the current categorization of attention disorder is too simplistic and much finer distinctions are required than those in the present diagnostic classifications.

Overview of behavioural measures used to assess attention and executive functions

We first describe three attention rating instruments that include scales to evaluate attention and hyperactivity and two attention task batteries designed to test more specific aspects of attentional performance. We consider to what extent the results from these instruments can provide an insight into the precise nature of attentional weaknesses in developmental disorders. See Cornish and Wilding[3] for a more detailed review of the full range of attention rating scales and measures.

Secondly, these five methods of evaluating attention will be discussed in relation to ADHD itself and a further two disorders that present with intellectual delay alongside comparable levels of ADHD behaviours: fragile X syndrome and Down syndrome. Age-related changes in attention performance will also be discussed to highlight the importance of recognizing early signs of inattention in terms of both inattentive behaviours and cognitive weaknesses.

RATING SCALES OF INATTENTIVE BEHAVIOURS

Although there is an increasing number of rating scales currently available to assess severity of inattentive behaviours in children and adolescents, space permits us to highlight only three of the most commonly used: the Child Behavior Checklist (CBCL), the Behavior Rating Inventory of Executive Function (BRIEF) and the Conners Rating Scales (CRS).

Child Behavior Checklist (CBCL)

Overview and purpose
The CBCL rating scales provide a measure for parents and teachers to assess a variety of problem behaviours in preschool- and school-age children. A core advantage is the diversity and wide range of behaviour problems that the scale covers.

Scales
There are two main types of scales:
- *'Syndrome'* scales comprise the following subscales: attention problems, emotional reactive (preschool version only), anxious/depressed, somatic complaints, withdrawal, sleep problems (parent versions only), aggressive problems, social problems and rule-breaking behaviour; and two general categories, namely internalizing behaviours (relating to problems that are mainly within the individual or self) and externalizing behaviours (relating to problems that result in conflict with others).
- *DSM*-orientated scales are based on the DSM-IV criteria and comprise the following subscales: affective problems, anxiety problems, pervasive developmental problems (preschool version only), attention-deficit–hyperactivity problems, oppositional defiant problems, somatic problems (school-age version only) and conduct problems (school-age version only).

Advantages
- It is standardized on a large normative, heterogeneous sample of children.
- It has strong cultural validity and has been translated into numerous languages; thus it has wide community appeal.
- It allows comparisons of ratings of inattentive behaviours across multiple settings, for example the classroom and home.
- There is significant congruence between the attention problem subscale and a clinical diagnosis of ADHD.

Disadvantages
- The lack of agreement between parent and teacher ratings suggests that the items on the scale reflect behaviour specific to only some situations, rather than pervasive cognitive weaknesses.

- The CBCL appears to have considerable difficulty in distinguishing between ADHD subtypes, specifically clinically diagnosed ADHD 'inattentive' versus 'combined' subtypes.

Behaviour Rating Inventory of Executive Function

Overview and purpose
The BRIEF focuses on ratings of executive function

CHILD BEHAVIOR CHECKLIST (CBCL)	
Purpose	Assessment of problem behaviours in preschool- and school-age children; teacher and parent rating forms
Population	1y 6mo–5y; 6–18y
Administration and test format	Preschool version: ratings of behaviour within the last 2mo on 99 items
	School-age version: ratings of behaviour within the last 2mo (teacher version) or 6mo (parent version) on 112 items
	Ratings on a three-point Likert scale; subscale scores are summed and converted to a T-score (>69 is regarded as within the clinical range)
Psychometric properties	*Normative samples* Preschool teacher version, n=1192; parent version, n=700
	School-age teacher version, n=319; parent version, n=1753
	Normative data by sex for age groups: 1.5–3, 6–7, 8–9, 10–11, 12–13, 14–15, 16–18y
	Syndrome scales Preschool teacher scales, internal consistency: 0.52–0.97; parent scales: 0.66–0.95
	Preschool teacher scales, test–retest reliability: 0.68–0.91; parent scales: 0.69–0.92
	Preschool attention problems, teacher subscale, internal consistency: 0.89; parent subscale: 0.68
	Preschool attention problems, teacher subscale, test–retest reliability: 0.84; parent subscale: 0.78
	School-age teacher scales, internal consistency: 0.7–0.97; parent scales: 0.78–0.98
	School-age teacher scales, test–retest reliability: 0.60–0.96; parent scales: 0.82–0.92
	School-age attention problems, teacher subscale, internal consistency: 0.95; parent subscale: 0.86
	School-age attention problems, teacher subscale, test–retest reliability: 0.95; parent subscale: 0.92
	DSM-orientated scales Preschool teacher version, internal consistency: 0.68–0.93; parent version: 0.63–0.86
	Preschool teacher version, test–retest reliability: 0.57–0.87; parent version: 0.74–0.87
	Preschool ADHD, teacher subscale, internal consistency: 0.92; parent subscale: 0.78
	Preschool ADHD, teacher subscale, test–retest reliability: 0.79; parent subscale: 0.74
	School-age teacher version, internal consistency: 0.72–0.97; parent version: 0.78–0.98
	School-age teacher version, test–retest reliability: 0.60–0.96; parent version: 0.82–0.92
	School-age ADHD, teacher subscale, internal consistency: 0.94; parent subscale: 0.84
	School-age ADHD, teacher subscale, test–retest reliability: 0.95; parent subscale: 0.93
References and sources	Achenbach TM (1991) *Manual for Child Behavior Checklist 4–18*. Burlington, VT: University of Vermont, Research Center for Children, Youth, and Families.
	Achenbach TM, Rescorla LA (2000) *Manual for the ASEBA Preschool Forms & Profiles*. Burlington, VT: University of Vermont, Research Center for Children, Youth, and Families.

behaviours in the everyday context as defined by parents and teachers for both preschool- and school-age children; hence, it focuses on the control aspect of attention that we have described above.

BEHAVIOR RATING INVENTORY OF EXECUTIVE FUNCTION (BRIEF)	
Purpose	Ratings of everyday executive function behaviour in preschool- and school-age children; teacher and parent rating forms
Population	2–5y and 5–18y
Administration and test format	Preschool version: ratings of behaviour on 63 items
	School-age version: ratings of behaviour on 86 items (different for teacher and parent versions)
	Ratings on a three-point Likert scale; subscale scores summed and converted to a T-score and centiles (T-scores >65 are regarded as indicating a problem)
Psychometric properties	*Ethnically diverse normative samples*
	Preschool teacher version, *n*=302; parent version, *n*=460
	School-age teacher version, *n*=702; parent version, *n*=1419
	Normative data for 2–3, 4–5, 5–6, 7–8, 9–13, 14–18y
	Internal consistency and reliability
	Preschool teacher scales, internal consistency: 0.90–0.97; parent scales: 0.80–0.95
	Preschool teacher scales, test–retest reliability: 0.65–0.94; parent scales: 0.78–0.90
	Preschool inhibit, teacher subscale, internal consistency: 0.94; parent subscale: 0.90
	Preschool working memory, teacher subscale, internal consistency: 0.94; parent subscale: 0.88
	Preschool plan/organize, teacher subscale, internal consistency: 0.97; parent subscale: 0.80
	Preschool inhibit, teacher subscale, test–retest reliability: 0.94; parent subscale: 0.90
	Preschool working memory, teacher subscale, test–retest reliability: 0.88; parent subscale: 0.85
	Preschool plan/organize, teacher subscale, test–retest reliability: 0.85; parent subscale: 0.78
	School-age teacher scales, internal consistency: 0.90–0.97; parent scales: 0.80–0.97
	School-age teacher scales, test–retest reliability: 0.83–0.92; parent scales: 0.76–0.86
	School-age inhibit, teacher subscale, internal consistency: 0.96; parent subscale: 0.91
	School-age working memory, teacher subscale, internal consistency: 0.93; parent subscale: 0.89
	School-age plan/organize, teacher subscale, internal consistency: 0.91; parent subscale: 0.90
	School-age inhibit, teacher subscale, test–retest reliability: 0.91; parent subscale: 0.84
	School-age working memory, teacher subscale, test–retest reliability: 0.86; parent subscale: 0.85
	School-age plan/organize, teacher subscale, test–retest reliability: 0.88; parent subscale: 0.85
	Validity
	Supported: correlates with other related scales
References and sources	Gioia GA, Isquith PK, Kenworthy L, Barton RM (2000) Profiles of everyday executive function in acquired and developmental disorders. *Child Neuropsychol* 8: 121–137.
	Gioia GA, Espy KA, Isquith PK (2003) *Behavior Rating Inventory of Executive Function – Preschool Version*. Odessa, FL: Psychological Assessment Resources, Inc.

Scales

There are five scales for preschool children: ability to inhibit, ability to shift attention, emotional control, working memory and ability to plan ahead. For school-age children, there are eight scales, comprising the same scales as above plus three additional scales – ability to initiate action, ability to organize materials and ability to monitor the environment for important information.

Advantages

• The BRIEF was standardized on a moderate-sized heterogeneous sample of children.

• It provides a broader assessment of executive function in addition to attention.

• It is used extensively to assess atypical variations in executive behaviours across a range of developmental disorders including ADHD and autism.

CONNERS TEACHER RATING SCALE, REVISED (CTRS-R), AND CONNERS PARENT RATING SCALE, REVISED (CPRS-R)	
Purpose	To provide ratings of a range of symptoms relating to attention-deficit–hyperactivity disorder and a global scale of attention-related behaviours
Population	3–17y
Administration and test format	Ratings on a four-point Likert scale can be summed and converted to standardized T-scores (mean 50, standard deviation 10) Behaviour is rated over the preceding month T-scores >65 are considered to be in the clinical range
Psychometric properties	*Normative samples from ethnically diverse populations in USA and Canada* CTRS-R long form, *n*=1973; CPRS-R long form, *n*=2482 CTRS-R short form, *n*=1897; CPRS-R short form, *n*=2426 *Overall internal consistency ranges:* CTRS-R long form: 0.77–0.96; CPRS long form: 0.73–0.94 CTRS-R short form: 0.88–0.95; CPRS-R short form: 0.86–0.94 *Cognitive problems/inattention subscale, internal consistency* CTRS-R long form: 0.91; CPRS-R long form: 0.93 CTRS-R short form: 0.89; CPRS-R short form: 0.69 *DSM-IV symptoms – inattentive subscale, internal consistency* CTRS-R long form: 0.95; CPRS-R long form: 0.92 *Overall test–retest reliability* CTRS-R long form: 0.47–0.88; CPRS-R long form: 0.47–0.85 CTRS-R short form: 0.72–0.92; CPRS-R short form: 0.62–0.85 *Cognitive problems/inattention subscale, test–retest reliability* CTRS-R long form: 0.47; CPRS-R long form: 0.69 CTRS-R short form: 0.92; CPRS-R short form: 0.73 *DSM-IV symptoms – inattentive subscale* CTRS-R long form: 0.70; CPRS-R long form: 0.67 *Validity supported* Cognitive problems/inattention subscale correlates with several other similar rating scales
References and sources	Conners CK (1997) *Conners Rating Scales – Revised*. North Tonawanda, NY: Multi-Health Systems. Conners CK (2008) *Conners Third Edition (Conners 3)*. North Tonawanda, NY: Multi-Health Systems.

Disadvantages
• It is rarely used in children with intellectual impairment.

Conners Rating Scales

Overview and purpose
The CRS [Conners Teacher Rating Scale – Revised (CTRS-R) and Conners Parent Rating Scale – Revised (CPRS-R)] are perhaps the most widely used scales for evaluating a range of attention-related behaviour at school and in the home. They are used principally to aid in judging whether a child should be rated as falling outside the normal range of behaviour and assigned to one of the types of ADHD.

Scoring
There are long and short forms of both teacher and parent rating scales. The *long form* can be used to calculate scores on six subscales (cognitive problems/inattention, hyperactivity, oppositional behaviour, anxious/shy, perfectionism and social problems), which can be combined to form the global index. Alternatively, these forms can be used to calculate scores only on the DSM-IV categories of inattention and hyperactivity/impulsivity, which in turn can be combined to form a total ADHD score. The *short form* generates three subscales (cognitive problems/ inattention, oppositional behaviour, hyperactivity) and an ADHD total score. There are also self-report versions for adolescents in both long and short forms.

Advantages
• The CRS were standardized on large normative, heterogeneous samples of children.
• They have strong cultural validity and have been translated into numerous languages; thus they have wide community appeal.
• They allow comparisons of ratings of inattentive behaviours across multiple settings (e.g. classroom and home).
• There is significant congruence between the attention problem subscale and a clinical diagnosis of ADHD.
• It is well established that the CRS represent valuable clinical and research tools for differentiating young children and adolescents with inattentive behaviours and ADHD from non-clinical peers.

Disadvantages
• The CRS demonstrate less sensitivity in discriminating children with ADHD from children with other clinical diagnoses and in discriminating ADHD as a distinct disorder in children with differing degrees

of intellectual impairment or specific developmental disorders, such as fragile X syndrome or Down syndrome.

MEASURES OF COGNITIVE COMPONENTS OF ATTENTION
There exists a wide range of paradigms that attempt to tap underlying cognitive processes in childhood and adolescence. Here we highlight two of the most commonly used measures: the Developmental Neuropsychological Assessment (NEPSY) and the TEA-Ch.

The NEPSY

Overview and purpose
The NEPSY comprises a battery of tasks designed for use as a clinical tool to identify weaknesses in a variety of components of cognitive functions, including attention and executive function. A second edition, NEPSY-II, has recently been published, with several changes in the component tasks. However, there is little published evidence using this revision and, accordingly, our comments are by necessity confined to the earlier version.

Functions tested
Twenty-seven subtests cover five cognitive domains: attention and executive function, language, sensorimotor, visuospatial ability, memory and learning. In the attention and executive function domains there are three 'core' tests for which there has been extensive research (planning, visual attention, inhibition). Subtests are specifically designed for children aged 3 to 4 years, with a more extensive range available for children aged 5 to 12 years.

Advantages
• It is a clinical tool that can differentiate attention and executive function problems in children with typical development from those with atypical development.
• There is some discrimination ability to differentiate attention and executive function profiles across differing developmental disorders.

Disadvantages
• It is time-consuming to administer the entire battery of tasks.
• There are some doubts about the ability of tasks to tap a single cognitive function and hence concerns regarding the validity of combining scores into a single overall score for the construct.
• There is a lack of substantial data as yet from the second edition.

Test of Everyday Attention in Children

Overview and purpose

The TEA-Ch battery comprises tasks that are expressly tests of *everyday* attention. It aims to employ tasks with some face validity that demand similar abilities to those required in daily life and cover the three most widely accepted aspects of attention: selection, maintenance and control.

Functions tested

Scores from the tasks are claimed to provide measures of ability in selective attention, maintenance of attention and control of attention. The threefold division was obtained from confirmatory factor analysis on data from 293 children aged 6 to 16 years. Wilding[5] has since criticized the validity of this analysis on the grounds that the factors that were derived may have depended on differences in the measures of performance (speed or accuracy) rather than differing attentional demands.

Advantages

- The TEA-Ch was designed primarily as a clinical tool to identify children with possible impairments in attention and has been used extensively to document attention profiles in children with ADHD, but also in children with other developmental disorders such as autism, fragile X syndrome and Down syndrome.
- It is easy to administer, with subtests presented in a 'real world' format.

Disadvantages

- It is time-consuming to administer the whole battery.
- There are concerns about validity regarding distinctions between subcategories of attention and assignment of tasks to these categories.

Atypical development of attention and executive function

ATTENTION-DEFICIT–HYPERACTIVITY DISORDER

The majority of research on attention disorders has been concerned with attempting to identify precisely which components of attention are impaired in ADHD. Groups defined by ratings on one of the available scales as impaired or normal are compared on one or more cognitive tasks in order to discover which tasks best discriminate between the groups. Essentially, these studies are attempting to develop more precise indices of the nature of ADHD, but progress has been slow because differences between ADHD and typically developing groups occur on a very wide range of tasks and it has proved difficult to

identify consistent and specific discriminating features. Thus, at present, overall rating scales, rather than diagnostic tasks, are widely used as the main means of diagnosing ADHD, with each instrument offering a cut-off point at which a clinical disorder is to be identified.

There are some limited data from subtests of the NEPSY indicating differences between children with specific neurodevelopmental disorders and control groups, but there has been no systematic analysis of possible differences between different subtests, particularly for the disorders listed above. There have been several studies employing the TEA-Ch (or some subtests of it) to compare children with a diagnosis of ADHD and a control group, and the Score! test of sustained attention emerges as the most reliable discriminating measure. See Cornish and Wilding (especially chapter 6)[3] for detailed discussion of these issues.

Recent findings by the present authors provide a more detailed analysis of the key distinctions between different disorders and suggest directions for future task design and research. A visual search task (a measure of selective attention) devised by Wilding (VISEARCH)[a] was used, in which the child was asked to scan a computer display and click on target 'holes' of a specified shape and colour. The child was told that monsters were hiding in these holes and their task was to find the hole in which the monster king was hiding. In a related test of maintained attention (VIGILAN), targets appeared intermittently in a similar display and a response was required within 7 seconds.

A difficult version of the search task in which the child is required to alternate between two target shapes has consistently discriminated between children with good attention (as shown by rating scales) and children with poor attention. The key finding has been that performance is poorer only in terms of the number of erroneous responses made to non-targets. Speed and other characteristics of performance did not differ between groups. Speed did improve markedly with increasing age, but the number of errors only declined slowly as age increased. These two aspects of performance were therefore largely independent, and we have argued that control of responses to non-targets depends on executive function.[5–11]

However, this is not to argue that all occurrences of attentional impairment should be attributed simply to a deficit in executive function without further differentiation. Studies of other developmental syndromes have confirmed that subtle differences in the nature of attentional problems, which are picked up only by specific

---

[a] There is at the time of writing no easily administered publicly available version of the VISEARCH and VIGILAN tasks used in these studies, so they were not included in the previous section. The current version can be obtained on request from the present authors.

DEVELOPMENTAL NEUROPSYCHOLOGICAL ASSESSMENT (NEPSY) AND NEPSY-II	
Purpose	A clinical tool to permit brief screening for different disorders and identify dysfunction in different components of cognitive functions
Population	NEPSY 3–12y; NEPSY-II 3–16y
Administration and test format	Subtests have a mean of 10; the combined score for each domain has a mean of 100 and a standard deviation of 15 *Attention and executive function subtests* Tower (ages 5–12y only): coloured balls are displayed on three vertical pegs and have to be moved one at a time between the pegs from an initial position to end up matching a target position; only the top ball on a peg may be moved. This transformation is to be achieved in a prescribed number of moves (which in some cases exceeds the minimum possible and thus requires suppression of a move towards the goal in favour of a 'detour'). A time limit is imposed of 30s on the first four problems and 45s per item on the remainder, and the test closes if failure occurs on four successive trials. This task is generally regarded as a test of planning, although it has been argued that an important factor is the ability to inhibit moves that make the display more similar to the target display but are not the correct moves required to eventually attain the goal Statue (ages 3–4y only): a motor position has to be adopted following instructions (such as standing still while pretending to hold a flag) then maintained for 75s. This task assesses control and maintenance of attention Design fluency (ages 5–12y only): in this task, dot patterns are presented and have to be connected by straight lines to make a new design in each case. A structured and a random array are given, each for 60s. This task assesses various aspects of attentional control, including planning and checking Knock and Tap (ages 5–12y): this task requires children to knock with their knuckles on the table when the examiner taps with a flat palm and do nothing when the examiner knocks with his or her knuckles. This pattern is then reversed. This is a go/no-go task that requires first the inhibition of the prepotent direct imitation then a reversal of the newly learned response pattern
Psychometric properties	Normative data for children aged 5–12y; n=800 *Reliability* Split-half, test–retest and generalizability methods used For attention and executive function, average reliability: 0.70 (ages 3–4y) and 0.82 (ages 5–12y) For individual tests: Visual attention: 0.76; Statue: 0.50 (ages 3–4y); Tower: 0.82; Design fluency: 0.59; Knock and Tap: not given (ages 5–12y) *Validity* No formal data are available to support claims that the tasks test the listed functions or that they are independent of each other in their cognitive demands
References and sources	Korkman M, Kirk U, Kemp S (1998) *NEPSY: A Developmental Neuropsychological Assessment*. San Antonio, TX: The Psychological Corporation. Korkman M, Kirk U, Kemp S (2007) *NEPSY II. Clinical and Interpretive Manual*. San Antonio, TX: The Psychological Corporation.

characteristics of task performance, can be identified. Although rating scales have been widely used in attempts to specify the cognitive weakness in a range of genetically caused developmental disorders, recent research has suggested that such usage is at best imprecise and at worst actually misleading. Similar global scores on a rating scale that are obtained from different disorders can conceal very specific differences in the nature of the

TEST OF EVERYDAY ATTENTION IN CHILDREN (TEA-CH)	
Purpose	To test selective attention, maintenance of attention and control of attention
Population	6–16y
Administration and test format	*Selection: Skysearch and Map Mission* Sky Search: the child has to search for 'target' spaceships placed in pairs; targets are defined as pairs when the two spaceships are identical. The mean time to find a target pair is recorded Map Mission: the child has to identify as many target symbols as possible (knife and fork signs) found on a map in a fixed short time span (1min) *Maintenance of attention: Score!, Score Dual Task (DT), Code Transmission, Walk/Do Not Walk, Skysearch DT* Score!: the child is required to keep count of a number of 'scoring' sounds on a tape over a period of 10 trials comprising between 9 and 15 tones at variable intervals (500–5000ms) Score DT: the child has to count specific tones as well as listen for an animal name read as part of a news bulletin. After each trial, they name the animal and the number of target tones Code Transmission: the child has to listen to monotonous sequences of digits, one every 2s, listening for two fives in a row. When they hear the specified sequence, they have to recall the preceding digit Walk/Do Not Walk: the child has to 'walk' along a paper pathway, one step at a time, each time he or she hears a specific tone. Unpredictably, the children hear a tone that is different from the rest and they must inhibit the next step and not continue walking until the target tone resumes. In essence, this requires them to listen carefully to the tones and to maintain attention and not get carried away Sky Search DT: a complex task in which, the child has to combine skills required for the two previous tasks: finding spaceships (Sky Search) and keeping a count of scoring sounds (Score!) *Control of attention: Creature Counting, Same World–Opposite Worlds* Creature Counting: a child is shown a picture of 'aliens' in their burrows and has to count the aliens; however, at intervals, an arrow is inserted pointing upward, in which case the incremental counting has to continue, or downward, when decremental counting is required. The task tests switching ability Same World–Opposite Worlds: the child has to follow a path scattered with the digits 1 or 2 and name each one in the order they are named on the pathway ('same world' condition). In the 'opposite world' condition, they do the same task, but this time when they see 1, they have to say 'two' and if they see 2 they have to say 'one'. This task measures the ability to reverse an established habit
Psychometric properties	Normative data for children aged 6–16y; n=293 (Australian children) *Reliability* Test–retest For individual tests: Sky Search attention score 0.75; Score! 0.76; Creature Counting accuracy 0.71; Sky Search DT 0.81; Map Mission 0.65; Score DT 0.71; Walk–Do Not Walk 0.71; Same World time 0.87; Opposite World time 0.85; Code Transmission 0.78 *Validity* Correlations were obtained with other tasks ($p<0.01$) as below, after chronological age had been considered, but demonstrate no clear separation of the hypothesized three factors:

Psychometric properties	*Selection tasks (Map Mission and Sky Search)* Stroop task (selection/control), Trails A task time (selection), Trails B task time (selection/ control), the Matching Familiar Figures Task (MFFT) errors (control)
	Maintenance of attention Score! and Score DT – MFFT errors (control)
	Code Transmission – Trails B time (selection and control), MFFT errors (control) Walk/Do Not Walk
	Sky Search DT – Trails A time (selection)
	Control of attention Creature Counting – Stroop (selection and control), MFFT errors (control)
	Opposite Worlds – Trails A time (selection)
Reference and source	Manly T, Anderson V, Nimmo-Smith I, Turner A, Watson P, Robertson IH (2003) The differential assessment of children's attention: The Test of Everyday Attention for Children (TEA-Ch), normative sample and ADHD performance. *J Child Psychol Psychiatry Allied Dis* 42: 1065–1081.

different impairments, as we will now demonstrate in the discussion of our two selected genetic disorders: fragile X sydrome and Down syndrome.

FRAGILE X SYNDROME

Fragile X syndrome is a well-recognized cause of hereditary developmental delay in males and to a lesser extent in females. It is one of the most widely studied genetic disorders worldwide, affecting an estimated 1 in 2500 males and females.[12]

In a series of studies using the visual search paradigm described above, the present authors and colleagues have compared toddlers and school-age children with fragile X syndrome with developmental age-matched children and with other groups of developmental disorders (Down syndrome and Williams syndrome; Williams syndrome is a relatively rare genetic disorder with cognitive impairments including attention and some aspects of visual perception). These studies revealed consistent and characteristic differences between groups in the patterns of impairment.[13–16] The most prominent weakness in the fragile X groups was repetition on already located (and clearly marked) targets together with difficulty in switching attention from one target type to another. In the study by Munir et al[13] (see also Wilding et al[14]), a typically developing group with poor rated attention matched to that of the group with fragile X syndrome was included, yet performance on the task differed between these two groups. Thus, matching on overall behaviour did not produce matched cognitive performance on this task. A more dramatic discrepancy between two syndromes was demonstrated by Scerif et al,[15] who found that while toddlers with fragile X syndrome performed poorly on a visual

search task because they tended to continue responding on already located targets, toddlers with Williams syndrome performed equally poorly owing to frequent responses to non-targets. So, different mechanisms were involved in these cases, which rating scales could not reveal. The authors argued that the problems characteristic of the group with fragile X syndrome are due to a weakness in inhibiting a successful response or previously correct target definition in order to look for a new target. This implies a problem in the control of attentional switching, which is one aspect of executive function. No problems were apparent in the fragile X syndrome group in discriminating targets from non-targets, suggesting relatively unimpaired visual perceptual abilities. Williams syndrome, on the other hand, involves a problem in discriminating targets and non-targets, but not in switching attention.

The weakness in inhibitory control is pervasive, beginning in infancy and persisting into adulthood, and serves to differentiate fragile X syndrome from other developmental disorders even when ADHD behaviour profiles measured by rating scales are similar. Problems in switching to a new target in the Wilding VISEARCH task were apparent from the age of 2 years onwards.[13,15,16] It seems, therefore, that the impairment in inhibition, which is another aspect of executive function, is early and prolonged in this disorder.

DOWN SYNDROME

Down syndrome, or trisomy 21, is the most common genetic cause of mental retardation.[a] The disorder has

---

[a] UK usage: learning disability.

an estimated frequency of 1 in 730,[17] and in most cases results from an additional copy of chromosome 21.

Munir et al,[13] in the study discussed above, also included a group with Down syndrome matched on behavioural ratings. Although this group showed some of the characteristics of the group with fragile X syndrome, their weakness in inhibition was much less severe than that of the group with fragile X syndrome. No problem in visual discrimination between targets and non-targets was apparent, compared with typically developing groups. Performance on the VIGILAN task was not significantly different from a typically developing group with poor attention as rated by teachers.

Overall, studies of attention in children with Down syndrome suggest a widespread impairment across attention and executive function measures compared with typically developing children matched on attention level as well as cognitive age, but no specific disorder-specific signature has emerged.

Evidence on changes over age in Down syndrome is meagre and lacking empirical support. Cornish et al[18] found that as chronological age increased, children with Down syndrome improved in the speed of visual search, the speed of detecting sporadically occurring targets in the VIGILAN task and the number of times they successfully inhibited responses in the 'Walk/Do Not Walk' subtest

from the TEA-Ch battery. Thus, the overall picture is of improvement with age on a range of aspects of attentional performance, including executive function.

Conclusions

The prevailing finding from the evidence that we have reviewed is that rating scales for attention, while useful in providing a coarse assessment for matching groups or discriminating between typically developing children and those with weaknesses of attention and executive function, provide rather little information on the precise nature of the deficit underlying poor ratings. Consequently, such scales have also consistently failed to discriminate between groups with different genetic disorders. As we have demonstrated, in order to pinpoint more precisely the causes of attentional disorders in such cases, more specific testing of well-defined cognitive processes is required. Our chapter has outlined some of those possibilities, but there is as yet only limited information from currently available cognitive tasks about their ability to pinpoint the precise weaknesses that may distinguish different developmental disorders. Without a greater body of data from these tasks, it is not yet possible to decide whether these tasks will eventually be shown to be adequate for this purpose or whether new, more effective batteries need to be developed.

REFERENCES

1. Conners CK (1997) *Conners Rating Scales – Revised*. North Tonawanda, NY: Multi-Health Systems.
2. Conners CK (2008) *Conners 3rd Edition (Conners 3)*. North Tonawanda, NY: Multi-Health Systems.
3. Cornish K, Wilding J (2010) *Attention, Genes and Developmental Disorders*. New York: Oxford University Press.
4. Manly T, Anderson V, Nimmo-Smith I, Turner A, Watson P, Robertson IH (2003) The differential assessment of children's attention: The Test of Everyday Attention for Children (TEA-Ch), normative sample and ADHD performance. *J Child Psychol Psychiatry Allied Dis* 42: 1065–1081.
5. Wilding J (2005) Is attention impaired in ADHD? *Br J Dev Psychol* 23: 487–505.
6. Wilding J, Munir F, Cornish K (2001) The nature of attentional differences between groups of children differentiated by teacher ratings of attention and hyperactivity. *Br J Psychol* 92: 357–371.
7. Wilding J (2003) Attentional difficulties in children: weakness in executive function or problems in coping with difficult tasks. *Br J Psychol* 94: 427–436.
8. Wilding J, Burke K (2006) Attentional differences between groups of preschool children differentiated by teacher ratings of attention and hyperactivity. *Br J Dev Psychol* 24: 283–291.
9. Wilding J, Pankhania P, Williams A (2007) Effects of speed and accuracy instructions on performance in a visual search task by children with good or poor attention. *Br J Psychol* 98: 127–139.
10. Wilding J, Cornish K (2007) Independence of speed and accuracy in visual search: evidence for separate mechanisms. *Child Neuropsychol* 13: 510–521.
11. Cornish KM, Wilding JM, Hollis C (2008) Visual search performance in children rated as good or poor attenders: the differential impact of DAT1 genotype, IQ and chronological age. *Neuropsychology* 22: 217–225.
12. Hagerman PJ (2008) The fragile X prevalence paradox. *J Med Genet* 45: 498–499.
13. Munir F, Cornish KM, Wilding J (2000) A neuropsychological profile of attention deficits in young males with fragile X syndrome. *Neuropsychologia* 38: 1261–1270.
14. Wilding J, Cornish K, Munir F (2002) Further delineation of the executive deficit in males with fragile-X syndrome. *Neuropsychologia* 40: 1343–1349.
15. Scerif G, Cornish K, Wilding J, Driver J, Karmiloff-Smith A (2004) Visual search in typically developing toddlers and toddlers with fragile X or Williams syndrome. *Dev Sci* 7: 116–130.
16. Scerif G, Cornish K, Wilding J, Driver J, Karmiloff-Smith A (2007) Delineation of early attentional control difficulties in fragile X syndrome: Focus on neurocomputational changes. *Neuropsychologia* 45: 1889–1898.
17. Canfield MA, Honein MA, Yuskiv N, et al (2006) National estimates and race/ethnic-specific variation of selected birth defects in the United States, 1999–2001. *Birth Defects Res Part A Clin Mol Teratol* 76: 747–756.
18. Cornish K, Scerif G, Karmiloff-Smith A (2007) Tracing syndrome-specific trajectories of attention across the lifespan. *Cortex* 43: 672–685.

10
SPECIFIC MENTAL FUNCTIONS: EMOTIONAL FUNCTIONS, EXPERIENCE OF SELF AND TIME (B152, B180)

Andrea Lee

This chapter focuses on conducting an assessment of two International Classification of Functioning, Disability and Health for Children and Youth (ICF-CY) codes which describe specific cognitive functions associated with subjective personal experiences, namely emotional functions (b152) and the child or young person's experience of self and time (b180). The chapter begins with an overview of terminology related to constructs associated with these codes. It continues with measurement considerations when assessing subjective personal experiences (such as emotion, self and time) with children and young people, and identifies challenges in documenting functioning given existing measures. The author proposes an assessment approach consistent with the ICF-CY and the specified codes, and provides detailed information on three measures which are consistent with the ICF-CY. The chapter concludes with recommendations for enhancing the measurement of functioning related to the ICF-CY codes for emotional functions and experiences of self and time functions in children and young people.

What is the construct?

The goal of this section is to clarify the codes describing emotional functions (b152) and experience of self and time functions (b180) by providing potential definitions of constructs embedded in the wording of each set of codes. When reading this section, it is important to consider the complexity of these codes and to balance this complexity with a need for definitions which may capture the underlying processes in a more concrete manner.

EMOTIONAL FUNCTIONS

In the ICF-CY, 'emotional functions' is defined as 'specific mental functions related to the feeling and affective components and processes of the mind.'[1] Included considerations are the appropriateness of emotion (b1520), the

regulation of emotion (b1521) and the range of emotion (b1522). Additionally, the ICF-CY emotions include 'sadness, happiness, love, fear, anger, hate, tension, anxiety, joy, sorrow; lability of emotion; flattening of affect'.[1]

In order to understand the nuances of the ICF-CY definition of 'emotional functions', it is important to describe and differentiate terminology utilized by researchers and practitioners. The first task, and perhaps the most daunting, is to discuss the concept of 'emotion'. There is no consensus definition of emotion[2,3] as it varies by theoretical orientation and those aspects of emotion which most interest a researcher or clinician. Because emotions are internal, how they are defined and described is based on what one believes drives human experience and what can be documented in studies or clinical practice. The most current definitions incorporate cognitive, behavioural, physiological, and learning and motivational aspects to markedly different degrees; however, most definitions highlight the internal, subjective personal experience of emotion.

At a basic level, emotion can be understood as referring to 'subjective feeling states' reflecting internal processes within an individual.[4] Emotions also can be defined so as to include the external (behavioural) reactions to events or experiences.[5,6] Most definitions are not quite so concise, however, and demonstrate the complexity underlying the human experience of emotion. Nesse and Ellsworth[7] provided a minimum definition of emotion including 'modes of functioning…that coordinate physiological, cognitive, motivational, behavioral, and subjective responses in patterns that increase the ability to meet the adaptive challenges of situations that have recurred over evolutionary time'.[7] This more complex definition suggests that emotions and regulation of emotion are not exclusively controlled by cognitive processes or functions, but rather are human experiences or modes of functioning which require integration of responses across various systems of functioning. More cognitively based theorists state a relationship between cognition (exclusively) and complex emotions, such as remorse and shame, by noting the cognitive evaluation involved in interpreting a situation, thus implying the role of cognitive or cognitive processes on emotional states and their expression.[8]

As defined in the ICF-CY, 'emotional functions' relate *only* to the specific *cognitive* functions which contribute to an individual's awareness of emotions, ability to experience diverse emotions and ability to exert some control over emotional expression. The focus on the specific cognitive processes associated with emotional functions suggests that the codes are most consistent with a cognitive framework, although a reliance on this theoretical perspective would not be necessary to understand the codes. For the purposes of this chapter, the author proposes that a definition of 'emotion' in the ICF-CY probably reflects a relatively basic concept referring to the experience and use of cognitive functions which contribute to the understanding of subjective, internal feeling states and their expression as affect. It is important for readers to understand that there are a number of theories which would suggest this definition is too simplistic and does not adequately capture emotional functioning.

The words 'feeling' and 'affect' also require an expanded definition. Like 'emotion', there are not consistent definitions of these concepts as they also vary depending on the theoretical perspective regarding emotion. Utilizing the language of the ICF-CY 'emotional functions' code (b152), 'feeling' is probably defined as the internal experience of an emotion with corresponding physiological responses. The ICF-CY also describes cognitive processes related to 'affect'. The definition of affect has been considered a broad psychological construct which references any cognitive state required to evaluate feelings,[4] a definition which closely mirrors definitions of emotion. Affect also has been considered synonymous with feeling. Applied to an individual, researchers and clinicians reference an individual's affective display, or the outward expression of underlying, internal feeling states. These external displays are often captured in facial expressions and other forms of body language, such as posture, and behaviours, such as rate of speech and motor activity. For the purposes of this chapter, 'feeling' will be considered as the internal physiological response or feeling state associated with an emotion. 'Affect' will be considered synonymous with feeling except when describing the affective display of an individual or his or her external, observable expression of feeling or affect.

Those interested in emotion will note that several commonly used words are absent in the 'emotional functions' codes. These include the concepts of 'mood' and 'internalizing' concerns or problems. Code b1263, psychic stability, provides the option of coding an individual's functioning and characteristics related to being 'moody' under the broader code of b126, temperament and personality functions. Internalizing problems are distinguished from externalizing problems and are considered as difficulties in internal processes, such as emotional experiences. The concept of internalizing problems may be captured in the fact that the ICF-CY further distinguishes aspects of emotional functions (b152) with three descriptive codes, including appropriateness of emotions (b1520), regulation of emotions (b1521) and range of emotions (b1522).

b1520: Appropriateness of emotions

This code is defined as 'Mental functions that produce congruence of feeling or affect with the situation, such as happiness at receiving good news'.[1] While this code may seem straightforward, there are actually many components which contribute to the congruence of affect with a situation. It is commonly agreed that certain emotions are useful and appropriate only in certain situations;[9] however, which emotions are appropriate under what circumstances is defined by social rules and cultural constructions as well as prior experience. Like the human experience of emotion, determination of congruence is subjective, and therefore must be determined at a case-by-case level.

As an example, consider a child who is known to enjoy a particular type of sweet. The child usually smiles and laughs when presented with this sweet – an affective display which would appear congruent with what seems to be a subjectively happy or good moment. However, the child's teacher notices a change in the child's behaviour, as he or she becomes prone to crying or other displays of distress when presented with the sweet. At first glance, this new affective display appears inappropriate or incongruent with the situation. When relaying concerns to the parent, the teacher discovers that the grandparent who used to give the child this sweet has recently passed away. Thus, with more information, the child's behaviour and affective display in the face of the situation may be understood as appropriate. The presented example is simplistic, but demonstrates the importance of having a full, clear understanding of the events and situations surrounding an individual's life when attempting to capture functioning related to appropriateness of emotion.

There are two complementary cognitive processes in producing or experiencing congruent feelings with a given situation. The first process is the ability to understand the situation, including the nuances and context surrounding an event. A child or young person must be able to identify the salient aspects of a particular situation in order to process or experience an appropriate affective response. This ability is founded in general cognitive abilities, which may be unrelated to the actual experience of emotion. The second complementary cognitive process is the ability to identify the emotional salience of the situation given its particulars and to then 'translate' this information into an affective experience congruent or adaptive to the situation. Whether the emotional experience is 'appropriate' to the situation will depend on the accuracy of the perception of the actual situation, as well as the emotional valence assigned to the event and the final emotional experience resulting from this process.

In summary, determining whether an emotional experience is 'appropriate' or 'congruent' ultimately requires a judgement by the researcher or clinician. This judgement must incorporate a number of important considerations. A measure of appropriateness of emotion will need to incorporate information on the context and prior experiences related to the child and the situation and the child or young person's understanding of the situation, and then give consideration to the child's ability to recognize the emotional salience of a situation. The process is even more complex when considering that measuring the child or young person's experience of the emotion requires an estimate of a subjective, internal experience. Such an endeavour necessitates a comprehensive approach to assessment, which probably is not easily accomplished through a single tool or measure.

b1521: Regulation of emotions
This code is defined as 'Mental functions that control the experience and display of affect'.[1] This code centres on the ability of the individual to utilize cognitive processes to regulate emotional experience and in turn affective display, which can be facial expression and other forms of body language. It speaks to an attempt to regulate or change internal feelings of arousal subsequent to exposure to stimuli evoking emotion, and in turn to alter affective display. The link between emotional experiences and subsequent affective display are quite clear.[10] There is consistent correlation between self-reported emotion or feeling and facial expressions; there are similar patterns of facial expression for emotions in infants across cultures.[11,12] The link is easily observable when working with an adolescent who is experiencing depressive symptoms or anxiety and presents with a 'flat' affect or facial expressions denoting worry or distress.

Increased regulation of emotions is associated with the general developmental progression of cognitive abilities, as it requires the use of cognitive processes to override the relatively involuntary experience of an emotion

and the impulse for affective display. The first process is an appraisal of the emotion-eliciting event, and possible cognitive re-appraisal, or an alteration in the way that the event is perceived as modifying the impact of the situation. The second process involves modifying or altering the actual emotional experience, for example by suppression, as a mechanism for regulating emotion.[13] The cognitive process of regulating emotion also involves identifying socially acceptable emotions and responses. The child or young person must recognize the need or importance of attempting to regulate emotion within the context of social display rules about regulating affective display.[14] As children and young people develop, they gain an increasing awareness and competence in utilizing these processes to identify a variety of emotional experiences, process them internally and then regulate their response to conform to social norms. When documenting functioning within these codes, researchers and clinicians should bear in mind social rules and an understanding that strength or valence of emotion may vary as a function of culture.[15]

b1522: Range of emotions
This code is described as the 'Mental functions that produce the spectrum of experience of arousal of affect or feeling such as love, hate, anxiousness, sorrow, joy, fear, and anger'.[1] The ICF-CY code 'range of emotion' appears to go beyond simple awareness of emotions and emotional variability. Instead, the code describes the 'experience of arousal' related to feelings. Thus, this code appears to speak predominantly to the ability to cognitively recognize the array of emotions or feeling states and then to experience a subsequent internal, physiological arousal. Arousal can be considered the degree or extent to which an individual experiences emotion,[10] and is considered a primary aspect of emotion that is important in emotional development.[16]

There is not agreement among professionals about the number of emotions that exist, and what these emotions may be. Some researchers describe only two basic emotional states, positive and negative, whereas others posit a spectrum of almost infinite emotions, with positive and negative emotions extending away from each other. Most theories of emotion include 'fear' and 'anger', and most include 'joy' and 'sorrow'.[7] These emotions are included in the ICF-CY examples of 'the spectrum' of emotional experiences; however, there may be considerable variability in how this code is utilized until a more definitive statement is made regarding the 'range' of emotions which should be considered.

It is not clear whether or how to utilize this code when one particular emotion dominates an individual's affective experience, but the individual has the cognitive capability of recognizing, understanding and experiencing arousal from other feeling states. For example, would b1522, range of emotions, be an appropriate code for documenting impairments in emotional functions described as mood disorders or anxiety disorders in the *Diagnostic and Statistical Manual of Mental Disorders*, fourth edition, text revision (DSM-IV-TR)?[17] The most likely answer to this question is that one may denote problems in functioning related to these disorders in b1522, but specifics of these disorders should be documented in disease-specific taxonomies, such as in chapter 5, 'Mental and behavioral disorders', of the *International Statistical Classification of Diseases and Related Health Problems*, 10th edition (ICD-10).[18] Considering the ICF-CY's definition of functioning, the author posits that the ICF-CY is not an appropriate tool for documenting particular emotionally related diseases or disorders (such as mood or anxiety disorders), and any measure devoted to diagnostics or measurement exclusively of problems related to these disorders is incongruent with the codes described within this chapter.

EXPERIENCE OF SELF AND TIME FUNCTIONS

As defined in the ICF-CY, code b180 describes 'Specific mental functions related to the awareness of one's identity, one's body, one's position in the reality of one's environment and time'.[1] Three subcodes include experience of self (b1800), body image (b1801) and experience of time (b1802). This group of codes relates to the subjective experiences of oneself, including identity and body image, as well as experiences of the passage of time. It may be helpful to distinguish b180 from the orientation functions, b114, in the ICF-CY. The orientation functions describe orientation of one's self in time, place and space, and they are more closely related to consciousness. They could be assessed by a cognitive status examination asking individuals to denote or acknowledge their understanding of who they are, where they are and the time in which they exist.

The experience of self and time functions are the more subjective, internal experience of understanding of one's self and are more difficult to measure. They describe the subjective experience of being a particular individual, and the possible maladaptive impairments in difficulty in perceiving oneself in a manner that would be consistent with others' 'reality'-based views of the individual and time. Experiences associated with these codes require self-awareness and self-reflection. Like the codes within emotional functions, codes within experience of self and time functions can be related to specific diagnostic criteria found within the DSM-IV-TR and the ICD-10. Impairments in specific cognitive functions can be documented using the ICF-CY codes, but any 'disorder' should

be coded elsewhere. The subjectivity of the experience of self and time codes is perhaps best demonstrated through details of the specific subcodes.

b1800: Experience of self
Examples within b1800, experience of self, include depersonalization and derealization. Depersonalization is a cognitive, internal phenomenon of feeling as though one is watching oneself act, without control over one's own actions. These feelings can be brought on by drug use, or experienced during panic attacks or as part of other DSM-IV-TR syndromes, such as dissociative disorder.[19] Experience of self, b1800, additionally provides derealization as an example, which is sometimes linked with depersonalization but can also be described separately. Derealization is the feeling of the external world being strange, unreal or altered in some way such that it is subjectively experienced by the individual as feeling abnormal.[20] Thus, experience of self is probably best described as the specific cognitive functions which create an internal sense of the self as being based in a world which feels real and in a way in which the individual perceives him- or herself as acting from within, with control over his or her actions. These experiences are completely internal, and impairments in functioning in these areas are only understood through individuals' verbal descriptions of their own experience, and possibly through observations of behaviour which seem 'odd'.

b1801: Body image
This code is defined as the 'specific mental functions related to the representation and awareness of one's body'.[1] Code b1801 refers to the perception of one's body's proportions and physical appearance, and whether this perception is congruent with others' 'reality'-based descriptions. The ICF-CY includes the experience of 'phantom limb' within this code, which suggests that the underlying basis for this code is the ability to accurately perceive aspects of one's body. Body image is a topic that is frequently discussed in literature related to eating disorders, and it should be noted that descriptions and perceptions of one's body may vary as a function of social rules and cultural norms, particularly in relation to sex and socialization.[21]

b1802: Experience of time
This code is described as the 'specific mental functions of the subjective experiences related to the length and passage of time'.[1] Inclusions are the feelings of jamais vu and déjà vu. Jamais vu is the subjective experience of suddenly not recognizing a situation or stimuli which would be considered common or easily recognizable to

the individual. Déjà vu is the subjective feeling of experiencing or seeing something which one has experienced or seen before, although logic would dictate this to be impossible. Like all of the codes considered in this chapter, this subcode is not directly observable and speaks to the subjective interpretations of experiences. Jamais vu and déjà vu have been described as occurring in populations without significant pathology related to dissociation, and are probably experienced at some point in most individuals within the general population.[22] When frequently occurring, these experiences can be disruptive to the individual and impair functioning, such that impairments coded in b1802 would probably represent challenges owing to the frequency of these experiences.

OVERLAPPING CHARACTERISTICS

In the current literature, one does not often find isolated descriptions of the specific constructs in the codes for functioning related to emotions or experiences of self and time. These aspects of functioning are often described within a larger context or in conjunction with other aspects of functioning. For example, it is common to read about a child's 'socioemotional' functioning or to find 'behavioural and emotional disorders' grouped together within a textbook. Because subjective experiences, like those described by the ICF-CY codes of interest, deal with similar issues in measurement and intervention, it is also common to find descriptions of emotional development coupled with descriptions of the development of the concept of self, or self versus others, and the development of identity and self-concept. Within this chapter, the concepts embedded in the ICF-CY codes for emotional functions and experience of self and time functions are maintained as distinct concepts, but considering these aspects in terms of functioning and in isolation from other concepts or aspects of functioning is atypical in existing measures.

General factors to consider when measuring this domain

At this point it should be clear that the codes b152, emotional functions, and b180, experience of self and time functions, are quite subjective in nature. Adding to this complexity is the fact that these codes are specific cognitive functions, which are internal and therefore not directly observable. Thus, approaches to measuring the constructs within these codes are attempts to infer internal processes.

METHODS OF MEASUREMENT

Measuring emotional functioning and experience of self and time functions is a challenging endeavour. Many of the constructs are abstract, and many of the experiences are subjective and internal. Measuring or capturing these

constructs will depend partly on theoretical perspective. For example, measuring emotional functions will necessarily vary as a function of one's beliefs about what emotions are and what aspects of emotion are of interest to study or clinical practice.[23] For this reason, measures related to emotion vary from measuring heart rate when shown various images, to estimating brain activity through electrophysiological recordings when presented stimuli, to an individual rating his or her emotional experience at various points in the day. Regardless of theoretical perspective, however, the literature is clear: assessment of subjective experiences requires a complex approach that is multimethod,[24] multi-informant[25] and across multiple settings and contexts.[26]

Multiple methods or modes of assessment

Multimethod assessment incorporates various assessment approaches, such as observations, interviews, record reviews, norm-referenced measures and informal assessment procedures. Direct observations of the child or adolescents are very important, as many subjective, internal experiences are believed to be expressed in observable behaviour. Interviews provide accounts of the child or adolescent's functioning across time and contexts and allow for information about development, the family's culture and beliefs, and the child or adolescent's past and current experiences to surface for incorporation into considerations of functioning. Record reviews serve a similar function, as they provide additional information regarding the child or adolescent's everyday context, history and overall functioning.

When selecting norm-referenced measures to capture subjective experiences, it is important to select measures which were normed on populations reflecting the child's characteristics. Researchers and clinicians should also be cautious in selecting measures which provide descriptions of child functioning or development as opposed to measures which exclusively capture whether a child's behaviour is problematic or consistent with specific diagnostic criteria for disorders discussed in other taxonomies. Ideally, these measures will also allow for the child's strengths and competences to be apparent and measurable as areas of concern. Informal approaches, which ask the child or young person to complete a task which has no norms or standardization, can complement the other approaches by providing further descriptive information regarding the child's functioning and internal experiences.

Multiple Informants

Data should also be gathered through interviews and ratings scales from multiple informants. Self-reports and self-ratings are considered integral to assessing emotions and experiences of self and time because of their subjective nature. That is, it is the individual's report which instigates further investigation or review of functioning. It may be challenging for children and young people to describe or rate their own experiences because of their relative lack of life experience, the developmental quality of their language skills and their ability to understand abstract concepts such as emotion. Nonetheless, it is important to gather information from the child about his or her own thoughts, feelings and experiences.

In an attempt to estimate the accuracy of children's reports and to consider more 'objective' views of child functioning, data should also be gathered from other informants who know the child well. For children and young people, these informants may be family members, teachers or caregivers, recreational leaders or coaches, and other adults in the children and adolescents' lives. Information from multiple informants is particularly important in determining the appropriateness of the child's subjective experiences, as full descriptions will be needed concerning the context and situations surrounding the child's functioning.

Multiple Settings
Children and young people experience life across many settings and locations. It is important to consider children's functioning across these locations, as impairments in one setting and not another suggest the salience of factors in the environment as negatively impacting the child's functioning as opposed to a disturbance in the child's overall functioning for a particular area. Given the salience of family members in children's development, it is imperative to include observations and information of children's functioning in the home.[27] Children and young people exist and interact with others across many settings, however, so it is equally important to consider their emotional functions in school or day care and other important locations in the community (such as the playground or libraries).

FACTORS RELATING TO FUNCTIONING VERSUS DISABILITY OR SPECIFIC DISORDER
Before conducting an assessment to gain insight into a child's functioning in regards to emotion or experience of self and time, researchers and clinicians need to first identify the goals of the assessment. The ICF-CY is a person- and functioning-orientated taxonomy based on a social model of health and disability. It is not a diagnostic taxonomy of disorders and does not focus on disease-specific or diagnostic criteria, as is the role of the ICD-10 or the DSM-IV-TR. This distinction is crucial to a discussion of assessment goals and measurement selection. If the assessment goal is to describe children's functioning and development in general – an approach congruent with the ICF-CY – then the researcher or clinician will need to utilize an assessment approach consistent with the one described above and discussed later in this chapter.

If the researcher or clinician is more interested in describing the child's problems in relation to a specific disability or disorder, however, then the approach will probably utilize measures based on the criteria described in other taxonomies, such as the DSM-IV-TR or the ICD-10. There are many existing tools that measure symptoms or experiences consistent with criteria for specific disorders which negatively impact an individual's functioning. More specifically, there are many existing measures designed to identify whether a child or young person experiences clinical or subclinical levels of problems related to emotional (mood or anxiety) disorders, dissociative disorders or eating disorders (which incorporate problems with body image). These are problem-orientated measures with the goal of determining whether a child may or may not meet diagnostic criteria for specific DSM-orientated disorders. For example, the Children's Depression Inventory[28] is a screen for assessing whether a child may meet the diagnostic criteria for a mood disorder, and depressive experiences specifically, according to the DSM-IV-TR. Other measures look specifically at anxiety disorder issues, and others are used to estimate the child's functioning in relation to criteria for disorders of dissociation or schizophrenia. These measures are specific to problems associated with distinct diagnostic criteria found in another taxonomy (the DSM-IV-TR) and are not consistent with an approach based on the ICF-CY.

AGE AND DEVELOPMENT
Overviews of emotional development and the developing understanding of self provide important information for assessing outcomes in the ICF-CY codes of interest in this chapter. As previously mentioned, there is a large emphasis on self-report in assessing the subjective experiences described in this chapter. However, the ability to identify and describe experiences and emotion develops over time and in tandem with the development of a greater understanding of self and self in relation to others. The ICF-CY codes for emotional functions and experiences of self and time also require a judgement of the relative appropriateness of the child and adolescent's subjective experiences. In order to make this determination, the researcher or clinician must first understand developmentally appropriate experiences and milestones related to emotional development and understanding of the self. Additionally, it is commonly believed that developmental considerations must be included in assessing the

appropriateness of children and adolescents' subjective experiences, including their emotional development.[27,29–30] This section reviews key developmental considerations and emotional milestones across phases of development, from infancy through adolescence.

Infancy through early childhood

Emotional milestones in infants include an emerging awareness of variable emotional states. Infants move from generalized affective states (i.e. experiences of happiness, fear, anger, sadness, and sometimes interest, surprise and disgust) to more specific emotional experiences[31] over the first 2 years of life as they gradually develop an understanding of the self, as differentiated by others, and use self-experience as a tool for understanding others and their experiences.[32] This new understanding provides the foundation for self-conscious emotions,[33] such as shame, embarrassment, guilt, envy and pride. It also sets the stage for greater awareness about one's own experiences, although the constructs found in the codes for experience of self and time have not been frequently discussed in literature regarding such young children. Emotional regulation also develops in stages, from reliance upon and use of caregivers to facilitate regulation of emotions[34] to more obvious attempts to control (or regulate) emotion as children approach 3 years of age[31] and they develop and use greater attentional and inhibitory control.[14] Preschool children also begin to mask emotions by altering facial expressions as a result of increasing awareness of the need to manage emotions to meet social standards or social display rules.[35] As children cannot accurately or reliably express their inner thoughts, as would be required to adequately describe their emotions or experiences of self and time at this phase of development,[36] parent report and direct observations are considered the most appropriate assessment approaches for measuring competences in infants, toddlers and young children.[27]

Middle and late childhood

Regulating and managing emotions and affective display is one of the most important competences of mid- to late childhood. Emotions are increasingly regulated as neurophysiological systems mature along with more sophisticated language, cognitive abilities and the development of emotional understanding.[37] In attempts to be more socially desirable or acceptable, children develop strategies to better suppress behaviours while experiencing a particular emotion, and can use strategies, often developed on their own, to redirect feelings. With greater emotional understanding, and more specifically an understanding of emotions as internal cognitive states, children

and adolescents employ a cognitive avoidance and confrontation approach as opposed to a physical one through behaviour.[38] Developing self-awareness also allows children in this stage of development to become more reliable informants of their internal experiences and to appreciate variability in their experiences of self and time. Coupled with their advancing language skills, young people in mid- to late childhood become capable of describing their internal experiences in a manner that conveys their experiences of self and time.

Adolescence

Identity development is a large task in mid- to late adolescence. Attuning to one's identity allows for greater reflection on subjective experiences of self, which are integral to adolescents' understanding of who they are. Emotional highs and lows are also hallmarks of adolescence and are developmentally appropriate in many ways, although the intensity and duration of emotions seems out of proportion given the demands in adolescents' lives and their previous management of emotions and affective display.[36] Adolescents possess the cognitive and language skills to adequately describe their internal, subjective experiences, but may choose to not do so for a variety of reasons. For example, adolescents become more adept at hiding their true emotions to observers, and they also may express internal discomfort through behaviour as opposed to using expressive language to describe uncomfortable internal states. At this phase of development, apparent emotional dysregulation, as observed through behaviour, can occur apart from or concurrent with atypical development and impairments in functioning.[36] Thus, adolescents are able to more accurately describe their internal experiences and experiences of time, but caution should be used in taking their statements at face value. To prevent misrepresentations of adolescents' functioning and any potential impairments, care must be taken in determining teenagers' motivations to describe their experiences as well as their relative ability to understand 'reality' and their experiences relative to this 'reality'.

MEASUREMENT CHALLENGES

'It is no easy matter to assess subjective experience, especially if what is wanted is something more than simply the amount of positive or negative emotion.'[2] This quote from Paul Ekman about capturing subjective experiences, and emotion in particular, is at the heart of the discussion of how to accurately assess or measure outcomes for emotional functions and experience of self and time functions. There are numerous conceptual, methodological and theoretical concerns in researchers' and clinicians' attempts to infer subjective emotional experiences with the existing measures.[3] Accurate measurement requires clearly defined constructs which are linked to quantifiable, concrete objective, observable phenomena. The mere idea of measuring a subjective experience is a bit of an oxymoron, as it insinuates an attempt to quantify something which may not be objectively definable.

There are few existing measures which seem to capture the spirit of functioning in these codes, as most related measures provide estimates of psychopathology consistent with the DSM-IV-TR or ICD-10. In assessing these subjective experiences, it is best to consider qualitatively describing an individual's experience, using a variety of methodologies, and quantitatively measuring any aspects which can be defined objectively and directly observed. Research utilizing outcomes on these codes poses a challenge because measurement of these constructs requires a complex, integrated approach to assessment. Such an approach is time-intensive and costly, and there are no guidelines on ways to integrate information to establish estimates of functioning. Thus, as currently defined and described in the ICF-CY, emotional functions and experiences of time and self may not be feasibly measured in a manner which is reliable and replicable for the purposes of research. It is not impossible to estimate functioning for constructs within these codes, however, and clinicians with sufficient time and resources can benefit their clients and patients by describing their functioning in these important areas. For those wishing to capture a description of a child or adolescent's functioning, the ICF-CY codes provide an opportunity to describe these internal experiences and functions with a broad stroke without resorting to diagnostic labels or criteria.

Overview of recommended measures

To measure emotional functions and experience of self and time in a manner consistent with the ICF-CY, clinicians and researchers need to use a complex approach incorporating facets of best practice in general assessment and factors specific to the study of emotion. There are few existing measures which can contribute data for 'emotional functions' and 'experience of self and time functions' consistent with the spirit and approach of the ICF-CY. In addition, there are special considerations for conducting assessments of subjective experiences with children and young people. Therefore, a qualitative description of children's functioning and development must be integrated with quantitative data based on the multimodal, multi-informant, multisetting approach previously described. It is imperative that the assessment approach provides the opportunity to describe areas of strength and weakness in the child's development and functioning.

This section elaborates on approaches which can contribute information for the purpose of describing children's functioning. Described first is the use of the interview as a tool for capturing important data related to children and adolescents' functioning. The section continues with a review of three existing measures, which provide estimates of functioning through three approaches: observations, self-report rating scales and questionnaires, and parent/caregiver rating scales and questionnaires. These measures were selected as those which probably best represent the constructs found in the ICF-CY definitions of emotional functions, as they appear consistent with describing functioning as opposed to specific psychopathology. Readers will note that the measures emphasize emotional functions, as there do not appear to be resources and tools for considering those experiences described as related to self and time in isolation – that is, apart from estimates of specific pathologies. Readers should bear in mind that these measures are *not* sufficient on their own to describe functioning in these areas, and information from these measures should be integrated with information from other approaches to describe children and young people's emotional functioning and experience of self and time functioning.

Finally, an additional section is provided that acknowledges the existence of many rating scales which have been developed for the purposes of identifying whether young people may exhibit the symptoms of specific disorders, such as depression or anxiety. A common measure utilized within this context is reviewed, and a list of other available measures is provided in Appendix 10.1 for readers who are interested in such measures, although their framework is not necessarily consistent with the language of the ICF-CY.

THE INTERVIEW

The interview may be the most versatile and useful tool for collecting information regarding human functioning. How the interview is designed and used will vary, partly as a function of an individual's professional role and responsibilities, but the ultimate goal of an interview for assessment purposes is to 'obtain relevant, reliable, and valid information about the interviewee'[39] and his or her functioning. This chapter is not geared towards a comprehensive review of interview purposes, goals and techniques; there are a number of excellent books and guides regarding interviewing, such as the comprehensive guide to interviewing youth authored by Jerome Suttler.[40]

For the purposes of gaining information regarding a child or adolescent's emotional functioning and experience of self and time functions, the clinician or researcher will need to incorporate a number of important considerations. Interviewers should begin by defining the constructs of interest and develop questions which address functioning on these constructs. How these questions are formulated, and which aspects of functioning are explored, will depend on the child or adolescent's age and developmental level. The age and developmental considerations discussed earlier in this chapter should help the interviewer to formulate meaningful questions around those milestones, skills and abilities which are integral to a child or adolescent's functioning. The interview should incorporate questions regarding the child's functioning across contexts and time, as well as with different individuals in their lives. Because of the subjective nature related to such issues as 'appropriateness', the interviewer additionally should ask about family routines, beliefs, values, expectations, attitudes and

rules. Areas of strength and concern should be explored in terms of how frequently these skills or behaviours occur, and the interviewee's perception of severity of any problems. The structure and language used in the interview will depend on the interviewee. It is important for interviews to be conducted with salient individuals in the child or adolescent's life, including the child or adolescent as much as is feasible.

OBSERVATIONS

Observations are often considered to be attempts to capture emotional functioning without having to rely on self-reports of internal experiences. These may include observations of motor behaviour, behaviours following emotional elicitation or arousal, and rate and tone of

FACIAL ACTION CODING SYSTEM (FACS)	
Purpose	To measure, describe and categorize facial behaviours
Population	All ages, all populations. Infant FACS is available for use with infants
Description of domains (subscales)	Facial behaviours are described on facial action units in the upper and lower face
Administration and test format	Time to complete: administration time will depend on the number of expressions to be recorded. Coding and measuring facial units will depend on familiarity with FACS, physiology and the software Testing format: facial expressions are video-recorded Scoring: recorded facial expressions are coded according to facial action units and measured accordingly Training: extensive training is required. Training can occur alone or in groups and with or without an expert leader or adviser. Workshops sponsored by FACS are also available. A 370-page self-instructional text is available on CD, which comes with the investigator's guide. A certification test is available
Psychometric properties	Normative sample: children without disabilities; children with disabilities *Reliability* Extensive data suggest good to excellent interobserver agreement across each facial action unit (for the half-second tolerance window, kappa coefficients range from 0.56 to 0.97) with moderate stability *Validity* There appears to be good concurrent validity across five approaches, detailed more specifically in Cohn et al (2007) (see Key references)
How to order	FACS 2002 is available on CD-ROM, which can be ordered from www.paulekman.com Cost is US$260 per CD-ROM
Key references	Cohn JF, Ambador Z, Ekman P (2007) Observer-based measurement of facial expression with the facial action coding system. In: Coan JA, Allen JJB, editors. *Handbook of Emotion Elicitation and Assessment.* New York: Oxford University Press, pp. 203–221. Ekman P, Friesen WV, Hager J (2002) *Facial Action Coding System Investigators' Guide* [E-book]. Salt Lake City, UT: Research Nexus.

speech. Some observational methodology may be quite simple and require only a well-developed technique, without the need for any particular measure. For example, observing delay of gratification would require set rules for when gratification is achieved, and a timing device to measure the amount of time from presentation of the desired stimulus and start of gratification.

There are, however, measures which incorporate observation and provide a measurement of a particular behaviour or experience. Observing emotional expressiveness in terms of facial expression has been of interest to many researchers for over a hundred years.[41] In the ICF-CY, congruence of affect with a situation and the regulation of emotional expression could feasibly be documented through behavioural observations of facial expression in given situations, along with a description of the expected affective experience given the child or adolescent's age and relative abilities and sociocultural rules. There are many systems for coding emotional expression, but the Facial Action Coding System (FACS) has been considered 'the most comprehensive, psychometrically rigorous, and widely used'.[41]

Overview and purpose
The FACS is a comprehensive system for describing and coding facial expressions as a mechanism for inferring underlying emotional experiences or feeling states. The FACS system describes facial action units, described and based on the fact that almost all people have the same facial muscles, which allow the face to make only certain expressions. The FACS allows researchers or clinicians to capture and document physiological responses to specific stimuli, so that the import of these facial actions can be defined and understood. How or why facial actions are being observed may vary substantially, depending on the question in consideration. Facial actions for an individual could potentially be compared with those of others or what was expected given existing research, cultural and social expectations, and the assumed appropriate affective response for the situation or stimuli.

Administration and scoring
The FACS involves video-recording facial expressions and then coding these expressions on nine action units in the upper face and 18 action units in the lower face. These units all relate to expressions of facial features, such as actions made by the eyebrows, eyelids, lips, nose, cheeks, chin and jaw, and as seen in head position. The facial action units are scored on a number of possible dimensions which are too complex to fully describe here. The action units can be coded using a comprehensive or selective coding system; a presence/absence or intensity

coding system; and the coding of multiple events or single events. Multiple methods may be employed and integrated for a single study. To make inferences regarding an individual's underlying emotion, based on their facial expression, researchers or clinicians must utilize a number of resources. Available resources include the FACS instructional text on compact disk, including the investigator's guide.[42]

Psychometric properties
Reliability information for the FACS stems primarily by a study by Sayette et al,[43] but other studies have provided further evidence of reliability. Reliability information is reported as interobserver agreement for each facial action unit, and so is quite extensive. Overall, there appears to be average reliability across all facial action units. There are also reliability estimates for aspects of coding, such as occurrence and temporal precision, coding of intensity and coding for specific events, called aggregates. Concurrent validity has been supported across five approaches, including performed action criterion and electrical activity criterion. Moderate stability has been reported for the actions, units and predictive validity in regards to personality-based and clinical outcomes.[41]

SELF-REPORT RATING SCALES AND QUESTIONNAIRES
Because emotional functions and experiences of self and time relate to subjective experiences, great importance is placed on self-reports of functioning. Self-report measures have a number of advantages and disadvantages, and when working with children and young people even more caution must be used when interpreting information from self-report measures. As discussed in previous sections, children are not as aware or insightful of their feelings, expressions and general functioning, so their perceptions as reported on self-report questionnaires must be understood for what they are: the child's own understanding and report of subjective experiences. The greatest advantage of self-report questionnaires is their ease of use and their time and cost-effectiveness. One promising measure for eliciting estimates of a child's perceptions of his or her regulation and range of emotions is 'How I Feel' (HIF).[10]

Overview and purpose
The HIF measure is a 30-item multidimensional self-report of arousal (range of emotion) and control (regulation of emotion) for 8- to 12-year-old children. It includes dimensions of intensity and frequency for both positive and negative emotions, and an estimate of emotional control.

How I Feel (HIF)	
Purpose	To provide a quantitatively based estimate of positive and negative emotional arousal (range of emotions) and control (regulation of emotion) in children
Population	Ages 8–12y
Description of domains (subscales)	Provides self-estimates on frequency and intensity of positive emotion, negative emotion and emotion control
Administration and test format	Time to complete: 10–15min to administer; about 10min to score Testing format: 30-item self-report measure; each item is responded to using a five-point Likert-style rating scale (where 1 represents the lowest score and 5 represents the highest) Scoring: subscale scores are the sum of items constituting the subscale; higher scores represent a greater amount of the construct describing the subscale Training: requires relatively little training, although an understanding of the role and purpose of self-report measures and the constructs in question would be integral
Psychometric properties	Normative sample: although thousands of children completed HIF in studies, the one described sample consisted of only 349 children approximating national proportions of sociocultural diversity *Reliability* Strong internal consistency (alpha coefficients from 0.84 to 0.90). Good stability over time (test–retest correlations 0.37–0.63) *Validity* Very strong construct validity with other emotion-based measures using convergent and discriminative validity
How to order	Provided at no charge. A copy of the measure can be found in the appendix of the key reference. Dr Tedra Walden can be contacted at tedra.walden@vanderbilt.edu
Key reference	Walden TA, Harris VS, Catron TF (2003) How I Feel: A self-report measures of emotional arousal and regulation for children. *Psychol Assess* 15: 399–412.

Administration and scoring

Children complete HIF by rating 30 sentence prompts for 'how true each was of you in the past three months'. The rating scale includes: 1 (not at all true of me), 2 (a little true of me), 3 (somewhat true of me), 4 (pretty true of me) and 5 (very true of me). Scores are summed to determine values on three subscales: positive emotion, negative emotion and emotion control. Higher scores indicate greater amounts of the construct describing that subscale, that is the higher the score on emotion control, the greater the amount of emotional control perceived and described by the child. Based on studies conducted by HIF developers, there are means and standard deviations for items and subscales by sex and age (≤10y or >10y).

Psychometric properties

The HIF measure was developed and reviewed using samples of children in the USA from diverse sociocultural backgrounds approximating national proportions of race and ethnicity. Item development and selection occurred across two pilot administrations, with a total sample of over 650 children in grades 3 to 6. Ten experts reviewed the items, and there was 96.4% agreement for item selection, suggesting strong content validity. Internal consistency was very strong, with alpha coefficients from 0.84 to 0.90. The reliability and validity of the three-subscale model was confirmed in studies using over 1500 children. Results from the studies suggested moderate longitudinal stability and established excellent construct validity using both convergent and discriminative validity.

PARENT/CAREGIVER RATING SCALES AND QUESTIONNAIRES

Rating scales completed by family members and teachers are also very important in measuring emotional functioning and experience of self and time functions. Rating scales and questionnaires can not only supplement information provided by parents and caregivers during the interview, but when they are standardized and normed they can provide estimates of the child's functioning in relation to children of similar age, sex, race/ethnicity and background. As noted previously, there are many rating scales related to children and young people's emotions and experiences of self and time, but they are orientated towards determining the presence of specific disabilities or disorders. One measure which appears to provide an estimate of child functioning, as well as pathology-orientated problems, is the Infant–Toddler Social and Emotional Assessment (ITSEA).[44]

Overview and purpose

The ITSEA is a comprehensive questionnaire providing a profile of 1- to 3-year-old children's strengths and weaknesses in the socioemotional domain. Not all of the domains and subscales of this measure are a fit with the ICF-CY; however, the information gathered and developmentally appropriate questions for infants and toddlers provide an opportunity to estimate some aspects of emotional functions and functioning of the self. Note this measure incorporates the concept of 'social–emotional' functioning, so its use for 'emotional functions'

INFANT–TODDLER SOCIAL AND EMOTIONAL ASSESSMENT (ITSEA)	
Purpose	To profile strengths and weaknesses of children's socioemotional functioning
Population	Children aged 1–3y
Description of domains (subscales)	166 items determining subscales within four broad domains: externalizing, internalizing, dysregulation and competences. Three additional indices of clinically significant behaviours include maladaptive behaviour, atypical behaviour and social relatedness
Administration and test format	Time to complete: 25–30min to administer/complete; 30min to score
	Testing format: 166-item questionnaire provided to parent or caregiver; can be administered as an interview
	Scoring: three-point rating scale (not true/rarely true; somewhat true/sometimes true; very true/often true) with the option to indicate behaviours not previously observed
	Training: administration requires minimal training; interpretation requires knowledge of standardized tests and knowledge specific to young children's development
Psychometric properties	Normative sample: national sample of 600 children, including children who were preterm at birth, those who had language delay and children with other diagnosed disorders
	Reliability Strong internal consistency (0.78–0.92 across domains) and test–retest reliability (0.61–0.91 across scales) established
	Validity Acceptable, moderate criterion-related validity established
How to order	The ITSEA kit with Scoring Assistant can be purchased for US$219 from Pearson Education, Inc. Details and orders can be found or made through http://pearsonassess.com
Key references	Briggs-Gowan MJ, Carter AS (1998) Preliminary acceptability and psychometrics of the Infant–Toddler Social and Emotional Assessment (ITSEA): A new adult-report questionnaire. *Infant Mental Health* 19: 422–445.
	Carter AS, Little C, Briggs-Gowan M, Kogan N (1999) The Infant–Toddler Social and Emotional Assessment (ITSEA): Parent ratings and observations of attachment, mastery motivation, emotion regulation and coping behaviours. *Infant Mental Health* 20: 1–18.
	Carter AS, Briggs-Gowan MJ, Jones SM, Little TD (2003) The Infants Toddler Social and Emotional Assessment: Factor structure, reliability, and validity. *J Abnorm Child Psychol* 31: 495–514.
	Carter AS, Briggs-Gowan MJ, Ornstein-Davis N (2004) Assessment of young children's social–emotional development and psychopathology: recent advances and recommendations for practice. *J Child Psychol Psychiatry* 45: 109–134.

in the ICF-CY requires some extrapolation or isolation of constructs.

Administration and scoring

Parents or caregivers complete a 166-item parent or caregiver form regarding the functioning of the infant or toddler. T-scores are calculated for 17 subscales within the four domains, including the externalizing domain (subscales of activity/impulsivity, aggression/defiance, peer aggression), internalizing domain (subscales of depression/withdrawal, general anxiety, separation distress, inhibition to novelty), dysregulation (subscales of sleep, negative emotionality, eating, sensory sensitivity) and competence (subscales of compliance, attention, imitation/play, mastery motivation, empathy, prosocial peer relations). There are three additional indices to describe clinically severe behaviour, associated with social relatedness and maladaptive and atypical behaviours. A Scoring Assistant® software program is available (http://shop1.mailordercentral.com/aseba/), which provides domain and subscale scores with a parent report.

Psychometric properties

Three studies have reviewed the reliability and validity of the ITSEA,[45–47] with the most recent study[47] using a large cohort of children born healthy to families in either urban or suburban areas in order to confirm the structure of the scales and domains. Acceptable internal consistency (0.78–0.92 for the domains) and test–retest reliability (0.61–0.91 across scales) have been found,[45] with moderate criterion-related validity.[27]

MEASURES CAPTURING SYMPTOMS OF DISORDERS

One of the challenges of authoring this chapter was to avoid the temptation to rely upon measures which are probably more in tune to the ICD-10 or DSM-IV-TR as opposed to the ICF-CY. There are a large number of rating scales and rating scale systems which are held in high regard by clinicians for the purposes of supporting the process of considering whether adolescents may exhibit the symptoms of specific cognitive health disorders, such as depression and anxiety – specific disorders described and listed within the ICD and DSM-IV-TR, but not within the ICF-CY (the ICF-CY describes functioning and not diagnostic criteria for disorders). These rating scales are very useful and helpful for diagnostic endeavours and they should not be ignored. As such, Appendix 10.1 provides a list of common measures utilized for the purposes of aiding diagnostic decision-making when considering the possibility that a child or adolescent may suffer from depression, anxiety and/

or disorders related to difficulties with the experience of self and time. It should be noted that the list is not exhaustive and that the exclusion of these measures from the main text of this chapter is not meant to suggest that their psychometric properties are lacking; in fact, the measures listed in Appendix 10.1 have been validated within the research literature for their utility in exploring whether adolescents may have various cognitive health disorders.

One of the measures listed in Appendix 10.1 is actually an entire system of rating scales, the Achenbach System of Empirically Based Assessment (ASEBA).[48] The ASEBA system includes rating scales designed to capture adaptive and maladaptive functioning across the lifespan, from 18 months to 90 years of age. Direct observation forms are also available, but are not discussed here. The ASEBA system's focus on functioning is at times consistent with the ICF-CY framework, as its goal is to enhance in-depth assessment; however, there is a clear slant towards establishing whether a child or adolescent meets the diagnostic criteria for a specific cognitive health disorder.

There are two ASEBA systems for children and adolescents. The Preschool Forms and Profiles[49] are for children aged 18 months to 5 years, and each rating scale comprises 99 questions plus the option of rating one or more additional respondent-identified concerns. The School-Age Forms and Profiles[50] are for children aged 6 to 18 years, and each rating scale comprises 112 questions plus the option of rating one or more additional respondent-identified concerns on the forms completed by respondents who are not the individuals in question. There are parent- or primary caregiver-completed Child Behavioral Checklist Language Development Surveys for children aged 18 months to 5 years (CBCL-LDS) and adolescents aged 6 to 18 years (CBCL); care-provider or teacher rating scales for children aged 18 months to 5 years (C-TRF) and teacher-completed rating scales (TRF) for adolescents aged 6 to 18 years; and a self-report measure for adolescents aged 11 to 18 years (YSR). The CBCL-LDS for children aged 18 months to 5 years includes an LDS, and the school-age series provides an opportunity to describe a child's competences on various activities and academic domains. Respondents rate each problem item as not true of the child (score of 0), somewhat or sometimes true of the child (score of 1) or very true or often true of the child (score of 2). Items are grouped into 'syndrome scales' and 'DSM-orientated scales', and the sum of the raw scores of items within a scale are converted into T-scores based on either a national sample (USA) or a multicultural sample.[51,52] Computerized scoring is available.

ACHENBACH SYSTEM OF EMPIRICALLY BASED ASSESSMENT (ASEBA): PRESCHOOL-AGE FORMS AND PROFILES AND SCHOOL-AGE FORMS AND PROFILES	
Purpose	To obtain and summarize information on young people's competences and specific behavioural and emotional challenges
Population	Preschool age: 18mo–5y School age: 6–18y
Description of domains (subscales)	*Preschool age* 'Syndrome scales': emotionally reactive, anxious/depressed, somatic complaints, withdrawn, attention problems, aggressive behaviour and sleep problems (CBCL-LDS only) 'DSM-orientated scales': affective problems, anxiety problems, pervasive developmental problems, attention-deficit–hyperactivity problems and oppositional defiant problems *School age* 'Syndrome scales': anxious/depressed, withdrawn/depressed, somatic complaints, social problems, thought problems, attention problems, rule-breaking behaviour and aggressive behaviour 'DSM-orientated scales': affective problems, anxiety problems, somatic problems, attention-deficit–hyperactivity problems, oppositional defiant problems and conduct problems
Administration and test format	Time to complete: respondent completion takes 15–20min Testing format: for the preschool age system, 100 problem items are rated by the respondent (caregiver or care-provider) with the option of completing a Language Development Survey. For the school-age system, 118 problem items are rated by the respondent (caregiver, teacher or self-report for children age 11–18y) and information is provided by a respondent to describe a child's competences in activities and school Scoring: three-point rating scale (not true; somewhat or sometimes true; very true or often true) of each problem item, resulting in calculated T-scores for subscales. Computer scoring is available. Cross-informant comparisons can be completed if multiple forms are completed for a particular individual Training: administration requires minimal training; interpretation requires knowledge of standardized tests and knowledge specific to development, child and adolescent psychopathology, emotional regulation and behavioural challenges
Psychometric properties	Normative sample: normative sample varies by form. For preschool-age forms, the CBCL was normed on a national sample of 700 children and scales' scores are based on ratings of 1728 children, while the care-provider form was normed on 1192 children and scales' scores are based on ratings of 1113 children. For school-age forms, the CBCL was normed on 1753 children with scales' scores based on ratings of 4994 refereed children; the TRF was normed on 2319 non-referred children and scales' scores are based on ratings of 4437 refereed children; and the YSR was normed on 1057 non-refereed young people with scales' scores based on 2581 high-scoring young people. Multicultural norms are available for both the preschool-age and school-age forms *Reliability* For preschool-age forms, strong test–retest reliability (0.80–0.90s) established on all scales across forms. On school-age forms, problem-focused scales' test–retest reliability has been varied but robust across forms (CBCL: 0.90s; TRF: 0.90s; YSR: 0.80s). The DSM-orientated scales across forms have demonstrated moderately strong test–retest reliability (0.79–0.88) as well *Validity* For both the preschool-age and school-age systems, strong content validity, strong criterion-related validity and construct validity have been established

How to order	The ASEBA system can be purchased in whole or as parts, such as the preschool-age system, school-age system or measures within a system. The cost depends on the number of components purchased and whether hand- or computer-scoring is selected. ASEBA products can be viewed and ordered through the website (www.aseba.org)
Key references	Achenbach TM (2000) *The Achenbach System of Empirically Based Assessment (ASEBA): Development, Findings, Theory, and Applications.* Burlington, VT: University of Vermont Research Center for Children, Youth, and Families.
	Achenbach TM, Rescorla LA (2000) *Manual for the ASEBA Preschool Forms & Profiles.* Burlington, VT: University of Vermont, Research Center for Children, Youth, and Families.
	Achenbach TM, Rescorla LA (2001) *Manual for the ASEBA School-Age Forms & Profiles.* Burlington, VT: University of Vermont, Research Center for Children, Youth, and Families.

Final thoughts and recommendations

The goal of this chapter was to provide an overview of emotional functions and experience of self and time functions as they exist in the ICF-CY, and to identify an approach to assessment that can provide estimates of children and adolescents' functioning on the constructs in these codes. To date, there do not appear to be many measures that provide estimates of functioning in these important areas, whereas there are many measures that do result in estimates of pathology. Because of the complexity of the constructs of interest and their subjective nature, measurement is further complicated by the need for a multimethod, multi-informant approach that considers multiple contexts.

The challenges which arose in writing this chapter suggest a few recommendations which could enhance the ICF-CY and its use in research and clinical settings. First, given the lack of consensus in emotion-based research, more specific definitions of 'emotional functions' in the ICF-CY would be very helpful. Second, there is a need for clearer distinctions between functioning in emotion and experience of self and time, as compared with the presence of specific disorders. That is, what is the role of documenting functions related to emotions and subjective experiences of self and time, and what do these functions look like more specifically compared with the disorders associated with these functions? Third, there is a need for measures which can capture estimates of functioning for these constructs, allowing for profiles of strengths and impairments in functioning to be documented.

REFERENCES

1. World Health Organization (2007) *International Classification of Functioning, Disability, and Health for Children and Youth (ICF-CY).* Geneva: World Health Organization.
2. Ekman P (1999) Basic emotions. In: Dalgleish T, Power M, editors. *Handbook of Cognition and Emotion.* Chichester: John Wiley & Sons, Ltd. Available at: www.vhml.org/theses/wijayat/sources/writings/papers/basic_emotions.pdf (accessed 12 February 2009).
3. Nielsen L, Kaszniak AW (2007) Conceptual, theoretical, and methodological issues in inferring subjective emotion experience: Recommendations for researchers. In: Coan JA, Allen JJB, editors. *Handbook of Emotion Elicitation and Assessment.* New York: Oxford University Press, pp. 360–377.
4. Gray EK, Watson D (2007) Assessing positive and negative affect via self-report. In: Coan JA, Allen JJB, editors. *Handbook of Emotion Elicitation and Assessment.* New York: Oxford University Press, pp. 171–183.
5. Meece JL, Daniels DH (2008) *Child and Adolescent Development for Educators*, 3rd edition. New York: McGraw-Hill.
6. Dworetsky JP (1985) *Psychology.* St Paul, MN: West Publishing Co.
7. Nesse RM, Ellsworth PC (2009) Evolution, emotions, and emotional disorders. *Am Psychol* 64: 129–139.

8. Williams JMG, Watts FN, MacLeod C, Matthews A. *Cognitive Psychology and Emotional Disorders,* 2nd edition. Chichester: John Wiley & Sons Ltd.
9. Underwood G (1954) Categories of adaptation. *Evolution* 8: 365–377.
10. Walden TA, Harris VS, Catron TF (2003) How I Feel: A self-report measures of emotional arousal and regulation for children. *Psychol Assess* 15: 399–412.
11. Cohn JF, Kanade T. Use of automated facial image analysis for measurement of emotional expression. In: Coan JA and Allen JJB, editors. *Handbook of Emotion Elicitation and Assessment.* New York: Oxford University Press, pp. 222–238.
12. Izard C (1977) *Human Emotions.* New York: Plenum.
13. John OP, Gross JJ (2004) Healthy and unhealthy emotion regulation: personality processes, individual differences, and life span development. *J Pers* 73: 1301–1333.
14. Henderson HA, Fox NA (2007) Considerations in studying emotion in infants and children. In: Coan JA, Allen JJB, editors. *Handbook of Emotion Elicitation and Assessment.* New York: Oxford University Press, pp. 349–360.
15. Ekman P (1992) An argument for basic emotions. *Cognition Emotion* 6: 169–200.
16. Thompson RA, Lewis MD, Calkins SD (2008) Reassessing emotion regulation. *Child Dev Perspectives* 2: 124–131.

17. American Psychiatric Association (2000) *Diagnostic and Statistical Manual of Mental Disorders*, 4th edition, text revision. Washington, DC: American Psychiatric Association.

18. World Health Organization (1992–1994) *International Classification of Diseases and Health Related Problems*, 10th revision, Vol. 1–3. Geneva: World Health Organization.

19. Radovic F, Radovic S (2002) Feelings of unreality: A conceptual and phenomenological analysis of the language of depersonalization. *Phil Psychiatry Psychol* 9: 271–279.

20. Hunter EC, Sierra M, David AS (2004) The epidemiology of depersonalisation and derealisation. A systematic review. *Soc Psychiatry Psychiatr Epidemiol* 39: 9–18.

21. Gilligan C (1982) *In a Different Voice. Psychological Theory and Women's Development.* Cambridge, MA: Harvard University Press.

22. Adachi N, Akanu N, Adachi T, et al (2008) Déjà vu experiences are rarely associated with pathological dissociation. *J Nerv Ment Dis* 196: 417–429.

23. Carlson JG, Hartfield E (1992) *Psychology of Emotion.* Fort Worth, TX: Holt, Rinehart, and Winston, Inc.

24. Larsen RJ, Prizmic-Larsen Z, Eid M, Diener E (2006) Measuring emotions: implications of a multimethod perspective. In: Eid M, Diener E, editors. *Handbook of Multimethod Measurement in Psychology.* Washington, DC: American Psychological Association, pp. 337–351.

25. Brandstatter H (2007) The time sampling diary (TSD) of emotional experience in everyday life situations. In: Coan JA, Allen JJB, editors. *Handbook of Emotion Elicitation and Assessment.* New York: Oxford University Press, pp. 318–331.

26. Ehrenreich JT, Fairholme CP, Buzzella BA, Ellard KK, Barlow B (2007) The role of emotion in psychological therapy. *Clin Psychologist* 14: 422–428.

27. Carter AS, Briggs-Gowan MJ, Ornstein-Davis N (2004) Assessment of young children's social–emotional development and psychopathology: recent advances and recommendations for practice. *J Child Psychol Psychiatry* 45: 109–134.

28. Kovacs M (1992) *The Children's Depression Inventory (CDI) Manual.* North Tonawanda, NY: Multi-Health Systems.

29. Zeman J, Klimes-Dougan B, Cassano M, Adrian M (2007) Measurement issues in emotion research with children and adolescents. *Clin Psychol Sci Pract* 14: 377–401.

30. Suveg C, Southam-Geraw MA, Goodman KL, Kendall PC (2007) The role of emotion therapy and research in child therapy development. *Clin Psychol Sci Pract* 14: 358–371.

31. Lewis M (2004) Overview of development from infancy through adolescence. In: Wiener JM, Dulcan ML, editors. *The American Psychiatric Publishing Textbook of Child and Adolescent Psychiatry,* 3rd edition. Washington, DC: American Psychiatric Publishing, Inc., pp. 13–44.

32. Meltzoff AN, Rechele R (2008) Self-experience as a mechanism for learning about others: A training study in social cognition. *Dev Psychol* 44: 1257–1265.

33. Saarni C, Mumme DL, Campos JJ (1998) Emotional development: Action, communication and understanding. In: Eisenberg N, editor. *Social, Emotional, and Personality Development: Handbook of Child Psychology,* Vol. 3. New York: John Wiley, pp. 237–309.

34. Santrock JW (2006) *Life-span Development,* 10th edition. New York: McGraw Hill.

35. Denham SA (1998) *Emotional Development in Young Children.* New York: Guilford Press.

36. Oltmanns TF, Emery RE (2004) *Abnormal Psychology,* 4th edition. Upper Saddle River, NJ: Pearson/Prentice Hall.

37. Gross JJ (1999) Emotion and emotion regulation. In: Pervin LA, John OP, editors. *Handbook of Personality: Theory and Research.* New York: Guilford Press, pp. 525–552.

38. Steege H, Meerum Twerogt M (1998) Perspectives on the strategic control of emotions: a developmental account. In:

Fischer A, editor. *Proceedings of the Xth Conference of the International Society for Research on Emotions.* Würzburg: ISRE Publications, pp. 45–47.

39. Sattler J, Mash EJ (1998) Introduction to clinical assessment interviewing. In: Sattler JM, editor. *Clinical and Forensic Interviewing of Children and Families: Guidelines for the Mental Health, Education, Paediatric, and Child Maltreatment Field.* San Diego, CA: Jerome M. Sattler, Publisher, Inc., pp. 2–44.

40. Sattler JM (1998) *Clinical and Forensic Interviewing of Children and Families: Guidelines for the Mental Health, Education, Paediatric, and Child Maltreatment Field.* San Diego, CA: Jerome M. Sattler, Publisher, Inc.

41. Cohn JF, Ambador Z, Ekman P (2007) Observer-based measurement of facial expression with the facial action coding system. In: Coan JA, Allen JJB, editors. *Handbook of Emotion Elicitation and Assessment.* New York: Oxford University Press, pp. 203–221.

42. Ekman P, Friesen WV, Hager J (2002) *Facial Action Coding System Investigators' Guide* [E-book]. Salt Lake City, UT: Research Nexus.

43. Sayette MA, Cohn JF, Wertz JM, Perrott MA, Parrott DJ (2001) A psychometric evaluations of the Facial Action Coding System for assessing spontaneous expression. *J Nonverbal Behav* 25: 167–186.

44. Carter AS, Briggs-Gowan ML (2005) *The Infant–Toddler Social and Emotional Assessment (ITSEA).* San Antonio, TX: Pearson Education, Inc.

45. Briggs-Gowan MJ, Carter AS (1998) Preliminary acceptability and psychometrics of the Infant–Toddler Social and Emotional Assessment (ITSEA): A new adult-report questionnaire. *Infant Mental Health* 19: 422–445.

46. Carter AS, Little C, Briggs-Gowan M, Kogan N (1999) The Infant–Toddler Social and Emotional Assessment (ITSEA): Parent ratings and observations of attachment, mastery motivation, emotion regulation and coping behaviors. *Infant Mental Health* 20: 1–18.

47. Carter AS, Briggs-Gowan MJ, Jones SM, Little TD (2003) The Infants Toddler Social and Emotional Assessment: Factor structure, reliability, and validity. *J Abnorm Child Psychol* 31: 495–514.

48. Achenbach TM (2009) *The Achenbach System of Empirically Based Assessment (ASEBA): Development, Findings, Theory, and Applications.* Burlington, VT: University of Vermont Research Center for Children, Youth, and Families.

49. Achenbach TM, Rescorla LA (2000) *Manual for the ASEBA Preschool Forms & Profiles.* Burlington, VT: University of Vermont, Research Center for Children, Youth, and Families.

50. Achenbach TM, Rescorla LA (2001) *Manual for the ASEBA School-Age Forms & Profiles.* Burlington, VT: University of Vermont, Research Center for Children, Youth, and Families.

51. Achenbach TM, Rescorla LA (2010) *Multicultural Supplement to the Manual for the ASEBA Preschool Forms & Profiles.* Burlington, VT: University of Vermont, Research Center for Children, Youth, and Families.

52. Achenbach TM, Rescorla LA (2007) *Multicultural Supplement to the Manual for the ASEBA School-Age Forms & Profiles.* Burlington, VT: University of Vermont, Research Center for Children, Youth, and Families.

53. Farrington A, Waller G, Smerden J, Faupel AW (2001) The adolescent dissociative experiences scale: psychometric properties and difference in scores across age groups. *J Nerv Ment Dis* 189: 722–727.

54. Beck AT, Steer RA, Brown GK (1996) *Manual for the Beck Depression Inventory,* 2nd edition. San Antonio, TX: The Psychological Corporation.

55. Angold A, Cox A, Prendergast M, Rutter M, Simonoff E (2008) *Child and Adolescent Psychiatric Assessment, Version 4.2.*

Available at: http://devepi.duhs.duke.edu/capa.html (accessed 15 September 2009).

56. Kovacs M (1992) *The Children's Depression Inventory Manual.* New York: Multi-Health Systems.

57. Butcher JN, Williams CL, Graham JR, et al (1992) *MMPI-A Manual for Administration, Scoring, and Interpretation.* Minneapolis, MN: University of Minnesota Press.

58. March JS, Parker JD, Sullivan K, Stallings P, Conners CK (1997) The Multidimensionsal Anxiety Scale for Children: factor structure, reliability, and validity. *J Am Acad Child Adolesc Psychiatry* 36: 554–565.

59. Reynolds CR, Richmond BO (2008) *Revised Children's Manifest Anxiety Scale,* 2nd edition. Torrance, CA: Western Psychological Services.

APPENDIX 10.1

Tools and measures to describe symptoms of mood disorders, anxiety disorders and disorders related to experience of self and time

Tool/measure	Mood disorders	Anxiety disorders	Disorders related to experience of self and time
Achenbach System of Empirically Based Assessment[48]	X	X	(X)
Adolescent Dissociative Experiences Scale[53]			X
Beck Depression Inventory-II[54]	X		
Child and Adolescent Psychiatric Assessment[55]	X	X	X
Children's Depression Inventory[56]	X		
Minnesota Multiphasic Personality Inventory, Adolescent Version[57]	X	X	X
Multidimensional Anxiety Scale for Children[58]		X	
Revised Children's Manifest Anxiety Scale[59]		X	

(X) indicates information on this construct that can be gleaned from responses on the measure, but this construct may not be directly measured.

11
SPECIFIC MENTAL FUNCTIONS: PERCEPTUAL (B156)

Suzanne Woods-Groves and Dennis C. Harper

What is the construct?

Perception functions is included under Mental Functions: Specific Mental Functions (b140–b189). Perceptual functions are 'specific mental functions of recognizing and interpreting sensory stimuli'.[1] As further noted in the text on classification, the codes on perceptual functions include auditory perception, visual perception, olfactory perception, gustatory perception, tactile perception and visuospatial perception. Hallucinations or illusions are included in this array, but remain unclear at the time of writing and so will not be discussed. Exclusions are noted as consciousness, orientation, attention, memory, mental functions of language, seeing and related functions, hearing and vestibular functions, and additional sensory functions. This entire area is very broad and rather difficult to define. We will confine our comments to the perceptual function measures available and offer suggestions on alternative methods for measurements where possible and other professionals who can assist in evaluations.

A contemporary definition of perceptual functions is based on a long and varied history in several bodies of literature, for example neuropsychology, neurology, occupational therapy and otolaryngology. Perception is the process of attaining an awareness or understanding of particular sensory information.[1] Evaluation of perception is a very complicated measurement task with many components, and we will offer comments and descriptions and, finally, assessment measures and strategies in several discrete areas. Four of the areas (auditory, visuospatial, olfactory, gustatory) will be noted separately. Visuospatial perception will also be discussed separately. Assessment of tactile and sensory measures appears in Chapter 13.

General factors to consider when measuring this domain

The screening of perceptual functions can be completed by proxy report, usually from a parent or a teacher, as an initial step. However, detailed assessment is often completed on an individual basis by a knowledgeable professional examiner. The validity and reliability of measures need to be reviewed as they are applied to the child/adolescent age group, and their feasibility with regard to the particular individual needs to be assessed. The majority of instruments and measures are designed based on and for individuals with 'average' or 'normal' physical, cognitive, sensory and perceptual skills. As an example, many instruments include questions, items or rankings based on normative skills and common experiences. In some instances, limitations due to a particular disability or functional limitation may result in an inappropriate and possibly inaccurate outcome score, reflective only of the inability of the individual to complete or respond to the item. This is a test-related limitation. This is often common in tests that did not include children with particular disabilities in the original development and norming of the test battery. Deficits for children and adolescents on such measures may give faulty interpretations and only document that the test is not a suitable measure for the specific test characteristic and the particular disability. Children and adolescents with developmental disabilities display variable, and in some instances idiosyncratic, rates of growth in many developmental areas. These growth rates can affect perceptual and sensory function. In some situations, skill development is hampered by a lag or a delay and may emerge at a later time in varying degrees. In other instances, children may reach a plateau in their development in particular domains, with no further change. Caution is therefore required in understanding and interpreting test results across a wide range of disabilities and age groups.

Generally, few perceptual measures have been developed for children and adolescents with developmental disabilities. Consequently, interpretation of results should be approached with caution. The child's age, developmental levels and ability to complete the measures are all key issues in this process. The use of multiple evaluation methods and multiple sources are always recommended. Proxy screening methods, when used, should be evaluated in reference to the particular respondent completing the proxy rating. Direct contact and review with the individual child is always useful in validating findings at some point. Knowledge of specific child/adolescent activity limitations is always useful in understanding their particular impact on measurement results and subsequent interpretation.

Several factors about subgroups of children with particular disabilities should be noted when using perceptual measures. Some children/adolescents are known to display behaviour patterns reflective of 'hypersensitivity' to touch, sound or other environmental and kinaesthetic stimuli. These behaviours can make assessments and their interpretation very challenging and may prevent the valid use or interpretation of particular perceptual measures. Individuals with neuromotor and neuromuscular disorders (e.g. cerebral palsy, muscular dystrophy) also display unique deficits in their ability to complete assessments, often invalidating some perceptual and sensory measures. Further, another subgroup of individuals with developmental disabilities may display unique behavioural phenotypes to include variable tempos, temperaments, activity levels and repetitive actions.[2] There may be an impact on the ability to complete the perceptual/sensory measure, and such behaviour is often very difficult to diagnose and accommodate. Aetiological evidence of these behavioural phenotypic patterns are often linked to genetic disorders.[3] For example, such behavioural patterns are recognized in children with Down syndrome, autism and Williams syndrome. Given the challenges of evaluating children with sensory, motor or behavioural difficulties, evaluation requires multiple measures to clearly elucidate abilities and deficit areas.

Assessment of visuospatial skills represents a combination of evaluating particular skills, their integration, their expression, and their impact on a child's functioning. Visuomotor and visuoperceptual dysfunction (delays or deficits) may have a significant and usually adverse impact on a child's functional skills. Aylward,[4] in his useful practitioner guide, notes the complexity in understanding visuomotor–visuoperceptual function:

A child with visual-motor impairment may not exhibit a visual-perceptual deficit; similarly, the reverse is also true. If a child can draw rapidly (without excessive effort) but is unable to recognize that the reproduction differs from the shape being copied, there is a strong likelihood that an underlying perceptual deficit exists. Conversely, if the child can recognize errors or discrepancies, but is unable to correct them, the likelihood of

having a visual-motor problem is high. Finally, a child who displays immature visual reproductions may have difficulty with the integration of perceptual and motor functions.

Aylward[4] (p. 189)

This statement defines the obvious complexity in evaluating and interpreting these common impairments in children and adolescents with disabilities. Additional complexity is also possible because these performances may reflect a delay, an emerging skill or a deficit in visuoperceptual/motor functioning. Time-referenced repeated evaluations are particularly important to clarify the need for intervention.

Particular evaluation of certain perceptual and sensory functions often requires a number of measurement tools. Such assessments may be performed by occupational therapists, paediatric neurologists, clinical neuropsychologists, speech/language therapists or audiologists. More specific evaluation of olfactory or gustatory skills may be accomplished by a paediatric otolaryngologist.

Overview of recommended measures
We recommend several key online resources for locating and reviewing tests. By far the most well-known site is the Buros Institute of Mental Measurements (www.unl. edu/buros/bimm./index.html). This institute produces a comprehensive review of numerous tests on a regular basis, reviewed by professionals in the field, and produces an extensive text for a fee. The American Psychological Association has a site that may assist as well, APAPsycNet (http://psycnet.apa.org/), which lists a variety of resources and journals. Finally, the Cochrane Library (www. cochrane.org/reviews/) is a resource for evidence and may also be helpful in the review of measures.

Auditory Perception

SCAN-3 for Children: Tests for Auditory Processing Disorders (SCAN-3:C) and SCAN-3 for Adolescents & Adults: Tests for Auditory Processing Disorders (SCAN-3:A)

Overview and purpose
The SCAN-3:C and SCAN-3:A are individually administered assessments designed to provide an appraisal of auditory processing abilities for the following areas: temporal processing, listening to noise, dichotic listening and listening to degraded speech.[5,6] The SCAN-3:C is intended for use with children who are 5 to 12 years of age. The SCAN-3:A is intended for use with adolescents and adults who are 13 to 50 years of age.

Administration and scoring

The manuals for the SCAN-3:C and SCAN-3:A are well written and provide extensive instructions for the administration, scoring and interpretation of assessment results. The SCAN-3:C and SCAN-3:A each comprise three screening tests, four diagnostic tests and three supplementary tests. Examinees are instructed to listen to sounds and to repeat words or sentences presented via a CD-ROM.[5,6] The SCAN-3:C and SCAN-3:A contain the following three screening tests: Gap Detection, designed to identify temporal processing problems; Auditory Figure-Ground (+8dB, SCAN-3:C; and 0dB, SCAN-3:A), designed to measure one's ability to understand words within the context of background noise; and Competing Words – Free Recall, designed as a dichotic listening measure that presents a different stimulus (a word) to each ear simultaneously and requires the examinee to repeat words in any order. According to the manual, the screening tests can be administered in 10 to 15 minutes.

The SCAN-3:C and SCAN-3:A comprise the following four diagnostic tests: Auditory Figure-Ground (+8dB, SCAN-3:C; 0dB, SCAN-3:A); Filtered Words, designed to measure the ability of an individual to process speech in the presence of distorted sounds or poor acoustics within the environment; Competing Words – Directed Ear, a dichotic listening measure that presents a different stimulus (a word) to each ear simultaneously and requires the examinee to repeat words in a certain order; and Competing Sentences, a dichotic task that appraises an individual's ability to process auditory information in the form of competing sentences presented simultaneously and requires the examinee to repeat the sentence for a particular ear. The following supplementary tests are included: Auditory Figure-Ground, which has a signal-to-noise ratio of 0:12dB for the SCAN-3:C and 8:12dB for the SCAN-3:A; Competing Words – Free Recall; and Time Compressed Sentences, which provide an appraisal of an individual's ability to process speech presented at a rapid rate.[5,6] The diagnostic and supplementary tests can be administered within 20 to 30 minutes.[5,6]

The SCAN-3:C and SCAN-3:A yield standardized assessment results which include standard scores, confidence intervals and centile ranks. For the screening tests, the examinee's responses are summed and a pass/fail criterion is employed. According to the manual, if an examinee fails one or more of the screening tests, then the diagnostic tests are administered.[5,6]

Raw scores are converted to scaled scores with a mean of 10 and a standard deviation of 3 for the SCAN-3:C and SCAN-3:A diagnostic and supplementary tests. The auditory processing composite is derived by adding the scaled scores for the four diagnostic tests, which results

in a standard score with a mean of 100 and a standard deviation of 15. In addition, an Ear Advantage Summary is also derived. Tables are provided in the manual for converting raw scores to scaled scores and for determining the auditory processing composite score. The manual also provides 90% and 95% confidence intervals, centile ranks and descriptive classifications. According to the manual, audiologists, speech/language pathologists, school psychologists, neuropsychologists and educational diagnosticians can administer and interpret SCAN-3:C and SCAN-3:A results.

Psychometric properties

The SCAN-3:C was standardized with 525 children ranging in age from 5 years to 12 years 11 months. The sample consisted of 49.7% females and 50.3% males. The SCAN-3:A was standardized with 250 individuals, who ranged in age from 13 years to 50 years 11 months. The sample was evenly divided for females and males. A stratified sampling plan was employed for both instruments, which incorporated the following demographic variables: age, sex, ethnicity, region and parent education level.[5] The normative samples adequately represented the 2004 US census data.[7]

The internal consistency, test–retest stability and interscorer reliability were investigated for the SCAN-3:C and SCAN-3:A. With regard to internal consistency, split-half reliability coefficients across six age groups for the SCAN-3:C ranged from 0.89 to 0.93 for the auditory processing composite and 0.50 to 0.94 for the eight tests.[5] The SCAN-3:A yielded reliability coefficients across four age groups that ranged from 0.92 to 0.93 for the auditory processing composite and 0.41 to 0.96 for the eight tests.[6] In order to examine test–retest stability, 48 children were administered the SCAN-3:C and 58 adolescents and adults were administered the SCAN-3:A. Participants were each tested twice by the same examiner, within an interval of 1 to 29 days.[5,6] Stability coefficients for the SCAN-3:C ranged from 0.54 to 0.73 across the eight tests and 0.77 for the auditory processing composite.[5] The SCAN-3:A yielded stability coefficients that ranged from 0.54 to 0.80 for the eight tests and 0.78 for the auditory processing composite.[6] According to the manual, all the SCAN-3:C and SCAN-3:A standardization tests were scored by two independent scorers. For both of the instruments, interscorer agreement was very high and ranged from 0.98 to 0.99.[5,6]

The validity of the SCAN-3:C and SCAN-3:A were investigated. As evidence of content validity, the SCAN-3:C and SCAN-3:A provide an appraisal of the auditory processing skills that are addressed by the American Speech–Language–Hearing Association, the American

SCAN-3 FOR CHILDREN: TESTS FOR AUDITORY PROCESSING DISORDERS (SCAN-3:C) AND SCAN-3 FOR ADOLESCENTS & ADULTS: TESTS FOR AUDITORY PROCESSING DISORDERS (SCAN-3:A)	
Purpose	To provide an appraisal of auditory processing abilities for the following areas: temporal processing, listening in noise, dichotic listening and listening to degraded speech[5,6]
Population	SCAN-3:C is designed for children aged 5–12y SCAN-3:A is designed for individuals aged 13–50y
Description of domains (subscales)	Both instruments comprise three screening tests, four diagnostic tests and three supplementary tests
Administration and test format	Time to complete: 10–15min to administer the screening tests and 20–30min to administer the diagnostic tests Testing format: tests are presented via CD and are individually administered Scoring: raw scores are used to derive norm-referenced standardized scores Training: audiologists, speech/language pathologists, school psychologists, neuropsychologists and educational diagnosticians can administer and interpret these assessments[6,7]
Psychometric properties	Normative sample: SCAN-3:C: n=525; SCAN-3:A: n=250 *Reliability* The SCAN-3:C and SCAN-3:A split-half reliability coefficients for the auditory processing composite scores across six and four age groups ranged from 0.89 to 0.93 and 0.92 to 0.93, respectively. For the SCAN-3:C and SCAN-3:A, stability coefficients ranged from 0.54 to 0.73 and 0.54 to 0.80 across the eight tests, and 0.77 and 0.78 for the auditory processing composite, respectively. Interscorer agreement was high for both instruments *Validity* The SCAN-3:C and SCAN-3:A provide an appraisal of the auditory processing skills addressed by the American Speech–Language–Hearing Association, the American Academy of Audiology and the British Society of Audiology For the SCAN-3:C and SCAN-3:A, intercorrelations for the auditory processing composite and for the individual tests provided support for the convergent validity for the two instruments The SCAN-3:C and SCAN-3:A mean scores differentiated between children with and without auditory processing disorders and revealed moderate to large effect sizes for the majority of the test and composite scores The sensitivity and specificity of the SCAN-3:C and SCAN-3:A were examined and revealed that when specific cut-off scores are employed, both instruments exhibited impressive rates of correctly identifying individuals who have auditory processing disorders
How to order	The SCAN-3:C and SCAN-3:A complete kits are available for US$255 each from Pearson Assessments (www.pearsonassessments.com) and include the examiner's manual, 25 record forms and a CD
Key references	Keith RW (2009) *SCAN-3 for Adolescents & Adults: Tests for Auditory Processing Disorders*. San Antonio, TX: Pearson. Keith RW (2009) *SCAN-3 for Children: Tests for Auditory Processing Disorders*. San Antonio, TX: Pearson.

Academy of Audiology and the British Society of Audiology. For the SCAN-3:C and SCAN-3:A, intercorrelations for the auditory processing composite and for the individual tests provided support for the convergent validity for the two instruments. For the SCAN-3:C and SCAN-3:A, children with auditory processing disorders were compared with a matched sample of individuals without auditory processing disorders. The mean scores were examined for each group and revealed moderate to large effect sizes for the majority of the test and composite scores for the SCAN-3:C and SCAN-3:A. This indicated that the instruments effectively discriminated between individuals with and without auditory processing disorders. The sensitivity and specificity of the SCAN-3:C and SCAN-3:A were examined and revealed that when specific cut-off scores were employed, both instruments exhibited impressive rates of correctly identifying individuals who had auditory processing disorders.[5,6]

VISUAL PERCEPTION

Wide Range Assessment of Visual Motor Abilities

Overview and purpose

The Wide Range Assessment of Visual Motor Abilities (WRAVMA)[8] is designed to measure visual motor ability in children and adolescents through three broad areas: visuomotor ability, visuospatial ability and fine motor ability.[8] As part of a comprehensive assessment process, the WRAVMA can be used in conjunction with other norm-referenced tests (e.g. academic achievement, intellectual and clinical assessments); teacher, parent and/or child interviews; and systematic observations. For the evaluation of children and adolescents, the WRAVMA is to be administered to individuals between the ages of 3 and 17 years.

Administration and scoring

The WRAVMA employs three subtests that can be administered within 14 to 24 minutes. The Drawing Test is designed to measure visuomotor ability. It consists of 24 items that can be administered within 5 to 10 minutes. Examinees are instructed to copy a design and continue forward to the next item until three consecutive items are failed.[8] The Matching Test is designed to measure visuospatial ability and consists of 46 items that can be administered within 5 to 10 minutes. The examinee is instructed to look at an item and mark or point to one out of four choices that 'goes best' with the item.[8] Testing continues until six errors occur within eight consecutive items. Both subtests use raw scores to derive standard scores with a mean of 100 and a standard deviation of 15.

The Pegboard Test is designed to measure fine motor ability. It consists of a square pegboard with 80 holes and pegs. The total administration time is approximately 4 minutes. As a trial, the examiner inserts three pegs and then asks the examinee to use his or her dominant hand to insert as many pegs as he or she can within 90 seconds. The total number of pegs inserted by the dominant hand is used to derive a fine motor standard score with a mean of 100 and a standard deviation of 15. A visuomotor composite standard score with a mean of 100 and a standard deviation of 15 is derived by summing the standard scores of the three subtests then consulting the manual's composite standard score table. The authors cautioned against using the composite score when a significant difference exists between any of the subtests; a table lists significant differences at 0.05 and 0.10.[8]

Regarding administration of the WRAVMA, the authors asserted that although each test could be administered separately, by administering the tests together a more comprehensive assessment is achieved. The manual reported that the Drawing Test and the Matching Test may be administered in a group format; however, only an individual administration format was used in the standardization of the instrument. Individuals familiar with administering standardized instruments to children and adolescents may administer the WRAVMA; however, only individuals with graduate training and experience, such as school psychologists, speech–language pathologists or occupational therapists, should interpret the results.[8]

Psychometric properties

The manual reported that the norms for each subtest were derived from the same standardization sample of 2600 children and adolescents ranging in age from 3 to 17 years. The authors employed a national stratified sampling plan that included several demographic components – age, sex, ethnicity, regional residence and socioeconomic level – that adequately reflected the 1990 US census data.[8,9] The total sample consisted of 49.8% males and 50.2% females. The norms were presented in 6-month intervals for ages 3 to 12 years and 1-year intervals for ages 13 to 17 years.

Information regarding the reliability of the WRAVMA for the normative sample included internal consistency and test–retest and inter-rater reliability. For each age group, the manual provided alpha coefficients and corrected split-half reliabilities. Reliability coefficients ranged from 0.69 to 0.89 for the Drawing Test and 0.65 to 0.92 for the Matching Test. Reported test–retest reliabilities ranged from 0.82 to 0.89 for the three subtests and 0.86 for the composite score. Finally, the inter-rater reliability of the Drawing Test was investigated using 39

WIDE RANGE ASSESSMENT OF VISUAL MOTOR ABILITIES (WRAVMA)	
Purpose	To assess visuomotor ability in three broad areas: visuomotor ability, visuospatial ability and fine motor ability
	May be used with other assessments for screening and diagnostic decisions for eligibility for special education services
	Occupational therapists use this assessment as part of a comprehensive evaluation
Population	For use with individuals aged 3–17y
Description of domains (subscales)	The following subtests can be used individually or together: the Drawing Test, the Matching Test and the Pegboard Test
Administration and test format	Time to complete: 14–24min to administer
	Testing format: individually administered to the examinee
	Scoring: raw scores are used to derive standardized scores for each subtest and a visuomotor total score, norm-referenced
	Training: occupational therapists, speech/language pathologists, diagnosticians and psychologists can administer and interpret these assessments
Psychometric properties	Normative sample: 2600 children and adolescents ranging in age from 3 to 17y
	Reliability
	For each age group, alpha coefficients and split-half reliabilities ranged from 0.69 to 0.89 for the Drawing Test and 0.65 to 0.92 for the Matching Test
	Test–retest reliabilities ranged from 0.82 to 0.89 for the three subtests and 0.86 for the composite score
	The inter-rater reliability of the Drawing Test for three examiners ranged from 0.96 to 0.97
	Validity
	As evidence of construct validity, items increased as developmental age increased
	Correlations between the subtests: 0.38 for Drawing/Matching, 0.28 for Drawing/Pegboard and 0.31 for Matching/Pegboard. These are modest correlations but maintain a degree of specificity
	Concurrent validity was supported by the following comparisons: the Drawing Test correlated 0.76 with the Developmental Test of Visual Motor Integration;[11] the Matching Test correlated 0.54 with the Motor Free Visual Perception Test;[12] and the Pegboard Test (dominant hand) correlated 0.35 with the Grooved Pegboard Test (dominant hand)[13]
How to order	A WRAVMA complete kit is available for US$300 from Psychological Assessment Resources, Inc (www.parinc.com). The kit includes the manual, 25 drawing forms, 25 visual matching forms, 25 examiner record forms, pegboard and pegs, pencils, markers and sharpener, in a soft canvas case
Key reference	Adams W, Sheslow D (1995) *Wide Range Assessment of Visual Motor Abilities.* Wilmington, DE: Wide Range, Inc.

protocols that were scored by three examiners and resulted in inter-rater reliability coefficients of 0.96, 0.97 and 0.97.

As evidence of content validity, the authors reported the range of item separation indices across age groups as 0.92 to 0.99 for the Drawing and Matching Tests. As evidence of construct validity, the authors noted that raw score means and age ranges are positively correlated. The authors purported that, although related, the three subtests of the WRAVMA still maintain a degree of specificity and as such should be moderately correlated. Intercorrelations were significant between the three subtests across all ages with the following average correlations between the subtests: 0.38 for Drawing/Matching, 0.28 for Drawing/Pegboard and 0.31 for Matching/Pegboard.

The concurrent validity of the WRAVMA subtests was examined by comparing the WRAVMA with popular tests that measure comparable constructs. The Drawing Test correlated 0.76 with the Developmental Test of Visual Motor Integration,[10] whereas the Matching Test correlated 0.54 with the Motor Free Visual Perception Test (MVPT).[11] The Pegboard Test (dominant hand) correlated 0.35 with the Grooved Pegboard Test (dominant hand).[12] Overall, the WRAVMA subtests correlated moderately to strongly with popular instruments that measure similar constructs.

Motor-Free Visual Perception Test, Third Edition

Overview and purpose

The MVPT-3 is designed to assess an individual's visuoperceptual ability without requiring a motor response from examinees. The authors noted that the MVPT-3 'serves as an important first step in the evaluation of visual perception' but encouraged professionals to conduct comprehensive assessments that include information from multiple sources.[13] The MVPT-3 can be administered to individuals aged 4 to 95 years and older.

Administration and scoring

The MVPT-3 is the third version of the MVPT[11] and consists of 65 items, is individually administered and can be completed within 20 to 30 minutes. The authors state that the items are designed to measure aspects of visual perception and address the following processes: spatial relationships, visual discrimination, figure-ground, visual closure and visual memory.[13] The items are presented in a spiral-bound easel. For each item, the examinee is shown a black-and-white line drawing with four choices of stimuli displayed underneath. The examiner poses a question and instructs the examinee to select from one of the four choices ('A', 'B', 'C' or 'D') by pointing to or saying the letter of their answer choice. For items designed to address visual memory, the four answer choices are presented after the line drawing has been presented and removed. The examiner records the answer on the provided record form.[13]

The total score can be derived by subtracting the number of errors made from the number of the last item administered. The total score is converted to a standard score with a mean of 100 and a standard deviation of 15, with a possible range of 55 to 145. The manual provides centile ranks, age equivalents, normal curve equivalents, stanines, scaled scores and T-scores. The authors note that although the MVPT-3 can be administered by individuals who do not have a background in assessment, the results should be interpreted by individuals who have been trained in psychometric testing.[13]

Psychometric properties

The standardized version of the MVPT-3 was administered to 2005 individuals. The normative sample consisted of 1856 individuals, with the remaining cases included in validity samples. The manual reported that 166 examiners, consisting of occupational therapists, school psychologists and educational specialists, were asked to randomly select their examinees from K-12 schools and hospitals. The following demographic components were reported: age, sex, ethnicity, regional residence and disability status. Data were collected in 118 cities in 34 states.

The authors reported that, although overall the sample was representative of the 2000 US census[14] demographic data, when the sample was classified into age groups, a statistical weighting procedure was applied to compensate for over- and under-representation in some of the demographic categories.[13] The total weighted sample consisted of 48.2% males and 51.8% females. The manual reports disability status data in the sample for ages 6 to 18 years: 92.9% no disability; 3.5% intellectual disability; 3.0% developmentally disabled; and 0.6% speech/language disorder.

The manual includes information on the internal consistency and test–retest reliability of the MVPT-3 for the total standardization sample. Alpha coefficients are reported for each age group for ages 4 to 10 years and range from 0.69 to 0.87. For individuals aged 11 years and older, alpha coefficients range from 0.86 to 0.90. The examiners retested 103 examinees after an average interval of 34 days. The corrected test–retest reliability coefficient was 0.87 for individuals aged 4 to 10 years and 0.92 for individuals 11 to 84+ years of age, thus indicating the stability of the MVPT-3.

The authors referred to their analysis of the MVPT-3 item difficulties and item bias as evidence of content validity. The manual reported that items were not biased with regard to sex, place of residence or ethnicity.[13] As evidence of construct validity, the authors asserted that, developmentally, age and visuoperceptual skills have a positive correlation. However, after the age of 39 years, as chronological age increases, visuoperceptual skills decrease. Correlations between ages and raw scores for the standardization sample were 0.72 for ages 4 to 10 years, 0.37 for ages 11 to 39 years and –0.46 for ages 40 years and above.

To further investigate construct validity, the authors purported that the MVPT-3 should have a low correlation with intelligence. This hypothesis was supported when approximately 18 individuals were administered the MVPT-3 and the Wechsler Intelligence Scales for Children, third edition[15] and no significant correlations were found. The authors explored the clinical utility of the

MOTOR-FREE VISUAL PERCEPTION TEST, THIRD EDITION (MVPT-3)	
Purpose	To assess an individual's visuoperceptual ability without requiring a motor response from examinees
	May be used with other measures to identify individuals who are at risk or who have visuoperceptual difficulties
	Can be used as part of an assessment battery for screening and diagnostic decisions for eligibility decisions for special education
Population	Can be administered to individuals aged 4y and older
Description of domains (subscales)	The items are designed to measure spatial relationships, visual discrimination, figure-ground, visual closure and visual memory, and result in a total score
Administration and test format	Time to complete: 20–30min to administer
	Testing format: individually administered to the examinee
	Scoring: raw scores are used to derive standardized scores, norm-referenced
	Training: can be administered by trained examiners but interpreted by individuals trained in psychometrics
Psychometric properties	Normative sample: 1856 individuals with and without disabilities
	Reliability
	Internal consistency alpha coefficients for the total score ranged from 0.69 to 0.87 for ages 4–10y and 0.86 to 0.90 for ages 11y and older
	Test–retest reliability coefficients were 0.87 for ages 4–10y and 0.92 for ages 11–84y after an average 34-day interval
	Validity
	As evidence of content validity, items were examined and found to be non-biased and to exhibit acceptable item difficulties
	Construct validity was supported by the correlation of developmental ages and item scores
	The clinical utility was supported by comparing the standard score mean differences of examinees diagnosed as having developmental delay, individuals suffering from traumatic brain injury or specific learning disabilities with the average population mean. Each of the three group means were significantly lower than the norm
How to order	An MVPT-3 complete kit is available for US$144 from Western Psychological Services. The kit includes the manual, one set of test plates in a spiral-bound easel and 25 recording forms
Key reference	Colarusso RP, Hammill DD (2003) *Motor-Free Visual Perception Test*, 3rd edition. Novato, CA: Academic Therapy Publications.

MVPT-3 by comparing the standard score mean differences of examinees that were diagnosed as having developmental delay, individuals suffering from traumatic brain injury or specific learning disabilities with the average population mean. The manual reported that each of the three group means were significantly lower when they were compared with the average population mean of 100. The group classified as developmentally delayed fell below two standard deviations when compared with the population mean.

OLFACTORY AND GUSTATORY PERCEPTION

Odor Identification Test, Wholemouth Taste Test and Regional Taste Test

Overview and purpose

The purpose of the Odor Identification Test is to assess olfactory loss in children. The Wholemouth Taste Test and Regional Taste Test are designed to assess gustatory loss in children. These assessments require individuals to identify odours or tastes. Laing et al[16] examined the psychometric properties of the three instruments and noted that the tests have a promising future for use as assessments of gustatory and olfactory performance in children. The instruments are currently used in research and clinical settings. The authors investigated the use of this assessment battery with individuals ranging in age from 5 to 7 years.[16]

Administration and scoring

The Odor Identification Test consists of the following 16 odorants: floral, orange, strawberry, fish, chocolate, infant powder, paint, cut grass, sour, minty, onion, Vicks Vapo-rub, spicy, dettol, cheese and petrol. The authors noted that each odorant is diluted and presented in a 250-ml flip-top squeeze bottle that contains a cotton ball saturated with the odorant solution.[16] The examiner presents a squeeze bottle containing a certain odour and three photographs of an object to the examinee. He or she is instructed to smell the odorant. The examiner reads the name of each photograph and asks the examinee to choose the photograph that represents the smell. The examiner records the response as incorrect or correct on a score sheet and waits 15 to 20 seconds before the next odorant presentation. The authors state that the test can be administered in 5 minutes.[16]

The Wholemouth Taste Test and the Regional Taste Test use the following tastants: (a) salty, analytical grade sodium chloride; (b) bitter, quinine hydrochloride; (c) sour, citric acid; and (d) sweet, sucrose.[16] The authors dilute the tastants with purified drinking water. For the Wholemouth Test, the tastants are placed in 30-ml plastic cups with 10ml of the solution. The examiner presents a set of photographs that consists of one photo of a glass of water and two photos of a tastant. The examiner reads the name of the tastant as each photograph is presented.[16] Examinees are instructed to sip a tastant from the plastic cup and identify the tastant from the three photographs. There is a 20- to 30-second interval between each trial, during which time the examinee is instructed to rinse his or her mouth with water.[16] The responses of the examinees are recorded on a score sheet as incorrect or correct.

For the Regional Taste Test, cotton buds saturated in each tastant solution are used to administer the flavours to small regions on both sides of the anterior and posterior tongue.[16] The examiner rolls the saturated cotton bud 1cm toward the posterior tongue at the designated region in order to produce a consistent taste sensation.[16] The examinee is instructed to extend his or her tongue while the tastant is applied and to maintain that position until he or she identifies the tastant by pointing to one

of three photographs. The same photographs are used in the Wholemouth Test. The examiner is instructed to present the three photographs and read the name of each tastant depicted for each trial. The examinee's responses are recorded as incorrect or correct on a score sheet.[16] The authors suggest that before the examinees begin each trial, they wait for 20 to 30 seconds and rinse their mouths with water.

Psychometric properties

The authors noted that their study provided 'normative data that can be used in the diagnosis of olfactory and gustatory impairment in school-age children'.[16] With regard to the sample employed in this study, the children attended public schools in Sydney, Australia, and the adults attended the University of Western Sydney, Australia. The Odor Identification test was administered to a sample of 232 children which included 5 year olds (*n*=70), 6 year olds (*n*=82), 7 year olds (*n*=80) and 56 adults ranging in age from 18 to 51 years. The Wholemouth Taste Test and the Regional Taste Test were administered to 266 individuals consisting of 107 males and 159 females. Seventy-two children were 5 years old, 71 were 6 years old and 69 were 7 years old. Fifty-four adults between the ages of 18 and 51 years also participated.

The Odor Identification Test data indicate that even though examinees aged 5 to 7 years did not correctly identify as many odorants as older participants, their 'mean correct scores were high, indicating the suitability of the odorants and photographs used'.[16] With regard to this sample, the authors asserted that a 5 year old with a correct score of 11 out of 16 odorants would be regarded as having a normal sense of smell, while a score of 4 correctly identified odorants out of 16 would indicate an impairment in olfactory ability.[16]

The Wholemouth Test data indicate that, with regard to this sample, typically developing individuals aged 6 to 7 years and adults 'could be expected to identify four of the five tests substances, whereas three should be identified by 5 year olds'.[16] The Regional Taste data indicate that individuals 'ages 5 years and older with a normal sense of taste can be expected to identify at least three of the tastants at each region'.[16] The authors report that this study indicates that children aged 5 to 7 years old could successfully identify the odorants and tastants addressed in this study.[16] The authors note that the difficulty with popular olfactory and gustatory measures currently in use is their length and complexity. The measures described in this research provided a non-complex, brief measure that could be completed by young examinees. The authors acknowledge the need for future studies that examine the specificity and sensitivity of the instruments.

The Sniffin' Sticks Test

Overview and purpose
The Sniffin' Sticks Test[17] is designed for use in clinical and research settings to assess olfactory function in children and adults. Olfactory measurement has historically encompassed a myriad of procedures in an attempt to assess olfactory function. Two such methods included absolute detection thresholds, described as a procedure designed to identify the lowest odorant concentration level that an individual can detect, and the differential thresholds procedure, designed to measure the smallest detectable difference in concentration of a chemical.[18] The Sniffin' Sticks Test could be construed as a psychophysical test because it 'provides a quantitative measure of sensory function and requires a verbal or conscious overt response on the part of the examinees'.[18]

Administration and scoring
The Sniffin' Sticks Test is described as a portable assessment with a shelf life of 6 to 12 months.[19] It is used to assess odour threshold, discrimination and identification, and can be administered in 20 to 30 minutes.[20] Pens containing material saturated in an odorant are employed. As the odorant is presented, the pen's cap is removed for 3 seconds and placed 2cm in front of the examinee's nostrils. For the odour threshold subtest, the examinee is blindfolded and presented with three pens: one pen contains the odorant and the remaining two contain a solvent. The examinee is asked to identify the pen with the odorant. For the odour discrimination subtest, the examinee is blindfolded and three pens are presented. Two pens contain the same odorant and one contains a different odorant.[21] The examinee selects the pen that smells different. For the odour identification subtest, the examinee is asked to identify an odorant that is presented by selecting from four descriptors. For all three tests, an interval of 20 to 30 seconds occurs between each trial. Possible scores for each subtest range from 0 to 16.[21] A total score is derived from summing the raw scores from the three subtests.

Psychometric properties
Kobal et al[21] investigated the psychometric properties of the Sniffin' Sticks Test. The sample consisted of 966 participants who were evaluated in 11 centres and were determined to have no clinically significant olfactory loss.[21] Individuals ranged in age from 6 years to over 55 years. The authors also investigated a sample of individuals diagnosed with olfactory problems. They noted that their study provided 'normative values for routine clinical use of the Sniffin' Sticks'.[21] As a result of this study, the total score centiles for clinical purposes were established. These scores can be used in conjunction with other assessments to determine whether a person has an olfactory loss.

COMPOSITE MEASURE OF SENSORIMOTOR AND VISUOSPATIAL PERCEPTION

NEPSY-II, second edition

Overview and purpose
According to the authors, the NEPSY-II is designed to provide a survey of cognitive skills in six neuropsychological domains that include attention and executive functioning, language, memory and learning, social perception, and sensorimotor and visuospatial processing. It is recommended that information provided by the NEPSY-II be used in conjunction with additional evaluations, direct observations and structured interviews in order to provide a comprehensive assessment.[22] The NEPSY-II is designed for individuals aged 3 years to 16 years 11 months.

Administration and scoring
The NEPSY-II is the second version of the NEPSY Developmental Neuropsychological Assessment[23] and consists of 32 subtests. The full battery can be administered within 90 minutes for preschoolers and 2 to 3 hours for older individuals. The authors recommend a General Referral Battery that addresses the following skills: basic language, visuomotor integration, inhibitory control, attention, working memory, visual and verbal memory, and visuoperceptual processing.[22] This battery can be administered within 45 to 75 minutes depending upon the age of the examinee. In order to allow examiners to tailor their assessments towards specific referral questions, the authors combined the subtests into the following batteries: learning differences – reading; learning differences – maths; attention/concentration; behaviour management; language delays/disorders; perceptual/motor delays/disorders; school readiness; and social/interpersonal.

The manual and administration guide provide detailed information concerning basal and ceiling rules, scoring criteria and the presentation of stimuli for each of the 32 subtests. The manual provides multiple scores for NEPSY-II subtests. These scores are classified by the authors as primary, process or contrast scores. Some subtests also provide behavioural observations. All of the subtests report primary scores, which provide a measure of the overall ability of the examinee with regard to the subtest.[22] According to the authors, process scores focus on the specific skills involved to complete the task. Contrast scores allow the examiner to score comparisons within or between subtests. Behavioural observations quantify common behaviours that an examinee may exhibit. Scores are presented as scaled scores, centile ranks, cumulative percentages or percentages of the normative sample.

The authors recommend that individuals who administer the NEPSY-II should be trained in psychometric assessments. For diagnostic purposes, the NEPSY-II should be administered and interpreted by school psychologists, clinical psychologists or neuropsychologists.[23]

Psychometric properties

According to the manual, the NEPSY-II was standardized using a stratified random sampling plan that included the following demographic variables: age, ethnicity, geographic region and parent education level. The sex of the sample was divided evenly. The normative sample included 1200 individuals who were between the ages of 3 and 16 years. The normative table was divided into 1-year intervals for age ranges between 3 and 12 years, while ages 13 and 14 years were combined, as were ages 15 and 16 years. This resulted in 100 participants for each age group. The demographic variables of the normative sample adequately reflected the October 2003 US Bureau of the Census data.[24]

The authors investigated internal consistency and test–retest and inter-rater reliability. The manual reports that the majority of the NEPSY-II subtests have adequate to high internal consistency or stability.[22] The following subtests were identified by the authors to have the highest alpha coefficients or split-half reliability coefficients when primary and process scaled scores were examined: comprehension of instructions, design copying, fingertip tapping, imitating hand positions, list memory, memory for names, phonological processing, picture puzzles and sentence repetition.

When test–retest reliability was examined, the authors reported the following subtests to have the lowest reliability coefficients: response set total correct, inhibition total errors, memory for designs spatial and total scores,

and memory for designs delayed total score. The manual reports that 1200 protocols were scored twice by two different raters, resulting in inter-rater and interscorer agreements with a range of 93% to 99%. The standard error of measurement was reported for each subtest and age group for all primary and process scaled scores.

The authors examined content and concurrent and construct validity. As evidence of content validity, the authors noted the theoretical underpinnings of Luria's work, current neuropsychological research and psychometric theory, all of which contributed to the construction of the NEPSY-II.[25] The authors also consulted experts in the field and users of the NEPSY, and conducted pilot and field studies. The examinees' responses to test items were examined for evidence of item bias.[22]

The manual addressed concurrent validity by examining the relationship of the NEPSY-II subtests with other popular measures of cognition, achievement, neurological functioning, behaviour and the previous version of the NEPSY.[23] The manual provides correlations for each comparison. Overall, the results support concurrent validity of the NEPSY-II. As evidence of construct validity, the authors refer to the concurrent validity studies. They also examined the NEPSY-II subtests and noted that when the relationships of the subtests were compared, one would expect a certain degree of correlation, while still maintaining some specificity. As expected, low to moderate correlations were revealed.[22]

In order to investigate the clinical utility and discriminant validity of the NEPSY-II, the mean subtest scores of individuals with the following clinical diagnoses were compared with a matched control group: attention-deficit–hyperactivity disorder, reading disorders, mathematics disorders, language disorders, intellectual disability, autistic spectrum disorder, Asperger syndrome, traumatic brain injury, hearing impairment and emotional disturbance. The manual provides detailed tables for each comparison. Overall, the studies support the clinical utility and discriminant ability of the NEPSY-II.[22]

REFERENCES

1. World Health Organization (2007) *International Classification of Functioning, Disability and Health Version for Children and Youth ICF-CY*. Geneva: World Health Organization.
2. Harris JC (2002) Behavioral phenotypes of neurodevelopmental disorders: Portals into the developing brain. In: Davis KL, Charney D, Coyle JT, Nemeroff C, editors. *Neuropsycholopharmacology: The Fifth Generation of Progress*. New York: Lippincott Williams & Wilkins, pp. 625–638.
3. Tome SA, Williamson N, Pauli R (1990) Temperament in Williams syndrome. *J Med Genet* 36: 345–352.
4. Aylward GP (1994) *Practitioner's Guide to Developmental and Psychological Testing*. New York: Plenum Medical Book Co.

5. Keith RW (2009) *SCAN-3 for Children: Tests for Auditory Processing Disorders*. San Antonio, TX: Pearson.
6. Keith RW (2009) *SCAN-3 for Adolescents & Adults: Tests for Auditory Processing Disorders*. San Antonio, TX: Pearson.
7. US Bureau of the Census (2004) *Current Population Survey, March 2004: School Enrollment Supplemental File*. Washington, DC: US Bureau of the Census.
8. Adams W, Sheslow D (1995) *Wide Range Assessment of Visual Motor Abilities*. Wilmington, DE: Wide Range, Inc.
9. US Bureau of the Census (1990) *Statistical Abstract of the United States: 1990*, 110th edition. Washington, DC: US Bureau of the Census.

10. Beery KE (1967) *Developmental Test of Visual-Motor Integration*. Chicago: Follett Educational Corporation.

11. Colarusso RP, Hammill DD (1972) *Motor-free Visual Perception Test*. Novato, CA: Academic Therapy Publications.

12. Grooved Pegboard. Lafayette, IN: Lafayette Instrument Company, Inc.

13. Colarusso RP, Hammill DD (2003) *Motor-free Visual Perception Test*, 3rd edition. Novato, CA: Academic Therapy Publications.

14. US Bureau of the Census (2000) *Statistical Abstract of the United States: 2000*, 120th edition. Washington, DC: US Bureau of the Census.

15. Wechsler D (1991) *Wechsler Intelligence Scale for Children*, 3rd edition. San Antonio, TX: The Psychological Corporation.

16. Laing DG, Segovia C, Fark T, Laing ON, Jinks AL (2008) Tests for screening olfactory and gustatory function in school-age children. *Otolaryngol Head Neck Surg* 139: 74–82.

17. Kobal G, Hummel T, Sekinger B, Bartz S, Roscher S, Wolf SR (1996) Sniffin' Sticks: Screening of olfactory performance. *Rhinology* 34: 222–226.

18. Doty RL, Laing DG (2003) Psychophysical measurement of human olfactory function, including odorant mixture assessment. In: Doty R, editor. *Handbook of Olfaction and Gustation*, 2nd edition. New York: Marcel-Dekker, pp. 203–238.

19. Eibenstein A, Fioretti AB, Lena C, Rosati, N, Fusetti M (2005) Modern psychophysical tests to assess olfactory function. *Neurol Sci* 26: 147–155.

20. Hummel T, Konnerth C, Rosenheim K, Kobal G (2001) Screening of olfactory function with a four-minute odor identification test: Reliability, normative data, and investigations in patients with olfactory loss. *Ann Otol Rhinol Laryngol* 110: 976–981.

21. Kobal G, Klimek L, Wolfensberger M, et al (2000) Multicenter investigation of 1,036 subjects using a standardized method for the assessment of olfactory function combining tests of odor identification, odor discrimination, and olfactory thresholds. *Eur Arch Otorhinolaryngol* 257: 205–211.

22. Korkman M, Kirk U, Kemp S (2007) *NEPSY-II, Second Edition: Clinical and Interpretive Manual*. San Antonio, TX: Harcourt Assessment, Inc.

23. Korkman M, Kirk U, Kemp S (1998) *NEPSY: A Developmental Neuropsychological Assessment*. San Antonio, TX: The Psychological Corporation.

24. US Bureau of the Census (2003) *Statistical Abstract of the United States: 2003*, 123th edition. Washington, DC: US Bureau of the Census.

25. Luria AR (1980) *Higher Cortical Functions in Man*, 2nd edition. (Haigh B, translator). New York: Basic Books. (Original work published 1962).

12
SPECIFIC MENTAL FUNCTIONS: LANGUAGE (B167)

Jane McCormack, Diane Jacobs and Karla Washington

What is the construct?

The mental functions of language (b167) domain relates to 'specific mental functions of recognizing and using signs, symbols and other components of a language'.[1] It includes mental functions underlying the reception of language (i.e. decoding messages to obtain meaning) and the expression of language (i.e. producing meaningful messages) in spoken, written, sign and gestural forms. It also includes integrative language functions, which are 'mental functions that organize semantic and symbolic meaning, grammatical structure and ideas for the production of messages'.[1] Thus, the mental functions of language chapter in the International Classification of Functioning, Disability and Health for Children and Youth (ICF-CY) broadly describes the mental functions that enable children to use and understand language (particularly grammatical and semantic aspects) successfully. It follows, then, that an impairment of these mental functions underlying language presents as an impaired ability to use and understand language; that is, difficulty with the activity of communication (d3).

For some children, impaired mental functions of language present as symptoms of another diagnosis. These may be congenital conditions, such as Down syndrome, neurofibromatosis, autism spectrum disorder or profound hearing loss, or acquired conditions (e.g. as a result of a traumatic brain injury [TBI]). The ICF-CY, in line with the ICF, identifies acquired language impairments (such as those involved in Broca and Wernicke aphasias) as 'inclusions' within the mental functions of language chapter; however, such impairments are rarely diagnosed in children.

Language development in childhood and adolescence is an ongoing process, with impaired mental functions of language more commonly reflecting slowed progression along the normal developmental trajectory rather than as an impairment that has been acquired. For affected children, impaired mental functions of language may occur independently of other conditions, and present clinically as diagnoses such as expressive/receptive language delay or specific language impairment.

The integrity (or impairment) of mental functions of language is determined according to a child's presenting language skills, which highlights the inter-relationship that exists between the body functions and activities and participation categories in the ICF-CY. Body functions form the basis for the range of communication skills and activities in which children engage. Despite conceptual differences (i.e. one relates to whether a body part functions correctly and the other to whether an activity can be performed), many body functions and activities and participation would be assessed using the same set of procedures.[2] In the case of mental functions of language, it is not typical to assess the mental functions that underlie the reception or expression of language, or indeed integrative language functions. Instead, the skills reliant on those functions are assessed, and a subsequent judgement is made about the integrity of the functions themselves. Consequently, assessments of mental functions of language need to incorporate assessments of skills and tasks that fall within the activities and participation component (particularly the learning and applying knowledge [d1] and communication [d3] chapters). For instance, in order to assess the reception of written language (b16701) (i.e. 'Mental functions of decoding written messages to obtain their meaning'), it is necessary to assess a child's performance of the activity of reading (d140). Impaired reception of written language will present as reading difficulties evidenced by poor decoding or reduced reading comprehension, or both. As a result, impairments of mental functions of language (functions underlying language production and understanding) often cannot be clearly delineated from limitations of activities related to language and communication (outcomes of those impairments).

A model of the mental functions underlying language

Cognitive neuropsychological models of language processing, such as those used in the assessment of language functions in adults with acquired language impairments,[3,4] are useful for considering the mental functions that underlie language expression and reception. There are no equivalent frameworks for evaluating language in child populations; however, researchers investigating child speech and language development and delays have suggested models of language processing which incorporate some of the same concepts.[5] An example of a cognitive neuropsychological model used for evaluating language processing in adults has been adapted for children and adolescents and is presented in Figure 12.1.

Cognitive neuropsychological models recognize the link between the functions that underlie language and the outcome of those functions (activities and participation). Furthermore, they recognize that effective communication is a process that involves being able to understand what others are communicating (reception of language), as well as being able to plan and produce one's own message (expression of language). Understanding the communication of others requires that information be received and analysed and that meaning is assigned. Expressing one's own message requires that the intended meaning of the message and the mode of communication be selected, the motor plan established and the message produced. In the sections that follow, the mental functions underlying the reception and expression of language are described in more detail, guided by the cognitive neuropsychological framework presented in Figure 12.1.

RECEPTION OF LANGUAGE (B1670)

Reception of language relates to the ability to decode and comprehend the messages produced by others (i.e. input). As shown in Figure 12.1, the first step in the reception of language involves mental functions relating to auditory phonological analysis (for the reception of spoken language) and visual analysis (for the reception of symbolic, signed, gestural or written language). That is, children need to distinguish sensory information (e.g. an auditory signal, orthographic symbol or gesture) that potentially communicates language meaning from other

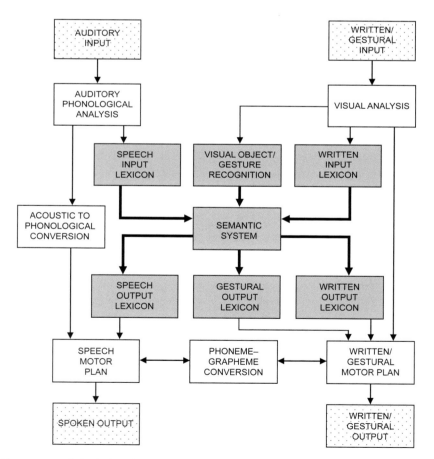

Figure 12.1 Cognitive neuropsychological model of the language processing system (adapted from Ellis and Young[3] and Kay et al[4]).

non-language sensory information (e.g. environmental sounds). The second step in the reception of language involves mental functions that identify whether or not the language-based sensory information (e.g. gestures, objects or spoken and written words) is familiar or unfamiliar. If familiar (present in the input lexicon), mental functions activate the third step, whereby meaning is attached to the auditory or visual stimuli (semantic system).

It is this final step that is evaluated in most assessments of the reception of language; however, the tasks used to assess this function vary according to age. For instance, the measurement of an infant's reception of language would consider whether or not he or she recognized and responded to his or her name (b16700), followed basic directions and understood gestures associated with commands such as 'stop' or 'come here' (16703). In the late preschool years, measurement would consider children's vocabulary knowledge and understanding of linguistic concepts and grammatical morphemes. For older primary school-aged children and adolescents, measurement would consider the mental functions that underlie more advanced decoding skills, such as complex vocabulary (synonyms, antonyms, multiple meanings), higher-level semantics (figurative language, ambiguity, sarcasm) and more advanced syntax (complex multistep instructions containing dependent/subordinate clauses, subordinating conjunctions, adverbial conjuncts). In addition, school commencement signals a transition in emphasis from spoken language skills to written language skills. As a result, the measurement of receptive language would also consider the mental functions that underlie the ability to decode written messages (b16701), such as reading a book. Finally, for some children, particularly those within the deaf community, sign language may be the predominant form of language they encounter. In such cases, this construct would consider the mental functions that underlie children's ability to decode messages expressed by signed hand movements (b16702).

EXPRESSION OF LANGUAGE (B1671)

Expression of language relates to the ability to produce meaningful messages. The first step in the expression of language comprises the mental functions that enable a speaker (for expression of spoken language), signer (for expression of sign or gesture) or writer (for the expression of written language) to conceptualize a message. Second, mental functions are activated, which enable access to, and retrieval of, stored representations of the conceptualized information (present in output lexicon) necessary to convey a message (in phonemic, gestural or graphemic

form). Finally, phonemes, gestures or graphemes are produced, resulting in a clear and coherent message (spoken language, sign/gesture or writing). This final step may be assessed alongside other components of the ICF-CY, as carrying out a motor plan is reliant on the integrity of other structures (e.g. structures involved in voice and speech [s3] or structures related to movement [s7]) and functions (e.g. voice and speech functions [b3] or neuromusculoskeletal and movement-related functions [b7]).

The tasks used to assess expression of language vary according to age and verbal ability. For some children (including infants), production of meaningful messages may take the form of gesture (b16713). Therefore, the measurement of expressive language would consider the mental functions that underlie gestural skills, including eye gaze, reaching, pointing and body movements towards or away from something. Alternatively, measurement may consider the mental functions that underlie the skills used in signing a meaningful message with hands and other movements (b16712).

For verbal children and adolescents, the measurement of expressive language would take into consideration the mental functions that underlie the spoken language skills required for activities such as oral narrative and contribution to class discussions and debates. In addition, for verbal school-aged children the construct would consider the mental functions that underlie the skills involved in producing meaningful written messages (b16711) in activities such as taking notes in class.

Children and adolescents with developmental disabilities, whether verbal or non-verbal, may express meaningful messages through a range of different forms. Most of these are covered by the categories outlined above – spoken, written, gestural or sign. However, some children and adolescents with developmental disabilities may be reliant on alternative and augmentative communication (AAC) in order to express their message. Often, AAC incorporates photos, pictures and/or symbols as the primary means for expression. The mental functions of language domain currently does not have a separate code to classify pictorial or symbolic modes of communication. Thus, they would be coded under 'Other mental functions of language – specified'. Even so, assessment of expressive language for children and adolescents utilizing AAC would need to consider the mental functions that underlie the skills required for the utilization of a specific AAC device. These include mental functions underlying global and specific mental areas, such as intellectual function, attention and concentration (b1), sensory and related functions such as hearing and vision (b2), voice and speech functions (b3) and movement-related functions such as muscle power, tone and reflex (b7).

INTEGRATIVE LANGUAGE FUNCTIONS (B1672)

Integrative language functions relate to the ability to assign meaning (phonological, syntactic and semantic) to information received and to generate meaningful messages in spoken, written or other forms of language. In Figure 12.1, integrative language functions are those that link the input and output lexicon with the semantic system (shaded boxes). Integrative language functions are inherent to receptive language. It is possible to receive a message, but it is not possible to *understand* a message without assigning meaning to the message. Consequently, any assessment of the reception of language will evaluate the individual's ability to access stored representations in order to assign meaning to the input received and then formulate an appropriate response (e.g. carry out an instruction, respond to a question or identify a picture corresponding to a given word). In contrast, it is possible to produce language (expression of language function) without the language being meaningful. For instance, individuals may be able to verbally repeat or write non-words, a task which does not require them to access their semantic system and assign meaning to their output (progress from auditory phonological analysis to auditory–phonological conversion to oral or written output). When meaningful language is produced, integrative language functions (and the semantic system) are involved

General factors to consider when measuring this domain

CO-OCCURRING IMPAIRMENTS

Language impairment may co-occur with impairments of body structure, or with additional body function impairments, and these need to be considered when determining appropriate modes of assessment and when interpreting results. For example, individuals may not perform well on language assessments if they have uncorrected visual or auditory impairment, a previously diagnosed physical condition or illness that might depress performance (e.g. TBI, stroke, cerebral tumour, epilepsy, cerebral infection), or current treated (taking medication that might depress performance) or untreated mental health concerns. Those who are primarily non-verbal or uncommunicative and those who exhibit unintelligible or disordered speech may also experience difficulty on language assessments. In such cases, performance may be more representative of the impaired body structure or additional body function impairment than of impaired mental functions of language. Consequently, alternative methods of evaluating language skills, such as a non-verbal assessment task or a naturalistic observation, may be more appropriate.

FORMAL LANGUAGE MEASURES

Mental functions of language are typically assessed through evaluations of language skills (see discussion above), and these evaluations typically comprise standardized language tests that are decontextualized and norm-referenced. A delay in language ability is established by comparing the child's performance on the standardized task with the performance of their age-matched typically developing peers.[6] Impairment severity is determined by measuring the extent to which the child's performance differs from the mean or average score for his or her age. Eight properties have been identified as requirements for standardized assessments in order for accurate conclusions to be drawn.[7] These eight properties are clear administration and scoring criteria, validity, reliability, diagnostic accuracy, standardization (particularly normative data that reflect the current population demography), measures of central tendency and variability, standard error of measurement and norm-referenced scores. Consideration of these eight properties of standardized assessments should be published with the test and the normative data for critical scrutiny.[8]

There are limitations to using standardized assessments as the sole measure of language skills (or impairment). These include the lack of standardized tools available for evaluating language production and comprehension in very young children, and the decontextualized nature of standardized assessments. That is, performance on a standardized assessment may not accurately reflect a child's language skills (or language impairment) in real-life naturalistic settings.[6] In such cases, utilising informal or non-standardized assessment may be beneficial.

INFORMAL LANGUAGE MEASURES

Informal or non-standardized language assessment refers to the use of any assessment that does not have standardized procedures for administration and scoring.[9,10] This includes utilizing interviews, questionnaires or developmental scales (checklists that sample behaviours from a specified developmental period) with caregivers or teachers. Additionally, informal, subjective measures such as direct behavioural observation using diary accounts, descriptive notes, running records and observation schedules may be useful in some cases for investigating language skills. Language sampling in order to assess an individual's free speech is another useful method. Language sampling makes a child's speech and language accessible for analysis using a range of quantitative and qualitative measures, and allows for the checking and confirmation of clinical judgements regarding speech and language skills. However, it is important to consider the representativeness of a language sample by taking into account the context, nature, setting and material utilized within the interaction, the method used for recording the sample and the length of the sample. For most children, a combination of formal and informal evaluations of language functions and the impact of impaired functions will provide the most representative appraisal of language abilities and the best guidance for intervention to improve language skills.[11]

Overview of recommended measures

The measures outlined in the following section are formal, standardized tools used to measure expressive and receptive language, and as such provide information about the integrity of specific mental functions underlying the reception and expression of language. As highlighted in the preceding sections, clinical evaluations of mental functions typically rely on measurement of the outcome of those functions.

The reviewed measures have been selected to provide a broad overview of the tools available to assess mental functions of language; it is acknowledged that other measures are also available. The measures were chosen to reflect those often used in English-speaking countries; however, some tools have been adapted for use with other populations, and these alternative versions are also identified. Additional measures have been summarized and are included in charts at the end of the chapter. It should be noted that most of the assessments outlined in this section evaluate the reception or expression of spoken language.

RECEPTION OF LANGUAGE (B1670)

Peabody Picture Vocabulary Test, fourth edition

Overview and purpose

The Peabody Picture Vocabulary Test, fourth edition[12] (PPVT-4), measures understanding of the spoken word, and thus enables the assessment of vocabulary acquisition for individuals aged 2 years 6 months to 90+ years. The first edition of the PPVT was published in 1959; the fourth edition, published in 2007, has updated vocabulary items including a better representation of word types across all levels of difficulty and a selection of simpler items to enable improved measurement of receptive vocabulary skills in low-functioning preschool children. Another feature of the fourth edition is the inclusion of growth scale values to enable the measurement of progress in vocabulary knowledge over time.

The PPVT-4 has a range of clinical applications, including use as a screening tool for identifying receptive language impairment and as a means of screening the receptive vocabulary knowledge of individuals whose primary language is not English. It can be used with individuals with a range of developmental disabilities, including those with autism, cerebral palsy and moderate visual disabilities.[12]

Furthermore, the authors suggest that it can be used for research purposes, as a general measure of verbal mental age. The second edition of the PPVT was adapted for Spanish speakers, and a Spanish adaptation of the PPVT-4 is currently being developed.

Administration and scoring

The PPVT-4 is designed for use by allied health or special education professionals. There are two parallel forms (A and B), each of which contains 19 sets of 12 items (total number of items=228). The items represent a range of semantic categories (e.g. vegetables, tools) and parts of speech (e.g. verbs, nouns, adjectives). The alternate-form reliability is good (r ranged from 0.87 to 0.93 for different ages; mean r by age=0.89), which indicates that each form measures the same construct with the same degree of accuracy, and therefore derived scores can be interpreted in the same way.

During administration of the PPVT-4, children are shown a page with four items (pictures) and asked to point to a specific item. Children receive one point for each correct response, and testing continues until a ceiling is reached (when the child responds incorrectly to eight or more items in a single set). The assessment is untimed; however, the authors suggest that most individuals achieve a ceiling within 20 minutes. Once a ceiling has been reached, the examiner calculates the total number of errors in all sets administered and subtracts this number from the highest ceiling item. The number obtained is the child's raw score, which can then be converted to a standard score or centile rank.

Psychometric properties

The PPVT-4 was co-normed with the Expressive Vocabulary Test, second edition (EVT-2)[13] in 2005–6. Thus, the scale development sample is the same, which enables direct comparison between the two measures. The sample of 3540 individuals (aged 2y6mo–90+y) was designed to match the US population (as ascertained by 2004 census data) for demographic variables including sex, race/ethnicity, geographical region, socioeconomic status and clinical diagnosis (e.g. attention-deficit–hyperactivity disorder, specific language impairment, autism).

The internal consistency (or consistency of performance on different portions of the test) was determined through calculating split-half reliability (correlation of each individual's score on odd-numbered items with

PEABODY PICTURE VOCABULARY TEST, FOURTH EDITION (PPVT-4)	
Purpose	To measure understanding of the spoken (American English) word
Population	Individuals aged 2y6mo–90+y
Description of domains (subscales)	The PPVT-4 is solely a measure of receptive vocabulary (comprehension)
Administration and test format	There are two parallel forms (A and B). Each form has 19 sets of items with 12 items per set (total number of items=228). The items represent a range of semantic categories (e.g. vegetables, tools) and parts of speech (e.g. verbs, nouns, adjectives)
	Time to complete: 10–15min
	Testing format: children are tested individually. The examiner calculates the child's chronological age to determine the appropriate starting point for the assessment. The examiner shows the child a page with four items (pictures) and asks the child to point to a specific item. Training items are administered first, and the child is required to respond correctly to two items before commencing the test items. Testing continues until a ceiling is reached (when the child responds incorrectly to eight or more items in a single set)
	Scoring: children receive one point for each correct response. The examiner determines the basal set (the lowest set of items administered in which the child scores no or one errors) and the ceiling set (the highest set of items administered in which the child scores eight or more errors). The examiner calculates the total number of errors in all sets administered, and subtracts this number from the highest ceiling item. The number obtained is the child's raw score, which can then be converted to a standard score or centile rank
	Training: restricted to use by allied health or special education professionals
Psychometric properties	Scale development sample: normative data for the PPVT-4 were collected in 2005–6. The age norms (2y6mo–90+y) were standardized on 3540 individuals; the grade norms (kindergarten–grade 12) were standardized on 2003 individuals. The normative samples were designed to match the US population (as ascertained by 2004 census data) for demographic variables including sex, race/ethnicity, geographical region, socioeconomic status (including father's level of education) and clinical diagnosis (e.g. attention-deficit–hyperactivity disorder, specific language impairment, autism)
	Reliability Internal consistency: split-half reliability was high (ranging from 0.89 to 0.97 for different ages; mean by age=0.94–0.95) on both forms
	Test–retest: a sample (*n*=340) of participants (aged 2–60) was retested after an average of 4 weeks from the first administration. Test–retest reliability was high (*r* ranged from 0.92 to 0.96 for different ages; mean *r*=0.93)
	Validity Content validity: the stimulus words represented 20 content areas and were chosen based on a review of published reference works.
	Construct validity: the PPVT-4 was correlated with the following language assessments and showed strong agreement: EVT-2 (average *r*=0.82); Comprehensive Assessment of Spoken Language (*r*=0.41–0.79 depending on age and subtest); Clinical Evaluation of Language Fundamentals, fourth edition (*r*=0.67–0.75 depending on age and scale) and PPVT-3 (average *r*=0.84)
How to order	The PPVT-4 is available from Pearson Assessments. It can be ordered online at www.pearsonassessments.com/ (USA)
Key references	Dunn LM, Dunn DM (2007) *Peabody Picture Vocabulary Test, fourth edition: User Manual*. Minneapolis, MN: Pearson.
	Pearson Assessments (2010) PPVT-4 Technical specifications. Available at: www.pearsonassessments.com/

their score on even-numbered items). Both forms in the PPVT-4 were found to have high internal consistency (ranging from 0.89 to 0.97 for different ages; mean=0.94). The test–retest reliability (temporal stability of performance) was also high (*r* ranged from 0.92 to 0.96 for different ages; mean *r* by age=0.93). The PPVT-4 correlated well with four other measures of language skills (including the EVT-2[13] and the Clinical Evaluation of Language Fundamentals, fourth edition[14]), demonstrating good construct reliability. Furthermore, the fourth edition of the PPVT correlated well (mean *r*=0.84) with the previous edition of the assessment (PPVT-3), showing a high degree of continuity in the construct measured by both editions. Finally, the content validity of the PPVT-4 was established through the inclusion of stimulus items representing 20 content areas, which were chosen based on a review of published reference works.

EXPRESSION OF LANGUAGE (B1671)

Expressive Vocabulary Test, second edition

Overview and purpose
The EVT[13] was first published in 1997 as a measure of expressive vocabulary and word (spoken) retrieval. The second edition was published in 2007, with stimulus items updated to be more representative of the vocabulary used in the contexts in which children communicate (e.g. including more words that are part of oral directions in the classroom, or words learnt in the home environment). New normative data (for individuals aged 2y6mo–90+y) was collected for the second edition, using the same sample as the PPVT-4.[12] In addition, a parallel form was developed for the updated edition of the EVT, which enables examiners to retest individuals in order to monitor progress. Analysis of items on each form indicates that both forms span a similar range of difficulty and progress in difficulty at a similar rate.

The EVT-2 may be used as a clinical or research tool. The author identified that potential clinical applications of the EVT-2 include screening language development and recording growth in vocabulary knowledge across time. However, caution should be taken when reporting vocabulary scores, as they may be more representative of the nature of a language problem rather than an indicator of general language ability.[15]

The EVT-2 is a useful research tool given the wide range of age norms provided (thereby enabling collection of longitudinal data), the development of parallel test forms (enabling test–retest) and the co–norming of the EVT-2 with the PPVT-4, which enables comparison of expressive and receptive vocabulary skills.[13]

Administration and scoring
The EVT-2 contains two parallel forms (A and B), each of which contains a total of 190 items, arranged according to increasing difficulty. The items represent a range of semantic categories (e.g. vegetables, tools) and parts of speech (e.g. verbs, nouns, adjectives). During the administration of the EVT-2, children are shown an item (picture) and asked to provide an acceptable label, answer a specific question or provide a synonym for a word that matches the picture. They receive a point for each correct response, and testing continues until a ceiling is reached (when the child responds incorrectly to five consecutive items). The examiner calculates the total number of errors in all sets administered and subtracts this number from the highest ceiling item. The number obtained is the child's raw score, which can then be converted to a standard score or centile rank.

Psychometric properties
Normative data for the second edition of the EVT were collected in the USA during 2005–6 (see sample description for PPVT-4 in preceding section).

The internal consistency of the EVT-2 was calculated using split-half reliability. The EVT-2 was found to have high internal consistency reliability (ranging from 0.88 to 0.97 for different ages; mean=0.93–0.94), suggesting that performance on any subset of items within the test will accurately predict performance on other test items.[13] The EVT-2 was also found to have high test–retest reliability when re-administered to a sample of participants (*r* ranged from 0.94 to 0.97 for different ages; mean *r*=0.95), suggesting that performance on the EVT-2 was highly stable over time and was not greatly influenced by changes in an individual's mental or physical state.[13]

The content validity of the EVT-2 is demonstrated through the inclusion of vocabulary items representing 20 content areas and determined through extensive review of published reference works. According to the author, 'items were chosen on the basis of frequency and common usage' and included 'words of high or moderately high frequency that could be acquired through common life experiences', while 'words that required specialized knowledge were avoided'.[13] Evidence that the EVT-2 is a valid measure of expressive vocabulary (i.e. has construct validity) is shown by the correlation of this assessment with four other language assessments, as well as the previous edition of the EVT (mean *r*=0.81). The correlation scores indicate a similar pattern of performance when children were administered the EVT-2 as when they were administered other tests that also measure vocabulary knowledge. Furthermore, the normative data provided in the EVT-2 have been found to differentiate among special populations of individuals to whom the test was administered.

EXPRESSIVE VOCABULARY TEST, SECOND EDITION (EVT-2)	
Purpose	To measure expressive vocabulary and word retrieval of the spoken word (American English), and thus assess vocabulary acquisition
Population	Individuals aged 2y 6mo–90+y
Description of domains (subscales)	The EVT-2 is a measure of expressive vocabulary (production)
Administration and test format	There are two parallel forms (A and B). Each form contains a total number of 190 items, arranged according to increasing difficulty. The items represent a range of semantic categories (e.g. vegetables, tools) and parts of speech (e.g. verbs, nouns, adjectives). They include items corresponding to home and school vocabulary, at varying levels of difficulty
	Time to complete: 10–20min depending on child's age and language skills
	Testing format: children are tested individually. The examiner calculates the child's chronological age to determine the appropriate starting point for the assessment. The examiner shows the child a page with an item (pictures) and asks the child to provide an acceptable label, answer a specific question or provide a synonym for a word that matches the picture. Training items are administered first, and the child is required to respond correctly to these before commencing the test items. The examiner records the child's response and determines if it matches a correct/incorrect response on the response form. Testing continues until a ceiling is reached (when the child responds incorrectly to five consecutive items)
	Scoring: children receive one point for each correct response. The basal rule is five consecutive correct items; the ceiling rule is five consecutive incorrect items. The examiner determines the basal item (the first/lowest item from the basal set of five correct items) and the ceiling item (the highest item from the ceiling set of five incorrect items). The examiner calculates the total number of errors in all sets administered, and subtracts this number from the highest ceiling item. The number obtained is the child's raw score, which can then be converted to a standard score or centile rank
	Training: restricted to use by allied health or special education professionals
Psychometric properties	Scale development sample: normative data for the EVT-2 were collected in 2005–6. The age norms (2y 6mo–90+y) were standardized on 3540 individuals; the grade norms (kindergarten–grade 12) were standardized on 2003 individuals. The normative samples were designed to match the US population (as ascertained by 2004 census data) for demographic variables including sex, race/ethnicity, geographical region, socioeconomic status (including father's level of education) and clinical diagnosis (e.g. attention-deficit–hyperactivity disorder, specific language impairment, autism)
	Reliability
	Internal consistency: split-half reliability was high (0.88–0.97 for different ages; mean by age=0.93–0.94) on both forms.
	Test–retest: a sample (*n*=348) of participants (aged 2–60y) was retested 2–6 weeks after the first administration.
	Test–retest reliability was high (*r* ranged from 0.94 to 0.97 for different ages; mean *r*=0.95)
	Validity
	Content validity: the stimulus words represented 20 content areas, and were chosen based on a review of published reference works.
	Construct validity: the EVT-2 was correlated with the following language assessments and showed strong agreement: PPVT-4 (average *r*=0.82); Comprehensive Assessment of Spoken Language (*r*=0.50 to.84 depending on age and subtest); Clinical Evaluation of Language Fundamentals, fourth edition (*r*=0.68–0.80 depending on age and scale); and EVT (average *r*=0.81)

How to order	The EVT-2 is available from Pearson Assessments. It can be ordered online at www. pearsonassessments.com/ (USA)
Key references	Pearson Assessments (2010) EVT-2 Technical specifications. Available at: www. pearsonassessments.com
	Williams KT (2007) *Expressive Vocabulary Test, second edition: Manual.* Minneapolis, MN: Pearson.

INTEGRATIVE LANGUAGE FUNCTIONS

The MacArthur–Bates Communicative Development Inventories, second edition

Overview and purpose

The MacArthur–Bates Communicative Development Inventories[16] (CDI-II) were designed to assess early language development (comprehension and production) in children aged 8 to 30 months. There are two forms: one designed for children aged 8 to 18 months, which examines the development of words and gestures (CDI-WG), and the other designed for children aged 16 to 30 months, which examines the development of words and sentences (CDI-WS). They were first published in 1993, and the revised edition was published in 2006, with extended norms for the CDI-WG. The second edition also includes a short form (CDI-III), developed as an upward extension of the CDIs, which measures expressive vocabulary and grammar in children aged 30 to 37 months. However, all forms may be used with older children with developmental delays.[16]

The CDIs have been adapted for use with children from a range of English-speaking countries including New Zealand[17] and the UK.[18] There are also adapted versions for children who speak languages other than English, such as Spanish,[19] Hebrew[20] and Swedish.[21] Versions of the CDIs have been developed recently for children who use American Sign Language.[22]

According to the authors, the CDIs may be used for clinical and research applications, including screening for language delay, describing individual patterns of strength and weakness, and assisting in the formulation of intervention goals.[16] They have been used to assess the language skills of children with cochlear implants[23] and autism spectrum disorders,[24] as well as children who are late in beginning talking.

Administration and scoring

The CDIs are parent-completed records of the communication used and understood by their children. As such, no training is required for completion of the measure, and the time taken to complete the measure is dependent on the child's level of language development (approximately 20–40min is expected). Once completed, allied health or special education professionals score the forms.

The CDI-WG requires parents to identify from a given list the gestures and phrases which their child understands, as well as actions that their child may use to communicate. The largest portion of the inventory is a 396-item vocabulary checklist, organized into 19 semantic categories, on which parents are requested to mark the items that their child uses and/or understands. Ten of the semantic categories are composed of nouns (animals, vehicles, toys, foods), while additional categories cover other parts of speech, such as verbs, adjectives and pronouns. Examination of the parent's responses to the CDI-WG enables the calculation of raw scores for the following aspects of communicative development: children's comprehension of phrases, comprehension and production of vocabulary, and use of actions and gestures. Raw scores can be compared with normative data.

The CDI-WS contains a 680-item vocabulary production checklist, on which parents are requested to mark the words that their child uses. The checklist is divided into 22 semantic categories, of which 11 are composed exclusively of nouns. The second part of the CDI-WS is designed to assess the child's grammatical development, including his or her use of morphemes (e.g. regular and irregular plurals and past tense) and the complexity of his or her utterances. Examination of the parent's responses to the CDI-WS enables calculation of raw scores for the following aspects of communicative development: vocabulary production, use of grammatical structures, word combinations, and sentence length and complexity. Raw scores can be compared with normative data.

Psychometric properties

Normative data for the CDIs were collected from 1789 children (903 females and 886 males) aged 8 to 30 months. Children were excluded from the scale development sample when parents reported developmental conditions such as Down syndrome or serious medical

MACARTHUR–BATES COMMUNICATIVE DEVELOPMENTAL INVENTORIES, SECOND EDITION (CDI-II)	
Purpose	To assess language and communication skills in young children
Population	Infants and young children (8–30mo)
	A short form (CDI-III) has been developed as an upward extension of the CDI-II and is aimed at children aged 30–37mo
Description of domains (subscales)	Two versions: the Words and Gestures Inventory (CDI-WG) and the Words and Sentences Inventory (CDI-WS)
	The CDI-WG is designed for children aged 8–16mo and examines children's understanding of gestures and phrases, as well as their use of actions and words (from a 396-item vocabulary checklist) to communicate. The CDI-WS is designed for children aged 16–30mo and examines children's production of oral language, including their use of words (from a checklist of 680 vocabulary items) and grammatical structures, and the complexity of their utterances
Administration and test format	Time to complete: 20–40min depending on the child's level of development
	Testing format: parents identify their child's use and/or understanding of a range of gestures/actions, single words, phrases and sentences from a given list
	Scoring: the number of items checked by parents is calculated for each section completed (e.g. vocabulary production, use of grammatical structures, word combinations, sentence length and complexity). These raw scores can be compared with normative data
	Training: parents complete the CDI forms; scoring is conducted by an allied health or special education professional
Psychometric properties	Scale development sample: normative data were collected for 1789 children (659 infants and 1130 toddlers) at three sites in the USA. There were approximately the same number of males and females in each age group. Children with Down syndrome and meningitis were excluded, as were children with 'serious medical problems' and those born more than 6 weeks preterm. All children spoke English as their primary language; however, some children were from bilingual language environments. The education levels of parents completing the CDIs were above the national average (i.e. most had at least a high-school education)
	Reliability
	Internal consistency: on the CDI-WG, vocabulary production (Cronbach's α=0.96) and vocabulary comprehension (α=0.95) both demonstrated high internal consistency. However, the CDI-WG gesture scale showed much lower internal consistency (α=0.39). On the CDI-WS, both vocabulary production (α=0.96) and sentence complexity (α=0.95) demonstrated a high degree of internal reliability.
	Test–retest: parents' (n=500) test–retest correlation was high (r=0.8–0.9) for the CDI-WG and for the CDI-WS (r>0.9)
	Validity
	Content validity: the items within each form were based on developmental literature and parent suggestions and sample the major features of communicative development across the targeted age groups.
	Construct validity: correlations between the CDI-WS and two other language measures (Expressive One-Word Picture Vocabulary Test and Type Token Ratio) were moderate (r=0.53–0.73) correlation between the CDI–WS complexity scale and Mean Length of Utterance (100 word utterance language sample) was also high (r=0.76–0.88)
How to order	The manual and forms are available from Paul H. Brookes Publishing. Orders can be placed online at www.brookespublishing.com/cdi

Key references	The MacArthur–Bates Communicative Development Inventories website is:
	www.sci.sdsu.edu/cdi/cdiwelcome.htm
	The website contains information about adapted versions of the CDI-II, as well as updated lexical norms and ordering information.
	Fenson L, Marchman VA, Thal D, Dale PS, Reznick JS, Bates E (2006) *MacArthur–Bates Communicative Development Inventories: User Guide and Technical Manual*, 2nd edition. Baltimore, MD: Paul H. Brookes.

conditions such as meningitis. Children born more than 6 weeks preterm were also excluded from the sample. All children spoke English as their primary language; however, children from bilingual language environments were included, as this is reflective of the US population. The education levels of parents completing the CDIs were above the national average (i.e. most had at least a high-school education).

Both of the CDI forms demonstrated high internal consistency for most of the scales (Cronbach's α=0.95–0.96), suggesting that items included within the same categories were measuring the same skills.[16] The exception was the gesture scale on the CDI-WG, which achieved a lower internal consistency score (α=0.39). Further examination indicated that a low correlation between the first subscale (first communicative gestures) and two other subscales (games and routines, and pretending to be a parent) on the gesture scale may have contributed to the lower consistency score. The authors suggested that the low correlation may reflect the distinct nature and time of emergence of the various gesture categories.[16] The CDIs were found to have high test–retest reliability (r=0.80–0.90) when completed by a sample of 500 parents 6 months after their initial completion, suggesting that the measures provide stable scores across two test sessions.

Correlations between the CDI-WS and two other measures of language development (Expressive One Word Picture Vocabulary Test and Type Token Ratio) were substantial (r=0.53–0.73) for children with typically developing language skills and those with delayed language development.[16] The items within each form were based on developmental literature and parent suggestions, and sample the major features of communicative development across the targeted age groups.

Preschool Language Scale, fourth edition

Overview and purpose
The Preschool Language Scale, fourth edition[25] (PLS-4), examines comprehension and production of spoken language for children from birth to age 6 years 11 months. The Preschool Language Scale was first published in

1969. The current and fourth edition (PLS-4) was published in 2002, and a fifth edition is currently in production. Revisions to the fourth edition focused on improved psychometric properties (especially ceiling, floor and difficulty gradients) and refining the scoring criteria. Additionally, the standardization sample for the fourth edition included increased racial/ethnic diversity, children with identified developmental disorders and children who spoke other languages in addition to English or a dialect other than standard American English.

Administration and scoring
The PLS-4 is individually administered by an allied health or special education professional, most commonly a speech–language pathologist (SLP). Test materials comprise a picture manual containing coloured picture stimuli and objects that can be handled (e.g. blocks, cups, teddy bear) to facilitate examiner–child interactions. The PLS-4 comprises two scales: an auditory comprehension (AC) scale, which examines attention, semantics, structure and integrative thinking skills, and an expressive communication (EC) scale, which examines vocal development, social communication, semantics, structure and integrative thinking skills. Either scale may be administered first; however, scales must be completed within one session with tasks administered in the order outlined in the examiner's record booklet. Examiners cannot alternate testing between the two scales. No specific start point is identified; rather it is based upon information obtained regarding the child's current language abilities.

A basal level is obtained with three consecutive scores of '1' before a '0' score. The ceiling criterion is flexible, with the administrator able to select from a choice of three, five or seven consecutive '0' scores. All responses are recorded by the examiner on the test record form with scoring criteria for each item (e.g. pass: two correct) outlined on the record form. Each item is scored as being elicited (E) from the child using administration directions, as spontaneous (S) productions used by the child when interacting with another individual or as reported by the caregiver (C) as able to be performed within the home environment. The PLS-4 also comprises open-ended questions.

PRESCHOOL LANGUAGE SCALE, FOURTH EDITION (PLS-4)	
Purpose	To identify children who have a language disorder or delay
Population	Birth to 6y 11mo
Description of domains (subscales)	The PLS-4 is based on the language constructs of form (structure), content (meaning) and use
	Receptive language/auditory comprehension (AC) examines attention, semantics, structure and integrative thinking skills. Expressive language/communication (EC) examines vocal development, social communication, semantics, structure and integrative thinking skills. A task analysis profile is included for summarizing AC and EC abilities. A total language score is derived from the combination of the AC and EC scores
	Additional measures: articulation screener, Language Sample Checklist examining morpho-syntax, semantics, social language and a rating of speech intelligibility, and a caregiver questionnaire
Administration and test format	Time to complete: variable according to age. Birth to 11mo, 20–40min; 12mo–3y 11mo, 30–40min; 4y–6y 11mo, 25–35min
	Testing format: one-to-one administration; auditory comprehension or expressive communication scale may be administered first. Tasks are administered in the order outlined in examiner's record booklet. No specific start point is identified; rather it is based upon information obtained regarding the examinee's current language abilities. A basal level is obtained with three consecutive scores of '1' before a score of '0'. The ceiling criterion is flexible with the administrator able to select from a choice of three, five or seven consecutive '0' scores
	Once commenced, a scale must be completed within one session, with breaks provided as required. Examiners cannot alternate between the two scales. The PLS-4 is suitable for students who speak English and its dialects as well as students with developmental difficulties such as global developmental delay or speech sound disorders
	Scoring: The PLS-4 enables calculation of AC, EC and total language standard scores ($70 <$score< 130), centiles (1st to 99th) and age equivalents. It also provides descriptive terms for subtests and composites (very poor to very superior).
	A PLS-4 Measure of Progress is available to track therapy progression and to assist with the interpretation of additional administrations of the PLS-4
	A PLS-4 screener is also available, as well as a PLS-4 Spanish edition
	A new version, the PLS-5, has recently been released
	Training: typically administered by professionals (speech–language pathologists, early education specialists, psychologists, educational diagnosticians) with formal training in test administration and scoring and interpretation, statistics and evaluation of language abilities; however, paraprofessionals can administer the PLS-4 under supervision
Psychometric properties	Normative sample: n=1564 (0–6y 11mo) from 48 US states and the District of Colombia; approximately 50% male and 50% female. Standardization sample was based on the 2000 US Census of Population stratified for parental education, region and race. Ethnic minorities constituted 39.1% of the total sample, with 13.2% of the sample children with additional needs such as autism and language disorder. An unspecified 'small' percentage of the sample spoke languages in addition to English or a dialect other than standard American English
	Reliability Internal consistency: Fisher's z: subtests and composites ranged from 0.66 to 0.94 for AC, from 0.73 to 0.94 for EC and from 0.81 to 0.97 for the total language score.
	Test–retest (n=218): r=0.82–0.95 for AC and EC and r=0.90–0.97 for the total language score.
	Internal consistency reliability: r=0.66–0.96. Inter-rater reliability (n=100): r=0.99

Psychometric properties	*Validity* Content description: literature review, user survey, content, bias and task reviews were conducted. Internal consistency across the two subscales was *r*=0.74. Concurrent validity – uncorrected correlation of PLS-4 composites with other measures: Denver II and PLS-3 (*n*=37). Participants scored as within the average range on both assessments. Correlation between the PLS-3 and PLS-4: AE=0.65, EC=0.79. Sensitivity and specificity information for a sample of 150 children with specific language impairment are as follows:	
	AC	Sensitivity 0.80, specificity 0.92
	EC	Sensitivity 0.77, specificity 0.84
	Total language score	Sensitivity 0.80, specificity 0.88
How to order	Pearson assessments: www.pearson.com; US$305 (with manipulatives)	
Key references	Friberg JC (2010) Considerations for test selection: How do validity and reliability impact diagnostic decisions? *Child Lang Teach Ther* 26: 77–92. Qi CH, Marley SC (2009) Differential item functioning analysis of the Preschool Language Scale-4 between English-speaking Hispanic and European American children from low-income families. *Topics Early Child Special Ed* 29: 171–180. Zimmerman IL, Castilleja NF (2005) The role of a language scale for infant and preschool assessment. *Mental Retard Dev Disabil Res Rev* 11: 238–246.	

The targeted response for these questions is outlined on the test record form, while the manual includes examples of typical correct and incorrect answers. For the auditory comprehension (AC), expressive communication (EC) and total language score (derived from the combination of the AC and EC scores), age-based standard scores, centile ranks and age equivalents can be determined. Finally, the manual provides directions for accommodations (able to use norm-referenced scores) and modifications (unable to use norm-referenced scores) to test administration for specific populations, such as those with vision impairment, hearing impairment or autism.

Psychometric properties

Normative data for the PLS-4 were collected from 1564 children in 2001, with sampling based upon the US population (as ascertained by 2000 census data).

Internal consistency within subtests and composites was moderate to good (Fisher's *z*=0.66–0.94 for AC, 0.73–0.94 for EC and 0.81–0.97 for the total language score). Test–retest reliability (2–14d gap, mean=5.9 days) was examined using a sample of 218 randomly selected participants aged 2 years to 5 years 11 months, and was found to be acceptable for both scales. Internal consistency reliability as measured via Cronbach's alpha coefficient was moderate to strong (α=0.66–0.94 for AC, 0.73–0.95 for EC and 0.81–0.97 for the total language score). Inter-rater reliability, completed on a sample of 100 participants utilizing 15 different raters (predominantly elementary school teachers), was strong (*r*=0.99).

The authors reported good content validity with task development based on literature review, user survey, content, bias and task review.[25] Internal structure consistency between the AC and EC scales was *r*=0.74 for the entire sample. Concurrent validity was examined between the PLS-4 and the Denver-II for 37 participants from birth to age 11 months. All participants received a rating of 'normal' on the Denver-II and a standard score within one standard deviation of the mean (i.e. within normal limits) on the PLS-4, demonstrating good consistency of results. Correlation was conducted between the PLS-4 and the PLS-3 for 104 participants aged 2 months to 7 years. The correlation between the PLS-4 and the PLS-3 was *r*=0.65 for AC and *r*=0.79 for EC. Finally, sensitivity was 0.80 for AC, 0.77 for EC and 0.92 for total language score, specificity was 0.92 for AC, 0.84 for EC and 0.88 for total language score when used with children diagnosed with a specific language impairment. Mean and standard deviation data are also provided for children with developmental language delay, autism or hearing loss in specific age groups. All groups were compared with age-matched typically developing peers and found to perform worse than peers across all scales.

Clinical Evaluation of Language Fundamentals, fourth edition

Overview and purpose

The Clinical Evaluation of Language Fundamentals, fourth edition[14] (CELF-4) is a formal, standardized

CLINICAL EVALUATION OF LANGUAGE FUNDAMENTALS, FOURTH EDITION (CELF-4)	
Purpose	To evaluate the general language abilities of children, adolescents and young adults to establish whether or not a language disorder exists. Four flexible levels of assessment testing are provided to assist the assessor in making judgements about language performance
Population	Ages 5–21y. However, 'out of age range administration' is permitted. Raw scores for these children cannot be translated to standard scores, but age-equivalency scores can be obtained
Description of subtests	The CELF-4 subtests are: Concepts and Following Directions* (54 items), Word Structure* (Recalling Sentences* [32 items]), Formulated Sentences* (28 items), Word Classes 1 (21 items) and Word Classes 2* (24 items), Sentence Structure (26 items), Expressive Vocabulary (27 items), Word Definitions (24 items), Understanding Spoken Paragraphs (15 items), Semantics Relationships (21 items), Sentence Assembly (19 items), Phonological Awareness (85 items), Rapid Automated Naming, Word Associations, Number Repetitions (1 and 2), Familiar Sequences (1 and 2), Pragmatics Profile (52 items) and Observational Rating Scale (40 items) *=required for core language score
Administration and test format	Time to complete: administration time ranges from 30 to 60min depending on the child's age, motivation, language level and subtest being administered. Four specific subtests need to be administered to obtain a core language score Testing format: the examiner individually administers the test to each student. Students respond either verbally or non-verbally depending on the subtest being administered Scoring: scoring is primarily objective. Responses are scored primarily as correct (1) or incorrect (0). Subtest scores, composite/index scores, centile ranks, criterion scores and age equivalents are obtained Administrator eligibility: speech–language pathologists, school psychologists, special educators and diagnosticians trained in the administration and interpretation of standardized tests
Psychometric properties	Normative sample: >2500 children from the USA with representative characteristics for race/ethnicity, age, sex, geographic region and primary caregiver's education level *Reliability* Adequate to excellent reliability established based on test–retest, internal consistency and interscorer agreement *Validity* There is extensive evidence of validity for the CELF-4 based on test content, response process, internal structure, relationships with other variables (i.e. the CELF-3) and consequences of testing. The CELF-4 is reported to have good sensitivity and specificity
How to order	The CELF-4 is available from Pearson Assessments (www.pearson.com). The cost is approximately US$505 (base price)
Key reference	[Semel WA, Wiig EH, Secord WA (2003) *Clinical Evaluation of Language Fundamentals*, 4th edition. San Antonio, TX: The Psychological Cooperation]

assessment for determining the presence and nature of a language disorder or delay in students aged 5 to 21 years, and for evaluating how the disorder affects students in the classroom.[14] It has a number of clinical and research applications including (1) determining eligibility for language services, (2) identifying language strengths and weaknesses and (3) providing performance-based authentic assessment with a strong relationship to educational objectives and the curriculum.[14] The CELF-4 has been norm-referenced for other populations including Spanish, Australian, British and Canadian children and adolescents.

Administration and scoring

The CELF-4 is an individually administered assessment that can be used by SLPs, school psychologists, special educators and others trained in the administration and interpretation of standardized tests. The administration time for the four subtests required to obtain a core language score is approximately 30 to 45 minutes and is dependent on student age and level of responsiveness. The administration time for each of the remaining subtests is variable depending on age, language ability, level of motivation and selected subtests. Subtest starting items and discontinue rules are included to shorten potential testing times for each subtest, as well as to decrease student fatigue and/or boredom.[14] Each item is scored using a standard rubric '0' to indicate an incorrect response or '1' to indicate a correct response for most subtests. Types of performance information obtained from this measure include (1) subtest scaled scores (mean=10, standard deviation=3), (2) composite scores, using sums of various subtest scaled scores (standard score, mean=100, standard deviation=15), (3) criterion scores, (4) index scores, (5) centile ranks and (6) age equivalents. Specific scoring instructions are clearly stated for each subtest. Consideration of cultural and dialectal variation is provided in this version of the CELF.

Psychometric properties

The CELF-4 was standardized on a representative sample of >2600 children. The sample was representative of the US population in 2000, based on age, sex, race/ethnicity, socioeconomic status based on the primary parent's educational level, geographic region and children identified with specific conditions.[14] Reliability was estimated using test–retest stability, internal consistency and interscorer agreement. A sample of 320 children from the standardization sample was utilized to establish reliability. Test–retest reliability coefficients ranged from $r=0.71$ to 0.86 for subtests and from $r=0.88$ to 0.92 for composite scores. Internal consistency, evaluated using Cronbach's alpha coefficient, ranged from 0.69 to 0.91 for subtests and from 0.87 to 0.95 for composite scores. Internal consistency using the split-half reliability ranged from $r=0.71$ to 0.92 for subtests and from $r=0.87$ to 0.95 for composites scores. Interscorer agreement for subtests requiring subjectivity in scoring interpretation was high (ranging from 0.88 to 0.99). There is extensive evidence of validity for the CELF-4 based on test content, response process, internal structure, relationships with other assessments (i.e. the CELF-3) and consequences of testing. The CELF-4 was also found to have good diagnostic accuracy as evidenced by sensitivity (the percentage of students classified as having a language disorder) and specificity (the percentage of students without a language disorder) based on the core language score at 1, 1.5 and 2 standard deviations below the mean.

Oral and Written Language Scales

Overview and purpose

The Oral and Written Language Scales (OWLS)[26,27] are comprehensive measures of language achievement in children, adolescents and young adults aged 3 to 21 years. There are three co-normed language scales: oral expression (OES), listening comprehension (LCS) and written expression (WES). The LCS measures receptive language and the OES evaluates oral expression skills for answering questions, completing sentences and sentence generation. The WES assesses writing skills, particularly the use of conventions (e.g. handwriting, spelling, punctuation), use of syntactical forms (e.g. modifiers, phrases, sentence structures) and content (namely the ability to communicate organized, cohesive and relevant messages in written form).

Results obtained from the scales are useful for (1) determining eligibility for special educational services, (2) planning instruction to help address potential academic difficulties, (3) monitoring growth in language skills across a broad time span and (4) gathering longitudinal data for research purposes. The OWLS has been used in research studies to establish its usefulness in evaluating the level of language functioning in children with specific profiles.

Administration and scoring

The OWLS is administered primarily individually, although the WES can also be administered in a group setting.[26,27] Administration and interpretation of the OWLS is restricted to individuals with educational or psychological backgrounds who have graduate-level training. There are specific scoring instructions for each of the OWLS language scales.

For the LCS, examiners read aloud verbal stimuli and examinees identify the corresponding picture from a group of four. Items are scored '0' or '1' to indicate correct or incorrect responses, respectively. Basal rules (a score of '1' on seven consecutive items) and ceiling rules (a score of '0' on five out of seven consecutive items) are included for the LCS. A child's total raw score can then be converted to a standard score. For the OES, examiners read aloud a verbal stimulus and show a picture(s), and examinees provide verbal responses by answering a question, completing a sentence or generating more sentences. Administration and scoring is mostly similar to the LCS, with a few exceptions (e.g. the ceiling rule, a score of '0'

ORAL AND WRITTEN LANGUAGE SCALES (OWLS)	
Purpose	To measure receptive and expressive language achievement in children, adolescents and young adults aged 3–21y. The OWLS can assist in determining to what extent ability scores may have been influenced by delays or disorders in language. Three separate scales are provided: Listening Comprehension Scale (LCS), Oral Expression Scale (OES) and Written Expression Scale (WES)
Population	Ages 3–21y. However, 'out of level' administration (i.e. testing within an examinee's language skills age vs chronological age) is permitted
Description of scales	The OWLS does not contain subtests; instead, three language scales are utilized:
	(1) The LCS: The LCS (3–21y) evaluates comprehension of language (listening skills) in three categories – lexical, syntactic and supralinguistic. There are 111 task items
	(2) The OES (3–21y) evaluates expression of language (verbal skills) in four categories – lexical, syntactic, pragmatic and supralinguistic. There are 96 task items
	(3) The WES (5–21y) evaluates written language skills (writing) in three categories – conventions, linguistics and content. There are five group tasks (39 items) – dictated sentences, functional writing, story completion, descriptive writing and brief expository writing
Administration and test format	Time to complete: administration time ranges from 5 to 25min depending on the language scale administered: LCS (5–15min), OES (10–25min) and WES (10–30min). If all three are administered, the following order of administration is recommended: LCS, WES and OES
	Testing format: each scale is administered individually. Note that the WES may also be administered in a group format. Examiners administer the test to each examinee. Examinees respond verbally, non-verbally or in written form depending on the administered scale
	Scoring: scoring is primarily objective. Standard score rubric for '0' (indicating incorrect response) and '1' (indicating correct response) in addition to multiple-point scoring rules for various scales. OWLS scales score for LCS, OES and WES. Additional scores include oral composite score, language composite score, centile, age equivalent and stanine
	Administrator eligibility: speech–language pathologists, school and clinical psychologists, special educators, resource teachers, etc. trained in the administration and interpretation of tests
Psychometric properties	Normative sample: >3000 children from the USA with representative characteristics for race/ethnicity, age, sex, geographic region and mother's education level for all three language scales
	Reliability
	Moderate to excellent reliability established based on test–retest, internal consistency and inter-rater agreement for all three language scales
	Validity
	There is extensive evidence of validity for the OWLS scales based on content validity, construct validity and criterion-related validity. Applicability to special populations is reported
How to order	The OWLS is available from multiple sources including Superduper (www.superduperinc. com/products, US$555) and Pro-Ed Inc. (www.proedinc.com, US$399)
Key references	[Carrow-Woolfolk (1995) *Oral and Written Language Scales (OWLS) – Listening Comprehension and Oral Expression Manual*. Circle Pines, MN: American Guidances Service
	Carrow-Woolfolk (1996) *Oral and Written Language Scales (OWLS) – Written Expression Scale*. Circle Pines, MN: American Guidances Service]

on six out of seven consecutive items, is slightly different). The sum of the LCS and the OES standard scores are combined together for an oral composite which includes performance information for (1) standard score, (2) confidence interval, (3) centile rank, (4) stanine, (5) normal curve equivalent (NCE) and (6) test age equivalent.

For the WES, there are 39 items divided into four overlapping sets, which are organized according to age. Examiners read aloud instructions for each set and examinees have a response booklet to write the appropriate responses. Scoring rules, which relate to a specific aspect of the item response and are based on one of three writing skill categories (i.e. conventions, linguistics and content), are used for each response item. Detailed scoring rules (provided in the manual) are needed to obtain a total raw score. Performance information obtained from the WES includes (1) ability score, (2) standard score for age or grade, (3) standard score confidence interval, (4) centile rank, (5) stanine, (6) normal curve equivalent and (7) test age equivalent or grade equivalent. Comparisons are possible between the WES and the oral composite score (sum of LCS and OES) to obtain a language composite score (mean=100, standard deviation=15).

Psychometric properties (listening comprehension and oral expression)
Standardization for the OWLS was completed on a representative sample of 1985 children and young people aged 3 to 21 years across 74 testing sites in the USA.[26] The sample was stratified to match US census data within specified age groups according to sex, race, ethnic group, geographic region and socioeconomic level (mother's education). A random sampling procedure was utilized to recruit the representative sample of examinees. For internal reliability (split-half method), the mean coefficients (based on item response theory) were excellent ($r=0.84$ for LCS, $r=0.87$ for OES and $r=0.91$ for oral composite). Temporal stability of the OWLS was evaluated through test–retest reliability (ranging from 20 to 165d) with three of the age groups (4y–5y 11mo; 8y–10y 11mo; 16y–18y 11mo). Reliability coefficients ranged from $r=0.73$ to 0.80 for LCS, $r=0.77$ to 0.86 for OES and $r=0.81$ to 0.89 for the oral composite.

Evidence of content validity was demonstrated in the detailed construct and descriptions of the scales provided. Strict adherence to specific scale blueprints for both the LCS and OES was noted. Two types of construct validity

were reported: (1) developmental progression of scores (showed steady increases in mean raw scores throughout the age ranges noted) and (2) intercorrelations of the scales (moderate correlation between the LCS and the OES was found: range $r=0.54$–0.77; mean $r=0.70$). This information demonstrated that each scale scored unique information, and validity was deemed high enough to support the combination of the LCS and the OES to obtain the oral composite.[26]

Studies were completed to establish evidence of criterion-related validity. Evidence was provided for both convergent and discriminant validity, with higher correlations noted for the former and lower for the latter. The oral composite was found to be correlated with other tests of language skills (e.g. Test of Auditory Comprehension of Language – revised, PPVT – revised, CELF – revised). Evidence for correlations with measures of cognitive abilities and academic achievement was also noted. An additional sample of students with specific diagnoses (e.g. speech/language impairment, language delay, specific learning disabilities and hearing impairment) were also included in clinical validity studies to address their performance on the LCS and OES.

Psychometric properties (written expression)
The WES was standardized on 1373 individuals aged 5 to 21 years. Similar to the other two scales, the sample was stratified to match the US census data based on a range of variables (age, sex, mother's education, race/ethnicity and geographic region), and an additional 185 individuals with specific diagnoses (language impairments, mental retardation,[a] learning disabilities, hearing losses and reading delays) were tested for clinical validity studies. Internal consistency reliability coefficients ranged from $r=0.77$ to 0.94, test–retest reliability (completed over 18 to 165-day intervals) ranged from $r=0.83$ to 0.88, and inter-rater reliability (completed for the open-ended portions of the scale) ranged from $r=0.91$ to 0.98 across the ages tested.

Similar to the oral scales, content validity was established based on the detailed construct and descriptions of the scales provided.[27] Construct validity was based on extensive development efforts to match content and format of the scale to language theory.[27] Correlations to other measures of academic achievement, measures of cognitive ability and language were also reported.

---

[a] UK usage: learning disability.

Additional Measures

CLINICAL EVALUATION OF LANGUAGE FUNDAMENTALS – PRESCHOOL 2 (CELF-P2)	
Purpose	To evaluate preschool children's general language abilities towards the end goal of establishing whether or not a language disorder exists. The CELF-P2 permits evaluation of language aspects necessary for preschool children to successfully matriculate to the classroom
Population	Ages 3–6y. However, 'out of age range administration' for older children functioning at a notably lower mental age is permitted. Raw scores for these children cannot be translated to standard scores, but age-equivalency scores can be obtained
Description of subtests	There are 11 subtests administered according to four specific assessment levels. The subtests are sentence structure (22 items), word structure (24 items), expressive vocabulary (20 items), concepts and following directions (13 items), recalling sentences (13 items), basic concepts (18 items), word classes (20 items), recalling sentences in context (14 items), phonological awareness (24 items), preliteracy rating scale (26 items) and descriptive pragmatics profile (26 items)
Administration and test format	Time to complete: administration time ranges from 15 to 45min depending on the child's age, motivation and language level and on the subtest being administered
	Testing format: the assessor individually administers the test to each child. Children respond either verbally or non-verbally depending on the subtest administered
	Scoring: scoring is primarily objective. Reponses are scored as correct (1) or incorrect (0) for most subtests. Subtest scores, composite/index scores, centile ranks, criterion scores and age equivalents are obtained
	Administrator eligibility: speech–language pathologists, school psychologists, special educators and diagnosticians trained in the administration and interpretation of standardized tests
Psychometric properties	Normative sample: >1100 children from the USA with representative characteristics for race/ethnicity, age, sex, geographic region and primary caregiver's education level
	Reliability Adequate to excellent reliability has been established based on test–retest, internal consistency and interscorer agreement
	Validity Experts involved in establishing content validity. Noted intercorrelations between subtests and composite/index scores. Correlates with (1) Clinical Evaluation of Language Fundamentals – Preschool; (2) Clinical Evaluation of Language Fundamentals, fourth edition; (3) Preschool Language Scales, fourth edition (concurrent validity). The CELF-P2 is reported to have good sensitivity and specificity
How to order	The CELF-P2 is available from Pearson Assessments (www.pearson.com). The cost is approximately US$360
Key Reference	Semel WA, Wiig EH, Secord WA (2003) *Clinical Evaluation of Language Fundamentals*, 4th edn. San Antonio, TX: The Psychological Corporation.

THE TEST OF ADOLESCENT AND ADULT LANGUAGE, FOURTH EDITION (TOAL-4)®	
Purpose	To measure varying degrees of English language knowledge in the spoken and written domains. Three relevant dimensions of language described as features (semantics, grammar, graphology), modes (spoken or written) and systems (receptive, expressive, integrative) within the TOAL-4. It can be used to identify adolescents and young adults who score significantly below their peers; determine areas of relative strength and weakness among language abilities; and serve as a research tool to investigate language problems in studies

Population	Adolescents and young adults aged 12y–24y 11mo
Description of subtests	There are six subtests used to evaluate spoken and written language skills: word opposites (34 items), word derivations (51 items), spoken analogies (26 items), word similarities (40 items), sentence combining (30 items) and orthographic usage (47 items). Each of the six subtests captures a specific mode, feature or system
Administration and test format	Time to complete: 60min, administered individually or in a group
	Testing format: examiner administration to students. Students have response booklets to complete their responses using a pencil
	Scoring: scoring is primarily objective. Reponses are scored as correct (1) or incorrect (0). Entry items and ceilings described
	Administrator eligibility: administration is restricted to professionals with formal training in assessment who are (1) knowledgeable about testing, statistics and the general procedures governing test administration, scoring and interpretation and (2) trained in the evaluation of linguistic abilities
Psychometric properties	Normative sample: >1600 adolescents and young adults across 35 different states in the USA with representative characteristics for sex, region, ethnicity, Hispanic status, exceptionality status, family income and parents' educational level
	Reliability Reliability established: coefficient alpha, test–retest and scorer differences
	Validity Content description: minimal amount of item bias for sex, race and ethnicity.
	Criterion-prediction validity: correlation with other measures of spoken and/or written language (e.g. Woodcock Johnson III Word Identification; Test of Pragmatic Language, second edition)
	Construction identification: correlates with age and tests of intelligence, scores differentiate between normal and poor language profiles
How to order	The TOAL-4 is available through a number of providers including Pearson (www.pearson.com) for US$260
Key reference	Hammill DD, Brown VL, Larsen SC, Wiederholt JL (2007) *Test of Adolescent and Adult Language*, 4th edn. San Antonio, TX: The psychological corporation.

TEST OF LANGUAGE DEVELOPMENT: PRIMARY, FOURTH EDITION (TOLD-P:4)

Purpose	To identify children who present significantly below their peers in language proficiency; determine children's specific strengths and weaknesses; document language progression resultant from intervention programmes; and to measure language in research studies (Newcomer and Hammill, 2008). Assessment of oral language proficiency utilizes a two-dimensional framework comprising linguistic systems (listening, organizing and speaking) and linguistic features (syntax, semantics and phonology)
Population	Ages 4y 0mo–8y 11mo
Description of domains (subscales)	Six core subtests examine semantics or syntax (picture vocabulary, relational vocabulary, oral vocabulary, syntactic understanding, sentence imitation and morphological completion)
	Three supplementary subtests assess phonology (word discrimination, phonemic analysis and word articulation). Supplemental subtests are administered after ages 7y 0mo only when difficulties are apparent. The core subtests form six composites: listening, organizing, speaking, grammar, semantics and spoken language

Administration and test format	Time to complete: core subtests – 35–50min; supplementary subtests – 30min
	Testing format: one-to-one administration, administer in order outlined in examiner's record booklet. One repetition of a test item is allowed upon request by the examinee for all subtests except sentence imitation. Typically core subtests can be administered within one session. Supplementary subtests should be administered at the same time as the core subtests.
	Scoring: subtest scaled scores (1–20). Composite indexes (<70 to >130). Descriptive terms for subtests and composites (very poor–very superior). Centiles (1st to >99th). Age equivalents. Scoring and reporting software available
	Training: formal training in test administration, scoring and interpretation, statistics and assessment of language abilities is required for administration
Psychometric properties	Normative sample: n=1108 from 16 US states. Ages tested: 4y (n=166), 5y (n=182), 6y (n=268), 7y (n=266) and 8y (n=226); 52% male, 48% female. Standardization sample matched 2005 US school-age population reported in the Statistical Abstract of the United States (US Census Bureau, 2007)
	Reliability Internal consistency: Fisher's z: subtests and composites ranged from 0.84 to 0.97.
	Test–retest (n=89): r=0.78–0.92
	Inter-rater reliability (n=50): r=0.97–0.99
	Validity Content description: item description and rationale, point-biserial correlation, item discrimination and item difficulty analyses of test content were adequate. Logistic regression identified no test bias for sex, race or ethnicity
	Uncorrected correlation (interpretation based on Brace et al, 2006) of Test of Language Development: Primary, fourth edition (TOLD-P:4), composites with other measures: Pragmatic Language Observation Schedule (PLOS) (Hammill and Newcomer, 2009 (moderate: range r=0.50–0.64), Test of Language Development – Intermediate: Fourth edition (TOLD-I:4) (Newcomer and Hamill, 2008) (moderate, range r=0.42–0.55), and Wechsler Intelligence Scale for Children, fourth edition (WISC-IV) (Wechsler, 2004) verbal comprehension composite (very small to large, range r=0.09–0.76). Level II sensitivity, specificity and positive predictive value $\geq$0.70 achieved between TOLD-P:4 global spoken language composite and the PLOS and the TOLD-I:4. Adequate construct identification validity
How to order	Available in the USA from Pro-Ed, www.proedinc.com. Cost is approximately US$324
Key references	Newcomer PL, Hammill DD (2008) *Critical Reviews and Research Findings for TOLD-P: 1977–2007*. Austin, TX: Pro-Ed.
	United States Census Bureau (2007) *The 2007 Statistical Abstract. The National Data Book*. Accessed: http://www.census.gov/compendia/stabab/2007/2007edition.html
	Hamill DD, Newcomer P (2009) *Pragmatic Language Observation Scale*. Austin, TX: Pro-Ed.
	Wechsler D (2004) *The Wechsler Abbreviated Scale of Intelligence*, 4th Edition. San Antonio, TX: Harcourt Assessment.
	Brace N, Kemp R, Snelgar R (2006) *SPSS for Psychologists: A Guide to Data Analysis using SPSS for Windows*, 3rd edn. Mahwah, NJ: Lawrence Erlbaum & Associates.

TEST OF LANGUAGE DEVELOPMENT: INTERMEDIATE, FOURTH EDITION (TOLD-I:4)	
Purpose	To identify children who present with difficulty with oral language proficiency; determine linguistic strengths and weaknesses; document language progression resulting from prescribed remedial or intervention programmes; and be a statistically robust measure of oral language for research purposes (Newcomer and Hammill, 2008). Assessment of oral language proficiency utilizes a two-dimensional framework comprising linguistic systems (listening, organizing and speaking) and linguistic features (semantics and syntax)

Population	8y 0mo–17y 11mo
Description of domains (subscales)	Six subtests examine semantics or syntax (picture vocabulary, relational vocabulary, multiple meanings, morphological comprehension, word ordering and sentence combining). Of these six subtests, two subtests measure listening abilities, two measure organizing abilities and two measure speaking abilities. The subtests form six composites: listening, organizing, speaking, grammar, semantics and spoken language
Administration and test format	Time to complete: six subtests: 35–50min Testing format: one-to-one administration, administer in the order outlined in the examiner's record booklet. One repetition of a test item is allowed upon request by the examinee for all subtests. Typically the six subtests can be administered within one session. Young, immature or inattentive children may require more than one session. The test is suitable for students who speak English and its dialects as well as students with articulation difficulties Scoring: subtest scaled scores (1–20). Composite indexes (<70 to >130). Descriptive terms for subtests and composites (very poor to very superior). Centiles (1st to >99th). Age equivalents. Scoring and reporting software available Training: formal training in test administration, scoring, interpretation, statistics and evaluation of language abilities is required for administration
Psychometric properties	Normative sample: n=1097 from 14 US states (aged 8–17y); 49% male, 51% female. Standardization sample matched 2005 US school-age population reported in the Statistical Abstract of the United States (US Bureau of the Census, 2007) *Reliability* Internal consistency: Fisher's z: subtests and composites ranged from 0.85 to 0.99. Test–retest (n=103) across subtests and composites: r=0.80–0.98 Inter-rater reliability (n=50): r=0.92–0.98 *Validity* Content description: item description and rationale, point-biserial correlation, item discrimination and item difficulty analyses of test content were adequate. Logistic regression identified no test bias for sex, race or ethnicity. Uncorrected correlation (interpretation based on Brace et al, 2006) of Test of Language Development – Primary, fourth edition (TOLD-P:4) composites with other language measures: Pragmatic Language Observation Schedule (PLOS) (Hammill and Newcomer, 2009) (moderate: range r=0.48–0.62), Peabody Picture Vocabulary Test, third edition (PPVT-III) (Dunn and Dunn, 2007) (small to large: range r=0.19–0.72), TOLD-P:4 (Newcomer and Hammill, 2008) (small to large: range r=0.19–0.72) and Wechsler Intelligence Scale for Children, fourth edition (WISC-IV) (Wechsler, 2004) verbal comprehension composite (moderate to large: range r=0.27–0.70). Level II sensitivity, specificity and positive predictive value >0.70 achieved between TOLD-I:4 global spoken language composite and the PLOS, PPVT-III and the TOLD-P:4. Adequate construct identification validity. Uncorrected correlation (interpretation based on Brace et al, 2006) of TOLD-I:4 composites with literacy measures: Reading Observation Scale (ROS) (Wiederholt et al, 2008) (small to moderate range: r=0.25–0.64), Test of Orthographic Competence (TOC) (Mather et al, 2008) (small to large: range r=0.29–0.77), Test of Reading Comprehension, fourth edition (TORC-4) (small to moderate: range r=0.31–0.56), and Woodcock–Johnson, third edition (W-J III) (Woodcock et al, 2001) (small to moderate range r=0.21–0.65). Uncorrected correlation (interpretation based on Brace et al, 2006) of TOLD-I:4 composites with WISC-IV composites: verbal comprehension (small to large range r=0.22–0.71), perceptual reasoning (very small to small range r=0.06–0.34), working memory (small to moderate range r=0.17–0.64) and processing speed (small negative to small positive range r=–0.30–0.22). Intercorrelations between subtests ranged from r=–0.36–0.65. Factor analysis: subtests load onto a single factor as expected
How to order	Available in the USA from Pro-Ed, www.proedinc.com. Cost is approximately US$224

Key references	Newcomer PL, Hammill DD (2008) *Test of Language Development – Intermediate: Fourth edition (TOLD-I:4) Examiners Manual*. Austin, TX: Pro-Ed.
	Brace N, Kemp R, Snelgar R (2006) *SPSS for Psychologists: A Guide to Data Analysis Using SPSS for Windows*, 3rd edn. Mahwah, NJ: Lawrence Erlbaum & Associates.
	Wiederhdt JL, Hammill DD, Brown VL (2008) *Reading Observation Schedule*. Austin, TX: Pro-Ed.

ACTION PICTURE TEST

Purpose	To evaluate children's expressive language in terms of the information given and the grammatical structures used
Population	Ages 3y 6mo to 8y 5mo
Description of domains (subscales)	Two domains (information and grammar)
Administration and test format	There are 10 picture cards, each with a specific sentence printed on the back.
	Time to complete: 5–10min
	Testing format: children are tested individually. The speech–language pathologist (SLP) presents the pictures, one at a time, to the child and asks the question corresponding to each picture. The SLP records the child's response verbatim
	Scoring: children's responses are scored for grammar and information using the guidelines provided in the user manual. On the information scale, points are given if specified vocabulary items (e.g. nouns, verbs, prepositions) are included in the children's responses; on the grammar scale, points are given if specified grammatical structures are used (e.g. tenses, conjunctions). Scores may be compared with normative data
	Training: designed for use by SLPs; however, it may be used by other professionals (e.g. psychologists, general practitioners and teachers)
Psychometric properties	Scale development sample: normative data were collected using the third edition of the Action Picture Test (Renfrew, 1986)
	Testing of the measure occurred with 594 children in the UK (approximately equal numbers of males and females) (Renfrew, 1997)
	Children were aged 3y 6mo to 8y 5mo and were primarily from middle-class families. Children from non-English-speaking families and those with communication difficulties were excluded from the sample
	Reliability Internal consistency: no information reported.
	Test–retest: no large-scale test–retest has been carried out. Random testing revealed 'little difference in responses' if the retest was given within 1 month (Renfrew, 1997); however, sample size was not reported
	Rater: inter-rater reliability was examined by having four SLPs separately score the responses of 12 children. Initial differences in scores were corrected through increasing the specificity of the scoring guidelines. Full agreement between the therapists was achieved for the information scale; 98% agreement was achieved for the grammar scale
	Validity Construct validity: 'high correlations' were found between the RAPT grammar scale and the Carrow Elicited Language Inventory in a small, unpublished study of children aged 5–6y (Renfrew, 1997). The validity of the RAPT Information Scale has not been examined owing to the lack of a comparative measure

How to order	The Action Picture Test is available from Speechmark Publishing. It can be ordered online at www.speechmark.net/
Key references	Renfrew C (1997) *The Renfrew Language Scales: Action Picture Test*, 4th edition. Bicester: Winslow Press.
	Mather N, Roberts R, Hammill DD, Allen EA (2008) *Test of Orthographic Competence*. Austin, TX: Pro-Ed.
	Woodcock RW, McGrew KS, Mather N (2001) *Woodcock Johnson III Test of Cognitive Ability*. Rolling Meadows, IL: Riverside Publishing.
	Renfrew C (1986) *The Renfrew Language Scales: Action Picture Test*, 3rd ed. Bicester: Winslaw Press.

THE CHILDREN'S COMMUNICATION CHECKLIST, SECOND EDITION (CCC-2)

Purpose	To identify children requiring further investigation by a speech–language pathologist or psychologist; identify pragmatic language deficits in children with communication impairments; and aid identification of children requiring further investigation for a possible autism spectrum disorder (Bishop, 2002)
Population	4y to 16y 11mo
Description of domains (subscales)	The CCC-2 comprises a 70-item multiple-choice checklist divided into 10 scales, each with seven items. Four scales (A–D) investigate language structure, vocabulary and discourse (A: speech, B: syntax, C: semantics, D: coherence). Four scales examine pragmatic language (E: inappropriate initiation, F: stereotyped language, G: use of context, H: non-verbal communication). Two scales assess areas typically implicated in the diagnosis of autistic disorder (I: social relations, J: interests). A general communication composite (GCC) is formulated by combining scales A–H and identifies children at increased risk of communication impairment. A social interaction deviance composite (SIDC) derived from a mismatch between the sums of the scales E, H, I and J and the sum of the scales A, B, C and D assists with the identification of children presenting with communication traits akin to those found within the autism population
Administration and test format	Time to complete: 5–15min
	Testing format: a checklist should be individually completed by an adult who has regular interaction with the child and who has observed him or her across an extended period of time. Typically this is a parent but it can be another adult in regular contact (3–4d per week for at least 3mo) with the child, such as a teacher or speech–language pathologist
	Scoring: scaled scores for scales A to J (0–15). GCC and SIDC composite. Centiles (<1st to >99th). May be hand scored; however, this is complex and time-consuming. Automated computer scoring software is included with the checklist and is quick and efficient to use
	Training: designed for administration by speech–language pathologists, psychologists and paediatricians
	Related products Bishop DVM, Whitehouse AJO, Sharp M (2009) *Communication Checklist – Self Report (CC-SR)*. London: Pearson Assessment. For ages 10–80y
	Whitehouse AJO, Bishop DVM (2009) *Communication Checklist – Adult (CC-A)*. London: Pearson Assessment. For ages 17–79y
	The CCC-2 has been translated into other languages such as Norwegian, Finnish and Dutch

Psychometric properties	Normative sample: the UK standardization sample (*n*=542, aged 4–16y) was based on but not identical to geodemographic groups based on postcodes from the 2001 UK Census; 48% male, 52% female. The Australian standardization sample (*n*=147) comprised children from the metropolitan area of Perth in Western Australia. It is not stated whether or not this sample is representative of the typical Australian paediatric population. Exclusionary criteria for the standardization sample were sensorineural hearing loss, children with identified special educational needs and those from non-English-speaking backgrounds. *Reliability* Internal consistency: Cronbach's alpha values were at least 0.65 for scales A to J. Inter-rater agreement between parents and teachers (*n*=55) for scales A to J ranged from *r*=0.16 to 0.53, for the GCC was *r*=0.40 and for the SIDC was *r*=0.79 *Validity* Validity testing was conducted with three UK clinical groups: 74 children with communication problems, 26 children receiving current intervention by a speech–language pathologist and 34 consecutive referrals to a tertiary developmental paediatric clinic. This sample comprised children with a diagnosis of specific language impairment (*n*=16), pragmatic language impairment without autistic features (*n*=13), pragmatic language impairment with autistic features (PLI+) (*n*=18), high-functioning autism (HFA) (*n*=14), Asperger disorder (*n*=11) and a control group comprising typically developing age-matched peers of similar non-verbal ability (*n*=20). Diagnostic groups were differentiated across the scales A to J with each clinical group obtaining significantly different scores from the control group
How to order	The CCC-2 can be ordered online from Pearson assessments: www.pearson.com. The cost is US$173
Key references	Bishop DVM, Maybery M, Wong D, Maley A, Hallmayer J (2006) Characteristics of the broader phenotype in autism: a study of siblings using the Children's Communication Checklist-2. *Am J Med Genet Part B (Neuropsych Genet)* 141B: 117–122. Norbury CF, Nash M, Baird G, Bishop DVM (2004) Using a parental checklist to identify diagnostic groups in children with communication impairment: a validation of the Children's Communication Checklist – 2. *Int J Comm Disord* 39: 345–364. Helland WA, Biringer E, Helland T, Helland WA (2009) The usability of a Norwegian adaptation of the Children's Communication Checklist Second Edition (CCC-2) in differentiating between language impaired and non-language impaired 6- to 12-year-olds. *Scandinavian J Psychol* 50: 287–292.

REFERENCES

1. World Health Organization (2007) *International Classification of Functioning, Disability and Health – Children and Youth version (ICF-CY)*. Geneva: World Health Organization.
2. Reed GM, Lux JB, Bufka LF, et al (2005) Operationalizing the International Classification of Functioning, Disability and Health in clinical settings. *Rehab Psych* 50: 122–131.
3. Ellis AW, Young AW (1996) *Human Cognitive Neuropsychology*. Hove: Psychology Press.
4. Kay J, Lesser R, Coltheart M (1996) Psycholinguistic Assessments of Language Processing in Aphasia (PALPA): An introduction. *Aphasiology* 10: 159–215.
5. Stackhouse J, Wells B (1997) *Children's Speech and Literacy Difficulties: A Psycholinguistic Framework*. London: Whurr.
6. Westby C (2007) Application of the ICF in children with language impairments. *Sem Speech Lang* 28: 265–272.
7. Linn RL, Miller MD (2005) *Measurement and Assessment in Teaching*, 9th edition. Upper Saddle River, NJ: Pearson.
8. Fox N, Mathers N, Hunn A (1998) *New Horizons: GMH601 Research Methods*, 2nd edition. Sheffield: Institute of General Practice and Primary Care, University of Sheffield.
9. Coelho C, Ylvisaker M, Turkstra LS (2007) Nonstandardized assessment approaches for individuals with traumatic brain injuries. *Sem Speech Lang* 26: 223–241.
10. Leonard LB, Perozzi JA, Prutting CA, Berkley RK (1978) Nonstandardized approaches to the assessment of language behaviours. *Am Speech Hearing Assoc* 20:371 –379.
11. Washington KN (2007) Using the ICF within speech–language pathology: Application to developmental language impairment. *Int J Speech Lang Pathol* 9: 242–255.
12. Dunn LM, Dunn DM (2007) *Peabody Picture Vocabulary Test – fourth edition: User Manual*. Minneapolis, MN: Pearson.
13. Williams KT (2007) *Expressive Vocabulary Test – second edition: Manual*. Minneapolis, MN: Pearson.
14. Semel WA, Wiig EH, Secord WA (2003) *Clinical Evaluation of Language Fundamentals*, 4th edition. San Antonio, TX: The Psychological Corporation.
15. Dockrell JE (2001) Assessing language skills in preschool children. *Child Psychol Psychiatry Rev* 6: 74–85.
16. Fenson L, Marchman VA, Thal D, Dale PS, Reznick JS, Bates E (2006) *MacArthur–Bates Communicative Development*

Inventories: User Guide and Technical Manual, 2nd edition. Baltimore, MD: Paul H. Brookes.

17. Reese E, Read S (2000) Predictive validity of the New Zealand MacArthur Communicative Development Inventory: words and sentences. *J Child Lang* 27: 255–266.

18. Hamilton A, Plunkett K, Schafer G (2000) Infant vocabulary development assessed with a British Communicative Development Inventory: Lower scores in the UK than the USA. *J Child Lang* 27: 689–705.

19. Jackson-Maldonado D, Thal D, Marchman V, Newton T, Fenson L, Conboy B (2003) *MacArthur Inventarios del Desarrollo de Habilidades Comunicativas: User's Guide and Technical Manual*. Baltimore, MD: Paul H. Brookes.

20. Maital SL, Dromi E, Sagi A, Bornstein MH (2000) The Hebrew Communicative Development Inventory: language specific properties and cross-linguistic generalizations. *J Child Lang* 27: 43–67.

21. Berglund E, Eriksson M (2000) Communicative development in Swedish children 16–28 months old: The Swedish Early Communicative Development Inventory – words and sentences. *Scand J Psych* 41: 133–144.

22. Anderson D, Reilly J (2002) The MacArthur Communicative Development Inventory: normative data for American Sign Language. *J Deaf Studies Deaf Ed* 7: 83–106.

23. Thal D, DesJardin JL, Eisenberg LS (2007) Validity of the MacArthur–Bates Communicative Development Inventories for measuring language abilities in children with cochlear implants. *Am J Speech-Lang Path* 16: 54–64.

24. Charman T, Drew A, Baird C, Baird G (2003) Measuring early language development in preschool children with autism spectrum disorder using the MacArthur Communicative Development Inventory (Infant Form). *J Child Lang* 30: 213–236.

25. Zimmerman IL, Steiner VG, Pond RE (2002) *Preschool Language Scale*, 4th edition. San Antonio, TX: The Psychological Corporation.

26. Carrow-Woolfolk E (1995) *Oral and Written Language Scales (OWLS) – Listening Comprehension and Oral Expression Manual*. Circle Pines, MN: American Guidance Service.

27. Carrow-Woolfolk E (1996) *Oral and Written Language Scales (OWLS) – Written Expression Scale*. Circle Pines, MN: American Guidance Service.

13
SENSORY FUNCTIONS: GENERAL (B210–B270)

Erna Imperatore Blanche, Zoe Mailloux and Gustavo Reinoso

What is the construct?

Sensory processing functions include the ability to detect sensory input, modulate responses to input, discriminate the nature of the stimuli and store information about the experience so that it can be used as a basis for perception and action in the future.[1,2] The main sources for sensory information to the body and brain include the visual, auditory, tactile, proprioceptive, vestibular, gustatory and olfactory senses.[3] Other forms of sensation, such as vibration, kinaesthesia, interoception, pain and temperature, are commonly associated with aspects of these sensory systems. For example, the senses of vibration and kinaesthesia are associated with the proprioceptive system, and the senses of pain and temperature are associated with the tactile sense. All sensory information impacts perception, movement and emotions, and therefore this information provides a critical foundation for functional performance and social participation.

Deriving information from peripheral events in the environment requires the sensory receptors to detect a stimulus that is then processed through the peripheral and central nervous systems to obtain meaning from it. Throughout this process, a person's neurophysiological mechanisms help to regulate internal states and filter unnecessary external sensory events so that the cortex can discriminate and derive meaning from it. Thus, a comprehensive evaluation of sensory functions needs to incorporate the ability to modulate or filter sensory information along with the ability to discriminate input. At the present time, however, there are no comprehensive assessment tools that include measurement of the ability to both modulate and discriminate sensation. An important development in this area is the work of several researchers on the National Institutes of Health (NIH) Toolbox project.[4] Their aim is to create a comprehensive measure that assesses several domains of functioning known to affect function and participation.

In most cases, evaluation of sensory functions requires the use of several assessment tools. In paediatric practice, clinicians often use parent surveys to collect information about the impact of sensory processing on daily activities and participation, observations of the child in the natural setting to explore potential links between participation and impairment, and standardized clinical tools to obtain information on the child's impairments and activity limitations.[5–9] This chapter will focus primarily on the proximal sensory systems – tactile, proprioceptive and vestibular – including considerations for evaluating these systems in clinical care and research. The final section will provide recommendations for measures and methods for collecting data relevant to sensory functions.

TACTILE FUNCTIONS

Each sense contributes to daily functional performance in unique and varied ways. The sense of touch encompasses an awareness of passive touch, localization of light touch, two-point discrimination, stereognosis and thermal sensation. Tactile perception alone is responsible for the detection and localization of input, as well as the perception of texture and temperature. The perception of shape and size utilized in stereognosis requires a combination of cutaneous and kinaesthetic input, which constitutes haptic perception.[10]

The isolated sensation of touch and temperature has traditionally been evaluated in adult neurology. Ernst Weber, a German physiologist, was one of the first scientists to develop tests examining cutaneous or tactile sensation. In 1846 he described a two-point discrimination test, performed with a compass.[11] Later on, von Frey used horse hairs to measure the perception of pressure.[12] Cutaneous sensation assessments have evolved into the use of more refined tools, including the Semmes-Weinstein monofilaments, which consist of a series of nylon fibres that represent a unique force, the Wartenberg pinwheel measuring two-point discrimination and the temperature testing surface.[13,14] Tools developed in neurology tend to focus on impairment and do not necessarily provide information about the impact of sensory functions on activity limitations and participation.

Thermal sensations are classically measured by providing hot (40–45°C) and cold (5–10°C) input. Most thermal measures are based on the Peltier principle, which uses an electrical current passing through two different metals and results in a change of temperature.[15] Kenshalo and Bergen[15] first introduced this method for the study of thermal sensation in 1975. Among the most commonly reported measures of thermal sensation are the Marstock stimulator described by Fruhstorfer et al;[16] the CASE IV, which includes thermal testing; a portable system known as the 'Triple T' or Thermal Threshold Tester, which does not require water cooling;[17] the Middlesex Hospital thermal testing system; the Thermal Sensitivity Tester (Sensortek, Clifton, NJ); the Thermal Sensory Analyzer TSA-2001 (Medoc, Ramat Yishai, Israel); and the PATH-Tester MPI 100 (PHYWE Systeme GmbH, D3400 Göttingen, Germany). Research on the application of the above-mentioned measures has been conducted with adult populations with diabetic neuropathy and carpal tunnel syndrome, but thermal sensation is seldom systematically evaluated in children.

Clinicians evaluate the tactile system in children by using surveys, skilled observations in natural settings and standardized tools. The most popular surveys include the Sensory Profile and the Sensory Processing Measure (SPM).[7,8] These surveys focus primarily on increased sensitivity, although items focusing on decreased sensitivity and poor discrimination of touch are also included. Skilled observations in the natural setting include observations of increased sensitivity, mostly based on Ayres' original description of tactile defensiveness.[18] Standardized assessments include the Touch Inventory for Elementary School Children, which measures tactile sensitivity, and the Localization of Tactile Stimuli, Finger Identification, Graphesthesia and Manual Form Perception tests of the Sensory Integration and Praxis Tests (SIPT), which measure several aspects of tactile discrimination.[5,19] The NIH Toolbox project is under way and proposes to include brief but comprehensive measures of cognition, emotion, motor function and sensation. The last of these will include audition, olfaction, somatosensation, taste, vestibular balance and vision. This is a promising measure for clinicians who need to be able to quickly but reliably assess these functions.[4]

PROPRIOCEPTIVE FUNCTIONS

Proprioception, first identified by Sherrington,[20] is defined as the summation of neuronal input from the joint capsule, ligaments, muscles, tendons and skin. It includes the senses of muscle contraction, limb position, timing of movement, sense of force, sense of effort and vibration.[21–24] Research in proprioception is slowly increasing. Traditionally, the proprioceptive sense was considered to be separate from kinaesthesia. Current classifications consider the kinaesthetic sense as part of proprioception.

Proprioceptive functions are closely related to motor coordination and are difficult to evaluate with standardized measures. In research studies, proprioception is evaluated by tools that measure the sense of joint position and movement, which are specifically developed for a study. These tools often require the person to perform a motor response, making it difficult to distinguish between proprioceptive processing difficulties and problems in motor execution. Tools developed for research purposes include the intra- and intersensory modality matching tool, which, among other skills, measures the ability to match the position and movement of one arm with the other, and the Test of Kinesthetic Sensitivity, which measures the ability to sense joint position.[24–26] Other research tools include the Proprioceptometer and the Proprioception Testing device.[27–29] These tools measure different aspects of proprioception but are not commercially available and therefore can seldom be used in clinical paediatric practice. In general, there is little or no correlation between the different tests of proprioception as they focus on different proprioceptive functions. Therefore, proprioceptive ability cannot be inferred from one measurement of proprioceptive ability alone.[22] A new development in this area is the Comprehensive Observations of Proprioception (COP) scale, a valid and reliable criterion-referenced short observational tool that structures the clinician's observations. This instrument collects information on different areas including tone and joint alignment, postural motor and motor planning skills, as well as the behavioural manifestations of inefficient proprioceptive processing.[23]

Occupational therapy clinicians evaluate the impact of proprioception and movement on functional performance in conjunction with other sensory systems, such as the vestibular or tactile senses through skilled observations, surveys and norm-referenced tests. Observations may focus on muscle tone, joint stability and movement preferences.[6] Surveys often focus on movements as they relate to proprioceptive feedback.[7,8] Standardized tools that involve an aspect of proprioceptive assessment include the Kinesthesia, Standing and Walking Balance, Postural Praxis and Oral Praxis tests of the SIPT[5] and the Pediatric Clinical Test of Sensory Interaction for Balance.[30]

VIBRATION

The assessment of vibration, a proprioceptive-related sense, is less common in paediatric practice. Evaluation of this sense originated in adult neurology with the tuning fork, an instrument that continues to be used currently in adult clinical practice. More contemporaneous laboratory assessment tools that focus on vibration, and are commonly reported, include the Bio-Thesiometer (Bio-Medical Instruments, Newbury, OH, USA); the Vibrameter (Somedic AB, Hörby, Sweden); the CASE IV vibration stimulator (WR Medical Electronics, Stillwater, MN, USA); the Vibratron II (Physitemp Instruments, Inc., Clifton, NJ, USA);[31,32] the Vibratory Sensory Analyzer (Medoc, Ramat Yishai, Israel); and the Maxivibrometer (Pennsylvania State University, University Park, PA, USA). These tools are not generally used in clinical paediatric practice.

VESTIBULAR FUNCTIONS

The vestibular system comprises different receptors and neural connections that significantly influence human performance. Vestibular functions comprise three clearly defined, neurologically based categories: vestibulospinal functions, vestibulo-ocular functions and vestibuloperceptual functions.[30] Vestibulospinal functions influence postural control, extensor tone and neck stability, vestibulo-ocular functions influence the ability to maintain a stable visual field and ocular motor control and vestibuloperceptual functions influence spatial organization. Some researchers also suggest that vestibular functions influence visual perception, arousal modulation, reading ability, bilateral motor coordination, language development, the establishment of laterality and psychosocial growth.[30,33,34,35]

In paediatric practice, the evaluation of the vestibular sense is accomplished by using surveys, skilled observations and normed clinical tests. Surveys focus on the impact of the vestibular system on arousal modulation, anxiety when the relationship to gravity is challenged and activity choices. Surveys should never be used alone when evaluating the vestibular system, as evaluating spinal and vestibulo-ocular functions require a skilled clinician. Skilled observations of vestibulospinal functions include testing extensor tone, postural control under different conditions and joint stability in the shoulder girdle and neck areas. Vestibulo-ocular functions are evaluated by testing the ability to stabilize the visual field and through observing visual- or movement-elicited nystagmus, and vestibuloperceptual functions are evaluated through observations of motor performance.[36] The most commonly utilized clinical tests of the vestibular system include the Post-rotary Nystagmus Test and the Standing and Walking Balance Test of the SIPT.[5]

PAIN

The sensation of pain, although critical for survival, has been less explored in rehabilitation, and its brain mechanisms remain largely unknown.[37] The relationship of pain to sensory experiences has been explored in vulnerable populations and is considered to have important clinical implications. For example, oversensitivity to touch has been described as 'painful'; in the same way, oversensitivity to visual input or auditory input may also be experienced as painful. The International Association for the Study of Pain terminology has used the term 'allodynia' to refer to these phenomena.[38] Thus, it is important for clinicians to understand the differences between pain (an unpleasant sensory and emotional experience associated with actual or potential tissue damage, or described in terms of such damage), hyperalgesia (an increased response to a stimulus which is normally painful) and allodynia (pain due to a stimulus which does not normally provoke pain).[39] The neural circuits and areas involved in pain transmission and perception are somewhat controversial, although most studies highlight significant differences between acute and chronic pain conditions, and some conditions resulting from injury to sensory fibres or from damage to the central nervous system itself, which is often described as 'neuropathic pain'.[40] Pain is usually elicited by the activation of specific sensory receptors known as nociceptors. This complex phenomenon is often described as 'nociceptive pain'. Because of its importance in health and participation, researchers now recognize the 'nociceptive system' as a sensory system in its own right, from primary afferents to multiple brain areas,[41] and thus will be described in detail in Chapter 14.

OTHER SENSORY FUNCTIONS

Other senses commonly associated with paediatric practice are the visual, auditory and olfactory senses. Visual perception will be reviewed in Chapter 11. The evaluation of the auditory sense includes determining the degree of hearing loss, the type of hearing loss and the configuration of the hearing loss. Audiology is often the professional discipline that provides this type of assessment. Evaluation of the auditory sensory processing may also include measures of detection, perception, discrimination and oversensitivity. For example, the Slosson Auditory Perceptual Skill Screener screens a child's ability to perceive auditory information, including word discrimination, auditory figure-ground perception and the ability to 'filter' words;[42]

and the Wepman's Auditory Discrimination Test assesses auditory perception by determining a child's ability to recognize subtle differences between phonemes used in speech.[43] The audiology and speech–language professions use a variety of additional measurement tools to assess auditory and language comprehension.[44]

Occupational therapists often include responses to auditory sensory input through surveys as part of a comprehensive evaluation of sensory functions, but do not measure auditory perception or discrimination. Charts presenting information regarding measures commonly used to assess sensory functions in other disciplines are presented later in this chapter.

Other sensory functions often neglected in paediatric practice are the olfactory (smell) and gustatory (taste) sensory functions. Smell and taste are part of the chemosensory systems and respond to the chemical reactions that occur between particles in the air or in substances such as food or drink.[45] These senses are primal and important for core aspects of survival. Common tests used to evaluate the sensations of smell and taste include the presentation of various stimuli through sheets or tabs of paper containing small beads, which carry specific odours or tastes for identification. Such measures are described in Chapter 11. Occupational therapists seek information about an individual's responses to tastes and smells as part of overall sensory questionnaires, but olfactory and gustatory discrimination are not typically assessed in a comprehensive way in occupational therapy clinical practice.

General factors to consider when measuring this domain

Assessments of sensory functions originate from several disciplines including neurology, psychology and occupational therapy, the last of which is at the forefront in the development of paediatric sensory integration assessment tools. According to the method utilized to gather information, measurement tools can be classified as surveys and questionnaires (reports by proxy), direct skilled observation and clinical testing. These tools focus on different levels of the person's abilities. Surveys focus on the impact of sensory functions on activity limitations and participation restrictions, while skilled observations provide insight into activity limitations and participation, and standardized tools tend to focus on impairments and activity limitations. Most methods of assessing the senses are diagnostic, in that the clinician attempts to identify sensory deficits as they relate to occupational performance. Because the senses are often evaluated together, in this section we will present the measures according to the method utilized to collect the information.

In paediatric occupational therapy, surveys addressing sensory functions and their relationships to functional performance are common. These surveys cover several sensory systems at a time, tend to focus on modulation and hypersensitivity issues in ambulatory children and are answered by parents, caretakers or teachers. Sensory function surveys cover different ages, with most of them focusing on children between the ages of 3 and 11 years.

The most widely utilized surveys are the Sensory Profile and the SPM.[7,8] Therapists primarily utilize these measures when assessing ambulatory children with a diagnosis of intellectual disability, autism spectrum disorder, attention-deficit–hyperactivity disorder, developmental coordination disorder and other developmental disabilities. Surveys measuring sensory processing in children with cerebral palsy or other more severe disabilities are seldom utilized. Surveys provide a window into the impact of sensory functions on the child's activity limitations and participation in daily activities. The limitation of surveys resides in the reliance on parents' and teachers' subjective evaluation of the child's performance, and the results need to be supported by direct observation or standardized tools.

NON-STANDARDIZED DIRECT OBSERVATION (OR SKILLED OBSERVATIONS)

There are several non-standardized observational tools that relate sensory processing to motor performance. The most common, originally identified by Ayres,[34] are 'clinical observations' or skilled observations used to evaluate postural control and oculomotor responses, as well as aspects of motor planning and motor coordination. Clinicians use these observations as accompanying information to the SIPT or when standardized testing is not recommended. Over the years, these isolated measures of observation have been standardized[46–52] and expanded.[6,53] There are also observation tools used with young children and infants, such as that included in the Bayley-III, the Infant Toddler Symptom Checklist and the Sensory Rating Scale for Infants and Young Children.[54–56]

The benefit of using skilled observations of sensory functions is that they can be carried out in the natural environment and thus provide an insight to the child's activity limitations and participation in daily activities. The limitations of skilled observations lie in their subjective nature, although attempts have been made towards systematizing them.

CLINICAL TESTING

Clinical testing tools can be divided into tools used in research and tools for clinical use. Among the standardized clinical assessments, the most comprehensive and widely utilized tool is the SIPT, which includes measures of tactile, visual, auditory, proprioceptive and vestibular functions and their relationship to functional performance. This battery of tests will be presented later in this chapter.

Other assessment tools that include aspects of sensory functions include the Miller Assessment for Preschoolers, which contains an assessment of tactile discrimination,

and the Paediatric Clinical Test of Sensory Interaction for Balance, which is used to assess the contribution of the vestibular, proprioceptive and visual systems to balance and can be used to identify sensory issues in the paediatric population.[57–59]

The contribution of standardized tools to the evaluation of children lies in the possibility of comparing the child's performance with a normative sample. However, they provide a limited understanding of the child's impairments. Because of the lack of standardized clinical measures of sensory modalities in the paediatric population, this section focuses on standardized tools that use survey

SENSORY PROFILE	
Purpose	To measure children's responses to sensory events in everyday life through caregiver responses on a questionnaire. Using national samples of >1000 children, the author calculated cut-off scores which indicate when a child's scores are significantly different from his or her peers' responses
Population	Ages 3–10y. Versions available for infants and toddlers (ages 0–36mo), and adolescents and adults (ages 11y+)
Description of domains (subscales)	The Sensory Profile contains sections corresponding to (1) each sensory system, (2) the modulation of sensory input across sensory systems and (3) behavioural and emotional responses that are associated with sensory processing. Additionally, professionals can calculate scores from a factor structure (responsiveness to sensory input, sensory seeking, emotional reactive, low endurance/tone, oral sensory sensitivity, inattention/distractibility, poor registration, sensory sensitivity, sedentary and fine motor/perceptual) which reflects children's responsiveness to sensory input across sensory systems
Administration and test format	There are 125 items in the profile (a short version, for screening and research programmes, contains 38 items). Caregivers complete the questionnaire by reporting how frequently their child responds in the way described by each item with a five-point Likert scale (nearly never, seldom, occasionally, frequently, almost always)
Psychometric properties	Studies with children who have various disabilities (including autism, Asperger syndrome and attention-deficit–hyperactivity disorder) have shown that these children have significantly different patterns of sensory processing from their peers and from children in other disability groups. Findings thus far suggest that sensory processing patterns may both inform the diagnosis of disorders and provide guidance for intervention planning. The test–retest correlation coefficient for the sensory processing sections was 0.86 and for the quadrants was 0.74
How to order	The profile can be ordered from Pearson (email ClinicalCustomerSupport@Pearson.com)
Key references	Dunn W (1999) *The Sensory Profile Manual*. San Antonio, TX: The Psychological Corporation.
	Dunn W, Bennett D (2002) Patterns of sensory processing in children with attention deficit hyperactivity disorder. *Occup Ther J Res* 22: 4–15.
	Dunn W, Myles B, Orr S (2002) Sensory processing issues associated with Asperger syndrome: a preliminary investigation. *Am J Occup Ther* 56: 97–102.
	Ermer J, Dunn W (1998) The sensory profile: A discriminant analysis of children with and without disabilities. *Am J Occup Ther* 52: 283–290.
	Kientz M, Dunn W (1997) A comparison of children with autism and typical children using the Sensory Profile. *Am J Occup Ther* 51: 530–537.

methods and observations of sensory functions. In summary, evaluation tools of sensory functions focus on different aspects of the child's limitations; therefore, a comprehensive evaluation requires utilization of several observational and survey measures.

Overview of recommended measures

SENSORY PROFILE

Overview and purpose
The Sensory Profile includes a group of measures aimed at measuring sensory processing abilities and at profiling the effect of sensory processing on functional performance in daily life from birth to adulthood.[7-64] In this section we will describe the Sensory Profile for children aged 5 to 10 years. The reader should, however, remember that this measure is also available for younger children and adolescents/adults. The Sensory Profile is a judgement-based caregiver questionnaire; thus, items describe children's responses to various sensory experiences. The Sensory Profile consists of 125 items grouped into three main sections: sensory processing, modulation, and behavioural and emotional responses.

Administration and scoring
The Sensory Profile is given to a caregiver or a person who knows the child well, as it asks how frequently the child engages in the behaviours of interest. Some items encourage the caregiver to provide additional comments about the child's behaviour, which are then analysed in relation to the child's sensory functions and behavioural/emotional responses.

Psychometric properties
Reliability was calculated by estimating internal consistency for each section, which ranged from 0.47 to 0.91. Content validity was established by literature review to ensure that the test sampled the full range of children's sensory processing behaviours and by having a panel of eight therapists provide feedback on the items included in the Sensory Profile. A national sample of 155 experienced clinicians also selected categories for each item; 80% of these therapists agreed on the category placement of 63% of the items. With respect to construct validity, the Sensory Profile was compared with the School Function Assessment. The comparison of these two instruments demonstrated convergent and discriminant validity. Studies involving children with various disabilities (including autism, Asperger syndrome and attention-deficit–hyperactivity disorder) have shown significantly different patterns of sensory processing than typically

developing children. The test–retest correlation coefficient for the sensory processing sections was 0.86 and for the quadrants was 0.74. These coefficients indicate that the caregiver rating is somewhat stable over time and is acceptable for identifying target areas for intervention. Findings thus far suggest that sensory processing patterns may assist in the diagnosis of disorders and guide intervention planning.

SENSORY PROCESSING MEASURE

Overview and purpose
The SPM comprises a group of rating scales for the assessment of sensory processing issues, praxis and social participation in elementary school-aged children (ages 5–12y). The SPM is composed of three different forms including scales for the home, main classroom and the school environment.[65] The home and main classroom forms produce norm-referenced standard scores in the following areas: (1) social participation, (2) vision, (3) hearing, (4) touch, (5) body awareness, (6) balance and motion, (7) planning and ideas and (8) total sensory systems. Depending on the standard scores achieved on these scales, the child's functioning is classified into typical, some problems and definitive dysfunction. The school environment form can be used by school personnel in six different settings including art class, music class, physical education class, recess/playground, cafeteria and school bus.

Administration and scoring
The SPM is completed by a person who knows the child well (e.g. parent, primary classroom teacher, homecare provider, school staff member, teacher's assistant). Items on the scales are rated based on the frequency of the behaviour observed. The home and main school forms of the SPM require 15 to 20 minutes for completion by the respondent and an additional 5 to 10 minutes for scoring.

Psychometric properties
With respect to content validity, the SPM was based on two previous scales – the Evaluation of Sensory Processing (ESP) and the School Assessment of Sensory Integration (SASI) – and also expert reviews. A previous confirmatory factor analysis on a clinical sample using the ESP revealed a goodness of fit in relation to sensory systems, supporting construct validity. Exploratory factor analysis on the SPM (home form) standardization sample revealed similar findings. The factorial structure for the SPM main classroom form is similar to that of the home form. For the internal consistency of the standardization sample, seven of eight home scales and five of eight main

SENSORY PROCESSING MEASURE (SPM)	
Purpose	To assess sensory processing issues, praxis and social participation
Population	Ages 5–12y
Description of domains (subscales)	Home and main classroom forms comprise items in the following areas: (1) social participation, (2) vision, (3) hearing, (4) touch, (5) body awareness, (6) balance and motion, (7) planning and ideas and (8) total sensory systems
	School environments forms comprise items in the following areas: (1) art class, (2) music class, (3) physical education class, (4) recess/playground, (5) cafeteria and (6) school bus
Administration and test format	Time to complete: 15–20min is required for the form to be completed by the respondent
	Scoring: 5–10min
Psychometric properties	Normative sample: standardization sample of 1051 children aged 5–12y
	Reliability
	Internal consistency: standardization sample, seven of eight home scales and five of eight main classroom scales have alphas of ≥0.80; clinical sample, six of eight home scales and four of eight main classroom scales have alphas of ≥0.80.
	Test–retest reliability: the sample consisted of 77 typically developing children, aged 5–12y, who were assessed with both the home and classroom forms over a 2-week interval. The results indicated that the SPM scales scores were highly correlated across the 2-week retest interval with *r*-values ≥0.94
	Validity
	Content validity was based on two previous scales – the Evaluation of Sensory Processing (ESP) and the School Assessment of Sensory Integration (SASI) – and expert reviews
	Construct validity: a previous confirmatory factor analysis on a clinical sample using the ESP revealed a goodness of fit in relation to sensory systems. Exploratory factor analysis on the SPM (home form) standardization sample revealed similar findings. The factorial structure for the SPM main classroom from is similar to that of the home form
How to order	The SPM can be ordered from Western Psychological Services (WPS) at www.wpspublish.com
Key references	Miller Kuhaneck H, Henry DA, Glennon TJ (2007) *Sensory Processing Measure (SPM) Main Classroom Form*. Los Angeles, CA: Western Psychological Services.
	Miller Kuhaneck H, Henry DA, Glennon TJ (2007) *Sensory Processing Measure (SPM) School Environments Form*. Los Angeles, CA: Western Psychological Services.
	Parham LD, Ecker C (2007) *Sensory Processing Measure (SPM) Home Form*. Los Angeles, CA: Western Psychological Services.
	Parham LD, Ecker C, Miller Kuhaneck H, Henry DA, Glennon TJ (2007) *Sensory Processing Measure (SPM): Manual*. Los Angeles, CA: Western Psychological Services.

classroom scales have alpha coefficients of ≥0.80. Using a clinical sample, six of eight home scales and four of eight main classroom scales have alphas of ≥0.80. To evaluate test–retest reliability, a sample consisting of 77 typically developing children, aged 5 to 12 years, were assessed with both the home and classroom forms within a 2-week interval. The results indicated that the SPM scales scores were highly correlated across the 2-week retest interval, with *r*-values ≥0.94.

TEST OF SENSORY FUNCTIONS IN INFANTS

Overview and purpose
The Test of Sensory Functions in Infants (TSFI) provides an overall measure of sensory processing and reactivity in infants aged 4 to 18 months. The test comprises five subtests, including reactivity to tactile deep pressure, adaptive motor functions, visual tactile integration, oculomotor control and reactivity to vestibular stimulation.

TEST OF SENSORY FUNCTIONS IN INFANTS (TSFI)	
Purpose	Objective way to determine whether and to what extent an infant has sensory processing deficits
Population	Ages 4–18mo with regulatory disorders and developmental delays and those at risk for learning and sensory processing disorders
Description of domains (subscales)	1. Reactivity to tactile deep pressure 2. Visual tactile integration 3. Adaptive motor function 4. Ocular motor control 5. Reactivity to vestibular stimulation
Administration and test format	Time to complete: approximately 20min for administration and 5min for scoring Testing format: 24 items individually administered Training: none required
Psychometric properties	1. Standardization sample: 288 typically developing infants, 27 with delays (preterm birth with motor delay, mild to moderate motor delay, Down syndrome and developmental delay) and 27 with regulatory disorders 2. Content validity was achieved by using an expert panel, studies of item validity, discriminative validity and test structure. It was found that the total test scores could be used for screening decisions with a 14–45% false-negative error rate and a 7–19% false-positive error rate. Discriminative validity studies showed that the TSFI is most accurate for identifying typically developing infants aged 4–18mo and infants with sensory dysfunction aged 10–18mo 3. Reliability: Two observers were used for interobserver reliability in 41 infants. Intraclass correlations were computed with coefficients ranging from 0.88 to 0.99
How to order	The kit includes one set of test materials, 100 administration and scoring forms and a manual. The manual and administration and scoring forms can also be ordered separately The Test of Sensory Function in Infants can be ordered from Western Psychological Services (WPS) at www.wpspublish.com

The TSFI was designed as a research and clinical measure to assess infants with regulatory disorders and developmental delays and those at risk for learning and sensory processing disorders.[66]

Administration and scoring
The TSFI consists of 24 items that can be administered in about 20 minutes. Scoring takes about 5 minutes. The scoring of the TSFI follows a numerical rating scale designating 'abnormal', 'poorly developed' and 'normal' skill development.

Psychometric properties
The standardization sample included 288 typically developing infants, 27 with delays (preterm birth with motor delay, mild to moderate motor delay, Down syndrome and developmental delay) and 27 with regulatory disorders. Infants were grouped into four age categories to include 4 to 6, 7 to 9, 10 to 12 and 13 to 18 months for data analysis. A review of possible items was conducted using eight experts from child development centres, infant programmes and hospitals from five different states in the USA. The majority (75–85%) of the ratings of item behaviour congruence were high for all items on the TSFI. Eighty-seven per cent of ratings were high for all of the subtests except reactivity to vestibular simulation, which was rated as high at 75%. Construct validity was investigated at the item, subtest and test levels. The total test scores can be used for screening decisions with a 14% to 45% false-negative error rate and a 7% to 19% false-positive error rate. Criterion validity was tested by administering the TSFI, Bayley scales, the Bates' Infant Characteristics Questionnaire and the Fagan Test of Infant Intelligence to a sample of 72 typically developing infants. The correlations suggested that TSFI measures distinct functions unrelated to the above-mentioned scales.[66] The

TSFI is most accurate for identifying typically developing infants from 4 to 18 months of age and infants with sensory dysfunction from 10 to 18 months of age.

Inter-rater reliability was established with two observers and 41 infants. Intraclass correlations were computed with coefficients ranging from 0.88 to 0.99. Test–retest reliability was established by calculating Pearson Product Moment correlation coefficients between test and retest scores. Stability in test scores was found to be good for the visual tactile integration subtest, ocular motor control subtest and total test scores. In summary, the TSFI total tests scores are both reliable and valid for screening decisions.[66]

SENSORY INTEGRATION AND PRAXIS TESTS

Overview and purpose

The SIPT is a battery comprising 17 individual tests that evolved from a group of earlier measures used by Ayres in the 1960s, the Southern California Sensory Integration Tests (SCSIT) and the Southern California Postrotary Nystagmus Tests.[67–70] The SIPT was standardized based on the US census of 1980, with a final normative sample comprising 1997 children aged 4 years 0 months to 8 years 11 months.[5] The purpose of the SIPT battery is to assess children with suspected sensory integrative dysfunction, including assessments of several areas of praxis and the abilities of the vestibular, proprioceptive, kinaesthetic, tactile and visual systems to adequately process sensory information and guide the treatment of such dysfunctions.[5] The final battery of the SIPT was designed based on extensive field and pilot testing and took into consideration (1) the ability to discriminate between children with and without dysfunction, (2) the association of scores by means of factor analyses and (3) the reliability of individual tests and test items.[67]

Administration and scoring

The administration, scoring and interpretation of the SIPT battery require formal training. Each of the 17 tests of the SIPT is individually administered; the complete battery usually takes 2 hours to administer and it requires 30 to 45 minutes to score. All tests are scored using computer software that creates several reports comparing the performance of the child tested with that of the standardization sample. The SIPT battery comprises the following tests: (1) space visualization, (2) figure-ground perception, (3) standing and walking balance, (4) design copying, (5) postural praxis, (6) bilateral motor coordination, (7) praxis on verbal command, (8) constructional praxis, (9) postrotary nystagmus, (10) motor accuracy, (11) sequencing praxis, (12) oral praxis, (13) manual form perception, (14) kinaesthesia, (15) finger identification, (16) graphaesthesia and (17) localization of tactile stimuli. Individual tests of the

SIPT are grouped into (1) measures of tactile, vestibular and proprioceptive processing, (2) tests of form and space perception and visual motor coordination, (3) tests of praxis skills and (4) measures of bilateral integration and sequencing abilities.[70]

Psychometric properties

Several studies have considered the validity and reliability of the SIPT. Content validity for the SIPT was established through the development of the SCSIT, its use and refinement, and consultation with a group of experts in the field of sensory integration.[67] Construct validity of the SIPT has been extensively established by a series of factor analysis studies before its publication. In addition, the construct measured by the SIPT has been further studied by comparing scores from different populations. A principal component analysis of the 17 major SIPT scores from a national sample (n=1750; mean age 6y 9mo, standard deviation [SD] 1.13) yielded four factors as follows: (1) visuopraxis, (2) somatopraxis, (3) vestibular and somatosensory and (4) kinaesthesia/motor accuracy. Another factor analysis including a sample of children with learning disabilities matched on age, grade, sex, geographic region and parental education and occupation with a group of typically developing children (incomplete data for 59 children) resulting in a final sample of 293 children (117 children with learning disabilities and 176 children from the standardization sample; mean age 7y 4mo; SD 1y 0mo). This study identified the following factors: (1) somatopraxis, (2) visuopraxis, (3) vestibular functioning and (4) somatosensory processing. The SIPT has also been studied by means of cluster analysis. The results are described to a great extent in the SIPT manual with the main clusters being (1) low average bilateral integration and sequencing, (2) generalized sensory integrative dysfunction, (3) visuo- and somatodyspraxia, (4) low average sensory integration and praxis, (5) dyspraxia on verbal command and (6) high average sensory integration and praxis.[5]

Scores from the SIPT have been compared with scores on other developmental measures and have shown a strong correlation with tests utilized to measure cognitive functions. A study administered the Kaufman Assessment Battery for Children and the SIPT to a combined sample of typically developing children (n=47) and children who had learning disabilities (n=35) or exhibited a sensory integrative disorder (n=9).[71] In this study, the SIPT tests that measured sequencing skills showed high correlations with comparable domains on the tests of the Kaufman Assessment Battery for Children. Another study comparing a sample of children with and without learning disabilities using the SIPT and the Kaufman Assessment Battery for Children revealed that SIPT factors were

SENSORY INTEGRATION AND PRAXIS TESTS (SIPT)

Purpose	To assess sensory integration dysfunction and its effects on general development, learning and behaviour
Population	Ages 4y–8y 11mo
Description of domains (subscales)	Seventeen individual subtests: (1) space visualization; (2) figure-ground perception; (3) standing and walking balance; (4) design copying; (5) postural praxis; (6) bilateral motor coordination; (7) praxis on verbal command; (8) constructional praxis; (9) postrotary nystagmus; (10) motor accuracy; (11) sequencing praxis; (12) oral praxis; (13) manual form perception; (14) kinaesthesia; (15) finger identification; (16) graphaesthesia; and (17) localization of tactile stimuli
Administration and test format	Time to complete: approximately 2h Testing format: 17 tests, which are administered individually Scoring: tests are scored individually. Information needs to be entered into a computer program for analysis. Computer software provides a comprehensive report including a summary of test and major scores, a summary graph of SIPT results, estimated true scores, a complete listing of SIPT scores, a measure of lateral function, a comparison with diagnostic prototypes and an audit of recorded data Training: available through the University of Southern California (USC) and Western Psychological Services (WPS) through the USC/WPS Comprehensive Programme in Sensory Integration
Psychometric properties	Normative sample: 1997 children aged between 4 and 8.11y living in the USA, in addition to a subsample from Canada *Reliability* Test–retest reliability ranged from 0.48 to 0.93, but only five of the tests had coefficients <0.70; inter-rater reliability for all of the major SIPT scores was between 0.94 and 0.99 *Validity* (1) Content validity was established by a previous version of the SIPT (Southern California Sensory Integration and Praxis Tests), its clinical and research utilization and a panel of experts in the field; (2) construct validity was established by factor analysis studies on the normative sample and samples of children with developmental dysfunctions. Cluster analyses revealed six groups: low average bilateral integration and sequencing, generalized sensory integrative dysfunction, visuo- and somatodyspraxia, low average sensory integration and praxis, dyspraxia on verbal command and high average sensory integration and praxis; (3) criterion-related validity was determined by collecting information on several developmental disability groups including learning disability and minimal brain dysfunction, language disorders, sensory integrative disorders, reading disorders, intellectual deficits, traumatic brain injury, spina bifida and meningomyelocele, cerebral palsy, emotional disturbance, orofacial cleft and exposure to agent orange, and by comparing SIPT scores with other measures including the Kaufman Assessment Battery for Children. SIPTs that measured sequencing skills showed high correlations with the tests of the Kaufman Assessment Battery for Children, which measures similar domains of function. Other measures have also shown significant associations with the earlier version of the SIPT, including the tactile-kinaesthetic sections of the SCSIT and the Luria–Nebraska Neuropsychological Battery, which obtained a correlation of 0.73 ($p<0.001$) and the motor section, which obtained a correlation of 0.83; the Bruininks–Oseretsky Test of Motor Proficiency fine motor scale and 13 tests of the SCSIT were correlated at 0.37 ($p<0.1$). The Bender–Gestalt test correlated significantly with space perception measures ($r=0.65$; $p<0.01$) and with the combined tactile praxis tests ($r=0.61$; $p<0.01$), the subtests of Motor Accuracy and Design Copying reached correlations of 0.71 and 0.72 ($p<0.01$), the Position in Space test had a correlation of 0.50 ($p<0.01$)

How to order	The SIPT can be ordered from Western Psychological Services at www.wpspublish.com
	Format: 10-use scoring CD package (scores 10 complete test batteries or 150 individual tests)
Key references	Ayres AJ (1980) *Southern California Sensory Integration Tests*, revised edition. Los Angeles, CA: Western Psychological Services.
	Ayres A (1989) *Sensory Integration and Praxis Tests*. Los Angeles, CA: Western Psychological Services.
	Ayres AJ, Marr D (1991) Sensory Integration and Praxis Tests. In: Fisher AG, Murray EA, Bundy AC, eds. *Sensory Integration, Theory and Practice*. Philadelphia, PA: FA Davis Company, pp. 203–229.
	Mailloux Z (1990) An overview of the Sensory Integration and Praxis Tests. *Am J Occup Ther* 1990; 44: 589–594.

strongly related to arithmetic achievement at early ages, but the strength of the relationship decreased with time. The opposite pattern was found between praxis and arithmetic achievement.[72]

In a more recent study, SIPT and SPM scores were analysed in a sample of 273 children with diagnoses such as learning disabilities, speech and language disorders, sensory integrative problems and developmental delays. Findings revealed factors similar to those originally described by Ayres,[5] and, as in the earlier studies, the patterns were also closely related to each other.[73]

Test–retest reliability coefficients for the major test scores on the 17 subtests of the SIPT ranged from 0.48 to 0.93, with only five of the tests <0.70. The inter-rater reliability coefficients for all of the major SIPT scores were between 0.94 and 0.99.[5]

Conclusion

This chapter has presented a review of measurements of sensory functions that are relevant to paediatric practice. These tools cover a wide range of ages and diverse methods of collecting information, allowing for a comprehensive evaluation of sensory functions. This review focused on sensory functions and hence did not include measures primarily focusing on sensorimotor performance; however, measures of sensorimotor performance need to be included in any evaluation of sensory functions. Furthermore, measures of discrete sensory modalities were not described in detail (see Table 13.1). Clinicians evaluating sensory functions with these above-mentioned tools need to consider several factors. First, when using tools focusing on sensory functions, it is important to identify the level of functioning (i.e. body structures and functions or activity and participation) that is being assessed. A comprehensive evaluation will include gathering information at the level of impairment, activity and participation; therefore, several assessment tools are needed.

Another concern about tools measuring sensory functions is that many of the tests presented in this chapter were developed for ambulatory children without severe behavioural or neuromotor difficulties. When evaluating children with moderate to severe physical or psychological deficits, the clinician must rely on skilled observations and parental reports. In the absence of appropriate tools, an experienced clinician can also explore the use of tools developed for research purposes or others developed for use in clinical neurology.

It should be noted that most of the clinical tools described in this chapter are more than 10 years old, and other measures currently under development are not yet available for public review and access. For example, the Sensory Over-responsivity Scales, developed by Schoen et al[74] to measure oversensitivity, and the Gravitational Insecurity Assessment by May-Benson and Koomar[75] will offer the possibility of objectively measuring aspects of sensory functions that were previously subjectively observed or assessed by proxy. The SIPT, considered by most as the criterion standard in the evaluation of sensory integration, is also currently under revision and will continue to offer a comprehensive overview of sensory functions. The NIH Toolbox promises to be a comprehensive instrument to assess several aspects of sensation in clinical populations.[4]

Other measures of sensory functions currently utilized in research and promising a contribution to clinical practice are psychophysiological measures of autonomic nervous system response to sensory input.[76,77] These measures will provide a more accurate reading of the child's impairment in sensory functions which has been linked to participation. If these and other tools under development are made available to for public use, the next 5 years promises to bring a significant change in the way in which sensory functions are evaluated.

TABLE 13.1

Other measures (research measures commonly reported in the literature that may assist clinicians in elucidating the impact of sensation and pain perception in clinical populations)

Measure	Age group	Description	Reference sources
Multimodal sensory assessments			
Computer-assisted sensory examination	Children aged >8y, adolescents and adults who are rested, attentive and co-operative	Thermal perception (5–50°C) including cold, warm and heat pain perception[18,43] Vibration	Developed by the Mayo Clinic and available through WR Medical Electronics, Stillwater, MN, USA Dyck et al;[78,79] Gruener and Dyck[80]
Somatosensory system: vibration			
The Bio-Thesiometer/ Neurothesiometer	17–82y with diagnosis of diabetes	Hand-held electromagnetic vibrator with a stimulating probe (12-mm diameter) that vibrates at 100Hz	Available through Bio-Medical Instruments, Newbury, OH, USA Bertelsmann et al[81]
The Vibrameter	Reported in children as young as 3.3y and older	Vibration	Somedic AB, Sweden Goldberg and Lindblom;[82] Hilz et al[83]
The Vibratron II	Early detection of sensory loss from disease, drug therapy, nerve recovery and other conditions	Vibration	Gerr and Letz;[84] Gerr et al[85]
The Medoc Vibratory Sensory Analyzer	6–59y	Warm and cold sensations Vibration	Medoc, Ramat Yishai, Israel Meier et al;[86] Yarnitsky and Sprecher[87]
Maxivibrometer	Individuals at risk for sensory dysfunction	Vibration	Pennsylvania State University, University Park, PA, USA van Deursen et al[88]
Tactile system: thermal sensation			
The Marstock stimulator	It has been used in individuals with diabetes aged ≥10y	Thermal sensation (warm perception)	Somedic AB, Sweden Fruhstorfer et al;[89] Ziegler et al[90]
The automated Glasgow system	6–73y, at risk for sensory dysfunction	Device to measure warm and cool thresholds perception	Medelec/Oxford Instruments, Hawthorne, NY, USA Dyck et al;[78] Jamal et al[91]
Thermal Threshold Tester	18–66y, individuals with moderate neuropathy	Thermal testing system	Bravenboer et al[92]
The Middlesex Hospital Thermal Testing System	One study cites participants aged 14–56y	Thermal testing system: warm and cool thresholds	Middlesex Hospital, London, UK Siao and Cros;[93] Fowler et al[94]
The Thermal Sensitivity Tester	Not specified	Thermal testing system	Sensortek, Clifton, NJ, USA Arezzo et al[95]
The Thermal Sensory Analyzer TSA-2001	Not specified	Thermal sensation: no visual or auditory cues are given to signal stimulus onset	Medoc, Ramat Yishai, Israel Physitemp Instruments, Inc., USA Yarnitsky and Sprecher[87]
PATH-Tester MPI 100	Not specified	Thermal sensation	PHYWE Systeme GmbH, D3400 Gottinger, Germany Claus et al[96]

TABLE 13.1
Continued

Measure	Age group	Description	Reference sources
Sensory integration			
Sensory Integration and Praxis Tests (SIPT)	4y–8y 11mo	Complete assessment of sensory integration	Western Psychological Services, Los Angeles, CA, USA Ayres[5]
DeGangi–Berk Test of Sensory Integration	3–5y	Early detection of sensory processing difficulties	Western Psychological Services, Los Angeles, CA, USA DeGangi and Berk[97]
Test of Sensory Functions	4–18mo	Measures sensory reactivity, regulation and adaptive motor functioning in infants	Western Psychological Services, Los Angeles, CA, USA DeGangi and Greespan[66]
Observations based on sensory integration	Not specified	Specific tasks, postural responses and signs of central nervous system integrity associated with sensory integrative functioning	Pediatric Therapy Network, Torrance, CA, USA Blanche[6]
Tactile system			
Miller Assessment for Preschoolers	Children aged 2y 9mo–5y 8mo	Subtests of stereognosis and finger localization	Miller[57]
Sensory Integration and Praxis Tests	Children ages 4y–8y 11mo	Manual form perception Localization of tactile stimuli Finger identification Graphaesthesia	Western Psychological Services, Los Angeles, CA, USA Ayres[5]
Sensory processing (reports by proxy) or observations during testing			
Sensory Processing Measure	5–12y	Sensory processing difficulties at home and school	Western Psychological Services, Los Angeles, CA, USA Parham and Ecker[8]
Sensory Profile	Birth through adulthood	Sensory processing difficulties by proxy (children) and self-report (adolescents/adults)	Pearson, San Antonio, TX, USA Dunn[7,60]
Bayley Scales of Infant and Toddler Development, 3rd edition	1–42mo	The Behavior Observation Inventory considers the presence of tactile defensiveness	Psychological Corporation, San Antonio, TX, USA Bayley[54]
The Sensory Rating Scale for Infants and Young Children	Birth–3y	Parent-report measure that can be used to identify and quantify sensory responsiveness including sensory defensive behaviours	Provost and Oetter[56]
Proprioceptive system			
Sensory Integration and Praxis Tests	4y–8y 11mo	Kinaesthesia Manual form perception Standing and walking balance	Western Psychological Services. Los Angeles, CA, USA Ayres[5]
Observations based on sensory integration	Not specified	Specific tasks, postural responses and signs of nervous system integrity associated with sensory integrative functioning	Pediatric Therapy Network, Torrance, CA, USA Blanche[6]
Vestibular system			
Sensory Integration and Praxis Tests	Children ages 4y–8y 11mo	Postrotary Nystagmus Test Standing and walking balance	Western Psychological Services, Los Angeles, CA, USA Ayres[5]

REFERENCES

1. Busey TA, Loftus GR (1994) Sensory and cognitive components of visual information acquisition. *Psychol Rev* 101: 446–469.
2. Miller LJ (1998) The diagnosis, treatment, and etiology of sensory modulation disorder. *Sensory Integrat Spec Int Sect Quarterly* 21: 1–3.
3. *Mosby's Medical Dictionary*, 8th edition. (2009) Philadelphia, PA: Elsevier.
4. National Institutes of Health (2011) National Institutes of Health Toolbox: Assessment of Neurological and Behavioral Functions. Available at: www.nihtoolbox.org/default.aspx.
5. Ayres AJ (1989) *Sensory Integration and Praxis Tests*. Los Angeles, CA: Western Psychological Services.
6. Blanche EI (2002) *Observations Based on Sensory Integration Theory*. Torrance, CA: Pediatric Therapy Network.
7. Dunn W (1999) *The Sensory Profile Manual*. San Antonio, TX: The Psychological Corporation.
8. Parham LD, Ecker C (2007) *Sensory Processing Measure (SPM) Home Form*. Los Angeles, CA: Western Psychological Services.
9. Parham LD, Mailloux Z (2010) Sensory integration. In: Case-Smith J, editor. *Occupational Therapy for Children*, 6th edition. St. Louis, MO: Mosby, pp. 325–372.
10. Lederman SJ, Klatzky RL (2009) Haptic perception: a tutorial. *Attention Percept Psychophys* 71: 1439–1459.
11. Ross HE, Murray DJ (eds & transl.) (1996) *E.H. Weber on the Tactile Senses*, 2nd edn. Hove: Erlbaum (UK) Taylor and Francis.
12. Levin S, Pearsall G, Ruderman RJ (1978) Von Frey's method of measuring pressure sensibility in the hand: an engineering analysis of the Weinstein–Semmes pressure aesthesiometer. *J Hand Surg* 3: 211–216.
13. Voerman VF, van Egmond J, Crul BJ (1999) Normal values for sensory thresholds in the cervical dermatomes: a critical note on the use of Semmes–Weinstein monofilaments. *Am J Phys Med Rehabil* 78: 24–29.
14. Wartenberg R (1948) Sign of median palsy: sign of facial palsy for examination of the sensibility and of superficial reflexes. *Trans Am Neurol Assoc* (73 Annual Meeting) 31: 3.
15. Kenshalo DR, Bergen DC (1975) A device to measure cutaneous temperature sensitivity in humans and subhuman species. *J Appl Physiol* 39: 1038–1040.
16. Fruhstorfer H, Lindblom U, Schmidt WG (1976) Method for quantitative estimation of thermal thresholds in patients. *J Neurol Neurosurg Psychiatry* 39: 1071–1075.
17. Bravenboer B, van Dam PS, Hop J, van der Steenhoven J, Erkelens DW (1992) Thermal threshold testing for the assessment of small fibre dysfunction: normal values and reproducibility. *Diabet Med* 9: 546–549.
18. Bauer BA (1977) Tactile-sensitive behavior in hyperactive and non-hyperactive children. *Am J Occup Ther* 31: 447–453.
19. Royeen CB, Fortune JC (1990) Touch inventory for elementary-school-aged children. *Am J Occup Ther* 44: 155–159.
20. Sherrington CS (1907) On the proprioceptive system, especially in its reflex aspect. *Brain* 29: 467–485.
21. Gandevia SC, Resfshauge KM, Collins DF (2002) Proprioception: peripheral inputs and perceptual interactions. *Adv Exp Med Biol* 508: 61–68.
22. Grob KR, Kuster MS, Higgins SA, Lloyd DG, Yata H (2002) Lack of correlation between different measurements of proprioception in the knee. *J Bone Joint Surg Br* 84: 614–618.
23. Blanche E, Bodison S, Chang M, Reinoso G (2011) Development of the Comprehensive Observations of Proprioception Scale (COP): validity, reliability and factor analysis. *Am J Occup Ther*, in press.
24. Sigmundsson H, Ingvaldsen, RP, Whiting HTA (1997) Inter- and intra-sensory modality matching in children with hand–eye coordination problems. *Exp Brain Res* 114: 492–499.
25. Sigmundsson H, Whiting HTA, Ingvaldsen RP (1999) 'Putting your foot in it'! A window into clumsy behavior. *Behav Brain Res* 102: 129–136.
26. Laszlo JI, Bairstow PJ (1980) The measurement of kinaesthetic sensitivity in children and adults. *Dev Child Neurol* 22: 454–464.
27. Wycherley AS, Helliwell PS, Bird HA (2005) A novel device for the measurement of proprioception in the hand. *Rheumatology* 44: 638–641.
28. Roberts D, Ageberg E, Andersson G, Friden T (2003) Effects of short-term cycling on knee joint proprioception in healthy young persons. *Am J Sports Med* 31: 990–994.
29. Swanik CB, Lephart SM, Rubash HE (2004) Proprioception, kinesthesia, and balance after total knee arthroplasty with cruciate-retaining and posterior stabilized prostheses. *J Bone Joint Surg Inc* 86A: 328–334.
30. Deitz JC, Richarson P, Atwater SW, Crowe TK, Odiorne M (1991) Performance of normal children on the pediatric clinical test of sensory interaction for balance. *Occup Ther J Res* 11: 336–355.
31. Gerr FE, Letz R (1988) Reliability of a widely used test of peripheral cutaneous vibration sensitivity and a comparison of two testing protocols. *Br J Ind Med* 45: 635–639.
32. Gerr F, Letz R, Harris-Abbott D, Hopkins LC (1995) Sensitivity and specificity of vibrometry for detection of carpal tunnel syndrome. *J Occup Environ Med* 37: 1108–1115.
33. Bidel DC, Horak FB (2001) Behavior therapy for vestibular rehabilitation. *J Anxiety Disord* 15: 121–130.
34. Ayres AJ (1972) *Southern California Sensory Integration Tests*. Los Angeles, CA: Western Psychological Services.
35. deQuiros JB, Schrager OL (1978) *Neuropsychological Fundamentals in Learning Disabilities*. San Rafael, CA: Academy Therapy.
36. Blanche EI, Reinoso G (2008) The use of clinical observations to evaluate vestibular and proprioceptive functions. *Am Occup Ther Assoc Occup Ther Pract* 13: 45–51.
37. Luo F, Wang JY (2009) Neuronal nociceptive responses in thalamocortical pathways. *Neurosci Bull* 25: 289–295.
38. Merskey H, Bogduk N (1994) *Classification of Chronic Pain. Description of Chronic Pain Syndromes and Definitions of Pain Terms*, 2nd edition. Seattle: IASP Press.
39. Keizer D, Fael D, Wierda JMKH, van Wijhe M (2008) Quantitative sensory testing with von Frey monofilaments in patients with allodynia what are we quantifying? *Clin J Pain* 24: 463–466.
40. Millan MJ (1999) The induction of pain: An integrative view. *Prog Neurobiol* 57: 1–164.
41. Apkarian AV, Bushnell MC, Treede RD, Zubieta JK (2005) Human brain mechanism of pain perception and regulation in health and disease. *Eur J Pain* 9: 463–484.
42. Bradley TE (2005) *Slosson Auditory Perceptual Skill Screener (SAPSS)*. New York: Slosson Educational Publications.
43. Wepman JM, Reynolds WM (1986) *Wepman's Auditory Discrimination Test*. Los Angeles, CA: Western Psychological Services.
44. ASHA. Available at: http://search.asha.org/default.aspx?q=evaluationtools/ (accessed 17 January 2010).
45. Schiffman SS (2000) Taste quality and neural coding: Implications from psychophysics and neurophysiology. *Physiol Behav* 69: 147–159.
46. Denckla MB (1973) Development of speed and repetitive and successive finger movements in normal children. *Dev Med Child Neurol* 15: 635–645.

47. Dunn W (1981) *A Guide to Testing Clinical Observations in Kindergartners*. Rockville, MD: The American Occupational Therapy Association.
48. Grant WW, Boelsche A, Zin D (1973) Developmental patterns of two motor functions. *Dev Med Child Neurol* 15: 171–177.
49. Gregory-Flock JL, Yerxa EJ (1984) Standardization of the prone extension postural test on children ages 4 through 8. *Am J Occup Ther* 38: 187–194.
50. Haack L, Short-DeGraff M, Hanzlik JR (1993) Relationship of oculomotor skills to vestibular related clinical observations. *Phys Occup Ther Pediatr* 13: 1–13.
51. Harris NP (1981) Duration and quality of the prone extension position in four, six, and eight year old normal children. *Am J Occup Ther* 35: 26–30.
52. Magalhaes LC, Koomar JA, Cermark SA (1989) Bilateral motor coordination in 5-to 9-year-old children: A pilot study. *Am J Occup Ther* 43: 437–443.
53. Wilson BN, Pollock N, Kaplan BJ, Law M (2000) *Clinical Observations of Motor and Postural Skills*, 2nd edition. Framingham, MA: Therapro, Inc.
54. Bayley N (2005) *The Bayley Scales of Infant and Toddler Development, 3rd edition: Manual*. San Antonio, TX: Pearson.
55. DeGangi GA, Poisson S, Sickel RZ, Santman Wiener A (1995) *The Infant/Toddler Symptom Checklist, A Screening Tool for Parents. Manual*. San Antonio, TX: Pearson.
56. Provost B, Oetter P (1993) The Sensory Rating Scale for infants and young children: Development and reliability. *Phys Occup Ther Pediatr* 13: 15–35.
57. Miller LJ (1982) *Miller Assessment for Preschoolers*. Littleton, CO: The Foundation for Knowledge in Development.
58. Crowe TK, Deitz JC, Richardson PK, Atwater SW (1990) Interrater reliability of the Clinical Test of Sensory Interaction for Balance. *Phys Occup Ther Pediatr* 10: 1–27.
59. Westcott SL, Crowe TK, Deitz JC, Richardson PK (1994) Test–retest reliability of the Pediatric Clinical Test of Sensory Interaction for Balance (P-CTSIB). *Phys Occup Ther Pediatr* 14: 1–22.
60. Dunn W (2001) The sensations of everyday life: theoretical, conceptual and pragmatic considerations. *Am J Occup Ther* 55: 608–620.
61. Dunn W, Bennett D (2002) Patterns of sensory processing in children with attention deficit hyperactivity disorder. *Occup Ther J Res* 22: 4–15.
62. Dunn W, Myles B, Orr S (2002) Sensory processing issues associated with Asperger syndrome: a preliminary investigation. *Am J Occup Ther* 56: 97–102.
63. Ermer J, Dunn W (1998) The sensory profile: A discriminant analysis of children with and without disabilities. *Am J Occup Ther* 52: 283–290.
64. Kientz M, Dunn W (1997) A comparison of children with autism and typical children using the Sensory Profile. *Am J Occup Ther* 51: 530–537.
65. Parham LD, Ecker C, Miller Kuhaneck H, Henry DA, Glennon TJ (2007) *Sensory Processing Measure (SPM): Manual*. Los Angeles, CA: Western Psychological Services.
66. DeGangi GA, Greenspan ST (1989) *Test of Sensory Functions in Infants (TSFI) Manual*. Los Angeles, CA: Western Psychological Services.
67. Mailloux Z (1990) An overview of the Sensory Integration and Praxis Tests. *Am J Occup Ther* 44: 589–594.
68. Ayres AJ (1980) *Southern California Sensory Integration Tests*, revised edition. Los Angeles, CA: Western Psychological Services.
69. Ayres AJ (1975) *Southern California Postrotary Nystagmus Test Manual*. Los Angeles, CA: Western Psychological Services.
70. Ayres AJ, Marr D (1991) Sensory Integration and Praxis Tests. In: Fisher AG, Murray EA, Bundy AC, editors. *Sensory Integration, Theory and Practice*. Philadelphia: F.A. Davis Company, pp. 203–229.
71. Kauffman AS, Kaufman AS (1983) *Kaufman Assessment Battery for Children*. Circle Pines, MN: American Guidance Service.
72. Parham LD (1998) The relationship of sensory integrative development to achievement in elementary students: Four-year longitudinal patterns. *Occup Ther J Res* 18: 105–127.
73. Mailloux Z, Mulligan S, Smith Roley S, et al. (2011) Verification and clarification of patterns of sensory integrative dysfunction. *Am J Occup Ther* 65: 143–151.
74. Schoen SA, Miller LJ, Green KE (2008) Pilot study of the Sensory Over-Responsivity Scales: assessment and inventory. *Am J Occup Ther* 62: 393–406.
75. May-Benson TA, Koomar JA (2007) Identifying gravitational insecurity in children: A pilot study. *Am J Occup Ther* 61: 142–147.
76. Miller LJ, McIntosh DN, McGrath J, et al (1999) Electrodermal responses to sensory stimuli in individuals with fragile X syndrome: a preliminary report. *Am J Med Genet* 83: 268–279.
77. Schaaf R, Miller LJ, Seawell D, O'Keefe S (2003) Children with disturbances in sensory processing: A pilot study examining the role of the parasympathetic nervous system. *Am J Occup Ther* 57: 442–449.
78. Dyck PJ, Zimmerman IR, O'Brien PC, et al (1978) Introduction of automated systems to evaluate touch-pressure vibration, and thermal cutaneous sensation in man. *Ann Neurol* 4: 502–510.
79. Dyck PJ, Zimmerman IR, Johnson DM, et al (1996) A standard test of heat-pain responses using CASE IV. *J Neurol Sci* 136: 54–63.
80. Gruener G, Dyck PJ (1994) Quantitative sensory testing: methodology, applications and future directions. *J Clin Neurophysiol* 11: 568–583.
81. Bertelsmann FW, Heimans JJ, van Rooy JC, Heine RJ, van der Veen EA (1986) Reproducibility of vibratory perception thresholds in patients with diabetic neuropathy. *Diabetes Res* 3: 463–466.
82. Goldberg JM, Lindblom U (1979) Standardised method of determining vibratory perception thresholds for diagnosis and screening in neurological investigation. *J Neurol Neurosurg Psychiatry* 42: 793–803.
83. Hilz MJ, Axelrod FB, Hermann K, Haertl U, Duetsch M, Neundörfer B (1998) Normative values of vibratory perception in 530 children, juveniles and adults aged 3–79 years. *J Neurol Sci* 159: 219–225.
84. Gerr FE, Letz R (1988) Reliability of a widely used test of peripheral cutaneous vibration sensitivity and a comparison of two testing protocols. *Br J Ind Med* 45: 635–639.
85. Gerr F, Letz R, Harris-Abbott D, Hopkins LC (1995) Sensitivity and specificity of vibrometry for detection of carpal tunnel syndrome. *J Occup Environ Med* 37: 1108–1115.
86. Meier PM, Berde CB, DiCanzio J, Zurakowski D, Sethna NF (2001) Quantitative assessment of cutaneous thermal and vibration sensation and thermal pain detection thresholds in healthy children and adolescents. *Muscle Nerve* 24: 1339–1345.
87. Yarnitsky D, Sprecher E (1994) Thermal testing: normative data and repeatability for various test algorithms. *J Neurol Sci* 125: 39–45.
88. van Deursen RW, Sanchez MM, Derr JA, Becker MB, Ulbrecht JS, Cavanagh PR (2001) Vibration perception threshold testing in patients with diabetic neuropathy: ceiling effects and reliability. *Diabet Med* 18: 469–475.
89. Fruhstorfer H, Lindblom U, Schmidt WG (1976) Method for quantitative estimation of thermal thresholds in patients. *J Neurol Neurosurg Psychiatry* 39: 1071–1075.
90. Ziegler D, Mayer P, Gries FA (1988) Evaluation of thermal, pain and vibration sensation thresholds in newly diagnosed

type 1 diabetic patients. *J Neurol Neurosurg Psychiatry* 51: 1420–1424.

91. Jamal GA, Hansen S, Weir AI, Ballantyne JP (1985) An improved automated method for the measurement of thermal thresholds. 1. Normal subjects. *J Neurol Neurosurg Psychiatry* 48: 354–360.

92. Bravenboer B, van Dam PS, Hop J, van der Steenhoven J, Erkelens DW (1992) Thermal threshold testing for the assessment of small fibre dysfunction: normal values and reproducibility. *Diabet Med* 9: 546–549.

93. Siao P, Cros DP (2003) Quantitaive sensory testing. *Phys Med Rehabil Clin N Am* 14: 261–286.

94. Fowler CJ, Carroll MB, Burns D, Howe N, Robinson K (1987) A portable system for measuring cutaneous thresholds for warming and cooling. *J Neurol Neurosurg Psychiatry* 50: 1211–1215.

95. Arezzo JC, Schaumburg HH, Laudadio C (1986) Device for quantitative assessment of thermal sense in diabetic neuropathy. *Diabetes* 35: 590–592.

96. Claus D, Hilz MJ, Neundorfer B (1990) Thermal discrimination thresholds: a comparison of different methods. *Acta Neurol Scand* 81: 533–540.

97. DeGangi GA, Berk RA (1983) Psychometric analysis of the test of sensory integration. *Phys Occup Ther Pediatr* 3: 43–60.

14
SENSORY FUNCTIONS: PAIN (B280–B289)

Tim F. Oberlander, Chantel C. Burkitt, Frank J. Symons and Celeste Johnston

What is the construct?

Unique challenges arise when assessing pain in children with developmental or intellectual disabilities[a] for whom pain cues are often ambiguous and highly subjective. Clinicians, caregivers and family alike struggle to decipher pain cues (signs or symptoms) because they can be altered, blunted or potentially confused with general stress or arousal. This poses a serious problem as there is no reason to suspect that a child with developmental disability would have any less pain than a typical peer. More likely, pain in children (and adults) with developmental disability is underdiagnosed simply because their communication of pain is not always understood or recognized by others. While the focus of this chapter is on pain assessment in children with a significant neurological impairment, it is critical to recognize that it is the level of function, not age, that will influence pain assessment in this setting, and thus we have included measures that cover a wide age spectrum, including adulthood.

The difficulties described above have been compounded by the fact that children with developmental disability have been systematically excluded from most pain research; thus, there is little scientific literature dedicated to the assessment and management of pain specific to children with developmental disability. This may be because studying children who have multiple physical disabilities (e.g. quadriplegia) and other developmental challenges (e.g. lack of communication, cognitive impairments, behaviour problems) can be extremely challenging. There are signs that the exclusion of those

with developmental disability in research is beginning to change.[1] The International Association for the Study of Pain (IASP) originally defined pain as 'an unpleasant sensory and emotional experience associated with actual or potential tissue damage, or described in terms of such damage',[2] but because the emphasis on self-report assumed a capacity for verbal communication, the IASP clarified the definition of pain to recognize that 'the inability to *verbally* [emphasis ours] communicate in no way negates the possibility that an individual is experiencing pain and is in need of appropriate pain relieving treatment'.[3] Children with developmental disability – comprising children with complex developmental disabilities – are limited in their ability to self-report owing to mobility and communication limitations, which makes it especially difficult for clinicians and caregivers to detect pain. The range of physiological or behavioural responses available to the child should be thoughtfully considered, and changes within those available behaviours (increases or decreases) may indicate potential signs of discomfort or pain. Any reaction to a noxious event should be considered as pain regardless of the characteristics of the reaction, as some pain cues are paradoxical in nature (e.g. laughter). The aim is to develop multifaceted strategies to effectively manage the pain of children with developmental disability once accurately detected.

The purpose of this chapter is to provide an overview of a number of issues inherent to assessing pain among children with developmental disability and associated significant neurological impairments (SNIs). Whether the developmental disability/SNI is from multifactorial causes (cerebral palsy), genetic/metabolic disorders (Down syndrome), traumatic brain injury or disorders of unknown origin, it can be associated with multiple sources of acute and chronic pain. Given that the term developmental disability can be used to describe clinical conditions with diverse aetiologies, anatomic lesions

---

[a] We acknowledge that the terms intellectual disability and developmental disability are not synonyms; however, for simplicity the term developmental disability has been used in this chapter as an umbrella term to include children with intellectual disabilities. The term developmental disability is used to incorporate a broad spectrum of disorders including multiple physical disabilities (e.g. quadriplegia) and other developmental disorders (e.g. autism).

and functional limitations, a considerable research effort remains to define precise relationships between the neural substrate that constitutes the condition and its impact on the pain system. At this point in our evolving understanding of pain in this context, the chapter will focus on summarizing currently available options for assessing pain in children with developmental disability, focusing on understanding pain and arousal behaviour in the context of the functional impairments that arise from a spectrum of cognitive, motor and communication limitations. Readers will note that many of the issues cut across the lifespan (preverbal neonatal populations, geriatric populations) and other clinical populations (neurodegenerative diseases such as Alzheimer syndrome) in which access to an internal state is difficult because spoken language is absent, not developed or impaired. For more information about pain in individuals with an SNI, readers are directed to Oberlander and Symons[1] or Siden and Oberlander.[4]

THE CONSTRUCT OF PAIN

Although pain has always been part of the human experience, the construct of pain was defined exclusively as a reflexive physical experience by Descartes almost four centuries ago.[5] The Cartesian perspective of pain considered it simply as nociception; that is, the experience of a stimulus as being noxious. Early philosophers such as Epicurus and Aristotle considered pain philosophically as the opposite of pleasure. This notion of opposite ends of a continuum is supported by recent neuroscience studies that indicate that pain and pleasure may share underlying anatomical substrates.[6]

It was only in 1965, however, that the notion of pain having multiple dimensions was proposed.[7] This definition of pain did include the Cartesian component of pain intensity, but added a sensory component of pain that reflected such things as sharpness and temperature, and also an affective component related to the emotional evaluation of the pain, such as cruelty or punishment. Measures, in particular the McGill Melzack Pain Questionnaire, were developed to include these three components of pain: intensity, sensorial and affective.[5,7] In a subsequent attempt to simplify the definition of pain while acknowledging the dimensional but subjective features, Macaffery[8] proposed that 'pain is what the person says it is'.

The IASP adopted Merskey's[9] definition of pain, emphasizing sensory and emotional experience dimensions related to 'tissue damage', and thus reflecting the definition proposed by Melzack and Wall.[5] McGrath and Dade[10] further elaborated the construct of pain focused on children to include the context (such as family, setting), the child's age and past experiences, as well as the actual nature of the painful stimulus.

In this model, the painful stimulus results from tissue damage, although the damage may have occurred well into the past and be related to chronic pain in as of yet not well-understood ways. This stimulus enters into the peripheral nervous system, reaching the spinal cord via the dorsal root ganglia, travelling up through the thalamus into higher regions of the brain, including the somatosensory cortices where the intensity and sensory components are deciphered, as well as into the amygdala and prefrontal and frontal cortices, where the emotional component of pain is perceived. For the purposes of this chapter, the child may be at varying ages, have varying degrees of neurological intactness and, as will be discussed below, will have different means of communication. Furthermore, the context in which this signal is processed – whether or not parents are present, whether the setting is known and whether that knowledge is positive or negative – provides some of the contextual factors that will influence how the pain is experienced emotionally. Furthermore, the three components may interact – for example, the greater the emotion of anxiety, the greater the perceived intensity. Given the complex interplay between intensity, sensory, emotional and evaluative components of pain, the construct of pain will be child-specific and will thus always require a thoughtful, comprehensive evaluation, including the use of measures such as those described below.

THE NATURE OF PAIN IN CHILDREN WITH DEVELOPMENTAL DISABILITIES

There is an increased risk of multiple pain experiences (acute and chronic) associated specifically with having an intellectual disability because of the high rate of co-occurring developmental and related physical impairments. A great deal of pain is associated with major events such as surgery, invasive medical procedures, dislocated hips, and splinting and casting, which are often necessary for children with developmental disability. Just as troubling can be ongoing pain associated with the difficulties of daily living and medical conditions. Daily pain may result from difficulties with positioning, communication and mobility devices, for example when children with developmental disability use aids such as walkers, augmentative communication devices, seating systems and wheelchairs. Medical conditions are often associated with pain caused by high tone, pressure sores due to skin breakdown, constipation, and eating and swallowing issues, which can require special techniques or enterostomy feeds. Feeding tubes can cause daily pain because of gastric distention, pulling and tugging, and skin breakdown around the tube site.

A neurological impairment may be associated with increased muscle tone, spasms, weakness and loss of function necessitating physical therapy, orthopaedic surgery, neurosurgery and pharmacological management, which collectively may introduce multiple sources of everyday frequent pain. High muscle tone/spasticity may be treated through surgical intervention (selective dorsal rhizotomy) or by surgical implantation of an intrathecal baclofen pump. Pharmacological management of muscle tone may include an intramuscular injection of botulinum toxin A, which may successfully relieve hypertonia; there is some evidence that it may be associated with a corresponding reduction in reported pain.[11] Pain in this setting is typically thought to be nociceptive in origin; however, after repeated injury or surgery, neuropathic pain may also occur. There are limited reports of neuropathic pain in children with cerebral palsy, accompanied by typical signs of swelling, redness and extremity tenderness, though, in the absence of a clear history of nerve injury. However, the diagnosis frequently remains elusive and challenging.

EFFECTS OF PAIN ON OUTCOMES FOR CHILDREN WITH DEVELOPMENTAL DISABILITIES

There has been limited work on the outcomes associated with pain among children with intellectual disabilities. Breau and colleagues[12] examined the impact of pain on the functional capacity of children with developmental disability.[12] This 2-year diary study completed by caregivers analysed the functional abilities of 63 children with developmental disability on a subset of days with pain compared with similar pain-free days. Children showed deficits during painful days in all functional domains including communication, daily living skills, and social and motor skills as assessed by the Vineland Adaptive Behavior Scales.[13] Children with the most severe disabilities were the most impeded by pain. Given these initial results, it would seem especially important for clinicians and caregivers to recognize the impact that pain can have on a child with developmental disability. Considering that children with developmental disability are limited to different degrees in functional capacity, this decline is especially troubling. Further, these data suggest that when in pain, children with developmental disability are at an even greater disadvantage because of limited abilities both to communicate conventionally about pain and to cope with it.

EPIDEMIOLOGY OF PAIN IN CHILDREN WITH DEVELOPMENTAL AND INTELLECTUAL DISABILITIES

The only relatively large-scale epidemiological study conducted to date examining pain incidence in children with severe developmental disability was gathered during a year-long cohort study by Breau et al.[14] This study included 94 children who experienced a total of 406 painful episodes during the year of study. During a specific 4-week period, 78% of children experienced some type of pain and 62% experienced non-accidental pain. Children with better motor ability were more likely to experience accidental pain, whereas children with more limited motor ability experienced more non-accidental pain, which was rated as more intense in nature. During each week of the study, 35% to 52% of children experienced pain, as reported by their caregivers. Based on the 4 weeks of parental reporting, the children had pain on 18% of the days. The pain reported was of a significant severity, with accidental pain scored on average as 3.8 out of 10 and non-accidental pain scored as 6.1 out of 10. Pain is usually medicated at a score of 3 out of 10. Thus, the pain reported in this sample is extremely disturbing. Pain was long in duration and was experienced on average for up to 10 hours a week. Pain did not vary by demographics, but the authors noted that children with more severe developmental disability experienced more pain.[14] Stallard[15] conducted a 2-week-long diary study to examine the detailed everyday occurrence of pain in children with developmental disability who were unable to communicate verbally. Of the 34 participants, 25 experienced some form of pain over the 2-week period, with 23 participants experiencing moderate to severe pain during that time. Four of the children studied experienced moderate to severe pain for more than 30 minutes for five or more of the days studied, and none of the children was receiving any type of pain management.[15] Taken together, the findings of these two studies suggest that children with developmental disability experience a great deal of pain.

General factors to consider when measuring this domain

How can pain be assessed and managed when typical means of verbal or non-verbal communication or cognition are altered or absent? In the absence of easily recognized verbal or motor-dependent forms of communication, it remains uncertain whether the pain experience itself is different or whether only the expressive manifestations are altered. Indeed, without easily understandable means of communication or motor skills, pain may remain under-recognized or untreated. Effective assessment of pain is an essential step towards establishing a diagnosis, selecting an appropriate treatment plan, assessing treatment efficacy and ultimately relieving pain. Given that pain assessment in children without disabilities needs to be calibrated to age-specific language and cognitive skills, a similar approach is required to assess pain for children with developmental disabilities.

TABLE 14.1

Pain assessment tools for children with intellectual and developmental disabilities

Pain scale	Brief description	No. of items	Psychometric properties	Recommendations
Child Pain Scales				
Pain Indicator for Communicatively Impaired Children Stallard et al[27]	200 pain cues derived from caregiver interview narrowed to four main cues	6	Accuracy demonstrated Not tested for validity or reliability	Short and simple Possible preliminary measure of pain
Pediatric Pain Profile Hunt et al[33]	Semi-individualized measure providing predetermined categories of behaviours which are then added to by the caregiver	20	Valid, reliable and sensitive measure for individual children Does not provide generalizable measures across children	May distinguish individual child's good days from bad days May be well suited for monitoring pain for an individual across long time scales
Non-Communicative Children's Pain Checklist – revised (NCCPC-R) Breau et al[28]	Assessment tool quantifies pain responses observed by clinicians, parents or caregivers Postoperative version available	30	Inter-rater reliability and internal consistency supported Consistent scores over time Sensitive and specific to pain Scores significantly related to parent pain rating	Useful across populations and settings Consistently accurate with short observation times and by those unfamiliar with the child
Faces Legs Activity Cry Consolability Scale – revised Malviya et al[36]	Behavioural categories scored based on pain descriptors for each Caregiver may add to list of pain descriptors for his or her child	5	Showed good inter-rater reliability and test–retest reliability Correlation between observer scores and parent's global pain rating	Shows clinical utility Individualized for each child
University of Wisconsin Children's Hospital (UWCH) pain scale for preverbal and non-verbal children Soetenga et al[39]	Observational assessment of five pain domains, with one overall rating	5	High internal consistency and inter-rater reliability Showed sensitivity to pain Low correlation with Wong–Baker Faces Scale	Designed to be simple and clinically useful Used with preverbal infants in addition to those with intellectual deficits
Adult Pain Scales				
The Pain and Discomfort Scale Bodfish et al[40] Phan et al[41]	Measures pain and discomfort during a standardized physical examination (pain examination procedure)	18	High inter-rater reliability Sensitivity to pain	Useful in isolating the location/ source of pain
Chronic Pain Scale for Non-verbal Adults with Intellectual Disabilities (CPS-NAID) Burkitt et al[42]	Adapted version of the NCCPC-R for adults with intellectual disability experiencing chronic or recurring pain	24	Strong internal consistency, inter-rater reliability and construct validity and sensitive to pain Cut-off score was established	The CPS-NAID is best suited for assessing chronic pain
Non-communicating Adult Pain Checklist (NCAPC) Lotan et al[43]	Adapted version of the NCCPC-R to assess acute pain in adults with intellectual disability	21	High internal consistency Sensitive to pain	The NCAPC is currently recommended for assessing acute or procedural pain in adults with intellectual disability

The ability to communicate pain and distress is fundamental to seeking and obtaining health care, regardless of the presence of developmental disabilities and the motor, cognitive, language and social barriers imposed by that disability on the objective evaluation of the pain system. Measurement involves assigning numerical values to a construct.[16] When measuring a construct such as pain, which is a subjective experience that only the person experiencing it truly knows, several questions arise. A fundamental question is whether or not it is even possible to measure a subjective experience. While there is some shared understanding of what pain is, it remains purely subjective and some would argue that it can never be accurately measured. Among other challenges is that pain is not static and can change very rapidly, so a measurement at one point in time may no longer be accurate a short time later.

Craig and others[17,18] proposed a sociocommunicative model of pain, with important implications regarding the way in which to think about the function of observational and self-report measures of pain. The first step in this model is that the pain signal needs to be encoded: it needs to be interpreted as pain and then encoded either automatically, for example through crying or facial grimacing, or in higher-order levels such as word finding to report the pain verbally. The second step is to express the pain, and this will be a reflection of the child's repertoire of pain expressions, be they automatic or more cognitive. The next step, however, is as important as the encoding and expression elements for the child experiencing pain, and that is the observer's interpretation of the expression. This is influenced by multiple observer characteristics including belief systems, experience, training and context, among others.

There is the possibility of inaccuracies throughout the communication of the pain process, which collectively influence the final measurement of pain in children. In examining measures, traditional considerations of psychometric properties need to be placed in the context of measuring pain in children. Here additional considerations must be reflected in the underlying model and construct of pain (e.g. how does the child's past experience with pain influence encoding and expression) and in the sociocommunicative aspects of pain (e.g. the observer's belief system about pain). Most measures of pain in children, including in children with developmental disabilities, do not address these issues, but rather the traditional psychometrics of reliability and validation processes, and occasionally feasibility and clinical utility. Although reliability and validity have traditionally been considered separately, and validity has typically been divided into the three 'C's of content, criterion and construct validity, some psychometricians have suggested that the most important evaluation of a measure is the extent to which it can inform us about the construct being measured in a person in a particular situation. Thus, in the following sections we will consider measures of pain in children with developmental disabilities in terms of what we can tell about a particular child's pain in a given situation.

EFFECTIVE USE OF PAIN MEASURES

Considering the limited knowledge base of how to assess pain to capture its multiple dimensions, the best recommendation we can give for pain assessment for children with developmental disability is the use of a comprehensive approach using multiple observational tools, parent report[44] and clinical judgement. It may be helpful for a clinician to collaborate with the parent to decipher what aspects of the child's behaviour and functional abilities have been impacted by the onset of pain. Self-report is not readily available, as verbal children with developmental disability seem to have difficulty reporting their own pain,[22] which may reflect an age effect (i.e. young children learn to report on pain) and/or a disability effect.

FEASIBILITY OF PAIN MEASURES IN CLINICAL SETTINGS

The most validated and reliable pain measures currently used may seem cumbersome, time-consuming and impractical to clinicians. Because of this, user groups may be tempted to create or adapt pain scales to satisfy clinical utility. This is a laudable objective, but caution must be exercised in ad-hoc scale changes as alterations may negatively impact the assessment tool's psychometric properties and decrease the tool's sensitivity to pain. Clinicians are urged to take the necessary time to use measurement tools to facilitate accurate pain assessment, which may result in reduced hospital stays and a reduction in medical complications associated with pain. On the other hand, additional research is needed that addresses more directly issues of clinical use(s) and adaptation in relation to effective implementation of existing pain scales.

Overview of recommended measures (Table 14.1)

SELF-REPORT PAIN MEASURES

Although self-report is often the method of choice for pain assessment in other populations, there is scarce evidence regarding the usefulness and accuracy of this method for use with children with developmental disability.[19] Two research studies have assessed the ability of those with developmental disability to rate pain intensity based on vignettes depicting common accidents or injuries (e.g. falling off a bicycle, a burn from a casserole). Zabalia and Duchaux[20] found that the rating of pain by children with intellectual disabilities differentiated according to the cause/type of pain, and the children were able to describe the pain using similar wording as would be expected by typically developing children. Bromley et al[21] conducted a similar study with adults with developmental disability and asked them to localize and rate the intensity of pain situations presented in photographs. Compared with a control group, participants were 93% accurate at localizing the pain source. Participants with developmental disability rated the intensity of pain as more severe than the control group in every case where images of 'mild' pain were presented and in 36% of cases where images of 'severe' pain were presented. Pain intensity ratings were consistent over time and were unrelated to the severity of developmental disability. Interestingly, when Benini et al[22] asked children with developmental disability to self-report on their own pain intensity and location following immunization, only half of the children with developmental disability were able to give self-reports that were fitting. This inability to report was despite an hour of instruction on how to use the various self-report tools, some of which were modified for simplicity. The limited and conflicting evidence for or against the use of self-report is potentially the consequence of diminished cognitive ability during the actual pain experience. Thus, the abilities that individuals with developmental disability show during training or hypothetical situations may not hold up during self-reports of actual pain.[12,19] The current evidence does not substantiate a recommendation for the use of self-report with individuals with developmental disability at this time.

OBSERVATIONAL RATING SCALE MEASURES OF PAIN BEHAVIOR

A child's limited repertoire of distress signals may become evident during a very painful event, or be difficult to discriminate from fear, sadness or even contentment. Emerging reports provide some description of the expression of pain in the case of certain disabilities and provide scales that have face validity, some empirical validity and perhaps clinical utility.

In a case report, Collignon et al[23] described the challenges of pain assessment in three children with cerebral palsy that led to the initial development of a 22-item scale. These focused on observations made during the response to physical examination that were thought to be indicative of pain.[24] Since then, a number of empirical studies have yielded important inventories of behaviours considered by observers to be related to pain among children with developmental disability.[25–27] Multidimensional instruments have been designed to assess pain in children and adults with communication and cognitive impairments.[28–32] These measures have focused on the identification of a variety of possible pain cues in children with intellectual impairment.[27,30,33,34] These include

vocalization (e.g. cry, scream, moan), facial expression, movement (both increased and decreased), change in muscle tone (increased and decreased), guarding/protection and changes in everyday activity (social interaction, eating and sleeping).

The Pain Indicator for Communicatively Impaired Children (PICIC) was created during semi-structured interviews with parents and caregivers.[27] A list of 200 pain cues was created, based on interview, and then narrowed to four cues of screaming, distressed face, tense body and difficulty consoling, which provided the best psychometric properties and were most frequently endorsed by interviewees. This tool showed accuracy; however, it has not been retested for validity or reliability. The PICIC is short, straightforward and simple, and may be an effective preliminary measure of pain.

An alternate approach has been offered by Hunt et al,[33] the Paediatric Pain Profile (PPP) (www.ppprofile.org.uk), which uses individual symptom clusters to develop an individual's pain assessment. This semi-individualized measure gives predetermined categories of behaviours, which are then added to by the parent/caregiver, and provides a base and ceiling for pain behaviours rated from 0 to 3 in severity scoring. This measure provides a highly valid, reliable and sensitive measure for each individual child, but does not provide measures that are generalizable across children of a similar condition. In this sense, the PPP measure gives the clinician and family a way of distinguishing an individual child's good days from bad days and so may be well suited for a clinical or home setting and for longitudinally monitoring the individual's pain.

Breau and colleagues[34] developed an observational assessment tool to quantify pain responses observed by parents and caregivers of cognitively and physically impaired children. The scale consists of seven domains including vocal, eating/sleeping, social/personality, facial expression, activity, body/limbs and physiological (with minor item adaptations in wording made to accommodate an adult vs paediatric sample). The Non-communicative Children's Pain Checklist (NCCPC) was initially developed using items from primary caregivers and professionals[32] and direct observation validation studies.[34] Intensity of items is scored on a four-point behavioural rating scale over a 10-minute observation period. The NCCPC has been shown to be a valid and reliable method of assessing everyday pain among children with developmental disabilities[28] and in postoperative settings.[29]

The NCCPC has good psychometric properties, including reliability and validity, for detecting pain in the child's natural setting. Later, two new versions of the NCCPC were created: the Non-communicative Children's Pain Checklist – Post-operative Version for pain assessment after surgery[29] and the Non-communicative Children's Pain Checklist – Revised (NCCPC-R),[28] which retested the NCCPC with a larger sample to further characterize the scale's psychometric properties.[28] The NCCPC-R has been used successfully with multiple populations within a variety of settings and is currently used in clinical settings internationally. It has proven to be useful when the assessor does or does not know the child and is consistently accurate when scored after short observation times. The score results on the NCCPC-R were internally consistent, significantly related to pain intensity ratings provided by caregivers, consistent over time, and sensitive and specific to pain. Analyses of children's individual scores indicated that up to 95% of their scores were consistent. Receiver operating characteristic curves suggested a score of seven or greater on the NCCPC-R as indicative of pain in children with cognitive impairments, with 84% sensitivity and up to 77% specificity. The scores of all items are summed to provide a total pain score. Inter-rater reliability and correlations between NCCPC-PV scores and Visual Analogue Scale of pain scores have been reported.

The FLACC (Face, Legs, Activity, Cry and Consolability) includes five categories of behaviour and is scored from 0 to 2, with total scores ranging from 0 to 10. Inter-rater reliability of the FLACC between two observers was established in 30 children in the postanaesthesia care unit (PACU) (r=0.94).[35] The FLACC assessment tool was developed to provide consistent approaches to pain assessment in non-verbal and preverbal children. A decrease in FLACC scores after analgesic administration has been reported, as well as agreement between FLACC scores, the PACU nurse's global rating of pain and other measures.[36] The reliability and validity of this tool has been established in diverse settings and in different patient populations.

Importantly, measures of agreement between observers were found to be acceptable using the face, cry and consolability scales; however, low agreement in the legs and activity categories have been reported.[35] This has led to the revised FLACC, which now includes behaviours specific to children with developmental impairments.[36] Although behavioural categories were left unchanged, descriptors of specific behaviours were added that were considered to be associated with pain in children with cognitive and other impairments. This enables parents/caregivers to record divergent or idiosyncratic pain behaviours. For studies on pain after postoperative analgesia, the FLACC offers a discrete number of pain-related behaviours; however, recent observations suggest that the 'legs' score may continue to be problematic in children with quadriplegia (the scores reach a 'ceiling' before the maximum possible) (Breau, personal communication, 2010).

Acceptable inter-rater reliability, intraclass correlation coefficients and measures of agreement between observers for each category, as well as total FLACC scores, test–retest reliability (repeated FLACC scores by observers viewing videotaped children following surgery) and moderate to high correlations between observers' FLACC scores and parents' global pain ratings have been reported.[37] The addition of parental pain descriptors adds an individual-specific dimension but may be problematic as there is no way to subject these highly individualized qualitative data to typical psychometric analyses, making comparisons across children challenging. There is also no way to know whether the unique descriptions have interval properties, which is a necessary condition for performing most quantitative statistics required to assess psychometrics for a tool designed to be used for more than one child. Clinical utility has also been studied, showing that clinicians rated the complexity, compatibility, relative advantage and overall clinical utility higher for the r-FLACC than for the NCCPC-PV.[38]

The University of Wisconsin Children's Hospital (UWCH) pain scale for preverbal and non-verbal children incorporates five domains: facial, vocal/cry, behavioural/consolability, body movements/posture and sleep. Each domain is observed and then a total score is given on a scale from 0 to 5 based on overall intensity. The UWCH pain scale was validated using a sample of 74 children (preverbal or non-verbal) over 124 observation intervals.[39] Seventy-six observations were made during an immunization or other painful procedure, 57 before analgesics were given and 49 after analgesics were given. Sixty-eight observations were made when another rater scored the Wong–Baker Faces Scale. Results showed high internal consistency and higher pain scores during painful procedures and before the delivery of analgesics than scores after analgesic delivery. Inter-rater reliability was high when two nurses scored pain using the UWCH pain scale; however, criterion validity was low when a nurse scored pain using the UWCH pain scale and another nurse or parent used the Faces Pain Scale. This discrepancy could be because of parent/nurse differences in scoring pain. Moreover, its application in a population of children with neurological impairments remains to be studied, and therefore its application in this setting may be limited.

OTHER PAIN ASSESSMENT TOOLS

Three additional pain assessment tools developed specifically for use with adults with developmental disability have emerged, providing additional assessment options. The Pain and Discomfort Scale (PADS) developed by Bodfish et al[40] was used by Phan and colleagues[41] to measure pain expression in adults with developmental disability during a dental scaling procedure. The PADS was completed at several time points before and after the painful procedure and once during the scaling. The PADS scores were significantly higher during the painful procedure compared with all other observations. The PADS showed high inter-rater reliability. The PADS is unique in that it measures pain and discomfort during a short standardized physical examination ('Pain Examination Procedure'), and therefore the assessor can isolate the location and potentially the cause of the pain.

Burkitt and colleagues[42] validated the NCCPC-R for use with adults (*n*=16) with developmental disability during chronic or recurring pain episodes. With six items discarded after analysis during pain and pain-free episodes, the revised scale (Chronic Pain Scale for Nonverbal Adults with Intellectual Disabilities [CPS-NAID]) showed strong internal consistency, inter-rater reliability and construct validity, and a cut-off score was established. The CPS-NAID is best suited for assessing chronic pain in adults with developmental disability.

Lotan et al[43] also adapted the NCCPC-R for use with adults with intellectual disabilities to assess acute pain (influenza immunization). The scale was modified to exclude 13 original items and include four new items. When rescored (*n*=89), the modified measure (Non-Communicating Adult Pain Checklist [NCAPC]) showed sensitivity to pain on all items and high internal consistency for use during acute pain across all levels of intellectual disability. The NCAPC is currently recommended for assessing acute or procedural pain in adults with developmental disability.

Biobehavioural issues and sensory threshold measurement

Basic Neurobiological Sensory Mechanisms

A critical challenge facing researchers is how to improve our understanding of whether and how the neurological damage associated with a developmental disability may disrupt the neural substrate that underlies the pain system. It is not well understood, in general, how injury or disruption to the development of one system may lead to the altered function of other systems (e.g. hypothalamic–pituitary–adrenal axis regulation and autonomic stress reactivity, learning and memory) that ultimately may alter the expression or experience of pain. The cumulative findings from multiple levels of inquiry (molecular, genomic, proteomic, cellular) continue to provide evidence of the remarkable plasticity in pain regulatory networks. How this plasticity works to moderate individual differences in pain sensation and response is an area of active inquiry. For example, in neuropathic pain, it appears that

peripheral or central nervous system injury can set up longlasting spinal and supraspinal reorganization through central sensitization.[45,46] Moreover, this reorganization can extend to higher cortical areas including the forebrain.[47] Casey et al[47] found that the forebrain of individuals with some forms of neuropathic pain undergoes pathologically induced changes that may impair clinical response to treatment because of reductions in the functional connectivity of subcortical pathways. What we do not know, however, is the relevance of work like that described above (neuropathic pain and brain/sensory system changes) as it relates to the somatosensory neurobiology of children with developmental disability. This issue is complex and will require integrative translational research approaches to be addressed successfully.[48]

Sensory Thresholds

Despite clinical impressions and anecdotal testimony, there is surprisingly little research specific to the issue of sensory thresholds and pain among individuals with developmental disability. Research by Biersdorff,[49] for example, suggested that those with developmental disability experience altered pain sensation and in many cases are insensitive or indifferent to pain.[49] The data, however, were based on incident reports of times when individuals with developmental disability (*n*=123) encountered a painful situation and their reaction to it. Seventy-seven per cent of those studied were reported to have normal or hypersensitive responses to pain, whereas 48% were reported to have hyposensitive responses. From these data, the conclusion was that many individuals with developmental disability have elevated pain thresholds. Surprisingly, those deemed to have a 'significantly elevated threshold' were those whose caregiver simply stated that they had to be 'very observant' in order to detect a pain reaction. Further, these results are based on the caregiver's subjective interpretations and there was no systematic control for the intensity, duration or context of the noxious stimuli. Rather than a study of thresholds, perhaps the findings are best understood in relation to reporter perceptions.

There are, however, only a few studies that have produced evidence that is directly related to sensory thresholds, per se, in developmental disability, suggesting, at least in part, the difficulty inherent in approaching work of this kind. In a study designed to examine sensory thresholds, Hennequin et al[50] compared the latency of detection of self-administered cold stimuli between a group (*n*=26) of individuals with Down syndrome and a disability-free comparison group (*n*=75). All participants were verbal. The first test used an ice cube applied to the wrist and temple, and the time between application and detection was measured in both groups. The second test used a cold cotton swab applied to several areas of the face, hand and mouth. This stimulus was not painful but was used to test the participant's ability to detect the location where the stimulus had been present, using their finger to point to the location once the swab was removed. The group with Down syndrome had significantly longer median detection latencies than the comparison group and more difficulties localizing the cold stimulus. The findings were ambiguous, however, with respect to sensitivity because several interpretations about the between-group differences are possible, including that individuals with Down syndrome were insensitive to pain or had higher cold stimuli perception thresholds, or that there was a processing speed delay because of differences somewhere along the sensory/motor pathway (afferent, decoding, vocal/motor output).

Symons et al[51] conducted a study of sensory functioning in individuals with moderate, severe and profound intellectual disabilities. Some participants were severely limited in verbal ability and most were completely nonverbal. The facial responses of the participants (*n*=44) were coded using the Facial Action Coding Scoring before, during and after five types of sensory stimulation (pin prick, light touch, deep pressure, cool, warm). A randomized sham-controlled sensory testing protocol was used to guard against observer bias. Participants showed significant sensitivity to sensory stimuli (all modalities) during active sensory trials ($p<0.05$) compared with sham trials, and females were more expressive than males ($p<0.05$). Surprisingly, participants with chronic self-injury showed significantly more pain expression ($p<0.05$) than those who did not self-injure. These results, although important from the perspective of documenting sensory detection capacity and perhaps a bias-free method for doing so, are still not specific to establishing thresholds.

In the one true pain threshold study to date, Defrin et al[52] addressed the issue of a reaction time confound. Defrin and colleagues[52] successfully completed a quantitative sensory testing study using two different quantitative measures examining heat-pain thresholds between a group of individuals with mild intellectual impairment (*n*=25) and a group without (*n*=14). Participant heat-pain threshold was measured using the method of limits and the method of levels (MLE). Heat-pain thresholds were significantly lower and the reaction time was significantly longer in the cognitive impairment group than in the comparison group when measured using MLE, independent of the reaction time. These results indicate that this sample of individuals with mild developmental disability were sensitive to heat pain, and more so than individuals without cognitive impairment.[52]

The studies described briefly above provide only clues to potential differences in sensory function in individuals with developmental disabilities. Sensation and sensory function appears to be intact in many individuals with intellectual and related developmental issues in the majority of study samples reported on to date, and, when reaction time is considered, there was evidence for lower thresholds and increased sensitivity to pain stimuli (not the converse). Apparent in this brief overview is that very little is known about sensory or pain thresholds among individuals with developmental disability. Further research building on the work of Defrin et al[52] is warranted and necessary.

Summary

While pain assessment in a child with a significant neurological impairment can be challenging, it is no less imperative than in all children. Pain-related behaviours can be ambiguous, and ratings subjective. Advances establishing valid and reliable tools for everyday and procedural/postoperative pain measures are emerging and offer clinically useful tools specific to this paediatric population. Moreover, recent research is advancing our understanding of unique somatosensory disturbances that might underlie links between central neurological lesions and altered pain experiences, and is offering important biobehavioural dimensions that should assist clinical pain assessment and management.

REFERENCES

1. Oberlander TF, Symons FJ (2006) *Pain in Children & Adults with Developmental Disabilities*. Baltimore, MD: Paul H. Brookes Publishing Co.
2. Merskey HE (1986) Classification of chronic pain: Descriptions of chronic pain syndromes and definitions of pain terms. *Pain* 3(Suppl): 51.
3. International Association for the Study of Pain (2001) http://www.iasp-pain.org/terms-p.html. [serial online].
4. Siden H, Oberlander TF (2008) Pain management for children with a developmental disability in a primary care setting. In: Walco GA, Goldschneider KR, editors. *Pain in Children: A Practical Guide for Primary Care*. Totowa, NJ: Humana Press, pp. 29–37.
5. Melzack R, Wall P (1996) *The Challenge of Pain*. New York, NY: Basic Books, Inc.
6. Leknes S, Tracey I (2008) A common neurobiology for pain and pleasure. *Nat Rev Neurosci* 9: 314–320.
7. Melzack R, Wall PD (1965) Pain mechanisms: a new theory. *Science* 150: 971–979.
8. Macaffery M (1972) *Nursing Management of the Patient with Pain*. Philadelphia: Lippincott.

9. Merskey H (1991) The definition of pain. *Eur Psychiatry* 6: 153–159.

10. McGrath PJ, Dade LA (2004) Effective strategies to decrease pain and minimise disibility. In: Price DD, Bushnell MC, editors. *Psychological Modulation of Pain: Integrating Basic Science and Clinical Perspectives*. Seattle, WA: IASP Press, pp. 73–96.

11. Rivard PF, Nugent AC, Symons FJ (2009) Parent-proxy ratings of pain before and after botulinum toxin type A treatment for children with spasticity and cerebral palsy. *Clin J Pain* 25: 413–417.

12. Breau LM, Camfield CS, McGrath PJ, Finley GA (2007) Pain's impact on adaptive functioning. *J Intellect Disabil Res* 51: 125–134.

13. Sparrow SS, Balla DA, Cicchettie DV (1984) *Vineland Adaptive Behavior Scales: Interview Edition Survey Form Manual*. Circle Pines, MN: American Guidance Service.

14. Breau LM, MacLaren J, McGrath PJ, Camfield CS, Finley GA (2003) Caregivers' beliefs regarding pain in children with cognitive impairment: relation between pain sensation and reaction increases with severity of impairment. *Clin J Pain* 19: 335–344.

15. Stallard P, Williams L, Lenton S, Velleman R (2001) Pain in cognitively impaired, non-communicating children. *Arch Dis Child* 85: 460–462.

16. Streiner D, Norman GR (2008) *Health Measurement Scales: A Practical Guide to their Development and Use*. Oxford: Oxford University Press.

17. Craig KD (2004) Social communication of pain enhances protective functions: a comment on Deyo, Prkachin and Mercer. *Pain* 107: 5–6.

18. Hadjistavropoulos T, Craig KD (2002) A theoretical framework for understanding self-report and observational measures of pain: a communications model. *Behav Res Ther* 40: 551–570.

19. Breau LM, Burkitt C (2009) Assessing pain in children with intellectual disabilities. *Pain Res Manag* 14: 116–120.

20. Zabalia M, Duchaux C (2007) Strategies de faire-face a la douleur chez des enfants porteurs de deficience intellectuelle. *Revue Francophone De La Deficience Intellectuelle* 17: 53–64.

21. Bromley J, Emerson E, Caine A (1998) The development of a self-report measure to assess the location and intensity of pain in people with intellectual disabilities. *J Intellect Disabil Res* 42: 72–80.

22. Benini F, Trapanotto M, Gobber D, et al (2004) Evaluating pain induced by venipuncture in pediatric patients with developmental delay. *Clin J Pain* 20: 156–163.

23. Collignon P, Giusiano B, Porsmoguer E, Jimeno MT, Combe JC (1995) Difficulties in identifying sources of pain in pediatric-patients with multiple disabilities. *Ann Pediatr (Paris)* 42: 123–126.

24. Giusiano B, Jimeno MT, Collignon P, Chau Y (1995) Utilization of neural network in the elaboration of an evaluation scale for pain in cerebral palsy. *Methods Inf Med* 34: 498–502.

25. Stallard P, Williams L, Velleman R, Lenton S, McGrath PJ (2002) Brief report: behaviors identified by caregivers to detect pain in noncommunicating children. *J Pediatr Psychol* 27: 209–214.

26. Stallard P, Williams L, Velleman R, Lenton S, McGrath PJ (2002) Intervening factors in caregivers' assessments of pain in non-communicating children. *Dev Med Child Neurol* 44: 213–214.

27. Stallard P, Williams L, Velleman R, Lenton S, McGrath PJ, Taylor G (2002) The development and evaluation of the Pain Indicator for Communicatively Impaired Children (PICIC). *Pain* 98: 145–149.

28. Breau LM, McGrath PJ, Camfield CS, Finley GA (2002) Psychometric properties of the Non-communicating Children's Pain Checklist – Revised. *Pain* 99: 349–357.

29. Breau LM, Finley GA, McGrath PJ, Camfield CS (2002) Validation of the Non-communicating Children's Pain Checklist – Postoperative Version. *Anesthesiology* 96: 528–535.

30. Collignon P, Giusiano B (2001) Validation of a pain evaluation scale for patients with severe cerebral palsy. *Eur J Pain* 5: 433–442.

31. Hadden KL, von Baeyer CL (2005) Global and specific behavioral measures of pain in children with cerebral palsy. *Clin J Pain* 21: 140–146.

32. McGrath PJ, Rosmus C, Canfield C, Campbell MA, Hennigar A (1998) Behaviours caregivers use to determine pain in non-verbal, cognitively impaired individuals. *Dev Med Child Neurol* 40: 340–343.

33. Hunt A, Goldman A, Seers K, et al (2004) Clinical validation of the Paediatric Pain Profile. *Dev Med Child Neurol* 46: 9–18.

34. Breau LM, McGrath PJ, Camfield C, Rosmus C, Finley GA (2000) Preliminary validation of an observational pain checklist for persons with cognitive impairments and inability to communicate verbally. *Dev Med Child Neurol* 42: 609–616.

35. Voepel-Lewis T, Merkel S, Tait AR, Trzcinka A, Malviya S (2002) The reliability and validity of the Face, Legs, Activity, Cry, Consolability observational tool as a measure of pain in children with cognitive impairment. *Anesth Analg* 95: 1224–1229.

36. Malviya S, Voepel-Lewis T, Burke C, Merkel S, Tait AR (2006) The revised FLACC observational pain tool: improved reliability and validity for pain assessment in children with cognitive impairment. *Paediatr Anaesth* 16: 258–265.

37. Voepel-Lewis T, Malviya S, Tait AR (2005) Validity of parent ratings as proxy measures of pain in children with cognitive impairment. *Pain Manag Nurs* 6: 168–174.

38. Voepel-Lewis T, Malviya S, Tait AR, et al (2008) A comparison of the clinical utility of pain assessment tools for children with cognitive impairment. *Anesth Analg* 106: 72–78.

39. Soetenga D, Frank J, Pellino TA (1999) Assessment of the validity and reliability of the University of Wisconsin Children's Hospital Pain scale for Preverbal and Nonverbal Children. *Pediatr Nurs* 25: 670–676.

40. Bodfish JW, Harper VN, Deacon JR, Symon FJ (2001) *Identifying and Measuring Pain in Persons with Developmental Disabilities: A Manual for the Pain and Discomfort Scale (PADS)*. Morganton, NC: Western Carolina Center.

41. Phan A, Edwards CL, Robinson EL (2005) The assessment of pain and discomfort in individuals with mental retardation. *Res Dev Disabil* 26: 433–439.

42. Burkitt C, Breau LM, Salsman S, Sarsfield-Turner S, Mullan R (2009) Pilot study of the feasibility of the Non-Communicating Children's Pain Checklist Revised for Pain Assessment for Adults with Intellectual Disabilities. *J Pain Manage* 2: 37–49.

43. Lotan M, Ljunggren EA, Johnsen TB, Defrin R, Pick CG, Strand LI (2009) A modified version of the Non-communicating Children Pain Checklist-revised, adapted to adults with intellectual and developmental disabilities: sensitivity to pain and internal consistency. *J Pain* 10: 398–407.

44. Spagrud LJ, von Baeyer CL, Ali K, et al (2008) Pain, distress, and adult–child interaction during venipuncture in paediatric oncology: an examination of three types of venous access. *J Pain Symptom Manage* 36: 173–184.

45. Woolf CJ, Salter MW (2000) Neuronal plasticity: increasing the gain in pain. *Science* 288: 1765–1769.

46. Kehl LJ, Goldetsky G (2006) Overview of pain mechanisms: neuroanatomical and neurophysiological processes. In: Oberlander TF, Symons FJ, editors. *Pain in Children and Adults with Developmental Disabilities*. Baltimore, MD: Brookes Publishing Company.

47. Casey KL, Lorenz J, Minoshima S (2003) Insights into the pathophysiology of neuropathic pain through functional brain imaging. *Exp Neurol* 184: S80–S88.

48. Mao J (2002) Translational pain research: bridging the gap between basic and clinical research. *Pain* 97: 183–187.

49. Biersdorff KK (1994) Incidence of significantly altered pain experience among individuals with developmental disabilities. *Am J Ment Retard* 98: 619–631.

50. Hennequin M, Morin C, Feine JS (2000) Pain expression and stimulus localisation in individuals with Down's syndrome. *Lancet* 356: 1882–1887.

51. Symons FJ, Shinde S, Clary J, Harper V, Bodfish JW (2010) Evaluating a sham-controlled sensory-testing protocol for non-verbal adults with neurodevelopmental disorders: self-injury and gender effects. *J Pain* 11: 778–781.

52. Defrin R, Pick CG, Peretz C, Carmeli E (2004) A quantitative somatosensory testing of pain threshold in individuals with mental retardation. *Pain* 108: 58–66.

15
VOICE AND SPEECH FUNCTIONS (B310–B340)

Elspeth McCartney

What is the construct?

The International Classification of Functioning, Disability and Health for Children and Youth (ICF-CY) domain 'voice and speech functions' (b3) includes production and quality of voice (b310), articulation functions (b320), fluency and rhythm of speech (b330) and alternative vocalizations (b340, such as making musical sounds and crying, which are not reviewed here). The underpinning construct is integrity or deviation of functional mechanisms of speech production. Overviews of ICF categories within this domain have been undertaken by Ma and colleagues[1] for voice impairments (without the CY update); by McLeod and McCormack[2] for child speech functions (including the CY update); and by Yaruss and Quesal[3] with respect to fluency (without the CY update). These authors list the many ICF codes relating to body structures (such as s240–260 structures of the ear and s3 structures involved in voice and speech), other body functions (such as auditory perception [b1560], mental functions of language [b167], hearing functions [b230] and respiratory system [b440–445]), activities and participation (particularly communication [d3]), and environmental factors that may be associated with voice, speech and fluency impairments (and see also relevant chapters in this text).

Those interested in the ICF-CY/b3 include speech–language pathologists (SLPs) offering clinical services to children diagnosed with voice or speech disorders or dysfluency. The ICF-CY does not consider the aetiology of health functions, which are classified by the International Classification of Diseases (ICD-10).[4] Voice or speech disorders or dysfluency may occur in isolation as a primary difficulty for a child, but clinicians are also interested in body functions secondary to known aetiologies. For example, children with Down syndrome often show difficulties in voice, speech and fluency.[5,6] An emphasis on clinical categories has tended to slant outcome measurement towards assessments that differentiate children

with impairments from typically developing children. For example, although it is possible to code fluency, rhythm, speed and melody of speech separately (b3300–b3303), and any of these may be relevant to an individual child, most research interest has centred on differentiating stuttering from normal developmental non-fluency, and in assessing reductions in stuttering after treatment. Fluency is therefore more likely to be assessed than speech melody. Features targeted in therapy are most frequently measured after research and clinical studies of treatment efficacy. Children are often assessed on entry to therapy and reassessed at the end of an episode of care using the same instruments, allowing 'before and after' comparisons.

Recent prevalence statistics from a survey of parents of nearly 5000 4- to 5-year-old children weighted to represent the Australian population reported that 2.2% of their children had voices that sounded 'unusual', 6.0% had speech 'not clear to the family', 12% had speech that was 'not clear to others' and 5.6% 'stuttered, stammered or lisped'.[7] Teachers of 10 425 children aged 4 to 12 years in 36 primary schools in Sydney, Australia, reported prevalence rates of 0.12% for voice disorders, 1.06% for speech disorders and 0.33% for stammering, using standardized descriptors and confirmed where possible by SLP reports.[8] Overall, prevalence estimates decreased with age. Children requiring investigation and intervention for voice, speech or fluency form a significant part of the caseload for some SLP services that deal with younger children. For example, a cohort of children mostly aged 2 to 4 years referred to a paediatric UK SLP service over a 16-month period showed 2.0% with voice or nasality disruption, 29.1% with speech difficulties and 5.3% with dysfluency.[9]

For young children, particularly those with primary voice, speech or fluency impairments, intervention is often directed towards improving function with either a curative (normalization) or a habilitative (improvement) care aim, anticipating communication benefits. Primary voice dysfunction may be associated with vocal mis-use and improve with therapy. Speech disorders typically manifest and are treated in the pre- and early school years, with intervention aimed towards the production of adult-language speech sounds. Developmental stuttering similarly is evidenced and treated in early childhood, although it may persist into adulthood, and for young children intervention aims to reduce moments of stuttering and improve fluency.

Where impairments persist into later childhood, however, intervention may move towards enabling, that is optimizing the use of existing functions, and activity and participation measures become increasingly relevant. These are reviewed under 'Communication' in Chapter 22.

General factors to consider when measuring this domain

One ICF code – articulatory functions (b320) – with no subcategories has to serve for all disorders of speech function. It includes functions of enunciation and articulation of phonemes; spastic, ataxic and flaccid dysarthria; and anarthria. As no other ICF-CY codes are available, no distinction is made between phonological substitutions and speech affected by motor impairments: McLeod[10] suggests additional codes that could usefully be added. Although speech terminology is far from standard,[11] 'articulatory' as the title of the ICF code for all speech difficulties may be confusing to some SLP practitioners.

CLINICAL AND RESEARCH APPLICATIONS OF
OUTCOME MEASURES

Two aspects of 'child talk' affect the measurement of voice, speech and fluency: inconsistency in the occurrence of disruption, and the ephemeral nature of the speech signal. Phonological output patterns are usually consistent at a whole-word level for typically developing children,[12] and only around 10% of referred children with primary speech impairments are reported to show inconsistent speech,[13] so a brief speech sample will either evidence a child's consistent level of functioning, and so form a valid basis for analysis, or show that further systematic sampling is needed (and see the review of the Diagnostic Evaluation of Articulation and Phonology [DEAP], below). Vocal function may be inconsistent depending upon fatigue and voice-use factors, and so will require repeated sampling. The occurrence of stuttering is highly inconsistent across talk samples, showing fluent speech or overt stuttering even within a brief time interval.[14] The amount and type of dysfluency may be influenced by child, linguistic and contextual factors that are highly

individual and may vary during a child's development. Obtaining a 'representative' sample of talk to assess fluency will therefore require careful thought, and several samples from a variety of contexts will be needed for analysis (and see a review of the Percentage Syllables Stuttered [PSS] below).

As talk is ephemeral, rapid transcription and data-gathering techniques are required, using either live or recorded speech samples. These have to be checked for reliability and subjected to detailed analyses. Data collection and analysis require a 'trained ear' and technical skills, for example in evaluating voice attributes or using the International Phonetic Alphabet (IPA). Such skills are acquired during SLP training, involving a considerable investment in time and expertise. Once acquired, inexpensive data-gathering and analysis protocols can show reliable and valid intra- and inter-rater results (see reviews below). Nonetheless, demonstrating rater reliability continues to be problematic for some measures, such as identifying moments of dysfluency, characterizing voice disorders or capturing fine-grained phonetic detail. As noted in reviews, some measures have been shown to be reliable with trained users or within research studies, but, although used in general clinical practice, their reliability in that context has not as yet firmly been established.

As well as data-analysis protocols, standardized measures and commercially published assessments have been developed that should offer psychometrically adequate standards of reliability and validity. However, these are not always demonstrated. Widely used measures of child speech and fluency were analysed, amongst other instruments, to determine their psychometric quality by the US Agency for Healthcare Research and Quality (HSTAT 52):[15] voice measures not specifically adapted for children were also included. In general, child assessment measures fared badly. The reviewers noted that reliability and validity data rarely came from peer-reviewed literature, but rather from publishers' manuals accompanying assessments. It is therefore not safe to assume that all published measures will show acceptable psychometric characteristics.

SUMMARY

Analysis of core voice and speech functions may be applied to naturalistic samples of child talk, and are thus applicable to a wide range of clinical contexts and are inexpensive to administer by trained SLPs. They do, however, have inbuilt reliability issues, associated with the ephemeral nature of speech and with sampling difficulties. As reliability is a precondition of validity and the measurement of change, this presents a continuing challenge to the development of clinical outcome measures. Standardized measures of core functions should have overcome reliability and validity problems before publication, but individual scrutiny is required to establish whether this is the case. In this chapter, two instruments are included for each of voice, speech and fluency functions: (1) one clinical data-collection and analysis protocol to assess core function and (2) one commercially packaged measure. These have been selected as illustrative only, but are measures currently in wide clinical use.

Overview of recommended measures

VOICE FUNCTIONS (B310)

Consensus Auditory-Perceptual Evaluation of Voice

Overview and purpose
The Consensus Auditory-Perceptual Evaluation of Voice, fifth edition (CAPE-V)[16,17] was developed by the American Speech–Language Hearing Association as a tool for clinical auditory-perceptual assessment of voice. It measures severity based on a minimal set of voice parameters determined by a conference of international voice scientists and SLPs to be meaningful for clinical use.[17] It is designed to obtain reliable results expediently while offering a refined analysis of vocal function. SLPs define and rate six vocal attributes that are salient in identifying voice dysfunction: overall severity, roughness, breathiness, strain, pitch and loudness. Additional features may also be noted as relevant.

Administration and scoring
Three child voice samples from different tasks are audio-taped using standardized procedures and, if possible, entered into a computer. Task 1 records 'vowels "a" and "i"' sustained for 3 to 5 seconds, each repeated three times. Task 2 involves the child reading (or younger children imitating) six standard 'sentences' to elicit (1) all vowel sounds, (2) easy voice onset using the phenome 'h', (3) only voiced phonemes, (4) hard glottal attack, (5) many nasal sounds and (6) many voiceless plosives. Task 3 records at least 20 seconds of natural 'speech' offered in response to a standard question.

All three tasks are performed by the child before the SLP enters a score. Severity is scored for each vocal attribute on a 100-mm visual analogue line, where 0 equates to normal and 100 to severe dysphonia. Other points are scaled in between as 'mildly deviant', 'moderately deviant' and 'severely deviant'. Severity judgements are made by the SLP and marked on the voice analogue line, and expressed both as a percentage and with the descriptive severity rating. If performance is uniform in severity across the three tasks, one severity rating is scored for each vocal attribute. If tasks show discrepant severity, each vocal attribute is recorded on the same scale but coded as Task 1, 2 or 3. Responses are also judged as either consistent or intermittent if the voice attribute does not occur on each task but is of equal severity when it does occur. CAPE-V ratings may be repeated to assess treatment outcomes.

Simulations and practice, including child voice disorder examples, can be accessed at http://engage.doit.wisc.edu/sims_games/showcase/speechpathology/index.html.

Psychometric properties
Validation studies are ongoing, and current psychometric information comes mainly from adults. Braden et al[18] found a weak correlation between CAPE-V and an institution-specific self-perception scale of voice impairment only for moderate to severe dysphonia in a retrospective study of 199 adult clients who had received BoNT-A injections, and Eadie and Baylor[19] found significant correlations with acoustic measures.

Establishing rater reliability has been an ongoing problem in developing adequate auditory-perceptual scales to evaluate voice quality.[20] Rater reliability measures of CAPE-V using adult voice samples show effects of training and prompting. Sixteen inexperienced SLP graduate students judged the ability to sustain the vowel 'a' and a pre-recorded speech sample from 54 speakers (48 dysphonic, six normal) using visual analogue scales. They were then trained using definitions, auditory 'anchor' examples of representative disorders and feedback on accuracy.[19] Inter-rater reliability improved with training. Karnell and colleagues[21] found intrarater Spearman's correlations of 0.88 to 0.93 and inter-rater reliability of 0.86 to 0.93 on overall severity ratings by four experienced SLPs who had listened to 'anchor' samples before commencing rating sessions. Forty inexperienced SLP undergraduate raters[22] compared written definitions ('written anchors') with auditory anchors. After 20 minutes of training, raters rated 36 sustained vowels exemplifying normal, breathy, hoarse or rough voices when randomly allocated to a no-anchor, written-anchor, auditory-anchor or combined auditory–written-anchor listening condition. Provision of anchors significantly improved inter-rater reliability. Auditory anchors allowed more improvement than written, but combined written–auditory examples offered the strongest measure of improvement. These studies suggest that inter-rater reliability is strongly affected by training and provision of external standard comparison measures.

Three SLPs with experience of using CAPE-V investigated inter- and intrarater reliability of CAPE-V

CONSENSUS AUDITORY-PERCEPTUAL EVALUATION OF VOICE (CAPE-V)	
Purpose	To provide an expedient clinical auditory-perceptual assessment of voice production and quality. To measure a minimal set of voice parameters and severity for clinical use
Population	Ages 4y to adults who are dysphonic or who are in the process of diagnosis
Description of domains (subscales)	One domain/six voice-quality subscales: severity, roughness, breathiness, strain, pitch, loudness. Additional features noted as relevant
Administration and test format	Time to complete: about 5min Testing format: child voice samples, audio-taped undertaking three tasks – sustained vowels, repeating standard sentences and natural speech Scoring: each voice quality feature is recorded on 100-mm visual analogue line from three tasks combined. (0) normal to (100) severe dysphonia. Any variation of attribute across tasks and any variation in severity should also be noted Training: designed for qualified Speech–Language pathologist use. No additional training
Psychometric properties	Normative sample: none *Reliability* Internal consistency: no item analysis; variation anticipated. Test–retest: no information retrieved; variation anticipated. Rater: shows effects of training and listening prompts (adult samples). Child samples: intrarater intraclass correlation coefficient 0.62 (strain) to 0.88 (breathiness), inter-rater intraclass corellation coefficient 0.35 (strain) to 0.71 (breathiness) *Validity* Content validity: expert consensus reported, with CAPE-V voice-quality features being those consistently assessed as 'clinically meaningful'. Construct/discriminant validity: correlations 0.89 (breathiness)–0.95 (severity) (adult voice samples) with Grade, Roughness, Breathiness, Asthenia, Strain: CAPE-V's visual analogue scale is probably more sensitive to small differences. Significant correlations with acoustic measures *Responsiveness* Showed positive change following laryngeal reinnervation, adults
How to order	Download from www.asha.org/uploadFiles/ASHA/SIG/03/affiliate/CAPE-V-Purpose-Applications.pdf or from Kempster et al (2009), below
Key references	Kempster GB, Gerratt BR, Verdolini AK, Barkmeier-Kraemer J, Hillman RE (2009) Consensus Auditory-Perceptual Evaluation of Voice: development of a standardized clinical protocol. *Am J Speech Lang Pathol* 18: 124–132.

sentences with children,[23] rating audio-taped samples of 50 children and young persons aged 4 to 20 years with airway conditions who had undergone at least one major laryngotracheal reconstructive surgery. No training was given, as the study aimed to generalize findings to the larger community of experienced voice-rater SLPs. Intrarater/inter-rater reliability interclass correlation coefficients were as follows: overall severity 0.86/0.67, roughness 0.86/0.68, breathiness 0.88/0.71, strain 0.62/0.35, pitch 0.86/0.68 and loudness 0.80/0.57. The low correlation for strain was considered to be due to the absence of visual evidence of excess vocal effort that would be available in live ratings of CAPE-V, and loudness may have been affected by listening conditions, despite standardization. The other four measures achieved moderate to strong correlations. On adult voice samples, comparison between CAPE-V and another widely used clinical measure of voice quality, Grade, Roughness, Breathiness,

Asthenia, Strain (GRBAS),[24] showed high correlations – Spearman's coefficients 0.89 (breathiness) to 0.95 (severity) – suggesting concurrent criterion-related validity.

Lee et al[25] showed CAPE-V scale improvements in severity, roughness and breathiness in 17 adult samples after reinnervation for unilateral vocal cord paralysis, suggesting responsivity.

Boone Voice Program for Children, second edition

Overview and purpose

The evaluation section of the widely used Boone Voice Program for Children[26] aims to provide a rapid voice screen to determine whether there is a problem, a detailed evaluation to plan therapy and a checklist to monitor improvements. The screen comprises a 'Voice Rating Scale' measuring eight voice parameters, and the 'S/Z ratio' that compares the length of time a child can sustain the unvoiced phoneme 's' and the voiced phoneme 'z' as an indication of laryngeal involvement.

If in-depth investigation is required after screening, the 'Voice Evaluation Form' assesses 10 aspects, four of which include voice. (Non-vocal aspects are not reviewed here.) The four voice-related functions measure nasal resonance, respiration, phonation and eight vocal parameters (breathing, pitch, pitch inflections, loudness, voice quality, horizontal focus, vertical focus and nasal resonance). If a therapy programme is undertaken, facilitating approaches are offered and changes in function are marked on a checklist to show outcomes.

Administration and scoring

The Voice Rating Scale assesses a speech sample elicited by telling a child a story with supporting pictures and asking for a re-tell. Two stories are provided, one for children up to 9 and the other for children aged 10 to 12 years. The SLP decides, on listening, whether the child's voice sounds like that of his or her peers. The eight voice parameters are scored as negative (–), normal (N) or positive (+). Negative (–) scores represent too few words on a breath, low pitch, monotonous pitch, inadequate loudness, breathy voice, anterior-focused voice ('baby' voice), laryngeal-focused voice and insufficient nasal resonance. Positive (+) scores are given for too many words on a breath, high pitch, excessive pitch variation, excessive loudness, harsh/tight voice, excessive oropharyngeal resonance, nasal-focused voice and excessive nasal resonance. Otherwise, the score is normal. Any non-normal score suggests further voice evaluation.

The S/Z ratio is assessed by demonstrating a prolonged 's' and then asking the child to sustain 's' for as long as possible, giving two trials. Prolongation time in seconds is recorded using a stopwatch, then the procedure is repeated using 'z'. The longer prolongation time for each consonant is used, dividing the longer 's' by the longer 'z', which is expressed as the S/Z ratio. An S/Z ratio >1.4 suggests laryngeal involvement.

Some sections of the Voice Evaluation Form are supported by or require the use of instrumental measures as available in specialist clinical settings. Only the three non-instrumental assessments are outlined here – see Colton et al[27] for a review of instrumental measurement. 'Section 5 – Nasal Resonance' uses two stories read aloud by the child (or repeated by younger children). One contains no nasal consonants, and therefore a child perceived as nasal is generally hypernasal. The other has many nasal consonants and includes 25 all-oral consonant words. Denasality will be evident, and also assimilative nasality, where the 25 all-oral consonant words will sound nasal in this context, although not if read in isolation. 'Section 6 – Respiration' uses clinical observation to assess respiration using a prepared checklist, and the S/Z ratio may be repeated. 'Section 8 – Voice Rating Scale' involves a more finely graded analysis of the Voice Rating Scale than the screen, with the '–/N/+' judgement replaced by a seven-point scale.

Psychometric properties

No psychometric data are given, and norms for children are not given in the manual. However, measures are validated from earlier voice assessments (and see CAPE-V above). Good test–retest and inter-rater reliability for S/Z ratios have been shown in typically developing 6- and 7-year-old children.[28] Ninety-five per cent of adults and children combined with vocal fold margin pathology (nodules and polyps) showed S/Z ratios >1.4, whereas normal and dysphonic speakers without pathology approximated 1.[29] This justifies the Boone Voice Program cut-off. However, for 123 dysphonic children aged 5 to 15 years, 69 with vocal cord nodules and 54 without, S/Z ratio performance did not discriminate those with fold margin pathology,[30] perhaps owing to typical differences in nodule characteristics and size between adults and children. This suggests that the S/Z ratio is not a safe indicator of vocal fold margin pathology in children.

ARTICULATION FUNCTIONS – PHONOLOGY (B320)

Percentage Consonants Correct – revised

Overview and purpose

Consonants are usually differentially affected in comparison to vowels in functional speech disorders. The 'percentage of consonants produced correctly' (Percentage

Consonants Correct measure [PCC[31]]) in a speech sample measures the severity of speech dysfunction and may be used repeatedly to track speech outcomes. The PCC acts as a major predictor of severity ratings made independently by SLPs[31] and can be calculated from brief talk samples by a qualified SLP.

However, the original version of the PCC devised by Shriberg and colleagues[32] marked subphonemic distinctions (consonant distortions) as errors. Such detailed analysis presents inherent difficulties for inter-rater reliability, and so limits clinical usefulness. The measure was therefore revised by defining clinically common and uncommon consonant distortions[33] and counting both types as correct realizations. The revised version (PCC-R)[33] showed increased inter-rater transcription reliability, owing to the broader level of analysis. Sensitivity to true speech impairment was also increased by ignoring subphonemic distortions, which are frequent in the speech of young children, but retaining phonemic substitutions and omissions that are salient markers of speech delay and disorder.

Administration and scoring

Administration has not changed from the original paper,[32] in which the procedures are detailed, although scoring procedures were altered from the PCC to the PCC-R, as noted above. Conversation with a child is tape-recorded to give a natural and representative speech sample. Around 3 minutes of continuous child speech is recorded using narrow phonetic transcription, omitting lengthy adult contributions and long silences. Knowledge of IPA symbols is required, as are phonetic transcription skills.

The unit of analysis is the consonant. The child's word productions are 'glossed' to give the correct adult consonant pattern. Only words that can be transcribed and glossed are scored. Although not part of Shriberg's procedures, a PCC count in some assessments is computed from single word elicitations checked against brief continuous speech samples as it can be difficult to gloss unintelligible continuous speech (see Diagnostic Evaluation of Articulation and Phonocology, below).

Target consonants are considered incorrect when they are either omitted, substituted by another consonant or glottal stop, inappropriately voiced or have extra phonemes added where these errors are not accounted for by dialectic variation or coarticulations associated with rapid speech. For the PCC, the response definition for children who obviously have speech errors is 'score as incorrect unless heard as correct',[32] but for the PCC-R, as noted, subphonemic distortions are counted as correct. Consonants in second or successive repetitions of an adjacent word or syllable are not scored unless they alter:

only the intended (adult-language) consonants in the first attempt. Calculation is a simple percentage: number of consonants correct/number of correct + incorrect consonants × 100. Severity ratings associated with percentage scores are: >85%, normal–mild; 65% to 85%, mild–moderate; 50% to 65%, moderate–severe; <50%, severe (*sic*: p. 115).[34]

Psychometric properties

In studies by Shriberg and colleagues,[31] the PCC-R averaged a standard error of measurement (SEM) of 2.4 from 33 speech samples of children and adults across all consonants: 1.7 for the eight early developing consonants, 2.9 for the next eight to develop and 5.7 for the later eight. The increase in SEM was ascribed to transcription difficulties for later-developing consonants on which distortion errors may still be evident. Inter-rater reliability measures showed that broad phonemic consonant transcription as used in the PCC-R achieved 92.7% agreement between two experienced transcribers. The authors concluded that the relative gain in transcription accuracy obtained by the PCC-R gave reliability measures that were adequate for clinical and research purposes (p. 718).[31] The PCC-R was considered to be the most appropriate metric from a list of alternative ways of counting phoneme realizations for comparison among 3- to 8-year-old children (p. 731),[34] giving sensitivity to true involvement through focusing on phonemic rather than subphonemic errors. The PCC-R distinguished children with typical speech from children with speech delays with no overlap, suggesting construct validity.

Further refinement of the PCC-R was undertaken by another research team using speech samples of typically developing children to compute a monthly performance growth curve for children from 18 to 172 months of age.[35] The aim was to track rapidly developing speech changes after childhood traumatic brain injury, and the initial results were successful, thus suggesting that high responsivity may be obtained.

The Diagnostic Evaluation of Articulation and Phonology

Overview and purpose

The Diagnostic Evaluation of Articulation and Phonology (DEAP)[36] aims both to identify subtypes of speech impairment by comparing a child's speech with developmental norms and to measure severity. Subtypes distinguish children using phoneme error patterns observed in typically developing children, albeit delayed or with developmentally early and later errors co-occurring, from children using developmentally unusual processes.

DIAGNOSTIC EVALUATION OF ARTICULATION AND PHONOLOGY (DEAP)	
Purpose	To assess child speech production, differentially diagnose types of speech disorder and assess severity
Population	Children aged 3y–6y 11mo with speech delay or disorder or who are in the process of diagnosis
Description of domains (subscales)	One domain/five subscales. Diagnostic Screen (10 pictures named twice; imitation of error phonemes); Articulation (30 pictures named; CV/VC syllable imitation); Oromotor (diadochokinetic [DDK] rates; isolated/sequenced oromotor movements); Phonology (50 pictures named; target words in connected speech); Inconsistency (25 pictures named three times)
Administration and test format	Time to complete: diagnostic screen 5min; full battery 30–40min
	Testing format: diagnostic screen then relevant subscales. Child names/describes stimulus pictures and carries out oral movements. Speech–language pathologist (SLP) transcribes using Institutional Phonetic Alphabet (IPA) symbols
	Scoring: standard scores/centile ranks for consonant inventory, DDK, isolated/sequenced oral movements, Percentage Consonant Correct (PCC), Percentage Vowels Correct, Percentage Phenomes Correct, single words vs connected speech and inconsistency. Qualitative analysis of typical and unusual error patterns
	Training: designed for qualified SLPs. Requires experience in speech transcription using IPA conventions. Restricted to purchasers with a formal qualification relevant to speech assessment
Psychometric properties	Normative sample: UK and Australia – 828 children, balanced for age, socioeconomic status and sex. USA – 650 children based on current US population. Also, 83 bilingual children with English as a second language and Punjabi/Mirpuri/Urdu as a first (separate analyses provided)
	Reliability Internal consistency: not applicable – complete range of consonants assessed.
	Test–retest: quantitative subscales Pearson correlations 0.666 (sequenced oral movement) – 0.939 (PCC). Production of consonants 87.50–100% agreement, error patterns 98.21–100%.
	Inter-rater: quantitative subscales Pearson correlations 0.315 (Percent Vowels Correct)–0.886 (Percent Phenomes Correct). Production of consonants and error patterns 94.2–100% agreement
	Validity Content validity: complete coverage of the phonological system of English language
	Construct validity: high correlation (r=0.95; p<0.001) between DEAP-PCC and Edinburgh Articulation Test
	Responsiveness Case studies show DEAP may detect changes in phoneme realization over short periods
How to order	The UK version is available from www.pearsonclinical.co.uk and costs £297. The US version is available from www.pearsonassessments.com and costs US$272.
Key reference	Dodd B, Hua Z, Crosbie S, Holm A, Ozanne A (2002) *Manual of Diagnostic Evaluation of Articulation and Phonology (DEAP), US edition*. London: Psychological Corporation.

A second distinction is between children whose error patterns are consistent across all instances of a word pronounced in the same linguistic context, and those who are inconsistent. These distinctions have significance for intervention. The DEAP is for children aged 3 years to 6 years 11 months.

Administration and scoring

The 'Diagnostic Screen' identifies which aspects of speech need further investigation using three tasks: (1) 'naming' 10 pictures representing words containing the most single English consonants and some consonant clusters and vowels; (2) 'imitating' any phonemes that show errors on the naming task; and (3) 're-naming' the 10 screening words to check for consistency. The SLP transcribes responses live using broad phonemic IPA symbols.

If the child fails to imitate error phonemes appropriate to his or her age, an 'Articulation' assessment is made of the vowels and consonants of English using a picture-naming task, with any incorrect productions later imitated, and an 'Oromotor' assessment is made of non-speech movements. If the child makes consonant errors but can correctly imitate the relevant speech sounds, a 'Phonological' assessment analyses error patterns in both single words and connected speech, again using picture elicitation and distinguishing developmentally typical from developmentally unusual errors. Where half or more words are produced differently on the two screening trials, a further 'Inconsistency' assessment uses a 25-word naming task to establish consistency of production, which is repeated three times with distracting activities between trials, and again the 'Oromotor' assessment is undertaken. The diagnostic screen takes around 5 minutes to complete, and the full assessment battery around 30 to 40 minutes.[37]

The unit of analysis is the syllable for the 'Phonological' assessment, the word for the 'Inconsistency' assessment and the phoneme for the 'Articulation' assessment. Picture and task materials for each assessment are included in the package. Standard scores/centile ranks are given for the consonant 'inventory' (the list of consonants used in speech at some time), 'diadochokinetic' rates, 'isolated oral movements', 'sequenced oral movements', PCC ('Percent Vowels Correct'), 'Percent Phonemes Correct' (consonants plus vowels), 'single words versus connected speech' and 'inconsistency'. Responses are recorded and scored on record forms. Qualitative analysis of error patterns compares the child with children of their own age, distinguishing among errors that would be used by at least 10% of typically developing children in the age band, delayed errors that would be used by at least 10% of younger children and unusual error patterns that would not be used by more than 10% of children in the normative sample at any age.

Psychometric properties

Information is taken from the DEAP manual.[36] A total of 1478 children were included in the standardization sample, with 828 balanced for age, socioeconomic status

and sex from the UK and Australia and 650 in a balanced US sample. Test–retest reliability for quantitative measures for 56 children showed Pearson's correlations of 0.67 (sequenced movement) to 0.94 (PCC). Per cent agreement on consonant production ranged from 87.50% ('–l') to 100% (13 consonants). Error patterns ranged from 98.21% to 100% agreement. Inter-rater reliability from 69 children and two raters showed Pearson's correlations from 0.32 (per cent vowels correct) to 0.89 (PCC). Consonant production and error patterns ranged from 94.2% to 100%. Sensitivity trials on a total of 57 age-appropriate children compared the Diagnostic Screen with the full DEAP assessment, giving 10% to 13% false positives, but no false negatives. Specificity assessed how accurately the Diagnostic Screen identified which further DEAP tests to use and gave 93% agreement between two SLPs blinded to DEAP test results.

Content validity was established by the complete coverage of the phonological system of the English language, and concurrent validity by comparing 50 children on the Edinburgh Articulation Test (EAT),[38] which showed a high correlation (r=0.95; p<0.001) between PCC measured by the DEAP and the EAT. Responsiveness is suggested by case study data.

FLUENCY AND RHYTHM OF SPEECH FUNCTIONS – STUTTERING (B330)

Percentage of Syllables Stuttered

Overview and purpose

Non-fluency is a feature of the speech of young children, and distinguishing normal non-fluency from stuttering can be problematic, with difficulties in collecting representative speech data and in establishing inter-rater reliability. However, a measured reduction in the number of moments of overt stuttering is a frequent intervention goal for young children. Percentage of Syllables Stuttered (PSS)[39] has been developed as a core measure of stuttering frequency to deal with these known measurement difficulties. The measure is the percentage of syllables unambiguously associated with stuttering in a sample of child speech, with a reduction in the PSS used as an outcome measure.

Administration and scoring

An adult engages the child in naturalistic conversation: at least 300 child syllables are needed for analysis.[39] A trained SLP unobtrusively presses one of two buttons on a commercially available tally counter as the child speaks: one button for every syllable judged as free of stuttering, the other for stuttered syllables. Such online judgements

PERCENTAGE OF SYLLABLES STUTTERED (PSS)	
Purpose	To assess core stuttering behaviour and severity
Population	Children of any age who stutter or who are in the process of diagnosis
Description of domains (subscales)	One domain, no subscales
Administration and test format	Time to complete: around 5min Testing format: around 5min of child speech (at least 300 syllables) is recorded Scoring: speech–language pathologist (SLP) observes and codes syllables as showing unambiguous stammering or not, live, using a push-button recorder Training: designed for SLP use. No training, but practice in accurate recording is needed
Psychometric properties	Normative sample: no normative sample *Reliability* Internal consistency: averages across syllables Test–retest: variation anticipated across samples Inter-rater: around 75% of instances of child stuttering/not stuttering agreed by 80% of highly experienced rates. Inter- and intrarater intraclass correlation coefficient 0.99, with experienced research raters *Validity* Content validity: dichotomous direct measure. Construct/discriminant validity: Spearman's correlation 0.91, with severity rating by adults. Case data show that PSS varies along with parental measures of severity *Responsiveness* Measured changes between pre-intervention and 1-year post-intervention follow-up
How to order	Published in book form as Onslow M, Packman A, Harrison E (2003) *The Lidcombe Programme of Early Stuttering Intervention*. Austin, TX: Pro-Ed Publishing.
Key reference	Bothe AK (2008) Identification of children's stuttered and nonstuttered speech by highly experienced judges: binary judgements and comparisons with disfluency-types definitions. *J Speech Lang Hear Res* 51: 867–878.

require training, but tape-recorded samples may be used. Where measurement is carried out online, the time taken is the few minutes needed to collect a sample of 300 syllables from a child. There is no age limit. The score is a simple percentage of stuttered syllables divided by stuttered plus unstuttered syllables.

Psychometric properties
Test–retest judgements are not appropriate, as the percentage of stuttering is expected to vary across samples. However, samples are taken and scored frequently and PSS is expected to decrease over time during intervention. Inter-rater measures of identifying stuttering have shown that 80% of highly experienced raters agreed on the presence or absence of stuttering in approximately

three-quarters of brief samples from children, aged 2 to 8 years, who stuttered.[40] Trained and experienced SLPs showed intraclass correlations of $r=0.99$ for both intra- and inter-rater reliability;[41] and the average differences between a researcher's pretreatment PSS measurement and an independent experienced blinded observer were 2.3 PSS, with no differences after treatment.[42] Measuring PSS reliably is therefore possible with training, but inexperienced users should test their standards of intra- and preferably inter-rater reliability before using the measure.

Comparison between the PSS and a nine-point severity scale showed a Spearman correlation of 0.91 for adults who stuttered, suggesting construct validity,[43] and case study data showed PSS reducing over time in line with parental judgements of severity.[39] Responsivity was shown by reductions in PSS from pre-intervention to 1-year follow-up, with interventions of varied durations.[42]

The Stuttering Severity Instrument for Children and Adults

Overview and purpose
The Stuttering Severity Instrument for Children and Adults (SSI-4)[44] instrument was first published in 1972[45] and is now in its fourth edition. It provides a standardized assessment of the quality and quantity of dysfluency for children aged 2 to 10 years and older. The subscales are 'frequency', 'duration', observable 'physical concomitants of stuttering' and a speech 'naturalness' scale.

Administration and scoring
Assessment takes 15 to 20 minutes. Pictures and conversation elicit child talk, which is tape recorded. At least 150 child words are needed. 'Frequency' of dysfluency is measured by PSS. 'Duration' is scaled using the average length of the three longest stuttering moments, measured to one-tenth of a second. Four observable distracting 'physical concomitants' of stuttering are scored: sounds which accompany stuttering, such as throat clearing; facial grimaces, such as eye blinks or tongue protrusion; head movements, such as head turning to avoid eye contact; and arm or leg movements, such as foot tapping. Scores are expressed as scale scores, and a total score may be calculated. There is the option of automatic computerized scoring of frequency and duration.

Psychometric properties
The normative sample for the SSI-4 was 72 preschool children, 139 school-aged children and 60 adults. The third edition of the instrument (SSI-3) showed an average inter-rater difference between a pretreatment measurement and a blinded expert comparison of 2.25 units, with no rater differences after treatment.[42] The SSI-3 was reviewed in HSTAT 52,[15] but did not meet relaxed validity or reliability criteria. SSI-3 scores showed change from pre-intervention to 1-year follow-up after intervention, with interventions varying in duration.[42]

REFERENCES

1. Ma EPM, Yiu EML, Abbott KV (2007) Application of the ICF in voice disorders. *Semin Speech Lang* 28: 343–350.
2. McLeod S, McCormack J (2007) Application of the ICF and ICF-children and youth in children with speech impairment. *Semin Speech Lang* 28: 254–264.
3. Yaruss JS, Quesal RW (2004) Stuttering and the International Classification of Functioning, Disability, and Health: an update. *J Commun Disord* 37: 35–52.
4. World Health Organization (2006) *International Classification of Diseases and Related Health Problems*, 10th edition. Geneva: World Health Organization.
5. Venail F, Gardiner Q, Mondain M (2004) ENT and speech disorders in children with Down's syndrome: an overview of pathophysiology, clinical features, treatments and current management. *Clin Pediatr* 43: 783–790.
6. Albertini G, Bonassi S, Dall'Armi V Giachetti I, Giaquinto S, Mignano M (2010) Spectral analysis of the voice in Down syndrome. *Res Dev Disabil* 31: 995–1001.
7. McLeod S, Harrison LJ (2009) Epidemiology of speech and language impairment in a nationally representative sample of 4- to 5-year old children. *J Speech Lang Hearing Res* 52: 1213–1229.
8. McKinnon DH, McLeod S, Reilly S (2007) The prevalence of stuttering, voice, and speech-sound disorders in primary school students in Australia. *Lang Speech Hearing Services Schools* 38: 5–15.
9. Broomfield J, Dodd B (2004) The nature of referred subtypes of primary speech disability. *Child Lang Teach Ther* 20: 135–151.
10. McLeod S (2006) An holistic view of a child with unintelligible speech: insights from the ICF and ICF-CY. *Adv Speech Lang Pathol* 8: 293–315.
11. Walsh R (2005) Meaning and purpose: a conceptual model for speech pathology terminology. *Int J Speech Lang Pathol* 7: 65–76.
12. Holm A, Crosbie S, Dodd B (2007) Differentiating normal variability from inconsistency in children's speech: normative data. *Int J Lang Commun Disord* 42: 467–486.
13. Broomfield J, Dodd B (2004) The nature of referred subtypes of primary speech disability. *Child Lang Teach Ther* 20: 135–151.
14. Yaruss JS (1997) Clinical implications of situational variability in preschool children who stutter. *J Fluency Disord* 22: 187–203.
15. Biddle A, Watson L, Hooper C, Lohr KN, Sutton SF (2002) *Evidence/Report Technology Assessment No. 52*. (Prepared by the University of North Carolina Evidence-based Practice Center under Contract No 290–97–0011). AHRQ Publication No. 02-E010. Rockville, MD: Agency for Healthcare Research and Quality.
16. Consensus Auditory-Perceptual Evaluation of Voice (CAPE-V) (2009) *ASHA Special Interest Division 3, Voice and Voice Disorders*.
17. Kempster GB, Gerratt BR, Verdolini AK, Barkmeier-Kraemer J, Hillman RE (2009) Consensus Auditory-Perceptual Evaluation of Voice: development of a standardized clinical protocol. *Am J Speech Lang Pathol* 18: 124–132.
18. Braden MN, Johns MM, Klein AM, Delguadio JM, Gilman M, Hapner ER (2010) Assessing the effectiveness of Botulinum toxin injections for adductor spasmodic dysphonia: clinician and patient perception. *J Voice* 20: 242–249.
19. Eadie TL, Baylor CR (2006) The effect of perceptual training on inexperienced listeners' judgments of dysphonic voice. *J Voice* 20: 527–544.
20. Oates J (2009) Auditory-perceptual evaluation of disordered voice quality: pros, cons and future directions. *Folia Phoniatrica Logopaedica* 61: 49–56.
21. Karnell MP, Melton SD, Childes JM, Coleman TC, Dailey SA, Hoffman HT (2007) Reliability of clinician-based (GRBAS and CAPE-V) and patient-based (V-RQOL and IPVI) documentation of voice disorders. *J Voice* 21: 576–590.

22. Awan SN, Lawson LL (2009) The effects of anchor modality on the reliability of vocal severity ratings. *J Voice* 23: 341–352.

23. Kelchner LN, Brehm SB, Weinrich B, et al (2010) Perceptual evaluation of severe pediatric voice disorders: rater reliability using the consensus auditory perceptual evaluation of voice. *J Voice* 24:441–449.

24. Hirano M (1981) Psycho-acoustic evaluation of voice. In: Arnold W, Wyke W, editors. *Disorders of Human Communication 5, Clinical Examination of Voice*. New York and Wien: Springer-Verlag, pp. 81–84.

25. Lee MD, Milstein C, Hicks D, Akst LM, Esclamado RM (2007) Results of ansa to recurrent laryngeal nerve reinnervation. *Otolaryngol Head Neck Surg* 136: 450–454.

26. Boone DR (1980) *The Boone Voice Program for Children: Screening, Evaluation and Referral Manual*, 2nd edition. Austin, TX: Pro-Ed.

27. Colton RH, Casper JK, Leonard R (2006) *Understanding Voice Problems*. Philadelphia, PA: Lippincott Williams & Wilkins.

28. Fendler M, Shearer WM (1988) Reliability of the S/Z ratio in normal children's voices. *Lang Speech Hearing Serv Schools* 19: 2–4.

29. Eckel FC, Boone DR (1981) The S/Z ratio as an indicator of laryngeal pathology. *ASHA* 46: 147–149.

30. Hufnagle J, Hufnagle KK (1988) S/Z ratio in dysphonic children with and without vocal cord nodules. *Lang Speech Hearing Serv Schools* 19: 418–422.

31. Shriberg LD, Austin D, Lewis BA, McSweeny JL, Wilson DL (1997) The Percentage of Consonants Correct (PCC) metric: extensions and reliability data. *J Speech Lang Hearing Res* 40: 708–722.

32. Shriberg LD, Kwiatkowski J (1982) Phonological disorders III: a procedure for assessing severity of involvement. *J Speech Hearing Disord* 47: 256–270.

33. Shriberg LD (1993) Four new speech and prosody-voice measures for genetics research and other studies in developmental phonological disorders. *J Speech Lang Hearing Res* 36: 105–140.

34. Shriberg LD, Austin D, Lewis BA, McSweeny JL, Wilson DL (1997) The speech disorders classification system (SDCS): extensions and lifespan reference data. *J Speech Lang Hearing Res* 40: 723–740.

35. Campbell TF, Dollaghan C, Janosky JE, Adelson PD (2008) A performance curve for assessing change in Percentage of Consonants Correct Revised (PCC-R). *J Speech Lang Hearing Res* 50: 1110–1119. [Erratum appears in *J Speech Lang Hear Res* 51: 301]

36. Dodd B, Hua Z, Crosbie S, Holm A, Ozanne A (2002) *Manual of Diagnostic Evaluation of Articulation and Phonology (DEAP)*. London: Psychological Corporation.

37. Leahy M, Dodd B. *DEAP test standardization*. Available at: www.tcd.ie/slscs/research/projects/current/deap.php (accessed 11 May 2012).

38. Anthony A, Bogle D, Ingram TTS, McIsaac MW (1971) *Edinburgh Articulation Test*. Edinburgh: Churchill Livingstone.

39. Onslow M, Packman A, Harrison E (2003) *The Lidcombe Program of Early Stuttering Intervention*. Austin, TX: Pro-Ed Publishing, pp. 59–63.

40. Bothe AK (2008) Identification of children's stuttered and nonstuttered speech by highly experienced judges: binary judgments and comparisons with disfluency-types definitions. *J Speech Lang Hear Res* 51: 867–878.

41. Jones M, Onslow M, Packman A, et al (2005) Randomised controlled trial of the Lidcombe Program of early stuttering intervention. *BMJ* 331(7518): 659.

42. Miller B, Guitar B (2009) Long-term outcome of the Lidcombe Program for early stuttering intervention. *Am J Speech Lang Pathol* 18: 42–49.

43. O'Brian S, Packman A, Onslow M, O'Brian N (2004) Measurement of stuttering in adults: comparison of stuttering-rate and severity-scaling methods. *J Speech Lang Hear Res* 47: 1081–1087.

44. Riley GD (2008) *Stuttering Severity Instrument for Children and Adults*, 4th edition. East Moline, IL: LinguiSystems.

16
NEUROMUSCULOSKELETAL AND MOVEMENT-RELATED FUNCTIONS (B710–B780)

F. Virginia Wright, Désirée B. Maltais, Heidi Marie Sanders and Patricia A. Burtner

What is the construct?

When thinking of early child development, one typically visualizes motor development unfolding in a rapid and remarkable manner from infancy through childhood. In the early twentieth century, developmentalists including Nancy Bayley,[1] Arnold Gesell[2] and Myrtle McGraw[3] began to study motor development in depth, producing a rich historical database of the appearance and sequence of motor milestones. Contributions from the disciplines of rehabilitation[4,5] and exercise science[6–9] have provided additional information about underlying body functions supporting motor development such as muscle strength, range of motion, body mechanics and motor control, as well as cognitive-based motor planning and motor learning.

According to the World Health Organization International Classification of Functioning, Disability and Health (ICF),[10] *body functions* are described as physiological functions of body systems and functions, with problems in this area considered to be impairments. In contrast, *activity* in the ICF is defined as the execution of tasks by actions of the individual. and *participation* is the involvement of the individual in life situations. For the purposes of this chapter, we have included body functions related to gross and fine motor development in measurement of muscle functions and the basic motor functions underlying motor skills (Table 16.1). Chapter 23 of this volume presents tests of motor functional skills that are considered to be activity and participation outcome measures. If measures included a combination of capacity and movement functions (often included in motor developmental tests), they were placed in Chapter 23.

In this chapter, we have included descriptions of measures of the various components of motor functions as outlined in the table below. Each section describes the constructs of each of these components, as well as factors to consider when measuring each of these domains.

Measuring muscle functions underlying gross and fine motor development and functional skill capacity

RANGE OF MOTION

Range of motion measurement is a mainstay of impairment level assessment in the clinic setting as well as in clinical trials (surgical and rehabilitation). The results are important for considerations related to orthopaedic management, spasticity management and decisions about orthotic devices. For children with neuromotor disorders and associated spasticity issues, passive range of motion is most commonly assessed, while active range of motion assessment is incorporated into evaluations of selective motor control. When considering measurement in cerebral palsy (CP), it is essential to use reliability estimates obtained with children with CP rather than with typically developing children so that the effects of spasticity and joint restriction on measurement accuracy are taken into account.[11] Spasticity makes the measurement technique more difficult, and variation in spasticity levels on different days may challenge test–retest reliability. Several studies have directly compared reliability in children with CP and typically developing children to study these issues, and the results are inconclusive (e.g. Kilgour et al[12] noted minimal differences in test–retest reliability between these two groups while Ten Berge et al[11] concluded that reliability was lower in the group with CP).

Goniometry

Overview and purpose

In the clinical context for children with neuromotor conditions, measurement approaches need to be efficient and of low cost. Thus, simple handheld goniometers are still the method of choice. Less common approaches include measurement mats[13] and inclinometers. Visual estimation techniques may be used rather than goniometry for ease

TABLE 16.1
Movement-related functions

Motor function areas	Components
Muscle functions underlying motor development and skills	Range of motion
	Spasticity
	Muscle strength
	Gait evaluation
	Observational gait assessments
	Muscle endurance and exercise tolerance
Motor functions underlying gross motor development	Gross motor development
	Balance tests
	Quality of movement
Motor functions underlying fine motor development	Manual dexterity
	Visual motor integration

of measurement, and there are several papers comparing visual and goniometric reliability; for example, a strong correlation was observed between visual and goniometric measurement for ankle dorsiflexion,[14] hip extension[15] and popliteal angle.[11] This comparison is relevant when thinking of tools such as the spinal alignment and range of motion (ROM) measures (below) as the scale is based on ROM estimation.

Psychometric properties
The focus of this section is on reliability work conducted since 2000. These studies have used more appropriate statistical techniques and larger sample sizes than the earlier ones, and provide estimates of measurement error as well as reliability coefficients. Evaluation of reliability of upper limb movements is notably lacking in the literature. Instead, ROM studies in CP have focused on hip abduction and hip extension, popliteal angle and ankle dorsiflexion. Intraclass correlation coefficient (ICC) estimates reported across reliability studies tend to be between 0.60 and 0.90 for inter-rater and test–retest reliability. Differences in ROM reliability are evident for different joints.[16] While there does not appear to be a single joint that has consistently inferior reliability, there are greater issues with measuring large two-joint muscles such as the hamstrings (popliteal angle and straight-leg raise measures).[12,17] While use of a helper to stabilize the non-tested leg during the popliteal angle measurement markedly improved reliability,[18] there was no evidence for hip extension that an assistant aided accuracy.[15]

Overall, it appears that changes of more than 10° to 20° are required (at 95% confidence level) for lower limb outcome evaluation,[12,19] although smaller changes can be detected (6–18°) if the same rater does the retest.[19] One other approach to reducing measurement error is to average several measures of the joint.[12] Measurement error may be higher in real-life clinical situations in which less attention to standardization is given.[12] A concluding comment in many of the research papers is that ROM should not be used on its own as the deciding factor for orthopaedic and other interventions given the challenges with reliability.[11]

Range of Motion Indices
Range of motion indices are intended to make the overall measurement process easier and more efficient. Two that were created for children with CP are described below.

Upper Extremity Rating Scale

OVERVIEW AND PURPOSE
For the upper limb, the Upper Extremity Rating Scale (UERS) was developed for children with CP to give a composite score of upper extremity active and passive ROM of the shoulder, elbow, forearm and wrist along with hand grasp/release scoring.[20]

ADMINISTRATION AND SCORING
Each of the measure's four joint motions is measured by goniometry and then rated according to a four-level response option format that is tied to ROM ranges. The score form for the UERS is provided in Koman et al's[20] publication. The UERS requires about 15 minutes to complete, and given its brevity it is easy to learn.

PSYCHOMETRIC PROPERTIES
Inter- and intrarater reliability were reported as good to excellent, and there was a fair correlation with the Melbourne Hand Assessment.[20] Test–retest reliability has not been evaluated.

The Spinal Alignment and Range of Motion Measure

OVERVIEW AND PURPOSE

The Spinal Alignment and Range of Motion Measure (SAROMM)[21] was designed as a discriminative tool to help provide benchmarks for assessing impairments in children with CP.[22]

ADMINISTRATION AND SCORING

The test incorporates active/passive measurement of lower extremity (10 movements tested bilaterally), spine (four movements) and upper extremity (one movement tested bilaterally) ROM. The 26 items are scored on a five-point scale related to ROM limitation increments. The SAROMM requires 15 to 30 minutes to complete, and the manual and score sheet can be accessed at www.canchild.ca/en/measures/saromm.asp.

PSYCHOMETRIC PROPERTIES

Intraclass correlation coefficients for the spine and extremities ROM scales were >0.80 for inter-rater and test–retest reliability (2-wk retest interval), when administered by trained raters. From a validity perspective, Gross Motor Function Classification System (GMFCS) and age contributed to the SAROMM score (r^2=0.41). It is important to stress that the impact of ROM estimation rounding error on the ability to detect change has not been studied. There is evidence that it also may be useful for evaluative purposes (i.e. reliability work indicates that a change of about nine points is needed on the 104-point scale to indicate change[21]).

SPASTICITY

Spasticity is one of three subtypes of neurologically mediated hypertonia. Measurement of the other two subtypes, rigidity and dystonia, are discussed in the next section. There are several approaches to measuring spasticity in the clinic setting. The Modified Ashworth Scale (MAS),[23] a passive movement test of spasticity, has been the standard clinical measure of resting tone and stiffness within surgical, medical and therapeutic intervention trials in CP, and until recently has been used in spasticity reduction studies with children with CP. However, reliability work with the MAS in CP emphasizes the need for caution in its use.[19,24–26] One weakness in using passive movement to indicate changes in spasticity is that resting muscle length is influenced by many factors in addition to spasticity reduction. There are concerns about its inability to account for the velocity-dependent aspect of spasticity, and its tendency to assess the intrinsic stiffness of the muscle.[27] The dynamic aspect of tone can be measured using complex instrumented approaches such as electrogoniometers during three-dimensional gait analysis,[28,29] or with mechanical instrumented techniques. However, a more practical clinical approach to the evaluation of dynamic spasticity is through the measurement of the initial resistance (R1) to rapid, dynamic stretch and then the assessment of its relationship to overall passive ROM (as indicated by an end-range resistance [R2]).

Tardieu scale

Overview and purpose

The consideration of both R1 and R2 within a single measure is known as the Tardieu Scale (as described by Boyd and Graham[30]). The score difference (window) between initial resistance (R1) and end-range resistance (R2) denotes the dynamic component of spasticity. The expectation after a spasticity-reducing intervention such as botulinum toxin-A (BoNT-A) is that the magnitude of this R1–R2 window should decrease because of the impact of BoNT-A on R2. Gracies et al[31] added a grading of muscle reaction during the fast stretch as a second component of the Tardieu Scale, resulting in what they renamed as the Modified Tardieu Scale.

Administration and scoring

Standardized positions for joint movement should be used. The angle of muscle reaction is determined by the fastest and slowest possible speeds of muscle stretch that the examiner can perform on the muscle being tested.[31] The joint angle of the muscle reaction where a velocity-elicited catch (i.e. the overactive stretch reflex) is first felt is called R1. The fast stretch is typically repeated three times with the angle of the catch from the third repetition taken as the R1.[19] When testing at the fast speed, signs of resistance, catches/releases or clonus are also scored on a five-point ordinal scale to provide a rating of muscle reaction. The extreme of the passive range (due to joint resistance or discomfort) on a slow stretch that is below the threshold of the stretch reflex is R2 (as described by Fosang et al[19] and Boyd and Graham[30]), with all other joints staying in a constant position for the test.[19,30] While measurement of R1 and R2 using a universal goniometer has been the usual approach taken, Gracies et al[31] determined that reliability is similar for visual and goniometric measurements with trained raters. The opportunity to do visual measurement might help to alleviate the challenges with goniometric measures, particularly for larger joints where stabilization in the full stretch position is difficult to maintain during measuring.

TARDIEU SCALE	
Purpose	To evaluate dynamic spasticity in a clinical setting without the use of instrumented equipment, by assessing resistance to rapid dynamic and passive stretch
Population	Children with cerebral palsy of all ages and Gross Motor Function Classification System levels
Description of domains (subscales)	Initial resistance (R1) to rapid dynamic stretch Passive range of motion (R2) as indicated by an end-range resistance
Administration and test format	Standardized positions for joint movement and stabilization should be used. Measurement of R1 and R2 is done with a universal goniometer, although visual measurement reduces the challenges associated with measuring large joints where stabilization in the stretch position is difficult to maintain during measuring R1: the joint angle of the muscle reaction where a velocity-elicited catch (i.e. the overactive stretch reflex) is first felt. The fast stretch is repeated three times with the angle of the catch from the third repetition recorded as R1. Signs of resistance, catches/releases or clonus are also scored on a five-point ordinal scale to provide a rating of muscle reaction R2: the extreme of the passive range (due to joint resistance or discomfort) on a slow stretch that is below the threshold of the stretch reflex
Psychometric properties	*Reliability* Intrarater reliability is excellent (intraclass correlation coefficient [ICC] 0.80) for lower limb, inter-rater reliability and test–retest reliability vary from fair to excellent (ICCs from 0.35 to 0.90) depending on the muscle group tested. Reliability was enhanced by in-depth training of the examiners. Increased leg length and weight of older children accentuate measurement difficulties. Minimal study to date of reliability for upper limb testing *Validity* While studies with the Tardieu scale with adults with spasticity have evaluated validity with instrumented techniques, paediatric validation studies have focused on reliability and assumed validity *Responsiveness* A change of >15–20° is required to demonstrate a true difference for hip, knee and ankle. Clinical trials with spasticity-reducing interventions have shown a change of this magnitude in Tardieu scores
How to order	Testing guidelines available in the appendices of Fosang et al (2003) and Maled and Graham (1999)
Key references	Fosang AL, Galea MP, McCoy AT, Reddihough DS, Story I (2003) Measures of muscle and joint performance in the lower limb of children with cerebral palsy. *Dev Med Child Neurol* 45: 664–670. Gracies J-M, Burke K, Clegg NJ, et al (2010) Reliability of the Tardieu Scale for assessing spasticity in children with cerebral palsy. *Arch Phys Med Rehabil* 91: 421–428. Maled RN, Graham HK (1999) Objective measurement of clinical findings in the use of botulinum toxin type A for the management of children with cerebral palsy. *Eur J Neurol* 6: S23–S35.

Psychometric properties
As a clinical tool, the Tardieu Scale is a more sensitive and relevant indicator of spasticity reduction than the MAS[19,30–32] and fits, in theory, with the velocity-dependent concept of spasticity.[33,34] While Gracies et al[31] found that intra- and inter-rater agreement was good to excellent (>80%) for ankle, elbow, hip and knee,[31] Yam and Leung[26] reported inter-rater ICCs of <0.75 with the lower limb.

One of the most important observations of Gracies et al's[31] work was that reliability was enhanced by in-depth training of the examiners.

Kilgour et al[12] provided evidence with typically developing children and those with CP that R1 and R2 scores both exhibit fair to excellent test–retest reliability when tested on two different days. According to this work, a change of more than 15° to 20° is required to demonstrate a true difference for knee and ankle R1/R2 measures in children with spastic diplegia. The increased leg length and weight of older children in the sample accentuated the measurement difficulties, that is the challenges in maintaining end-range positioning while measuring with the goniometer. In Fosang et al's[19] study in children with CP, test–retest ICCs varied from 0.38 (plantarflexors) to 0.97 (hamstrings). R1 changes ≥15° (ankle dorsiflexion) and 20° (popliteal angle), and R2 changes ≥10° (ankle dorsiflexion) to 20° (popliteal angle) can be detected. In the only test–retest reliability study for the upper limb, Mackey et al[35] noted large test–retest R1 differences (i.e. >15° in 5 of 10 children tested) in the measurement of biceps spasticity in children with CP, suggesting problematic issues with reliability across sessions.[35]

Selective Motor Control Test

Overview and purpose
The recent emphasis on discerning the functional implications of spasticity has led to the development of measures that quantify selective voluntary motor control, whereby greater spasticity is associated with less selective motor control/co-contraction issues in the related muscles. These measures are meant to be used alongside traditional measures of spasticity. The Selective Motor Control Test[30] (SMC) is a clinical measure that was developed to be used in BoNT-A trials to evaluate ankle dorsiflexor control.[30]

Administration and scoring
The child is positioned in long sitting and asked to dorsiflex their foot to touch the examiner's hand. If this is not possible with the knee extended, the child is then allowed to flex his or her knee and try again. The child is able to watch his or her foot action through the entire test. The knee and ankle muscle activity is scored on the SMC's five-level ordinal scale as outlined by Boyd and Graham.[30]

Psychometric properties
While SMC test–retest reliability was excellent in children with spastic CP, inter-rater reliability results demonstrate that retesting should be by the same assessor.[36] The SMC has been found to improve after BoNT-A injections

and to have a moderate association with ROM, and an even stronger link with Gross Motor Function Measure scores.[37,38]

Selective Control Assessment of the Lower Extremity

Overview and purpose
The Selective Control Assessment of the Lower Extremity (SCALE)[39] is similar to the SMC in its quantification of selective voluntary motor control of primary lower limb joints in children over 4 years of age with the spastic form of CP. It has greatest applicability to children in GMFCS levels I to IV. Factors that were used to develop the assessment and grading criteria were the ability to move each joint selectively, involuntary movement at other joints, the ability to reciprocate movement, speed of movement and generation of force, as demonstrated by excursion within the available ROM.

Administration and scoring
The child is asked to perform certain movement patterns in accordance with verbal cues (e.g. flex–extend–flex) and voluntary movement grading is on a three-point scale (unable, impaired or normal). The SCALE score for each limb is obtained by summing the points assigned to each joint to a maximum of 10 points per limb. Minimal training is required for use of the SCALE, and guidelines are provided in the paper by Fowler et al.[39]

Psychometric properties
Validation by the developers[39] has shown that inter-rater reliability was excellent, with ICCs varying from 0.88 to 0.91. Content validity was substantiated by strong overall agreement among 14 expert clinicians, with use of their feedback for amendments and clarifications to the tool. Construct validity was demonstrated by scores that were strongly inversely correlated with GMFCS levels (r=−0.83).

The Hypertonia Assessment Tool

Overview and purpose
When thinking of hypertonicity, it is also important to recognize that some children with CP have dystonic movement patterns, rather than spasticity, that need to be evaluated. Dystonia refers to involuntary intermittent or sustained muscle contractions, while rigidity involves bidirectional resistance (agonist/antagonist) that is independent of movement velocity.[40] While the Barry–Albright Dystonia Scale[41] was designed to specifically evaluate dystonic postures, and the modified Ashworth

Scale permits measurement of spasticity and rigidity, the Hypertonia Assessment Tool (HAT)[40] permits the differentiation of the subtypes of hypertonia within a single scale.

Administration and scoring

This clinical assessment tool contains seven items (three for dystonia, two for spasticity and two for rigidity) that allow the identification of different types of hypertonicity within the selected limb(s). The description of how to apply the HAT is provided in the paper by Jethwa et al[40] and also on the website of the centre where the senior author works (www.hollandbloorview.ca). In brief, the child is positioned supine in a comfortable supported position. The entire sequence of items is conducted on one involved extremity before progressing to the next extremity. For the first two items evaluating dystonia, the child is asked to carry out two of five purposeful movements listed in the HAT instructions (e.g. count to 10 slowly, open and close one hand repeatedly [not the one being examined], visually track a bright object). Any movements of the tested limb are observed during this purposeful movement. For the next four items evaluating spasticity or rigidity, a series of prescribed passive movements are carried out on the tested limb. During one of the sustained stretches, a purposeful movement of another limb is requested for one last item evaluating dystonia.

Psychometric properties

In the developers' validation work with children with CP, inter-rater and test–retest reliability and criterion validity were good to excellent for identification of spasticity (κ=0.57–1.00) and in the fair to good range for dystonia (κ=0.30–0.65). Reliability and validity were high for absence of rigidity (κ>0.90).[40] The authors of the HAT noted the presence of spasticity and dystonia in >75% of children in their study sample of 34 children. The developers note that further evaluation of the HAT is required in a heterogeneous group of children with hypertonia, and work is under way to enhance the instructions for scoring the dystonia items in particular.

MUSCLE STRENGTH

When conducting assessments of muscle strength, clinicians and researchers can choose between basic manual muscle testing, isometric and isokinetic testing methods using strength-measuring devices. While manual muscle testing is suitable for a quick screen of the strength of key muscle groups, it has well-documented challenges with respect to reliability and lacks the sensitivity needed for outcome evaluation. Either isometric or isokinetic test

protocols are suitable when assessing strength in children aged 6 years and over. Below this age, manual muscle testing and antigravity movement observation are the only practical options, given the need to be able to follow the instructions associated with isometric and isokinetic testing.

While there has been considerable research on isometric and isokinetic muscle strength testing reliability in typically developing school-aged children, along with establishment of normative scores, there is a relatively small body of literature that focuses on psychometric properties in children with physical disabilities. Further isometric and isokinetic reliability evaluation specifically in children with CP is warranted given the potential impact of underlying spasticity, ROM restrictions and co-contraction on psychometric properties. Isometric testing is more feasible than isokinetic testing in clinical practice,[42–44] but an understanding of isokinetic testing and its potential value is important, thus both are discussed in this review.

Isometric strength testing: dynamometer

Administration and scoring

Hand-held dynamometers are commercially available and provide a digital read-out of force in newtons. The assessor needs to use standard muscle test positions (as described in physical therapy texts or CP papers, e.g. Damiano and Abel[45]). One consideration is the technique applied, that is the 'break method' as used by Taylor et al[43] and Dodd et al[46] or the 'make method' as used by Berry et al,[47] Blundell et al,[48] Damiano et al[49] and Seniorou et al.[50] Consistency of approach is essential for follow-up evaluations with the child. For children with CP, the muscles of greatest functional relevance for testing are the hip extensors, flexors and abductors, and knee flexors and extensors. Testing of the ankle dorsiflexors may be more appropriately done using the selective motor control test described in the previous spasticity measurement section. Calibration of the dynamometer should be maintained according to the manufacturer's instructions to optimize reliability. The head of the dynamometer may need to be adapted with padding to fit small children. Adapted measurement positions or techniques may be necessary with neuromotor disorders and contractures to optimize reliability.[45] Alterations also may need to be made when testing larger muscle groups such as the hip extensors, which can be difficult to test because of positioning difficulties with children with CP.[51] Fixed dynamometers that are anchored on a table or wall can be helpful in these situations.

Psychometric properties

Much of the reliability work on isometric strength testing protocols using hand-held or fixed dynamometers in children with CP is embedded in publications about the effectiveness of muscle strength training protocols[50,52] rather than as specific reliability study publications.[53] For example, within their clinical trial, Vaz et al[52] demonstrated excellent test–retest reliability (1-wk interval) for muscle strength testing of wrist flexors and extensors in children with hemiplegic CP. Berry et al[47] determined that test–retest reliability (4- to 14-day retest) was excellent for muscle strength testing of the knee extensors and hip abductors and good for the knee flexors.[47] Standard error of measurement (SEM) estimates provided in this work may be of use to clinicians for the interpretation of change scores. Similarly, Crompton et al[53] noted good to excellent reliability for hip and knee muscle groups as well as ankle dorsiflexors, but noted that the SEM was different depending on the muscle group and test position and needs to be taken into account when interpreting change. A reliability study specifically in children with CP by Taylor et al[43] focused on five key lower limb muscle groups. While ICCs indicated excellent reliability (all >0.80), the authors expressed concern that unrealistically large amounts of change would need to occur for the hip extensors before change could be detected. A study of isometric strength of children with Down syndrome demonstrated excellent test–retest reliability (1-wk interval) of peak force for knee extensors and hip abductors as measured by hand-held dynamometry.[42] In contrast, while comparability of the 'make test' and 'break test' approaches in CP was verified by Verschuren et al[44], this study introduced concerns about hand-held dynamometry overall as, with either method, inter-rater reliability was not optimal (ICCs from 0.42 to 0.82).[44] Ultimately, the authors recommended the use of a 30-second maximum repetition time as a more reliable approach to functional strength testing.

Isokinetic strength testing: dynamometer

Overview and purpose

Isokinetic muscle strength is the force produced by the muscle through the entire range of motion at a preset, constant velocity. Muscle action may be either concentric (shortening) or eccentric (lengthening).

Administration and scoring

Testing is done by attaching the child to an isokinetic dynamometer, which controls the test position and speed of movement. The dynamometer supports may have to be modified to allow children (who are shorter than adults) to be properly tested.[54] A habituation session is recommended to enable children to learn how to reliably give a maximal effort.[55] The instructions should be standardized; for example, 'you need to push and pull as hard as possible'.[55] A minimum of two and a maximum of six repetitions are recommended to ensure maximal effort without fatigue.[54] Testing velocities are usually dictated by the research question and the skill level of the participants, with faster velocities being more difficult to perform. Velocities up to 240° per second have been used for typically developing children,[54] up to 180° per second for children with CP,[56] and up to 210° per second for children with developmental coordination disorder (DCD).[57] Common variables calculated are peak torque, the highest value during a trial, and mean torque, the mean value during a trial. Torque is typically measured in Newton meters (Nm). The higher the torque, the greater the isokinetic muscle strength. When movements used to evaluate strength are in the vertical plane, a gravitational torque contributes to the measured torque, and thus correction for the effect of gravity must be made.[58]

Psychometric properties

In typically developing children, test–retest reliability varies with the muscle group evaluated, with overall test–retest differences reported to be ≤10%.[59] van den Berg-Emmons et al[60] evaluated between-day test–retest reliability of knee flexor and extensor peak torques at 30°, 60° and 120° per second in 7- to 12-year-old children with CP, one-third of whom were non-ambulatory.[60] For the knee flexors, the correlations between test–retest peak torques were significant at all speeds (ρ=0.65–0.84), with the coefficient values increasing as velocity decreased. The authors interpreted this information as indicating that the peak knee flexor torque could be reliably measured at all three speeds, but that reliability may be somewhat affected by velocity. For the knee extensors, only the peak torques at 30° per second were reliable (r_s=0.71). Kramer and MacPhail[61] reported somewhat higher test–retest (1-wk interval) reliability coefficients (r≥0.87) for peak knee flexor and extensor eccentric and concentric torques at 90° per second for adolescents (mean age 15.8, SD 3.0y) with mild CP (all were ambulatory without assistive devices).[61] Taken together with the information from the van den Berg-Emmons et al[60] study, this suggests that reliability may increase with increasing age and decreasing motor impairment. Ayalon et al[62] also found the test–retest (1-wk interval) reliability of peak and mean knee flexor and extensor torques at 90° per second to be high (ICC ≥0.95) for 9- to 15-year-old children with CP, all of whom were ambulatory and most of whom were able to walk without assistive devices.[62] When compared with the results of van den Berg-Emmons et al, these findings again suggest that a younger age and a greater level of motor impairment may negatively affect reliability.

Convergent validity with the energy cost of walking estimated from heart rate (r=0.49–0.64) and with gross motor function related to walking as evaluated by the Gross Motor Function Measure Standing and Walking, Running and Jumping dimensions (r=0.58–0.68) has been shown for peak knee extensor but not peak knee flexor torque at 90° per second for children with CP.[61] Using the data of Ayalon et al,[62] an estimate of the minimal detectable change (95% confidence interval) in peak torque is about 13% for the knee extensors and 20% for the knee flexors, which is sufficient to detect change following an isokinetic strength training intervention in adolescents with mild CP.

Finally, in evaluations of strength training for children with CP[45,52,63,64] or strength-related outcomes after surgery,[50] isometric strength testing rather than isokinetic testing has typically been used alongside functional outcome measures.[45,48,52,64,65] Some investigators have omitted strength assessment altogether and instead used gait lab analysis,[66,67] muscle volume changes[64] or strength-related functional outcomes[64,66,67] with measures such as the Gross Motor Function Measure, Functional Assessment Questionnaire and Functional Mobility Scale as indicators of strength changes. Absence of strength measures in these studies may reflect investigators' concerns about the reliability and sensitivity of muscle strength testing to change.

Grip and pinch strength

Overview and purpose
Although grasp and pinch emerge functionally around 4 months of age with refinement to the finest pincer grasp at 12 months, neurophysiological structures and peripheral connections are present at birth.[68] Research using force transducers have documented sequential grip and load force in infants and young children.[69] Accurate and reliable measures of grip and/or pinch strength are limited to data collected in the 1980s on preschool-aged and older children.[70–73] Robertson and Dietz[73] used the Martin Vigorimeter to measure grip strength only in 380 white preschoolers aged 3 years to 5 years 6 months.[73] Standardized procedures were used to obtain a mean of three trials, resulting in group means and standard deviations reported in 6-month increments. Grip in the preschool children increased significantly with age, with right-hand grip significantly stronger than left and no sex differences found. The Jamar dynamometer and pinch gauges were used by Mathiowetz and colleagues[71] for data collection on 471 children aged 6 to 19 years residing in

Wisconsin and by Ager and colleagues[70] for 474 children aged 5 to 12 years in the greater Denver area.

Overall, results of studies have documented (1) increased strength with age, (2) comparable strength in males and females (males being somewhat stronger) until adolescence, when males showed a sharp increase in strength, (3) stronger right hand for right-handers but inconsistent for left-handers and (4) that height and weight of the children correlated with grip and pinch strength.[74]

The purpose of measuring grip and pinch is to document current function relative to peers of similar age and sex (descriptive, discriminative measure) and to detect change over time (evaluative measure). Normative data are used for comparison with individual performance expressed in z-scores.

Administration and scoring
Different authors have used different administration procedures when testing grip and pinch. However, guidelines outlined by the American Society of Hand Therapists (ASHT) are considered best practice for children as well as adults. Using an adapted version of the standard protocol for children aged 6 to 19 years, a calibrated hydraulic hand dynamometer[75] is used with the child seated (using height-appropriate chairs and tables), with the shoulder adducted and neutrally rotated, the shoulder flexed between 50° and 70°, the elbow flexed at approximately 90° and the forearm in a neutral position. The wrist is between 0° and 30° of extension and between 0° and 15° of ulnar deviation. The hand not being tested remains on the individual's lap during testing. The examiner says 'Ready? Squeeze as hard as you can'. Three trials are given with a 30-second rest period between each squeeze. The mean of the trials is recorded. A calibrated pinch gauge is used to measure finger grasp strength using a key (lateral) pinch, the three-jaw chuck and the two-point pinch. The child is seated as described above and with each pinch measure the examiner says 'Ready? Pinch as hard as you can'. The examiner holds the pinch meter, and with verbal encouragement, the child pinches three times with a 30-second rest period between each pinch. The mean of three trials is recorded. The time to administer grip and pinch strength is approximately 10 to 15 minutes.

Psychometric properties
As the procedures recommended by the ASHT were used by Mathiowetz and colleagues,[71] including reporting the mean of three trials, these norms are typically used. Group mean and standard deviation tables by sex and by age are included in this article. No studies have reported reliability statistics (inter-rater, test–retest) or validity studies for children. However, good to excellent test–retest reliability

GRIP AND PINCH STRENGTH (DYNAMOMETER AND PINCH GAUGE)	
Purpose	To measure hand strength in children so as to assist in identifying level of development and/or degree of impairment
Population	Ages 5–19y
Description of domains (subscales)	Measurements can be obtained for the following (both hands): Grip strength (dynamometer) Tip pinch (pinch gauge) Lateral pinch (pinch gauge) Palmar pinch (pinch gauge)
Administration and test format	Time to complete: approximately 10min Testing format: client completes one to three trials of each grip or pinch as demonstrated with maximal force Scoring: score is recorded in pounds of force and then compared with age and sex norms Training: specialized training is not required
Psychometric properties	Normative sample: 360 children aged 6–19y in original study. 471 children aged 5–12y in secondary study *Reliability* Test–retest reliability excellent – intraclass correlation coefficients ranged from 0.91 to 0.98 *Validity* Construct validity studies reported *Responsiveness* Study of 415 children with mild disability demonstrated improvement of scores with chronological age
How to order	Norms can be obtained from references
Key references	van den Beld WA, van der Sanden GA, Sengers RC, Verbeek AL, Gabreels FJ (2006) Validity and reproducibility of the Jamar dynamometer in children aged 4–11 years. *Disabil Rehabil* 28: 1303–1309. Daniels L, Backman C (1993) Grip and pinch strength norms for children. *Phys Occup Ther Pediatr* 13: 81–90. Mathiowetz V, Wiemer DM, Federman SM (1986) Grip and pinch strength: norms for 6- to 19-year olds. *Am J Occup Ther* 40: 705–711. Molenaar HM, Zuidam JM, Selles RW, Stam HJ, Hovius SE (2008) Age specific reliability of two grip-strength dynamometers when used by children. *J Bone Joint Surg A* 90: 1053–1059.

(r=0.88–0.93) has been reported for grip strength measurement in adults. Inter-rater reliability for pinch testing, following the recommended protocol for adults, was found to be 0.98, and test–retest reliability after 1 week was >0.81.[76]

Validity studies using adults have been found to be good when the dynamometer has been calibrated properly[30] and when standard positioning is utilized.[76] Updated normative data for children from national and international regions representing multiple ethnic/race populations with accompanying reliability and validity information are urgently needed to fill an obvious gap in the developmental and rehabilitation literature.

GAIT EVALUATION

Gait issues are common in children with physical disabilities, and optimizing gait pattern and endurance are key motor treatment goals. Functional implications of gait changes from the perspective of parents and clinicians include improved gait appearance, greater stability, improved speed and less tripping and falling. Computerized gait analysis (CGA), also known as three-dimensional gait analysis (3DGA), is considered to be the standard tool for assessing gait deviations in children with mobility restrictions, while observational gait scales (discussed later) are more practical clinically. CGA data provide a biomechanical understanding of pathological gait and are used to guide decisions on various orthopaedic, neurosurgical and orthotic interventions.[77] Despite widespread acceptance, few studies have documented the consistency of discrete gait parameters measured by CGA in children with CP. Instead, reliability work has tended to focus on the evaluation of underlying kinematic waveforms, and has demonstrated some issues with test–retest reliability.[78,79] Parameters measured in the sagittal and transverse planes generally displayed stronger reliability in children with CP (ICC ≥0.84) than those in the frontal plane, for which reliability was fair to good (ICCs 0.46–0.78). Sampling a minimum of four strides has been recommended for children in GMFCS level I and a minimum of six strides for children in GMFCS levels II and III.[80]

A pragmatic issue with CGA is that it is too costly for routine use, it is unsuitable for in-depth use with young children and it requires specialized gait laboratories that are unavailable to most clinicians. In the context of BoNT-A and other rehabilitation interventions, CGA is more appropriate as a second analytical level to explore deviations noted in observational gait analyses. There have been recent suggestions to use measures such as the Gillette Gait Index (GGI, known initially as the Normalcy Index[81]) to permit amalgamation of key CGA variables studied into a summary score.

Gillette Gait Index

Overview and purpose
The GGI incorporates 16 clinically pertinent kinematic variables measured using CGA, as well as several temporal parameters, into a single summary score.[81] Its purpose is to provide a simple summary of a child's gait to help the clinician consider the numerous variables collected in an instrumented gait assessment and the extent to which a child's gait deviates from the norm.

Administration and scoring
The 16 gait variables are extracted from the child's instrumented gait analysis that is conducted using standard protocols, and data from a single or a series of averaged gait cycles are processed, using the analytical

approach provided by Schutte et al,[81] into a single summary score. Scoring is based on principal component analysis for each of the GGI's 16 variables. The dimensionless summary score reflects the extent of deviation of the child's gait from an average profile of typically developing individuals. There are a number of data sets available that provide normal profiles, or gait laboratories can choose to use data sets from typically developing children tested in their laboratory. Individual GGI summary scores can vary from a mean value of 16 for able-bodied reference groups[82,83] to >660 for children with quadriplegia.[84]

Psychometric properties
Information about the GGI's reliability is scarce in the peer-reviewed literature. Perhaps reliability has been assumed because the GGI is based upon individual gait parameters that have been shown to have at least fair reliability with CGA. Bothner et al[85] determined excellent GGI summary score reliability between gait cycles (ICC >0.90) in children with CP, and that a single gait cycle can confidently be used for GGI calculation. A test–retest evaluation of the GGI[86] concluded that measurement error is about 12 points for typically developing children but could be 15 to 100 points for a child with CP, with more error associated with higher (more impaired) GGI scores, that is those in GMFCS level II and III.

The validity of reference group values (the foundation of GGI summary scores) has been the more common subject of evaluation. The similarity of reference group (control data) values was demonstrated by Romei et al,[84] while McMulkin and MacWilliams[87] concluded that reference group values from different data sets resulted in GGI differences within the same child (i.e. 250–1200 point spreads). They recommended that comparison of GGI values should be done by computing GGI scores from the same reference data set. The need for caution in describing a child's change in GGI score was stressed by Tulchin et al,[83] along with a recommendation to have at least 96 individuals in the reference data group to ensure <10% error in determining the principal components of the GGI value.

Discriminant validity evaluations verified score differences among GMFCS levels I to IV as well as differences among individuals with quadri-,di or hemiplegia.[81,84] Construct validity was demonstrated with strong correlation using the Gross Motor Function Measure (GMFM; $r=-0.75$)[88,89] and the Pediatric Orthopedic Society of North America scale,[82] and moderate correlations between the GGI and the GMFM, energy expenditure index and Functional Assessment Questionnaire (FAQ) in children with spastic diplegic CP.[90]

Minimal detectable change has been estimated to be at least 85 units in GGI, with higher changes required for children in GMFCS level IV who have greater walking impairment (minimal detectable change >300 points).[85] The GGI has been used in several clinical trials related to gait-based interventions with mixed results in terms of sensitivity to change (e.g. improvement in GGI scores after intrathecal baclofen,[91] multilevel orthopaedic surgery[92,93] or hamstring tenotomies[94]), while there was no GGI score difference between ankle–foot orthosis (AFO) and barefoot walking gait despite significant differences in walking efficiency in children with CP.[95]

As with most measurement areas, the evolution of new approaches continues. Two main criticisms of the GGI are the choice of parameters for evaluation and dependence on control data for scoring the GGI.[96] The Gait Deviation Index (GDI) has been introduced to address these issues.[97] It evaluates nine kinematic variables and uses joint rotation pattern recognition followed by a singular value decomposition analytical approach to arrive at a single index score (the scoring process is provided in an addendum to Schwartz and Rozumalski's paper[97]). The GDI has demonstrated construct validity when evaluated alongside the GGI, Gillette FAQ and GMFCS.[96,97] While the GDI appears to detect changes in status after surgery, like the GGI, the single summary score does not provide a full assessment of gait changes. Further descriptive analysis at each joint level is still necessary.[96]

Observational gait assessments
Several observational gait assessments (OGAs) have been created to quantify the process of visual gait assessment. These are typically variations on the original Physician Rating Scale (PRS)[98] designed for use with BoNT-A interventions. Although OGAs rank high as far as feasibility and economy of time/cost are concerned, there are reliability and responsiveness issues. Reliability studies with OGAs with children with CP[99,100] emphasize the strong potential of some items but stress that there are at least as many items that do not work well from the perspective of reliability and responsiveness. OGAs require that the observer simultaneously assesses body segment motion from different viewing angles as well as at many joint levels. It is recommended that OGAs be scored from video recordings since split-screen, slow-motion and playback features can be applied.[101] A second limitation is that most OGAs examine only the sagittal plane. The Edinburgh Gait Scale (EGS)[102] was developed specifically for children with CP to evaluate both coronal and sagittal planes. It shows more promise than other OGAs in terms of its reliability and validity. Details about the EGS are provided below.

Martin et al[103] created and validated an OGS to evaluate children with Down syndrome, stating that the existing scales for children with CP did not contain suitable items in terms of the gait deviations that children with Down syndrome have. Their pilot study demonstrated good intra- and inter-rater reliability, but stressed the need for validity evaluation.

As an extension of the OGA approach, new joint angle video-screen measurement computer programs that assist quantification of joint angles from recorded videos of walking have been developed. These demonstrate promise with respect to reliability for the evaluation of children with CP.[104]

Edinburgh Gait Scale

Overview and purpose
The EGS[102] was designed to assess the gait of children with CP within a setting that does not have an instrumented gait laboratory. Because it was designed expressly for evaluation in an orthopaedic surgery context, it evaluates kinematic variables in both coronal and sagittal planes.

Administration and scoring
There are 17 variables observed during the gait cycle at six levels (foot, ankle, knee, hip, pelvis and trunk). Each is measured using a three-point ordinal scale where higher scores indicate greater deviations. The EGS uses a video gait analysis format to enhance the accuracy of scoring. A large room and good lighting are essential, and it is ideal if two video cameras can be used to simultaneously capture anterior and lateral views. Scoring guidelines are available in the publication by Read et al.[102]

Psychometric properties
The developers of the EGS demonstrated good intra- and interobserver reliability with children with CP,[102] while other researchers found excellent intrarater reliability but poor inter-rater reliability.[105] While there is no specific training for the EGS other than review of published test guidelines, there is evidence that individuals with gait evaluation experience are more reliable in their scoring than novices to gait analysis.[101] From a concurrent validity standpoint, the EGS correlates strongly with the GGI (r=0.79), which is based on CGA data, and moderately with the FAQ (r=−0.52).[88] Ong et al[101] demonstrated concurrent validity by showing a 64% agreement of scores with those from CGA. Studies have demonstrated the ability of the EGS to detect change after intervention.[102,106] A change of three to four points per limb is considered to reflect change beyond measurement error.[102]

EDINBURGH GAIT SCALE (EGS)

Purpose	To assess the gait of children with cerebral palsy within a setting that does not have an instrumented gait laboratory. It evaluates kinematic variables in both coronal and sagittal planes
Population	Ambulatory children (with or without gait devices), ages 3y+; must be old enough to do repeated walks when asked
Description of domains (subscales)	Six anatomical levels assessed: foot, ankle, knee, hip, pelvis, trunk
Administration and test format	Time to complete: 15–20min for child's live assessment followed by 20–30min for video scoring
	Testing format: the child walks repeatedly across the floor in a large well-lit room. Video-taping of gait is done to enhance the accuracy of scoring. Marking key anatomical landmarks before testing aids scoring. The test can be done with the child barefoot or with orthoses. Gait aids can be used as required. It is ideal if two video cameras are used to simultaneously capture anterior and lateral views as well as close-up views of the feet and pelvis. Seventeen variables are observed during the gait cycle at six levels (foot, ankle, knee, hip, pelvis and trunk). Each is measured using a five-point ordinal scale where a higher score indicates a greater deviation. A summary score is computed for each leg (out of 17 points) with an EGS total score (out of 34 points)
	Training: self-training for the assessment is outlined by Read et al (2003). It is preferable if the assessor has experience of gait assessment
Psychometric properties	*Reliability* Intrarater reliability in children with cerebral palsy: for individual items, kappa varied from 0.17 for peak hip flexion to 0.94 for foot initial contact. Coefficient of repeatability was 5.15 for novice observers vs 4.21 for experienced observers
	Inter-rater reliability: for individual items, kappa varied from 0.00 for clearance in swing to 0.69 for foot initial contact for inexperienced raters and from 0.17 for peak hip flexion to 0.94 for foot initial contact. Coefficient of repeatability was 5.99 for novice observers vs 4.60 for experienced observers
	Test–retest reliability: not reported
	Validity Construct validity: comparing with three-dimensional gait analysis, total agreement with 52% of 10 numerical items for inexperienced observers and 64% for those experienced with children with cerebral palsy. Moderate to strong correlations for EGS total score with Gillette Gait Index (r=0.85), speed (r=–0.67) and Gillette Functional Questionnaire (r=–0.52)
	Responsiveness Able to detect change as small as four points (within limb total score) in an orthopaedic surgery trial
How to order	Scoring guidelines are available in Read et al (2003)
Key references	Hillman SJ, Hazlewood ME, Schwartz MH, van der Linden ML, Robb JE (2007) Correlation of the Edinburgh Gait Score with the Gillette Gait Index, the Gillette Functional Assessment Questionnaire, and dimensionless speed. *J Pediatr Orthop* 27: 7–11.
	Ong AML, Hillman SJ, Robb JE (2008) Reliability and validity of the Edinburgh Visual Gait Score for cerebral palsy when used by inexperienced observers. *Gait Post* 28: 323–326.
	Read HS, Hazlewood ME, Hillman SJ, Prescott RJ, Robb JE (2003) Edinburgh visual gait score for use in cerebral palsy. *J Pediatr Orthop* 23: 296–301.

MUSCLE ENDURANCE AND EXERCISE TOLERANCE:

Anaerobic Muscle Power and Endurance

Anaerobic muscle power is the rate of doing high-intensity, short-duration exercise such as pulling to stand, jumping or sprinting. Anaerobic muscle endurance is the ability to repeat or to maintain high-intensity muscular contractions over a short time (<2 min). The term 'anaerobic' refers to the energy systems which do not require oxygen. In general, the higher the intensity and the shorter the duration, the greater is the demand on the anaerobic versus the aerobic (oxygen-requiring) energy systems.

Wingate Anaerobic Test

OVERVIEW AND PURPOSE

The Wingate Anaerobic Test measures upper and lower limb anaerobic muscle power and endurance. The test is appropriate for children ≥5 years of age who can arm-crank or pedal continuously at a maximum effort for 30 seconds.[107]

ADMINISTRATION AND SCORING

An arm or cycle ergometer with a crank/pedal-rate counter and a braking force independent of the cranking/pedalling rate is required to perform the test. For children with motor impairments, the hands or feet may be secured to the handles or pedals, respectively, and for upper limb tests the trunk may be secured to the backrest. The test consists of cranking or pedalling for 30 seconds at a maximum velocity against a constant, individually determined braking force. This force must be high enough to produce fatigue (a slowing down of cranking/pedalling) within a few seconds. Equations based on body mass are typically used to calculate braking force as body mass is related to muscle mass.[107] For children and adolescents with CP, where the body–muscle mass relationship is not so clear, trial and error[60,108,109] or the force–velocity test have been used to determine the braking force.[110]

The Wingate Anaerobic Test is preceded by 3 to 5 minutes of cranking/pedalling at a moderate intensity (heart rate of 150–160 beats per min), followed by 1 to 2 minutes of rest.[107] The test is then followed by 2 to 3 minutes of arm cranking/pedalling against a very low resistance to minimize post-test symptoms of light-headedness or nausea.[107] The main Wingate Anaerobic Test variables are peak power (the highest mechanical power obtained during the test [typically obtained during the first few seconds]), and mean power (the average power over the entire 30 seconds). The latter is considered an indication of anaerobic muscle endurance. Power is measured in

watts (W). Higher values indicate greater anaerobic power or endurance.

PSYCHOMETRIC PROPERTIES

Upper and lower limb mean and peak power measured with the Wingate Anaerobic Test are reliable from test to test (between-day and within-day reliability coefficients ≥0.90) for children with CP.[60,109] After two to three sessions of habituation, Guerra et al[111] showed excellent between-day test–retest reliability (ICCs ≥0.86) for lower limb mean and peak power in children with Down syndrome. Peak, but not mean, power was, however, significantly lower on the first test than on the second (210.4 vs 236.3W). This suggests that two to three sessions of habituation may not be sufficient for obtaining stable values for individuals with cognitive impairment. Lower limb mean and peak power for children who were born preterm is also reliable from test to test (r=0.96).[112] For children with DCD, O'Beirne et al[113] showed convergent validity (r≥0.59) of lower limb mean and peak power with lower limb motor coordination as measured by the McCarron Assessment of Neuromuscular Development. Convergent validity (r≥0.73) with the GMFM-88 total score has also been shown for lower limb mean and peak power with children with CP.[114] For upper limb mean and peak power, the only significant correlations with the GMFM-88 were for the 'lying and rolling' and 'sitting' dimensions, as these dimensions rely more on upper limb rather than lower limb muscle function.

The Wingate Anaerobic Test discriminates between children with DCD and their typically developing peers[113] and between subgroups of children with CP (hemiplegia, diplegia, quadriplegia).[108] As might be expected, based on specificity of training for any population, aerobic exercise training does not affect anaerobic power or endurance in children with spastic CP.[115] The magnitude of change that can be expected after an intervention targeting anaerobic power has not been reported for children with developmental disabilities. Moreover, at present there is little information to guide clinicians in interpreting change scores for an individual child.

Muscle Power Sprint Test

OVERVIEW AND PURPOSE

Given that the Wingate Anaerobic Test requires specialized expertise and equipment, 'functional' tests to assess anaerobic muscle power and endurance have been developed. The Muscle Power Sprint Test is one example, as its measurement properties have been evaluated in children with a developmental disability (CP). The test is suitable for children ≥6 years of age who are able to walk without support. For an overview of various functional tests to assess anaerobic power that have been used with typically developing children, including their psychometric properties, see Chia.[116]

ADMINISTRATION AND SCORING

The test consists of six 15-m sprints, done as fast as possible, separated by 10-second rest periods. Sprint and rest periods are timed. Before the test, the child performs a practice at a comfortable walking speed to warm up, and then rests for 3 minutes.[117] While a cool down is not explicitly stated as part of the protocol,[117] it is prudent to follow the test with 2 or 3 minutes of walking at a comfortable pace to avoid dizziness or nausea. Power output (W) (force × velocity, where force=body mass × acceleration) is estimated for each sprint using the average velocity of the sprint and the child's body mass. Peak power is the highest value, derived from the sprint with the highest mean velocity. Mean power is the average power across the six sprints and is considered a measure of anaerobic muscle endurance. As with the Wingate test, higher values indicate greater anaerobic power or endurance. The power outputs derived from the Muscle Power Sprint Test probably underestimate the true power outputs that occur during the sprints because a constant, positive acceleration based on the average velocity is assumed to have occurred during sprinting, and the power calculation does not consider any mechanical work performed (power=work/time) not directly related to moving the body forward.[118] Although the test may lack the precision of laboratory measures such as the Wingate Anaerobic Test, it is more feasible to perform for clinicians who work outside of a specialized exercise testing facility.

PSYCHOMETRIC PROPERTIES

The test shows good between-day (two visits within 1 wk) test–retest reliability for peak and mean power (ICCs ≥0.98) for children with CP.[117] Convergent validity of test results with gross motor function has also been shown in that mean power (corrected for age, sex and GMFCS level) positively correlates with results from the standing (r=0.30) and the walking, running and jumping (r=0.60) dimensions of the GMFM.[119] Test results also discriminate between children at levels I and II on the GMFCS.[117] The minimal detectable change (90% confidence interval) is about 31% for peak power and about 27% for mean power.[117] Based on data from one training study,[120] where there was a significant increase in mean power of about 25% for the group, the test may detect change after an intervention in some children with CP.

Maximal aerobic exercise tests

Maximal aerobic exercise tests evaluate aerobic fitness – the capacity to perform exercise depending mainly on the body's aerobic or oxygen-requiring energy system. Unless performed as a sprint, walking, running, cycling, swimming and propelling a wheelchair are examples of 'aerobic' exercises. Individuals with high aerobic fitness will be able to perform submaximal aerobic exercise with less fatigue than those with lower levels of aerobic fitness.[121] With maximal aerobic exercise tests, the exercise intensity is progressively increased until the test is terminated, because (1) a plateau is reached where an increase in exercise intensity no longer leads to an increase in aerobic energy expenditure, (2) the individual can no longer maintain the desired exercise intensity or (3) it is no longer safe for the individual to continue because of irregularities in the physiological responses.[122] Verbal encouragement is usually given throughout the test. In the absence of a plateau in energy expenditure, objective indications of a maximal effort with children are a respiratory exchange ratio >1.1 and a peak heart rate close to the predicted maximum (≈200 beats per min for typically developing children).[122] Maximal aerobic exercise test protocols differ mainly in (1) the type of exercise performed (e.g. walking/running on level ground or on a treadmill, cycling or arm-cranking exercise) and (2) the length and intensity at each stage. Protocols are chosen based on the reason for the test and the child's fitness level and physical abilities. Tests generally last 8 to 12 minutes, although shorter and longer tests may also be valid.[123] Children should be well rested and should not consume caffeine on the testing day, and they should avoid eating a heavy meal during the 2 to 3 hours before testing.[122] For children, and especially for young children (aged 3–4y), treadmill protocols are preferable as long as the child is able to walk without support. Protocols using a cycle or arm ergometer or overground walking/running are generally suitable for children ≥6 years of age, assuming that they have the motor and cognitive skills necessary to perform the test.[122]

Maximum oxygen uptake, the highest value at the end of the test, is the 'criterion standard' measure of aerobic fitness. As maximal oxygen uptake is proportional to body size, the effect of body size is usually accounted for, often by normalizing for body mass (e.g. oxygen uptake measured in millilitres per minute per kilogram).[124] Higher normalized values mean greater aerobic fitness. Most tests, with the exception of clinical or field tests such as a shuttle run (see below), require specialized equipment to measure cardiorespiratory variables such as oxygen uptake and heart rate as well as the calibrated ergometer on which the child performs the test. Children should be familiarized with this equipment before testing begins.

For detailed information on the equipment, the variables measured, evaluator training and safety procedures, see Paridon et al.[122]

Treadmill ergometry

Overview and purpose
Maximal oxygen uptake values are about 10% higher with treadmill protocols than with cycling protocols.[122] Children should practise walking and running on the treadmill before the test.[122]

Administration and scoring
It is advisable that children do not hold on to the handrails during testing, except fleetingly for balance, as oxygen uptake decreases in proportion to the amount of body weight supported,[125,126] and use can render the test invalid. The most popular protocols to use are the Bruce protocol (3-min stages, exercise intensity increased at each stage by increasing the treadmill belt speed and the slope) and the modified Balke protocol (2-min stages, individually determined treadmill belt speed that is generally held constant and slope increased in equal increments at each stage, the amount depending on the treadmill belt speed).[122,127] The Bruce protocol is the more challenging of the two.[122]

The specific protocols that have been reported in the literature for children with developmental disabilities, and are thus known to be feasible for them, are as follows: Fernhall et al[128,129] used the modified Balke protocol (individualized starting speed from 3.2 to 6.4km/h, starting slope=0%, with 4% increments) to measure the aerobic fitness of children with mild to moderate global developmental delay. Hoofwijk et al[130] and Maltais et al[131] used another version of the modified Balke protocol (stage 1 speed=2.4–4.0km/h, increased to 0.2–0.5km/h below the fastest treadmill walking speed by stage 3, then held constant; 0% slope for stages 1–3, then increased in equal increments of 2.4–5% with each subsequent stage) to quantify the aerobic fitness of children with CP. Verschuren et al[132,133] also assessed aerobic fitness using a treadmill protocol for children with CP, but they used neither the Bruce nor the modified Balke protocol. Instead, those who were classified in GMFCS level I started at 5.0km/h, and those at level II began at 2.0km/h. The speed was increased by 0.25km/h every minute while the slope was constant at 2%. Wu et al[134] used the Bruce protocol (0.5–0.9km/h increase in speed and 2% increase in slope with each stage) to assess aerobic fitness in children with DCD.[134]

Psychometric properties
Maximum oxygen uptake using a treadmill protocol (test starting at 4.02km/h and a 0% slope, speed increased by 0.81km/h each minute until a speed of 9.5km/h, then the slope increased 3% every minute) can be reliably (ICC=0.93) measured from test to test (≥1-wk interval) with typically developing children.[135] Maximum oxygen uptake values for the modified Balke protocol as used by Fernhall et al[128] on children and adolescents with global developmental delay shows test–retest reliability (r=0.90; 2- to 7-d interval).[128] The reliability of maximum oxygen uptake determined using the above-mentioned treadmill protocols for young people with CP or developmental delay, however, is unknown, although these protocols show discriminant validity in that maximum oxygen uptake values are lower for those with CP[130,136] or developmental delay[134] than for their typically developing peers.

Shuttle run tests

Overview and purpose
Shuttle run tests are clinical or field tests of aerobic fitness where maximal oxygen uptake is not directly measured. To perform these tests, children walk or run back and forth between two lines a set distance apart. The pace is determined by a prerecorded signal. These tests are suitable for children ≥6 years old.[137]

Administration and scoring
The 20-m shuttle run test[137] is one of the most commonly used field tests to evaluate aerobic fitness. Children run between two lines 20m apart, at a starting speed of 8.5km/h, with the speed increasing by 0.5km/h each minute.[137] A variant of the test uses the same speed increase each minute but has a slightly slower start speed (8.0km/h).[138] Maximum oxygen uptake can be estimated based on the maximum running speed during the last stage of the test and the child's age.[137] It is debatable whether adding other variables such as sex and anthropometric factors to the prediction equation improves the precision of the estimate.[139] One can also score the test by the number of stages completed or the mean speed during the last stage. On average, typically developing 6-year-old children complete the test in about 4 minutes, and 17 year olds in about 9 minutes.[137]

Two shuttle run tests (SRT-I and SRT-II) have been developed for children, adolescents and young adults (aged 6–20y) with CP classified at levels I and II, respectively, on the GMFCS.[132] Both tests use a 10-m distance. The starting speed for the SRT-I is 5.0km/h and for the SRT-II is 2.0km/h. With both tests, the speed increases by 0.25km/h each minute.[132] Test completion time is 2 to 18 minutes.[133] The test is scored as the number of stages completed, the time to complete the test or the average speed for the final stage. No equations to estimate maximum oxygen uptake have been developed for these tests, although reference values for children with CP are available for the number of stages completed for a given height.[133] If children wear a heart rate monitor during the test, their maximum heart rate can be directly determined, thus avoiding the error inherent in predicting maximum heart rate based on age.[140] Aerobic exercise training intensity can subsequently be calculated as a percentage of the heart rate reserve – the difference between resting and maximum heart rate.

Psychometric properties
Test–retest (2–7d) results for the 20-m shuttle run with typically developing children and adolescents are reliable (r=0.89),[137] as are results for children and adolescents with mild–moderate global developmental delay (r=0.97).[129] Test–retest (2–7d) results for the SRT-I and the SRT-II are also reliable (ICC ≥0.87) for children with CP.[132] Results from the 20-m shuttle run show construct (concurrent) validity with maximum oxygen uptake measured (1) during a treadmill test with children and adolescents who are typically developing (r=0.76)[141] or who have mild–moderate global developmental delay (r=0.74)[129] and (2) during a cycling protocol with children with DCD (r=0.59).[142] The SRT-I and the SRT-II also yield results that show concurrent validity with oxygen uptake measured during a treadmill test (r=0.96) with children and adolescents with CP.[132] The test results from the 20-m shuttle run performed by children with DCD[142,143] and children born preterm[144,145] show discriminate validity in that they are lower than those of their typically developing peers.

The minimal detectable change (95% confidence interval) for the time to complete the SRT is 0.84 minutes for the SRT-I and 0.50 minutes for the SRT-II.[132] Based on one exercise training study,[132] the average increase in completion time on the SRT-I or SRT-II after such an intervention is 2.4 SD 1.9 minutes, meaning that at the individual level the SRT-I or the SRT-II may detect changes in aerobic fitness after an exercise intervention in some but not all children with CP classified at levels I or II on the GMFCS.

Cycle ergometry

Overview and purpose
Maximal aerobic exercise tests performed on a cycle ergometer are often used in studies that evaluate multiple physiological responses to exercise where the extensive instrumentation on the child would make treadmill protocols impractical. As noted above, maximal oxygen uptake

values are about 10% lower with cycling protocols than with treadmill protocols.[122]

Administration and scoring
Several well-accepted cycling protocols suitable for children exist.[122] With the exception of the modified McMaster protocol discussed below, they have not been used with children with developmental disabilities and thus are not discussed here. A modified version of the McMaster protocol[146] has been used to assess the aerobic fitness of children with CP (75% ambulatory) and that of their able-bodied peers.[60] This test uses the 2-minute stages of the original McMaster protocol. However, rather than impose a cadence of 50 revolutions per minute and use the exercise intensities based on body height of the original test (which results in a linear increase in power output from stage to stage), children are allowed to pedal at their own rhythm, and intensity at each stage is individually determined such that the test lasts the expected 8 to 12 minutes. Minute-to-minute cadence must be monitored for this protocol to allow for the calculation of power output at each stage. Cairney et al[142] evaluated aerobic fitness in children with DCD using a cycling protocol with a fixed pedalling cadence of 60 to 65 revolutions per minute.[142] The initial stage was 3 minutes with a power output of 20W. This was increased to 40W for the fourth minute, and then increased by 20W each minute thereafter until the final stages, when 15-W increases were used. The completion time was not reported.

Psychometric properties
Aerobic power (maximal power output) determined using the modified McMaster protocol is reliable (test–retest) in children with CP (ρ≥0.72) and in typically developing children (ρ≥0.90).[60] This protocol also has discriminant validity in that aerobic power is lower in those with CP than that in their typically developing peers.[60] The modified McMaster protocol is also able to detect changes in aerobic fitness following training at the group level with children with CP.[60] The reliability of the above-mentioned cycling protocol used in children with DCD is unknown, but the test shows discriminant validity such that maximum oxygen uptake was lower for those with DCD than for their typically developing peers.[142]

Arm ergometry

Overview and purpose
Arm-cranking protocols are useful in situations where lower limb protocols are not feasible owing to impairment(s) of the lower limbs. Maximum oxygen uptake determined with an arm-cranking protocol is

about 60% to 80% of that determined from a lower limb protocol.[147] While it is well accepted that arm-cranking protocols are an appropriate method to evaluate the effect on aerobic fitness of upper limb aerobic exercise training, it is less well known that arm-cranking protocols are also sensitive to changes in aerobic fitness after a lower limb exercise training protocol.[148–150] Thus, arm-cranking protocols can be used to evaluate the effects on maximum oxygen uptake of a walking exercise programme with children who are ambulatory but who cannot cycle or walk on a treadmill without support, as is the case with certain children with CP classified at levels II and III on the GMFCS.[148,150]

Administration and scoring

The McMaster arm-crank protocol has been used to evaluate aerobic fitness in children and young adults with CP.[148] With this test, the power output at each 2-minute stage and the cadence (standard cadence=50 revolutions per minute) are individually determined based on a series of at least three submaximal arm-cranking trials. Unnithan et al[150] used a different test to evaluate the aerobic fitness of adolescents with CP.[150] For their test, the cadence was set at 50 revolutions per minute and power output during the first 4 minutes was 2.5W, with increases of 2.5W each minute for the subsequent stages.

Psychometric properties

While the test–retest reliability of maximal oxygen uptake using the McMaster protocol is unknown in children, results from test to test are reliable (r=0.94; 2-wk interval) in adults without a disability.[151] The reliability of results determined using the protocol from the Unnithan et al[150] study is unknown. Both protocols, however, are able to detect changes in maximum oxygen uptake at the group level after aerobic training with children with CP.[148,150]

Muscle endurance and exercise tolerance: submaximal aerobic exercise tests

Submaximal aerobic exercise tests use the same exercise modalities as maximal tests (walking/running on level ground or on a treadmill, cycling, arm cranking) but at intensities below the individual's maximum intensity. Two types of tests have been developed: predictive tests, used to predict aerobic fitness (e.g. maximum oxygen uptake), and capacity tests, used to measure the individual's ability to perform the activity itself.[152] Only walking capacity tests (i.e. walking economy and time/distance walk tests) are discussed in this review, because there is little information in the literature on arm cranking and cycling capacity tests in children with developmental disabilities

and because predictive tests are generally not used with this group, as maximal tests are for the most part safe to perform, assuming that standard safety procedures are followed[122] and the individual does not have marked cardiorespiratory impairment. As with maximal aerobic exercise tests, children should be well rested and should not consume caffeine on the test day if cardiorespiratory measures are to be taken, and they should avoid eating a heavy meal during the 2 to 3 hours before testing.[122] These tests are suitable for children ≥4 years of age assuming that they have the motor and cognitive skills necessary to perform the test. Similar to that required for maximal aerobic exercise tests, specialized equipment will be required if cardiorespiratory variables such as oxygen uptake and heart rate are to be measured. A calibrated treadmill will also be required for treadmill walking protocols. Ideally, children should be familiarized with the equipment used during the test. For detailed information on the equipment, see Paridon et al.[122] Whether or not the child uses a walking aid or other assistive device during the evaluation depends on the purpose of the test.

Walking economy tests

Overview and purpose

Walking economy tests assess walking capacity by measuring metabolic energy expenditure during walking at a given absolute or relative speed. This is done by measuring oxygen uptake. Energy expenditure can also be estimated indirectly by using a surrogate measure such as heart rate. The lower the energy expenditure (after normalizing for body size and speed if necessary), the greater the walking economy and the greater the walking proficiency.[153,154] It is assumed that the more economical the walker, the more he or she will be resistant to fatigue during walking.[155,156] The term walking efficiency, although sometimes used interchangeably with walking economy, refers to a different construct: the ratio of mechanical power output to metabolic energy expenditure input.[155] Walking economy tests can be done on a treadmill or over ground. The primary advantage of using a treadmill is that the walking speed can be controlled more easily, which eliminates the need to later adjust the results for differences in speed. For some groups, such as children with CP, however, the gait pattern is altered when walking on a treadmill compared with walking over ground.[157] This may limit the generalizability of treadmill protocol results to the child's day-to-day environment.

Administration and scoring

It is important that children be familiar with testing procedures, such as walking on a treadmill or breathing through a mask or mouthpiece (for oxygen uptake measurements), before testing is carried out. If a treadmill protocol is used, children should not support their body weight on the handrails during the test, except fleetingly for balance, as this will underestimate energy expenditure.[158] The choice of the walking speed(s) usually depends on the reason for the test and the abilities of the child. Tests last at least 2 minutes[159] to ensure that the child has reached a 'steady state', that is a plateau in the physiological measures of energy expenditure. Oxygen uptake or heart rate can be expressed as a net value, which does not include energy expenditure at rest (i.e. oxygen uptake during walking – oxygen uptake at rest), or as a gross value, which does. If resting measures are taken, in addition to avoiding exercise and caffeine on the testing day, children should rest at the testing site for at least 15 minutes before data collection. About 5 minutes of resting data collection are usually sufficient to ensure a resting steady state. Children can watch a 'neutral' video to prevent boredom (and fidgeting) during a resting measures protocol.

The effect of body size on oxygen uptake is accounted for when comparisons are made between children or within a child over time, typically by dividing by body mass, yielding oxygen uptake in millilitres per minute per kilogram. When having to control or normalize for differences in walking speed, one can divide by speed in metres per minute, in which case oxygen uptake would be expressed in litres per metre or millilitres per metre per kilogram. Other, more complicated, methods to normalize for body size and speed have been proposed[160] but are not used in this review as most of the literature on children with developmental disabilities reports results using the above-mentioned simpler normalization methods. Oxygen uptake, normalized for body mass and, if necessary, for speed, can also be converted to energy expenditure in joules by employing equations that use the child's respiratory exchange ratio to account for differences in the oxygen uptake–energy expenditure relationship based on the fuel source. When the net heart rate during steady-state walking is normalized by walking speed in the above-mentioned manner, that is walking heart rate in beats per minute minus resting heart rate in beats per minute divided by walking speed in metres per minute, the resulting heart rate in beats per metre (walked) is termed the 'physiological cost index'[161] or the 'energy expenditure index'.[162] Only the term 'physiological cost index' will be used in this review because the term 'physiological cost index' predates the term 'energy expenditure index' by several years and because one does not actually determine energy expenditure with this index as oxygen uptake is not measured.

Psychometric properties

Treadmill and overground walking economy at various speeds is reliable from test to test with typically developing children[163–166] and in those with CP,[163,167–169] whether walking economy is quantified as gross or net oxygen uptake[164,166–168] or energy expenditure[163] or is quantified using the physiological cost index[165,168,169] (i.e. reliability coefficients ≥0.91 with the interval between the tests varying, depending on the study, from within the same day, to within a week or a month, to annually over 4y). Gross energy expenditure during overground walking is also reliable for children with spina bifida (ICC=0.91, 2-wk interval).[170] For all three of these populations, the reliability of net oxygen uptake appears to be slightly lower than that of gross oxygen uptake.[163,170,171] The reliability of oxygen uptake and of the physiological cost index is also lower than the above-mentioned range of values for children with CP who have the same topographic distribution of spasticity[172] or the same GMFCS level.[168] This is possibly because of the decreased variability between the individuals within these subgroups compared with the variability in the general population of ambulatory children with CP.

Construct (concurrent) validity with gross oxygen uptake has been shown for heart rate during treadmill walking over a wide range of speeds ($r \geq 0.91$) with typically developing children and for those children with CP.[173] This suggests that a heart rate-based walking economy measure such as the physiological cost index is a valid one for these populations. As the exact oxygen uptake–heart rate relationship is specific to the individual,[174] and as the strength of a correlation depends in part on the variability within the data, it is not surprising to find weaker relationships between oxygen uptake and the physiological cost index ($0.50 \leq r \leq 0.66$) when the correlations are between children with CP walking on the treadmill at the same absolute speed[175] or walking overground at the same relative speed.[168,176] For children with spastic CP walking on the treadmill at 3.0km/h, Unnithan et al[154,159] showed convergent validity of gross oxygen uptake with measures of walking proficiency, that is antagonist muscle co-activation at the thigh ($r=0.72$) and lower leg ($r=0.66$) and mechanical power output ($r=0.93$). Keefer et al[177] did not find a relationship between net oxygen uptake during treadmill walking at various speeds and antagonist muscle co-activation at the thigh for children with CP of the spastic hemiplegic type. This may be owing to the lower level of antagonist muscle co-activation of this group compared with that of the children in the Unnithan et al[154,159] study. It may also be because of the method Keefer et al[177] used to quantify co-activation, as the level of co-activation between the participants' 'involved' and 'uninvolved' thighs was similar. Gross oxygen uptake or energy expenditure discriminates between the treadmill[159] and overground[163,178] walking economy of children with CP and that of their typically developing peers. Both oxygen uptake[168,178,179] and the physiological cost index[168] discriminate between children with CP classified at different GMFCS levels. Running economy, measured as gross oxygen uptake during treadmill running at several speeds, however, was not different between males with DCD and their typically developing peers.[180]

For typically developing children and adolescents, Brehm et al[171] reported a minimal detectable change of 9.1% (95% confidence interval) for gross energy expenditure during overground walking. For children with CP, the minimal detectable change at a 95% confidence interval for this type of measure has been reported to be as low as 6.8%[163] to 15%[181,182] and as high as 33%.[168] Given the small sample sizes of the studies of Thompson et al[168](n=23) and of Brehm et al[163] (n=13) compared with that of Oeffinger et al[181, 182] (n=292), it may be that the results of 15% are the more generalizable. Detecting a difference of 15% in overground walking economy using gross oxygen uptake may be sufficient to detect differences in individual children with CP after lower limb orthopaedic surgery.[183] The minimal detectable difference at a 95% confidence interval for the physiological cost index has been reported to be between 26%[168] and 40%[176] when the same methods are used to calculate this statistic. However, significant changes in overground walking economy quantified using this index are about 11% on average after the use of ankle–foot orthoses[184] or after a lower limb strength training programme.[185] Thus, it is unlikely that the physiological cost index can detect changes in walking economy in individual children following these types of interventions. For the time being, until more is known about differences in the physiological cost index after other interventions, its utility in detecting intervention-related change appears to be limited to measuring differences at the group level.

Six-minute Walk Test

Overview and purpose
The Six-Minute Walk Test (6MWT) is a measure of functional walking capacity that was originally designed for use with adults with respiratory impairments.[186]

Administration and scoring
The child performs this test by walking along a level walkway over a 6-minute time period. Instructions to the child before and during the test are standardized.[186] The child is told to cover the greatest distance that he or she can in

6 minutes. Rests (sitting or standing) are allowed, with no limit as to their duration or frequency, but the child is informed before the test to return to walking as soon as he or she can after stopping to rest. Rest time is included in the 6 minutes, that is the clock does not stop even if the child stops. The 6MWT is scored as the total distance walked in metres.[186] Longer distances reflect greater walking capacity. The walkway is generally 30m in length, but shorter and longer distances have been used depending on what is available at the evaluation site.[186] Walkway lengths between 15 and 50m will not affect test scores, but oval tracks will result in higher scores (longer distances), at least in adults with respiratory impairments.[186]

It has been suggested that test results may improve with a practice walk for children with CP classified at level I on the GMFCS.[187] This, however, is not the case when both walks are done on the same day.[188] In general for typically developing children, those who are older and bigger will cover longer distances than their younger and smaller peers.[189–191] No such significant relationships were found for a small group (n=22) of children with a physical disability (spina bifida).[192] Given that the correlation coefficients in the study by Hassan[192] were not stated, however, it is uncertain whether or not the failure of these authors to find a significant relationship between the distance walked and age or anthropometric factors was due to low statistical power. Thus, although not done at present in the literature for children with developmental disabilities, it is probably prudent to control for the effects of age and height on the distance walked if one wishes to evaluate walking capacity in relation to a developmental disability and not to growth and maturation per se.

Psychometric properties
With typically developing children, the 6MWT distance is reliable from test to test (ICC=0.94; 2- to 4-wk interval).[193] Test scores are also reliable (ICC=0.98) for children with CP, whether the tests are done on the same day[188] or on different days (1- to 4-wk interval).[187] Test–retest reliability for children with CP within the same GMFCS level can be somewhat less,[187,188] probably because there is less variability within the subgroup than within the total group of ambulatory children with CP. Convergent validity ($0.44 \leq r \leq 0.62$) with maximum oxygen uptake (i.e. aerobic fitness) has been shown for typically developing children[193–196] and for those with spina bifida (r=0.46).[197] As the strength of the relationship between maximum oxygen uptake and the distance walked is modest, the 6MWT cannot be considered an evaluation of aerobic fitness for these groups. The 6MWT distance discriminates between children with CP classified at different levels on the GMFCS.[187]

SIX-MINUTE WALK TEST (6MWT)

Purpose	To evaluate functional walking capacity in a clinical setting without the need for specialized equipment. The test can also be performed over level ground outside (weather permitting)
Population	The 6MWT was originally designed for use with adults with respiratory impairments, but it is now used with children (age ≥4y) and adults with a wide range of impairments that could theoretically affect walking capacity. To perform the test, the individual has to be able to walk and follow test directions
Description of domains (subscales)	Single scale: the total distance walked in 6min. Optional scales include the number and duration of rest periods and the energy expenditure during walking
Administration and test format	Time to complete: approximately 20min (pretest rest period, test, recovery period). Completion time can be greater if physiological measures are taken simultaneously or if habituation to the protocol is required
	Testing format: the test can be administered by a therapist or another health professional in a quiet area. A physician is required only when the physiological responses may be unstable. The child walks up and down a 30-m walkway, with the distance marked off at regular intervals. Slightly shorter or longer walkways can also be used. Children are asked to cover the longest distance they can in 6min, with rests only if needed
	Scoring: the test is scored as the total distance (metres) covered in 6min
	Training: no specialized training is required unless children have unstable physiological responses, in which case certification in basic life support is desirable
Psychometric properties	Normative sample: normative data for children have been collected in the USA, Germany, Hong Kong and Tunisia
	Reliability Test–retest reliability with typically developing children and with those with cerebral palsy is good to excellent (intraclass correlation coefficient [ICC] ≥0.94). The lower test–retest reliabilities (ICC ≥0.59) reported for subgroups of children with cerebral palsy, i.e. grouped as per their Gross Motor Function Classification System level, may be due to decreased variability amongst the children within each level
	Validity Convergent validity ($0.44 \leq r \leq 0.62$) with maximum oxygen uptake has been reported for typically developing children and for those with spina bifida
	Responsiveness: In children with cerebral palsy, the minimal detectable change is 16% (54.9m). The test is probably not able to detect change in children classified in Gross Motor Classification System level III after interventions such as robotic-assisted gait training; based on data from young adults with cerebral palsy, the test may be sensitive to changes in walking capacity after lower limb strength training in individuals with cerebral palsy with less motor impairment
How to order	Test guidelines are reported in American Thoracic Society (2002)
	Modifications to the test for young children are reported in Thompson et al (2008).
Key references	American Thoracic Society (2002) ATS statement: guidelines for the six-minute walk test. *Am J Respir Crit Care Med* 166: 111–117.
	Ben Saad H, Prefaut C, Missaoui R, Mohamed IH, Tabka Z, Hayot M (2009) Reference equation for 6-min walk distance in healthy North African children 6–16 years old. *Pediatr Pulmonol* 44: 316–324.

Key references	Geiger RA, Strasak B, Treml K, et al (2007) Six-minute walk test in children and adolescents. *J Paediatr* 150: 395–399.
	Li AM, Yin J, Yu CC, et al (2005) The six-minute walk test in healthy children: reliability and validity. *Eur Respir J* 25: 1057–1060.
	Li AM, Yin J, Au JT, et al (2007) Standard reference for the six-minute-walk test in healthy children aged 7 to 16 years. *Am J Respir Crit Care Med* 176: 174–180.
	Thompson P, Beath T, Bell J, et al (2008) Test–retest reliability of the 10-metre fast walk test and 6-minute walk test in ambulatory school-aged children with cerebral palsy. *Dev Med Child Neurol* 50: 370–376.

The minimal detectable change for the 6MWT distance for an individual child with CP is 16% (54.9m).[187] When children in this latter study[187] were grouped according to their GMFCS level, the minimal detectable difference varied from level to level. The interpretation of these differences, however, can differ depending on the reference point. For example, the absolute minimal detectable change for children classified at level III was 47.4m and thus lower than that for children at level I, which was 61.9m. Relative to their walking capacity (6MWT distance), however, the pattern is reversed. A 13% change can theoretically be detected for those at level I, whereas for those at level III the change in walking capacity must be at least 20%. Based on the data available in the literature for changes in the 6MWT distance following an intervention, the ability of the test to detect change in walking capacity with an individual child is probably related to the degree of his or her walking limitation and possibly to his or her age and the type of intervention received. After 10 weeks of lower limb strength training, for example, young adults with CP, 50% of whom walked without support, showed an average increase of 86m (31%) in the 6MWT distance.[198] After 3 to 5 weeks of robotic-assisted locomotion training, children with CP who all walked with support (classified at level III on the GMFCS), on the other hand, showed only an 18m (14%) change in the distance walked.[199] Until more information is available, clinicians wanting to detect change in individual clients may wish to use the 6MWT in conjunction with other tests of walking-related skills, such as dimension E of the GMFM. The test can also be used to detect change at a group level, as noted above.

10-m Walk Test

Overview and purpose

The 10-m Walk Test was originally designed to measure walking capacity in adults who had survived a stroke.[200] Ten metres is considered to be the minimum distance for 'functional' walking,[201] although this has not been explicitly evaluated with children.

Administration and scoring

The child performs the test by walking at a self-selected comfortable speed towards a target that is at least 12m away.[201] The middle 10-m section of the walkway is marked. The test is scored as the average time (one to three trials) required to traverse this 10-m section,[187,201] although others have used the best time of the trials.[48] Shorter times are considered to reflect better walking capacity. Instructions given to the child are standardized[201] and a practice trial is recommended.[187] The effect of age and anthropometric factors should probably be considered when one is comparing the results between children and within a child over time, although information on the specific effects of these factors on test results is currently lacking in the literature.

Psychometric properties

No results are available to the best of our knowledge for the reliability of this test for typically developing children. For adults without a diagnosed health condition, test–retest reliability (within-day) is good to excellent ($0.75 \leq r \leq 0.90$).[201] Thompson et al[187] evaluated between reliability (1- to 4 week interval) and the minimal detectable difference of a modified version of the 10-m Walk Test for children with CP. For this study, children were asked to walk at their 'fastest' speed. While these authors reported an acceptable test–retest coefficient of reliability (ICC=0.81), due to the wide 95% confidence interval in the ICC (0.65–0.90) and the large coefficient of variation (37%), they did not feel that the (modified) 10-m Walk Test was sufficiently reliable to be used as an outcome measure for children with CP. That being said, results with this modified 10-m Walk Test discriminate between children with CP classified at different levels on the GMFCS.[187] The minimal detectable change of the modified version of the 10-m Walk Test was reported to be 107% for ambulatory children with CP as a group.[187] Significant changes in the 10-m walk time for the standard test with children with CP, after interventions such as lower limb strength training[48] or vibration therapy,[202] is 30% to 40%. Until more is known about reliability and the ability to detect change of the standard 10-m Walk Test, it might be prudent to restrict the use of this test to the evaluation of change at the group level.

Measuring basic motor functions underlying gross motor development

Evaluation of gross motor movement in the early developmental years for infants who are considered to be at risk for a movement disorder (e.g. preterm infants) can be done with screening measures such as the Battelle Developmental Inventory, Bayley Scales of Infant Development III and the Alberta Infant Motor Scale (AIMS). Several of these have been described in depth in Chapter 18. It has been recommended that several serial assessments be done during the first 12 to 24 months of the child's life to portray a valid picture of the child's emerging motor abilities.

MORE ADVANCED TESTS OF GROSS MOTOR DEVELOPMENT

Young children who subsequently have a movement disorder such as CP can then be assessed (once there is no further need for normative scores) by the GMFM to track their acquisition of gross motor skills. Alternatively, if the child's movement disorder is mild, a motor control test such as the Movement Assessment Battery for Children (MABC) or Test of Gross Motor Development (TGMD) is suitable for further evaluation as the child gets older. The MABC and TGMD are described below, while the GMFM is discussed in detail in Chapter 23. This section includes tests that evaluate basic motor functions supporting the ability to perform advanced motor skills required by school-aged children at home, at school and in the community, including balance, coordination and other aspects of quality of movement.

Movement Assessment Battery for Children

Overview and purpose

The MABC identifies children with DCD and other mild motor impairments (rather than disorders with mobility restrictions such as CP).[203] Even though the MABC was not intended to evaluate change, it is frequently used in that capacity. This internationally recognized test has a translated version[204–207] and has been restandardized in several countries to provide culture-specific normative scores.[208,209] While designed as a screening measure, it

is also used for outcome evaluation as described below. The original MABC was created for children aged 4 to 12 years with tasks organized within four age bands. It contains three performance subtests: manual dexterity (three items), static and dynamic balance (two items) and ball skills (three items). These are administered by a therapist or other health professional. There is a separate 40-item parent or teacher checklist rating the child's motor competence. It considers everyday situations in which the child has to function, as well as a child's attitudes about motor tasks.

A revised edition, known as the MABC-2, is described in depth by Brown and Lalor.[204] In brief, the age range was broadened to 3 to 17 years, the items were revised slightly and a new standardization sample from the UK was introduced. The checklist was shortened by 50%, scoring age bands were combined, and administration and scoring was made easier.

Administration and scoring

Gross motor testing requires 20 to 40 minutes. There is no special training.[210] The child is given several trials of each item and his or her highest score is used. Item scores (in seconds or number of correct trials) are converted into point scores between 0 and 5, with higher scores indicating greater impairment. The total impairment standard score is translated into age-related centile scores based on normative data. Children scoring under the fifth centile are classified as having 'definite' motor problems, while those between the fifth and thirtieth centile have 'mild to moderate motor impairment', that is they are clumsier than their peers without necessarily having a definite motor problem. There is evidence that normative scores established in the USA apply to Europe.[207] Qualitative observations accompany the score sheet and can guide the treatment actions taken. The 10-minute parent/teacher checklist is informative for goal planning but does not give scores for diagnosis or evaluation of change. The test kit is available for approximately US$1000 through Pearson Assessments.

Psychometric properties

The results that follow pertain primarily to the original MABC. Inter-rater reliability of classification (normal/ at risk/impaired or pass/fail) has been tested for children with diagnosed movement difficulties[207] and with preschool children[211] and support its use as a diagnostic test. Test–retest reliability of the MABC performance test with typically developing children was demonstrated (ICCs and kappas for total score and individual items >0.70)[211–213] and confirmed when tested with children who were the least motor skilled in their class.[209] A pilot

MOVEMENT ABC (MABC) AND REVISED VERSION (MABC-2)	
Purpose	To evaluate mild to moderate movement difficulties in children and identify children with developmental coordination disorder (DCD) and other mild motor impairments. MABC-2 is profiled by its developers as an outcome measure, to assist in planning an intervention programme in either a school or clinical setting
Population	Children with identified movement difficulties. Original MABC was for children age 4–12y, while MABC-2 expanded the age range to children ages 3–16y
Description of domains (subscales)	Three performance subtests: manual dexterity (three items), static and dynamic balance (two items) and ball skills (three items). A separate 40-item checklist rates the child's motor competence in everyday situations, including his or her attitudes and feelings about motor tasks
Administration and test format	Time to complete: 20–40min for performance test, and 10min for checklist
	Testing format: performance subtests are administered by a therapist or other health professional. The child is given several trials of each item and the highest score is used. The checklist is completed by the child's parent or teacher
	Scoring: item scores (in seconds or number of correct trials) are converted into point scores between 0 and 5 – higher scores indicate greater impairment. The total impairment standard score is then translated into age-related centile scores based on normative data. Children scoring below the fifth centile are classified as having 'definite' motor problems, while those between the fifth and fifteenth centile have 'mild to moderate motor impairment', i.e. they are clumsy compared with their peers without necessarily having a definite motor problem
	Training: no specialized training
Psychometric properties	Normative sample: normative data have been collected in the USA, Canada and the UK for the original MABC. The MABC-2 has updated normative data. New normative data are being established by various research groups for children who live outside the USA
	Diagnostic accuracy: sensitivity and specificity of diagnosis for children with DCD was examined in relation to the DCD Questionnaire and the Bruininks–Oseretsky Test of Motor Proficiency. MABC is better able to identify children with DCD. Inter-rater reliability of classification (normal/at risk/impaired or pass/fail) has been verified for children with diagnosed movement difficulties and with preschool children
	Reliability Test–retest reliability of the MABC performance test with typically developing children is good to excellent (>0.70). Reliability of the MABC qualitative observations section has been confirmed for two items with children who were typically developing or had DCD or cerebral palsy
	Validity Correlations between the MABC and other measures vary from moderate (Bruininks–Oseretsky Test of Motor Proficiency, $r=-0.53$) to strong (Peabody Developmental Motor Scales, $r=0.75$). Discriminant validity was demonstrated in children who were either typically developing, had DCD or cerebral palsy
	Responsiveness In children with poor coordination, a change of six to eight points on the 40-point scale is required to be considered clinically important. Subscale scores are not as sensitive as the total score. Mean changes of 8 to 10 points have been observed in clinical studies with children with attention-deficit–hyperactivity disorder or DCD. While normative scores and centiles have been used to show a change from impaired to typical range, these scores lack sensitivity within diagnostic categories
How to order	The MABC-2 is available to appropriately qualified professionals from Pearson Assessments (www.pearsonassessments.com/HAIWEB/Cultures/en-us/Productdetail.htm?Pid=015–8541–308&Mode=summary). The cost is US$1150 for the examiner's kit

Key references	Brown T, Lalor A (2009) The Movement Assessment Battery for Children – Second Edition (MABC-2): a review and critique. *Phys Occup Ther Pediatr* 29: 86–103.
	Leemrijse C, Meijer OG, Vermeer A, Lambregts B, Ader HJ (1999) Detecting individual change in children with mild to moderate motor impairment: the standard error of measurement of the Movement ABC. *Clin Rehabil* 13: 420–429.
	Livesey D, Coleman R, Piek J (2007) Performance on the Movement Assessment Battery for Children by Australian 3- to 5-year-old children. *Child Care Health Dev* 33: 713–719.
	Van Waelvelde H, Peersman W, Lenoir M, Engelsman BC (2007) Convergent validity between two motor tests: Movement-ABC and PDMS-2. *Adapt Phys Act Quart* 24: 59–69.

study[214] confirmed the reliability of the qualitative observations section for two items of the MABC with children who were either typically developing or had DCD or CP. Brown and Lalor's[204] overview of the MABC-2 describes some reliability and validity work with the pilot version of the MABC-2 and stresses the importance of replicating this work with the final MABC-2.

From a diagnostic standpoint, the sensitivity and specificity of diagnosis for children with DCD[215] has been examined in relation to the DCD Questionnaire and the Bruininks–Oseretsky Test of Motor Proficiency.[216] While the MABC is better able to identify children with DCD, the authors recommended that clinicians use more than one test to confirm a diagnosis of DCD. Discriminant validity was demonstrated in children who are typically developing or have a diagnosis of DCD or CP.[214] For construct validity, correlations between the MABC and other measures vary from moderate (MABC and the performance score of the Bruininks–Oseretsky Test, $r=-0.53$)[217] to strong (PDMS and MABC, $r=0.75$).[209]

Two studies[203,209] evaluating the SEM and minimal detectable change of the performance scale in children with poor coordination are important when considering the MABC as an outcome measure. According to this work, the total score needs to change by six to eight points[203,209] on the 40-point scale. Subscale scores are not as sensitive as the total score, but may still be acceptable. A learning effect was noted, and thus a double baseline is recommended with use of the second test's score. In clinical trials, mean changes of 8 to 10 points have been observed in children with attention-deficit–hyperactivity disorder (ADHD) and DCD after intensive physical therapy,[218] in a parent and teacher cognitive-motor intervention approach in a randomized crossover study[219] and in a trial of neuromotor task training of children with DCD.[220] While normative scores and centiles have been used to show change from the impaired range to the typically developing range, these scores lack sensitivity within diagnostic categories. Instead, the total standard score should be used to evaluate change.[218,221]

While the focus of the MABC is on its use for children with DCD or ADHD, there are several papers applying it to other developmental diagnoses to include children with CP[214,222] and autism spectrum disorder.

Test of Gross Motor Development

There are several more advanced tests that are used by kinaesiologists, general and special educators, psychologists and physical therapists within the school setting to identify school-aged children who have gross motor problems. One of these, the Test of Gross Motor Development (TGMD-2),[223] has 12 skills categorized as locomotor (run, gallop, hop, leap, horizontal jump and slide) or object control (striking a stationary ball, stationary dribble, kick, catch, overhand throw and underhand roll). The test takes 15 to 20 minutes to administer. Scoring primarily considers the quality of motor patterns. Reliability, validity and normative scores are reported by the test developers in the manual. There are concerns about the lack of validation studies by groups other than the developers, and about outcome measurement using a tool designed to diagnose (i.e. normative scores).[221] However, a motor learning intervention demonstrated that TGMD mean scores improved from the second (poor) to tenth centile (below average).[220] The test has also been successfully used to measure change in trials with children with ADHD[224] and DCD.[225]

Balance tests

Balance, defined as postural control for movement that supports performance of everyday tasks,[226] is a key factor affecting gait and other functional skills. Clinical trials on children with CP and other developmental disabilities often assess balance by means of instrument laboratory-executed techniques such as force platform measurement, sway evaluation or computerized balance systems. In clinical practice, the GMFM or a balance subtest of motor developmental scales such as the Bruininks–Oseretsky Test of Motor Proficiency (BOTMP) or MABC tend to be used to evaluate balance skills. It has been noted that balance subscales that are within gross motor measures such as BOTMP or MABC may be too brief or too difficult to be sensitive measures of balance.[227]

There are several options for balance-specific assessments that can be used within a therapy or school environment and that require minimal time and set-up. The Timed Up and Go Test (TUG), Berg Balance Scale (BBS) and Functional Reach Test (FRT) are the best known of these. Each requires that the child co-operate with the test instructions, and hence these tests are reserved for use with children >4 years of age. All have been imported from adult rehabilitation measures and tested with children with CP, and each is described in detail below. One other test, the Timed Up and Down Stairs (TUDS), was developed as a functional balance measure for children with CP.[228] There appear to be only two published studies using the TUDS: one was a preliminary validation study by its developers and the other was within a physical training programme for children with CP in GMFCS levels I and II.[229] In the latter, there was a 25% improvement in speed (*p*<0.001).

Timed Up and Go Test

Overview and purpose
The TUG was introduced for the frail elderly to determine their risk of falling.[230] This test of functional mobility integrates walking skills, transitions and functional balance, and is also used in the paediatric setting.

Administration and scoring
The individual gets up from a chair on the word 'go', stands, walks (not runs) forward for 3m, turns and goes back the chair. Timing ends when the person's buttocks touch the chair.[231] The test was adapted for children by adding a target to touch.[232] The child wears shoes but not orthotics in the test. Gait devices are permitted. The test takes 5 to 10 minutes to complete.

Psychometric properties
The TUG has demonstrated strong reliability and validity with adults. In children, Williams et al[232] evaluated it in a sample of typically developing children as young as 3 years of age, and also in a sample of children with CP or spina bifida. Reliability was high, with an ICC of 0.84 for test–retest reliability in typically developing children and an ICC of 0.99 for within-session reliability for children with a disability. Gan et al[231] found that both intersession test–retest and inter-rater reliability were excellent (ICCs >0.95) for children with CP.

From a validity standpoint, the TUG was moderately to highly correlated with the GMFM

($-0.055<r>-0.90$)[231,232] and highly correlated with walking speed ($r=-0.93$) and the FRT ($r=-0.77$).[231] Although the TUG differentiated between children in GMFCS levels II and III,[231,232] its inability to discriminate between children in GFMCS levels I and II was noted.[231] This might have been due to insufficient study power since there was a 5-second mean difference in TUG scores between these two groups. Regardless, the TUG may not be suitable for children in GMFCS level I, whose main challenges pertain to higher level running and jumping skills.[231] The TUG was able to detect mobility changes in children with CP undergoing a functional strengthening intervention[233] and also with children receiving a home exercise programme.[234]

Berg Balance Scale

Overview and purpose
The BBS was developed to assess balance in the elderly.[235] It evaluates balance during functional activities, focusing on skill performance rather than underlying balance-related impairments.[236] Its 14 items test functional skills that underlie everyday activities and include reaching, bending, transferring and standing postures. Items progress from static positions to balance-challenging manoeuvres. The Pediatric Balance Scale (PBS) was modified from the BBS by Franjoine et al[226] for ambulatory school-aged children with mild to moderate motor impairments. The modification included reordering of test items, reducing static posture item time criteria, modifying test equipment to make it more child-friendly and providing greater instructional clarity.[226]

Administration and scoring
The test requires 15 to 20 minutes to complete. While there is no specific training protocol, detail about PBS administration and the minimal equipment required are provided in the appendix of the PBS development paper.[226] The original BBS is available at www.aahf.info/pdf/Berg_Balance_Scale.pdf and also as an appendix in the paper by Kembhavi et al.[236] During the test, the evaluator can offer cues and assistance as needed to permit full comprehension of the task. A single practice trial of each item is allowed, and items can then be tested up to three times. If the child scores the full score, no further trials are required.[231] By the age of 7 years, a typically developing child is expected to obtain full scores on all items. Items are scored on a five-point ordinal scale (0 [cannot perform] to 4 [normal performance]) with a total score out of 56 points. Some tasks are rated according to performance quality and others by time required.

Berg Balance Scale (BBS)

Purpose	To evaluate balance during functional activities, focusing on skill performance rather than underlying balance-related impairments
Population	Children aged 3y+ who can follow simple gross motor instructions and who are able to stand independently for at least 3s (Gross Motor Function Classification System levels I–III)
Description of domains (subscales)	Single scale of 14 items. Some tasks are rated according to performance quality and others by time required. A small modification was done for use in paediatrics and is known as the Paediatric Balance Scale (PBS) (Franjoine et al, 2003)
Administration and test format	Time to complete: 15–20min Testing format: after a single practice trial, an item can be tested up to three times. If the child scores the full score, no further trials are required. Scoring uses a five-point ordinal scale (0 [cannot perform] to 4 [normal performance]) with a total score out of 56 points. By age 7y, a typically developing child is expected to obtain full scores on all items. Regular therapy department equipment is required Training: no specialized training is required, but administration specifications and the minimal equipment required are provided in the appendix of the PBS development paper
Psychometric properties	*Reliability* Inter-rater reliability for BBS and PBS: ICC=0.99. Test–retest reliability for BBS and PBS:ICCs >0.95 for BBS and PBS *Validity* Correlations with Functional Reach Test (r=0.84), Timed Up and Go Test (r=−0.88) and Gross Motor Function Measure (r>0.95) Discriminant validity: able to differentiate between children who are typically developing and children with cerebral palsy who walk without devices or who use gait aids. Not able to differentiate between children in Gross Motor Function Classification System levels I and II *Responsiveness* In children in Gross Motor Function Classification System level I, there is evidence of a ceiling effect. Clinically important change (eight points) has been identified for adults, but not established for children
How to order	Test form and guidelines for BBS available in the appendix of the papers by Kembhavi et al (2002), while PBS materials are available in the appendix of Franjoine et al (2003)
Key references	Franjoine MR, Gunther JS, Taylor MJ (2003) Paediatric Balance Scale: a modified version of the Berg Balance Scale for the school-age child with mild to moderate motor impairment. *Pediatr Phys Ther* 15: 114–128. Gan SM, Tung LC, Tang YH, Wang CH (2008) Psychometric properties of functional balance assessment in children with cerebral palsy. *Neurorehabil Neural Repair* 22: 745–753. Kembhavi G, Darrah J, Magill-Evans J, Loomis J (2002) Using the Berg Balance Scale to distinguish balance abilities in children with cerebral palsy. *Pediatr Phys Ther* 14: 92–99.

Psychometric properties

Gan et al[231] found excellent inter-rater and test–retest reliability (ICCs ≥0.95) with the BBS with children in GMFCS levels I to IV. Franjoine et al[226] had similar results for the PBS when used with children with known balance difficulties. Measurement error estimates are not available from either study. From a validity standpoint, while the BBS discriminated between children with CP who used gait aids and those who were typically developing or had CP but walked without aids, it did not differentiate between children in GMFCS level I and typically developing children.[231] Notably, while BBS scores showed a ceiling effect with children in GMFCS level I,[231,236] Gan et al[231] did not find signs of a ceiling effect for the FRT or TUG when used with these same children, perhaps because these other measures are time and distance based and thus have a full range of values available.[231] There was strong correlation between BBS total score and FRT (*r*=0.84), TUG (*r*=−0.88), GMFM total score and walk score (*r*>0.95) and timed walk (*r*=0.84).[231] A change of eight points is considered clinically important with adults (www.aahf.info/pdf/Berg_Balance_Scale.pdf), but paediatric values need to be established.

Functional Reach Test

Overview and purpose
The FRT was developed for adults but has been adopted as a simple test of balance in children. From use with typically developing children, the FRT appears to be related to functional mobility and balance and is reflective of strength.[228]

Administration and scoring
The child raises his or her arm to 90° alongside a measuring stick attached to the wall, and the distance to the third metacarpal is recorded. The child then reaches forward as far as possible with the body straight and without losing balance from a fixed standing position (feet positioned within a drawn area on the floor).[237] The third metacarpal distance for the full reach position is measured and the difference from baseline reach is the FRT distance. Loss of balance demands a retest. One practice and one test trial are recommended.[237] Children need to have at least 90° of shoulder flexion to perform this test so it is best for children without upper limb impairment. They also need to be able to stand on their own for at least 1 minute. The FRT has been revised and outlined in detail by Bartlett and Birmingham[238] (renamed the Pediatric Reach Test [PRT]) and should be more applicable to a wide group of children with motor impairments.[238] It evaluates stability in sitting and standing for both forward and lateral reach.

Psychometric properties
For the FRT, intrarater and test–retest reliability was excellent (ICCs >0.80) in children with diplegia, with an SEM of 3cm,[237] and for the PRT inter-rater and test–retest reliability was excellent (ICCs >0.80) with an experienced rater but lower with a novice assessor.[238] In validity evaluations, scores were 25% to 45% lower than with typically developing children of a similar age,[237] and there was strong correlation between measures of age and FRT/PRT score,[237,238] moderate to strong correlation between force platform measures of limits of stability and PRT, and

moderate negative correlation between GMFCS levels and PRT reach distance support validity.[238] Katz-Leurer et al[234] observed FRT changes of 3cm in the experimental group in a trial of the impact of a home programme on children with CP.

QUALITY OF GROSS MOTOR MOVEMENT
As gross motor dysfunction is the defining problem for children with CP, considerable attention is paid to optimizing both what the child is able to do (his or her functional skill set) and the way that they do it (quality of movement). Enhancement of movement quality is important in relation to gait-based skills and pertains to factors associated with the safety and ease of movement (i.e. economy and efficiency of movement). It encompasses attributes such as coordination (accuracy, timing, speed, smoothness of movement), balance/stability, effort, dissociated movement, ability to shift weight appropriately and postural alignment. Failure to measure quality of movement means that a key focus of interventions provided to children with CP is not evaluated. Furthermore, 'negative' outcome trials that did not assess quality of movement may have missed this important aspect of change. The Gross Motor Performance Measure (GMPM)[239] is the only published quality of movement measure that addresses multiple components of quality of gross motor skills for children with CP.[240] Other multi-attribute scales of quality of movement in CP have focused on the upper extremity, and one such scale is discussed below, under 'Manual dexterity'.

The Gross Motor Performance Measure

Overview and purpose
The GMPM was developed as a companion measure to the GMFM's assessment of how much a child (aged 5mo–18y) can do in terms of motor function skills (refer to GMFM description in Chapter 23). The GMPM was developed using consensus methodology, and its purpose was to provide a quantitative way of measuring key aspects of quality of movement and to evaluate change in children with neurological disorders (e.g. CP and acquired brain injury).[239,241] Its five key attributes of movement quality are alignment, coordination, dissociated movement, stability and weight shift.

Administration and scoring
Quality of movement is evaluated within 20 of the GMFM's 88 gross motor items (i.e. four in each of the GMFM's five dimensions of lying/rolling, sitting, crawling, standing and walking/running/jumping). Each item is evaluated on three predesignated quality of movement

attributes on a five-point scale (normal movement to severe pathology). Summary scores are then calculated for each quality attribute across the items tested. An overall total score is also computed. The child needs to be able to at least partially perform the gross motor skill (GMFM score of '2') before a quality score can be given. The GMPM can be rated while watching the child's live performance of the GMFM items. Given the complexity of scoring three quality attributes at once, it has been recommended that scoring from a video of the assessment is preferable.[242] Self-training and practice are essential, and the GMPM manual provides detailed guidelines,[243] although training videos and criterion tests are no longer available. Assessment should be done by an experienced paediatric therapist with knowledge of normal/abnormal movement.[242]

Psychometric properties

The GMPM has shown good to excellent intra- and inter-rater reliability (ICC >0.80) with GMPM-experienced raters,[242,244,245] and excellent test–retest reliability (ICC=0.96)[244] for a 2-week retest. Reliability is enhanced by increased practice with use.[245] The GMPM discriminated among children in mild, moderate and severe impairment categories[246] and those judged by therapists to be stable versus those rated as having quality of movement changes.[246] There is evidence of its ability to detect change in relation to interventions such as orthopaedic surgery versus rhizotomy[247] and use of ankle orthoses.[248]

Two criticisms of the GMPM are the lack of item-specific response option descriptions and the need for highly experienced raters. In addition, the original focus of the GMPM was to consider quality of movement across *all* aspects of motor function evaluated on the GMFM. However, from a clinical perspective, work on improvements in movement quality is typically associated with higher level skills, that is those related to standing and walking rather than on basic skills in the areas of lying, crawling and sitting. It is only when basic foundational skills are adequately consolidated for the child to have them in his or her repertoire that quality of movement becomes of interest. It is important to have a measure that can help therapists and physicians to identify strengths and deficits as far as movement quality so that they can use this information in both intervention planning and outcome evaluation.

Consensus methods were used to produce a new ambulation-specific version for children aged 4 years and up in GMFCS levels I, II and III, measuring quality of movement for all skills tested in the GMFM's stand and walk dimensions. The number of GMPM response options was reduced from five to four to bring the scoring in line

with the GMFM's four-point scoring system, use of the distinction between quality with and without performance cues replaced the GMPM's focus on the pathology/no pathology distinction and item-specific response option wording to make the rating easier and thus more accessible to less-experienced therapists. Initial validation work with the Quality Function Measure has revealed excellent intra- and inter-rater and test–retest reliability (ICCs >0.80) and an ability to discriminate among children in GMFCS levels I, II and III.[22] A training and criterion testing CD-ROM is under development by the Quality Function Measure's creators.

Measuring basic motor functions underlying fine motor development

Basic motor functions supporting manual dexterity include the individual's ability to grasp, lift and release objects with speed and accuracy with minimal object manipulation. As therapists often provide services to persons with deficits in manual dexterity, measures of speed and accuracy are needed to evaluate changes over time. Many tests used in paediatric practice were first developed to measure hand dexterity in adults receiving rehabilitation services. Nonetheless, these measures have been standardized using populations of children to establish normative data. Three tests are commonly used to measure manual dexterity changes and to document research outcomes in current literature. One other test that is described is used to evaluate the way in which the child performs the activities (quality of movement).

MANUAL DEXTERITY

Box and Block Test

Overview and purpose

The Box and Block Test (BBT) was originally created in the early 1950s by A Jean Ayres and Patricia Holser Buehler as a test that could be completed by persons with severe dexterity deficits. At that time, blocks and a bowl were used to test adults with CP. Later, the BBT was standardized and copyrighted in 1957.[249] The purpose of the test is to measure gross manual dexterity as well as prevocational skills. Normative data for children aged 6 to 19 years as well as for adults provide comparative age and sex data. As such, the test is descriptive/diagnostic as well as evaluative.

Administration and scoring

The test is a wooden box divided into two equal compartments with a high partition between them. Individuals sitting at a standard height table are instructed to transfer as many cubes as possible from one side of the partition to the other in 1 minute. A 15-second trial period precedes the test to allow the individual to adjust to the test. The hand being tested rests on the edge of the box until timing begins. The hand not being tested remains on its respective edge of the box for the duration of the test. Individuals have 1 minute to move as many blocks as possible to the opposite half of the box, first with the dominant and then the non-dominant hand. The time to administer the test is approximately 5 minutes.

Psychometric properties
The BBT was copyrighted and standardized for adults in the 1970s with reliability and validity studies reported.[250] Normative data for children for dominant and non-dominant hands were established in a sample of 471 children aged 6 to 19 years of age living in Wisconsin.[249] Test–retest and inter-rater reliability correlation coefficients are high for adults on the BBT ($r=0.97$ and $r=0.99$, respectively).[251] No psychometric testing has been completed with children.

NINE-HOLE PEG TEST

Overview and purpose
The Nine-hole Peg Test is a timed test in which nine pegs are inserted and removed from a 3×3 configuration of nine holes in a pegboard, and conducted with each hand separately. Original normative data were established with adults using a therapist-constructed pegboard.[252] Commercially available tests are now used with a plastic pegboard and pegs. The purpose of the Nine Hole Peg Test is to measure hand dexterity unilaterally and compare it with normative data by age and sex. The test has been used as a descriptive/diagnostic measure as well as an evaluative measure pre- and post intervention.

Administration and scoring
The participant completes a practice trial, removing three pegs, before the actual test, which is performed for the dominant and the non-dominant hand. After the practice trial, the participant inserts and removes all nine pegs as quickly as possible while being timed. The hand not being tested remains on the participant's lap during testing. The number of seconds from picking up the first peg to removal of the last peg is the score for the hand tested. The time to administer the test is approximately 5 minutes.

Psychometric properties
Normative data for children were established on 826 children aged between 5 and 10 years and on 406 children aged

between 4 and 19 years.[254] Normative data are presented by age and sex. High inter-rater reliability ($r>0.99$) and test–retest reliability ($r=0.81$ and $r>0.79$) were reported.[253] Correlations of -0.80 and -0.74 between the scores on the Nine-hole Peg Test and Purdue Pegboard Test for children aged 5 to 10 years indicated adequate concurrent validity of the measures and a significant difference in test scores between regular and special education groups provided further evidence of construct validity.[253] Korean normative data were published by Yim and colleagues.[255]

Purdue Pegboard Test

Overview and purpose
The Purdue Pegboard is a test of dexterity originally designed to aid in the selection of adults applying for assembly line factory work.[256] Adult normative data were originally established on college students and veterans and industry applicants[256] with good psychometric properties documented. A pilot study in 1958[257] investigated adolescent males only on the test and concluded that males over 15 years of age could be tested using adult normative data. A much larger study of 1334 school-age children of 5 to 16 years of both sexes from the greater New York City area were included to establish normative data.[258] Additional normative data for children were published in 1986 by Mathiowetz et al.[259] Normative data for preschool children were reported by Wilson and colleagues[260] on the peg subtest only while using the right hand, left hand and both hands.

The purpose of the Purdue Pegboard Test is to measure manual dexterity in children and it can be used as a diagnostic and evaluative tool. According to the manual, two types of dexterity are measured: dexterity involving gross movement of the arms, hand and fingers, and 'fingertip' dexterity. Four subtests are included: right hand, left hand, both hands and assembly. The last two subtests of this assessment tool measure unilateral and bilateral manual dexterity. Research results suggest that females perform faster on three of the four subtests and suburban participants scored better than urban peers.

Administration and scoring
The board consists of two parallel rows of 25 holes each. Pins, collars and washers used for the test are located in four cups at the top of the board. Mathiowetz et al[259] had children complete a total of three trials for each of the four subtests using the following sequence: right hand, left hand, both hands and assembly. The total number of pegs placed in the holes in a 30-second trial period is recorded. For the assemblies, the child is asked to insert the peg with

the right hand while the left hand picks up and places the washer on the peg, followed by the right hand placing the collar and the left hand placing a second washer on top. The time to administer the test is approximately 15 minutes. The mean of the three trials is computed for the final raw score. Raw scores are converted to standard scores based on normative age and sex data.

Psychometric properties
Validity was studied by Gardner and Broman,[258] comparing children with and without diagnosed minimal brain dysfunction and demonstrating significant differences ($p<0.01$) between groups. They therefore recommended the use of the Purdue pegboard in a diagnostic battery for children with suspected central nervous system deficits. Developmental trends of increased proficiency with age were documented in preschool children,[260] supporting construct validity for children ($n=206$). The authors also reported high test–retest reliability for the right hand ($r=0.85$) and left hand ($r=0.92$) in a sample of 104 children between the ages of 2 years 6 months and 5 years 11 months.

Quality of Upper Extremity Skills Test

Overview and purpose
The Quality of Upper Extremity Skills Test (QUEST) is a criterion-referenced test used to evaluate the quality of movement patterns and hand function in children with CP.[261] Items are designed to measure unilateral function (both arms, one at a time) including the four domains of dissociated movements, grasp, protective extension and weight bearing during play. Items are related to quality of movement, not chronological age. The measure is useful in describing quality of movement clinically and detecting changes in function before changes in skill level are apparent. As such, the QUEST is considered an evaluative assessment, but not a discriminative tool, and has been used as an outcome measure for intervention research investigations.

Administration and scoring
Items are administered in a play (non-standardized) format, requiring approximately 30 to 45 minutes to complete. Each of the 34 items are scored on a two-point scale (yes=2 points, no=1 point, not tested=1 point). Scores are then calculated as percentages, with a higher percentage representing better quality of movement. The QUEST manual is available free of charge at www.canchild.ca/en/measures/quest.asp. Test administration time ranges from 30 to 45 minutes.

Psychometric properties
Three reliability studies were completed with children aged 18 months to 8 years who had a diagnosis with CP. Interobserver reliability coefficients for the QUEST total score ranged from 0.90 to 0.96; however, individual item coefficients showed greater variability (0.51–0.93).[261] Test–retest reliability studies of QUEST total scores resulted in high (ICC: $r=0.95$)[261] and moderate to high (Spearman's rho: $r=0.85–0.94$) correlation coefficients.[262] There was concurrent validity with the Peabody Developmental Motor Scales (PDMS) – Fine Motor Scales ($r=0.84$), with correlations between QUEST domains and subscores of the PDMS ranging from 0.58 to 0.84. Concurrent validity of the QUEST total score with the Melbourne Assessment of Unilateral Upper Limb Function total score was 0.83.[263] Construct validity of the QUEST with the therapist's judgement of level of hand function in 71 children was 0.72 for left hand function and 0.58 for right hand function.[261]

VISUAL MOTOR INTEGRATION FOR UPPER LIMB

Beery–Buktenica Developmental Test of Visual Motor Integration, fifth edition

Overview and purpose
The Beery–Buktenica Test of Visual Motor Integration (Beery-VMI) was designed as a measure of the degree to which visual perception and motor behaviour (eye–hand coordination) are integrated in children.[264] The first edition was published in 1967, and it has been standardized five times between 1964 and 2003. In the manual the authors offer the reader a historical perspective of VMI test development over the decades. The Beery-VMI is a developmental sequence of geometric forms to be copied in the paper booklet with a pencil. The 30-item full form Beery-VMI was developed and standardized for children between 2 and 18 years of age. The Beery-VMI short form (for ages 2–7y) contains the six marking and scribbling items plus 15 Beery-VMI forms to copy for a total of 21 items. A 30-item adult form is also available for adults aged 19 to 100 years. Two optional standardized tests are also included in the Beery-VMI, fifth edition: the Beery-VMI Visual Perception Test, designed to measure non-motor visual perception, and the Beery-VMI Motor Coordination Test, designed to measure relatively pure motor performance. Formal training is not required. The Beery-VMI has been used extensively by numerous disciplines as a discriminative/descriptive measure, a screening/predictive measure and as an evaluative measure.

QUALITY OF UPPER EXTREMITY SKILLS TEST (QUEST)	
Purpose	Designed to evaluate the quality of movement patterns and hand function in children with cerebral palsy (CP)
Population	Children with CP aged 18mo–8y

Description of domains (subscales)	Quality of upper extremity function is measured in four domains:
	    Dissociated movement
	    Grasp
	    Protective extension
	    Weight bearing

Administration and test format	Time to complete: 30–45min to administer Testing format: 36 items assessing dissociated movements, grasp, protective extension and weight bearing administered in a play format Scoring: scores are calculated as percentages with a high score of 100. Higher scores represent better quality of movement Training: no specialized training is required
Psychometric properties	Normative sample: criterion-referenced assessment *Reliability* 71 children, ages 18mo–8y, in Ontario, Canada, diagnosed with spastic CP and with spasticity present in the wrist and hand during movement Test–retest: 0.75–0.95 Inter-rater: 0.51–0.96 with all coefficients except one >0.70 *Validity* Concurrent validity with the Peabody Developmental Motor Scales (PDMS): fine motor is 0.84. Correlations between QUEST domains and subscores of the PDMS range from 0.58 to 0.84. Construct validity with therapist's judgement of child's level of hand function – 0.72 for left hand function and 0.58 for right hand function *Responsiveness* QUEST was responsive to changes in quality of movement after upper extremity casting in a study of 72 children with CP
How to order	Available to download for free at: www.canchild.ca/en/measures/quest.asp
Key references	DeMatteo C, Law M, Russell D, Pollock N, Rosenbaum P, Walter S (1993) The reliability and validity of Quality of Upper Extremity Skills Test. *Phys Occup Ther Pediatr* 13: 1–18. Klingels K, De Cock P, Desloovere K, et al (2008) Comparison of the Melbourne Assessment of Unilateral Upper Limb Function and the Quality of Upper Extremity Skills Test in hemiplegic CP. *Dev Med Child Neurol* 50: 904–909.

Administration and scoring

The Beery-VMI may be administered in individual or group format. For children over 6 years of age, testing begins with copying tasks 7, 8 and 9, omitting the scribbling and marking items. The ceiling is reached after three consecutive forms have failed. The child's raw score is determined by the number of forms passed up to three consecutive failures. Raw scores may be converted to standard scores, stanines, age equivalents, centiles and scaled scores. Authors recommend the use of standard scores (mean 100, SD 15). Scores SD 20 points of the mean are considered high and low for score interpretation. Authors stress that age-equivalent scores are to be used with caution. The entire test takes 10 to 15 minutes to complete.

BEERY–BUKTENICA TEST OF VISUAL MOTOR INTEGRATION (BEERY-VMI)	
Purpose	Devised as a measure of the degree to which visual perception and motor behaviour are integrated in children
Population	Ages 2–18y. Designed primarily for children in preschool and early primary grades
Description of domains (subscales)	A series of 24 geometric forms are copied in a manual in a developmentally sequenced order
	The first forms are three types of marking or scribbling items for younger children only for a total of 30 items in the entire test
	Short form (for ages 2–7y) contains the six marking and scribbling items plus 15 Beery-VMI forms to copy for a total of 21 items
	Two supplemental tests, the Visual Perceptual Test and the Motor Coordination Test, are also provided for comparison of VMI with pure visual and motor performance of an individual
Administration and test format	Time to complete: 10–15min
	Testing format: 24 geometric forms are copied in the provided manual with direction from the administrator. May be used in a group format
	Scoring: basal for children over 6y, who begin with copying tasks 7, 8 and 9 (omit scribbling and marking items). Ceiling is reached after three consecutive forms have not been passed. Raw score is determined by the number of forms passed up to three consecutive failures. The test provides standard scores, stanines, age equivalents, centiles and scaled scores. The authors suggest the use of standard scores (mean=100, standard deviation=15). Scores ±20 points of the mean are considered high and low for score interpretation. Authors stress that age-equivalent scores should be used with caution
	Training: training is not required
Psychometric properties	Normative sample: normative data based on 2512 individuals, aged 2–18y. The majority of test items have been previously standardized five times with over 11 000 children between 1964 and 2003. Representation of geographic, ethnic and sex characteristics are representative of US census percentages
	Reliability Inter-rater: r=0.92 for VMI, 0.98 for Visual Perception, 0.93 for Motor Coordination, supporting high reliability
	Test–retest: r=0.89 for VMI, 0.85 for Visual Perception, 0.86 for Motor Coordination, within a 10-day window of time
	Split-half: r=0.88 for VMI, 0.85 for Visual Perception, 0.87 for Motor Coordination and coefficient alpha (r=0.82 for VMI, 0.82 for Visual Perception, 0.82 for Motor Coordination)
	Validity Content validity is highly supported with item analysis over decades; quantitatively assessed by Rasch–Wright and other item analyses. Concurrent validity with Developmental Test of Visual Perception resulted in r=0.75 for VMI; and 0.62 for Visual Perception; 0.62 for Motor Coordination. Predictive validity study reported by authors stated correct prediction of 85% of kindergarten children who had reading problem 7y later. Authors also cite numerous studies using the Beery-VMI in conjunction with other tests for predicting school performance
How to order	The test can be ordered from Academic Therapy Publications (www.academictherapy.com). The cost is US$160 for the starter kit
Key references	Alyward EH, Schmidt S (1986) An examination of three tests of visual-motor integration. *J Learn Disabil* 19: 328–330.
	Tseng MH (1994) Differences in perceptual-motor measures in children with good and poor handwriting. *Occup Ther J Res* 14: 19–36.

Psychometric properties

Normative data are based on 2512 individuals aged 2 to 18 years. The majority of test items have been previously standardized five times with over 11 000 children between 1964 and 2003. The normative sample was selected as a representation of geographic, ethnic and sex characteristics according to US census percentages. High inter-rater reliability has been reported for all versions of the Beery-VMI, fifth edition (r=0.92 for VMI; 0.98 for the Visual Perception Test; 0.93 for the Motor Coordination Test). Good test–retest reliability has also been reported (r=0.89 for VMI; 0.85 for the Visual Perception Test; 0.86 for the Motor Coordination Test) with testing completed within a 10-day window of time. Other measures of reliability include split-half reliability (r=0.88 for VMI; 0.85 for the Visual Perception Test; 0.87 for the Motor Coordination

Test) and coefficient alpha (r=0.82 for VMI; 0.82 for the Visual Perception Test; 0.82 for the Motor Coordination Test).

Content validity is highly supported with item analysis over decades, quantitatively assessed by Rasch and other item analyses. Concurrent validity with the Developmental Test of Visual Perception resulted in r=0.75 for VMI total score (0.62 for the Visual Perception Test; 0.62 for the Motor Coordination Test). The Beery-VMI has also been used as a predictive tool for children's future performance. A predictive validity study stated the correct prediction of 85% of kindergarten children who had reading problems 7 years later. Throughout this chapter the authors have also cited numerous studies using the Beery-VMI in conjunction with other tests for predicting school performance.[264]

REFERENCES

1. Bayley N (1935) The development of motor abilities during the first three years or life. *Monog Soc Res Child Dev* 1: 1–26.
2. Gesell A, Amatruda CS (1949) *Gesell Developmental Schedules*. New York: Psychological Corporation.
3. McGraw MB (1943) *The Neuromuscular Maturation of the Human Infant*. New York: Columbia University Press.
4. Campbell SK, Palisano RJ, Vander Linden DW (2006) *Physical Therapy for Children*, 3rd edition. St. Louis, MO: Sanders Elsevier.
5. Case-Smith J (2005) *Occupational Therapy for Children*. St Louis, MO: Mosby.
6. Haywood KM, Getchell N (2009) *Life Span Motor Development*. Champaign, IL: Human Kinetics.
7. Schmidt RA, Wrisberg CA (2004) *Motor Learning and Performance*. Champaign, IL: Human Kinetics.
8. Shumway-Cook A, Woollacott MH (2007) *Motor Control Translating Research into Clinical Practice*, 3rd edition. Philadelphia PA: Lippincott Williams & Wilkins.
9. Thelen E (1995) Motor development. A new synthesis. *Am Psychol* 50: 79–95.
10. World Health Organization (2001) *International Classification of Functioning, Disability and Health*. Geneva: World Health Organization. Available at: www.who.int/classifications/icf/en/ (accessed 1 October 2011).
11. TenBerge SR, Halbertsma JP, Maathuis PG, Verheij NP, Dijkstra PU, Maathuis KG (2007) Reliability of popliteal angle measurement: a study in cerebral palsy patients and healthy controls. *J Pediatr Orthop* 27: 648–652.
12. Kilgour G, McNair P, Stott NS (2003) Intrarater reliability of lower limb sagittal range-of-motion measures in children with spastic diplegia. *Dev Med Child Neurol* 45: 391–399.
13. Pott P, Selley A, Tyson SF (2008) The reliability, responsiveness and clinical utility of the Proximat: a new tool for measuring hip range of movement in children with cerebral palsy. *Physiother Res Int* 13: 223–230.
14. Allington NJ, Leroy N, Doneux C (2002) Ankle joint range of motion measurements in spastic cerebral palsy children: intraobserver and interobserver reliability and reproducibility of goniometry and visual estimation. *J Pediatr Orthop B* 11: 236–239.
15. Glanzman AM, Swenson AE, Kim H (2008) Intrarater range of motion reliability in cerebral palsy: a comparison of assessment methods. *Pediatr Phys Ther* 20: 369–372.

16. Mutlu A, Livanelioglu A, Gunel MK (2007) Reliability of goniometric measurements in children with spastic cerebral palsy. *Med Sci Mon* 13: 323–329.
17. McDowell BC, Hewitt V, Nurse A, Weston T, Baker R (2000) The variability of goniometric measurements in ambulatory children with spastic cerebral palsy. *Gait Post* 12: 114–121.
18. McWhirk LB, Glanzman AM (2006) Within-session inter-rater reliability of goniometric measures in patients with spastic cerebral palsy. *Pediatr Phys Ther* 18: 262–265.
19. Fosang AL, Galea MP, McCoy AT, Reddihough DS, Story I (2003) Measures of muscle and joint performance in the lower limb of children with cerebral palsy. *Dev Med Child Neurol* 45: 664–670.
20. Koman LA, Williams RM, Evans PJ, et al (2008) Quantification of upper extremity function and range of motion in children with cerebral palsy. *Dev Med Child Neurol* 50: 910–917.
21. Bartlett D, Purdie B (2005) Testing of the spinal alignment and range of motion measure: a discriminative measure of posture and flexibility for children with cerebral palsy. *Dev Med Child Neurol* 47: 739–743.
22. Wright M, Bartlett DJ (2010) Distribution of contractures and spinal malalignments in adolescents with cerebral palsy: observations and influences of function, sex and age. *Dev Neurorehabil* 13: 46–52.
23. Bohannon RW, Smith MB (1987) Interrater reliability of a modified Ashworth scale of muscle spasticity. *Phys Ther* 67: 206–207.
24. Clopton N, Dutton J, Featherston T, Grigsby A, Mobley J, Melvin J (2005) Interrater and intrarater reliability of the Modified Ashworth Scale in children with hypertonia. *Pediatr Phys Ther* 17: 268–274.
25. Patrick E, Ada L (2006) The Tardieu Scale differentiates contracture from spasticity whereas the Ashworth Scale is confounded by it. *Clin Rehabil* 20: 173–182.
26. Yam WK, Leung MS (2006) Interrater reliability of Modified Ashworth Scale and Modified Tardieu Scale in children with spastic cerebral palsy. *J Child Neurol* 21: 1031–1035.
27. Tuzson AE, Granata KP, Abel MF (2003) Spastic velocity threshold constrains functional performance in cerebral palsy. *Arch Phys Med Rehabil* 84: 1363–1368.
28. Baker R, Jasinski M, iag-Tymecka I, et al (2002) Botulinum toxin treatment of spasticity in diplegic cerebral palsy: a

randomized, double-blind, placebo-controlled, dose-ranging study. *Dev Med Child Neurol* 44: 666–675.

29. Boyd RN, Pliatsios V, Starr R, Wolfe R, Graham HK (2000) Biomechanical transformation of the gastroc-soleus muscle with botulinum toxin A in children with cerebral palsy. *Dev Med Child Neurol* 42: 32–41.

30. Boyd RN, Graham HK (1999) Objective measurement of clinical findings in the use of botulinum toxin type A for the management of children with cerebral palsy. *Eur J Neurol* 6: S23–S35.

31. Gracies JM, Burke K, Clegg NJ, et al (2010) Reliability of the Tardieu Scale for assessing spasticity in children with cerebral palsy. *Arch Phys Med Rehabil* 91: 421–428.

32. Love SC, Valentine JP, Blair EM, Price CJ, Cole JH, Chauvel PJ (2001) The effect of botulinum toxin type A on the functional ability of the child with spastic hemiplegia: a randomized controlled trial. *Eur J Neurol* 8 (suppl.): 50–58.

33. Scholtes VA, Becher JG, Beelen A, Lankhorst GJ (2006) Clinical assessment of spasticity in children with cerebral palsy: a critical review of available instruments. *Dev Med Child Neurol* 48: 64–73.

34. Haugh AB, Pandyan AD, Johnson GR (2006) A systematic review of the Tardieu Scale for the measurement of spasticity. *Disabil Rehabil* 28: 899–907.

35. Mackey AH, Walt SE, Lobb G, Stott NS (2004) Intraobserver reliability of the modified Tardieu scale in the upper limb of children with hemiplegia. *Dev Med Child Neurol* 46: 267–272.

36. Lowing K, Bexelius A, Carlberg EB (2010) Goal-directed functional therapy: a longitudinal study on gross motor function in children with cerebral palsy. *Disabil Rehabil* 32: 908–916.

37. Slawek J, Klimont L (2003) Functional improvement in cerebral palsy patients treated with botulinum toxin A injections – preliminary results. *Eur J Neurol* 10: 313–317.

38. Ostensjo S, Carlberg EB, Vollestad NK (2004) Motor impairments in young children with cerebral palsy: relationship to gross motor function and everyday activities. *Dev Med Child Neurol* 46: 580–589.

39. Fowler EG, Staudt LA, Greenberg MB, Oppenheim WL (2009) Selective Control Assessment of the Lower Extremity (SCALE): development, validation, and interrater reliability of a clinical tool for patients with cerebral palsy. *Dev Med Child Neurol* 51: 607–614.

40. Jethwa A, Mink J, Macarthur C, Knights S, Fehlings T, Fehlings D (2010) Development of the Hypertonia Assessment Tool (HAT): a discriminative tool for hypertonia in children. *Dev Med Child Neurol* 52: e83–e87.

41. Barry MJ, VanSwearingen JM, Albright AL (1999) Reliability and responsiveness of the Barry–Albright Dystonia Scale. *Dev Med Child Neurol* 41: 404–411.

42. Mercer V, Lewis CL (2001) Hip abductor and knee extensor muscle strength of children with and without Down syndrome. *Pediatr Phys Ther* 13: 18–26.

43. Taylor NF, Dodd KJ, Graham HK (2004) Test–retest reliability of hand-held dynamometric strength testing in young people with cerebral palsy. *Arch Phys Med Rehabil* 85: 77–80.

44. Verschuren O, Ketelaar M, Takken T, Van BM, Helders PJ, Gorter JW (2008) Reliability of hand-held dynamometry and functional strength tests for the lower extremity in children with cerebral palsy. *Disabil Rehabil* 30: 1358–1366.

45. Damiano DL, Abel MF (1998) Functional outcomes of strength training in spastic cerebral palsy. *Arch Phys Med Rehabil* 79: 119–125.

46. Dodd KJ, Taylor NF, Graham HK (2003) A randomized clinical trial of strength training in young people with cerebral palsy. *Dev Med Child Neurol* 45: 652–657.

47. Berry ET, Giuliani CA, Damiano DL (2004) Intrasession and intersession reliability of handheld dynamometry in children with cerebral palsy. *Pediatr Phys Ther* 16: 191–198.

48. Blundell SW, Shepherd RB, Dean CM, Adams RD, Cahill BM (2003) Functional strength training in cerebral palsy: a pilot study of a group circuit training class for children aged 4–8 years. *Clin Rehabil* 17: 48–57.

49. Damiano DL, Martellotta TL, Sullivan DJ, Granata KP, Abel MF (2000) Muscle force production and functional performance in spastic cerebral palsy: relationship of cocontraction. *Arch Phys Med Rehabil* 81: 895–900.

50. Seniorou M, Thompson N, Harrington M, Theologis T (2007) Recovery of muscle strength following multi-level orthopaedic surgery in diplegic cerebral palsy. *Gait Post* 26: 475–481.

51. van der Linden ML, Aitchison AM, Hazlewood ME, Hillman SJ, Robb JE (2004) Test–retest repeatability of gluteus maximus strength testing using a fixed digital dynamometer in children with cerebral palsy. *Arch Phys Med Rehabil* 85: 2058–2063.

52. Vaz DV, Mancini MC, da Fonseca ST, Arantes NF, Pinto TP, de Araujo PA (2008) Effects of strength training aided by electrical stimulation on wrist muscle characteristics and hand function of children with hemiplegic cerebral palsy. *Phys Occup Ther Pediatr* 28: 309–325.

53. Crompton J, Galea MP, Phillips B (2007) Hand-held dynamometry for muscle strength measurement in children with cerebral palsy. *Dev Med Child Neurol* 49: 106–111.

54. Gaul CA (1995) Muscular strength and endurance. In: Docherty D, editor. *Measurement in Pediatric Exercise Science.* Champaign, IL: Human Kinetics, pp. 225–258.

55. Baltzopoulos V, Kellis E (1998) Isokinetic strength during childhood and adolescence. In: Van Praagh E, editor. *Pediatric Anaerobic Performance.* Champaign, IL: Human Kinetics, pp. 225–240.

56. Patikas D, Wolf SI, Armbrust P, et al (2006) Effects of a postoperative resistive exercise programme on the knee extension and flexion torque in children with cerebral palsy: a randomized clinical trial. *Arch Phys Med Rehabil* 87: 1161–1169.

57. Raynor AJ (2001) Strength, power, and coactivation in children with developmental coordination disorder. *Dev Med Child Neurol* 43: 676–684.

58. Herzog W (1988) The relation between the resultant moments at a joint and the moments measured by an isokinetic dynamometer. *J Biomech* 21: 5–12.

59. Molnar GE, Alexander J, Gutfeld N (1979) Reliability of quantitative strength measurements in children. *Arch Phys Med Rehabil* 60: 218–221.

60. van den Berg-Emons RJ, van Baak MA, de Barbanson, Speth L, Saris WH (1996) Reliability of tests to determine peak aerobic power, anaerobic power and isokinetic muscle strength in children with spastic cerebral palsy. *Dev Med Child Neurol* 38: 1117–1125.

61. Kramer JF, MacPhail HE (1994) Relationships among measures of walking efficiency, gross motor ability, and isokinetic strength in adolescents with cerebral palsy. *Pediatr Phys Ther* 6: 3–8.

62. Ayalon M, Ben-Sira D, Hutzler Y, Gilad T (2000) Reliability of isokinetic strength measurements of the knee in children with cerebral palsy. *Dev Med Child Neurol* 42: 398–402.

63. Damiano DL, Arnold AS, Steele KM, Delp SL (2010) Can strength training predictably improve gait kinematics? A pilot study on the effects of hip and knee extensor strengthening on lower-extremity alignment in cerebral palsy. *Phys Ther* 90: 269–279.

64. McNee AE, Gough M, Morrissey MC, Shortland AP (2009) Increases in muscle volume after plantarflexor strength training in children with spastic cerebral palsy. *Dev Med Child Neurol* 51: 429–435.

65. Eek MN, Tranberg R, Zugner R, Alkema K, Beckung E (2008) Muscle strength training to improve gait function in children with cerebral palsy. *Dev Med Child Neurol* 50: 759–764.

66. Patikas D, Wolf SI, Mund K, Armbrust P, Schuster W, Doderlein L (2006) Effects of a postoperative strength-training program on the walking ability of children with cerebral palsy: a randomized controlled trial. *Arch Phys Med Rehabil* 87: 619–626.

67. Unger M, Faure M, Frieg A (2006) Strength training in adolescent learners with cerebral palsy: a randomized controlled trial. *Clin Rehabil* 20: 469–477.

68. Eyre JA, Miller S, Clowry GJ, Conway EA, Watts C (2000) Functional corticospinal projections are established prenatally in the human foetus permitting involvement in the development of spinal motor centres. *Brain* 123: 51–64.

69. Forssberg H, Eliasson AC, Kinoshita H, Johansson RS, Westling G (1991) Development of human precision grip. I: Basic coordination of force. *Exp Brain Res* 85: 451–457.

70. Ager CL, Olivett BL, Johnson CL (1984) Grasp and pinch strength in children 5 to 12 years old. *Am J Occup Ther* 38: 107–113.

71. Mathiowetz V, Wiemer DM, Federman SM (1986) Grip and pinch strength: norms for 6- to 19-year-olds. *Am J Occup Ther* 40: 705–711.

72. Newman DG, Pearn J, Barnes A, Young CM, Kehoe M, Newman J (1984) Norms for hand grip strength. *Arch Dis Child* 59: 453–459.

73. Robertson A, Deitz J (1988) A description of grip strength in preschool children. *Am J Occup Ther* 42: 647–652.

74. Daniels L, Backman C (1993) Grip and pinch strength norm for children. *Phys Occup Ther Pediatr* 13: 81–90.

75. Fess EE (1987) A method for checking Jamar dynamometer calibration. *J Hand Ther* 1: 28–32.

76. Mathiowetz V, Weber K, Volland G, Kashman N (1984) Reliability and validity of grip and pinch strength evaluations. *J Hand Surg [Am]* 9: 222–226.

77. Cook RE, Schneider I, Hazlewood ME, Hillman SJ, Robb JE (2003) Gait analysis alters decision-making in cerebral palsy. *J Pediatr Orthop* 23: 292–5.

78. Mackey AH, Walt SE, Lobb GA, Stott NS (2005) Reliability of upper and lower limb three-dimensional kinematics in children with hemiplegia. *Gait Post* 22: 1–9.

79. Steinwender G, Saraph V, Scheiber S, Zwick EB, Uitz C, Hackl K (2000) Intrasubject repeatability of gait analysis data in normal and spastic children. *Clin Biomech* 15: 134–139.

80. Redekop S, Andrysek J, Wright V (2008) Single-session reliability of discrete gait parameters in ambulatory children with cerebral palsy based on GMFCS level. *Gait Post* 28: 627–633.

81. Schutte LM, Narayanan U, Stout JL, Selber P, Gage JR, Schwartz MH (2000) An index for quantifying deviations from normal gait. *Gait Post* 11: 25–31.

82. Tervo RC, Azuma S, Stout J, Novacheck T (2002) Correlation between physical functioning and gait measures in children with cerebral palsy. *Dev Med Child Neurol* 44: 185–190.

83. Tulchin K, Campbell S, Browne R, Orendurff M (2009) Effect of sample size and reduced number of principle components on the Gillette Gait Index. *Gait Post* 29: 526–529.

84. Romei M, Galli M, Motta F, Schwartz M, Crivellini M (2004) Use of the normalcy index for the evaluation of gait pathology. *Gait Post* 19: 85–90.

85. Bothner KE, Fischer R, Alderink G (2003) Assessment of reliability of the normalcy index for children with cerebral palsy. *Gait Post* 18: S3–S4.

86. Assi A, Ghanem I, Lavaste F, Skalli W (2009) Gait analysis in children and uncertainty assessment for Davis protocol and Gillette Gait Index. *Gait Post* 30: 22–26.

87. McMulkin ML, MacWilliams BA (2008) Intersite variations of the Gillette Gait Index. *Gait Post* 28: 483–487.

88. Hillman SJ, Hazlewood ME, Schwartz MH, van der Linden ML, Robb JE (2007) Correlation of the Edinburgh Gait Score with the Gillette Gait Index, the Gillette Functional Assessment Questionnaire, and dimensionless speed. *J Pediatr Orthop* 27: 7–11.

89. Romei M, Galli M, Fazzi E, et al (2007) Analysis of the correlation between three methods used in the assessment of children with cerebral palsy. *Funct Neurol* 22: 17–21.

90. Viehweger E, Haumont T, de Lattre C, et al (2008) Multidimensional outcome assessment in cerebral palsy: is it feasible and relevant? *J Pediatr Orthop* 28: 576–583.

91. Brochard S, Lempereur M, Filipetti P, Remy-Neris O (2009) Changes in gait following continuous intrathecal baclofen infusion in ambulant children and young adults with cerebral palsy. *Dev Neurorehabil* 12: 397–405.

92. Gorton GE, III, Abel MF, Oeffinger DJ, et al (2009) A prospective cohort study of the effects of lower extremity orthopaedic surgery on outcome measures in ambulatory children with cerebral palsy. *J Pediatr Orthop* 29: 903–909.

93. Gough M, Schneider P, Shortland AP (2008) The outcome of surgical intervention for early deformity in young ambulant children with bilateral spastic cerebral palsy. *J Bone Joint Surg Br* 90: 946–951.

94. Gordon AB, Baird GO, McMulkin ML, Caskey PM, Ferguson RL (2008) Gait analysis outcomes of percutaneous medial hamstring tenotomies in children with cerebral palsy. *J Pediatr Orthop* 28: 324–329.

95. Brehm MA, Harlaar J, Schwartz M (2008) Effect of ankle–foot orthoses on walking efficiency and gait in children with cerebral palsy. *J Rehabil Med* 40: 529–534.

96. Molloy M, McDowell BC, Kerr C, Cosgrove AP (2010) Further evidence of validity of the Gait Deviation Index. *Gait Post* 31: 479–482.

97. Schwartz MH, Rozumalski A (2008) The Gait Deviation Index: a new comprehensive index of gait pathology. *Gait Post* 28: 351–357.

98. Koman LA, Mooney JF, III, Smith BP, Goodman A, Mulvaney T (1994) Management of spasticity in cerebral palsy with botulinum-A toxin: report of a preliminary, randomized, double-blind trial. *J Pediatr Orthop* 14: 299–303.

99. Mackey AH, Lobb GL, Walt SE, Stott NS (2003) Reliability and validity of the Observational Gait Scale in children with spastic diplegia. *Dev Med Child Neurol* 45: 4–11.

100. Wren TA, Rethlefsen SA, Healy BS, Do KP, Dennis SW, Kay RM (2005) Reliability and validity of visual assessments of gait using a modified physician rating scale for crouch and foot contact. *J Pediatr Orthop* 25: 646–650.

101. Ong AM, Hillman SJ, Robb JE (2008) Reliability and validity of the Edinburgh Visual Gait Score for cerebral palsy when used by inexperienced observers. *Gait Post* 28: 323–326.

102. Read HS, Hazlewood ME, Hillman SJ, Prescott RJ, Robb JE (2003) Edinburgh visual gait score for use in cerebral palsy. *J Pediatr Orthop* 23: 296–301.

103. Martin K, Hoover D, Wagoner E, et al (2009) Development and reliability of an observational gait analysis tool for children with Down syndrome. *Pediatr Phys Ther* 21: 261–268.

104. Grunt S, van Kampen PJ, van der Krogt MM, Brehm MA, Doorenbosch CA, Becher JG (2010) Reproducibility and validity of video screen measurements of gait in children with spastic cerebral palsy. *Gait Post* 31: 489–494.

105. Maathuis KG, van der Schans CP, van IA, Rietman HS, Geertzen JH (2005) Gait in children with cerebral palsy: observer reliability of Physician Rating Scale and Edinburgh Visual Gait Analysis Interval Testing scale. *J Pediatr Orthop* 25: 268–272.

106. van Schie PE, Vermeulen RJ, van Ouwerkerk WJ, Kwakkel G, Becher JG (2005) Selective dorsal rhizotomy in cerebral palsy to improve functional abilities: evaluation of criteria for selection. *Child Nerv Syst* 21: 451–457.

107. Bar-Or O (1995) Anaerobic performance. In: Docherty D, editor. *Measurement in Pediatric Exercise Science.* Champaign, IL: Human Kinetics, pp. 161–182.

108. Parker DF, Carriere L, Hebestreit H, Bar-Or O (1992) Anaerobic endurance and peak muscle power in children with spastic cerebral palsy. *Am J Dis Child* 146: 1069–1073.

109. Tirosh E, Bar-Or O, Rosenbaum P (1990) New muscle power test in neuromuscular disease. Feasibility and reliability. *Am J Dis Child* 144: 1083–1087.

110. Van ME, Schoeber N, Calvert RE, Bar-Or O (1996) Optimization of force in the Wingate Test for children with a neuromuscular disease. *Med Sci Sports Exerc* 28: 1087–1092.

111. Guerra M, Gine-Garriga M, Fernhall B (2009) Reliability of Wingate testing in adolescents with Down syndrome. *Pediatr Exerc Sci* 21: 47–54.

112. Keller H, Bar-Or O, Kriemler S, Ayub BV, Saigal S (2000) Anaerobic performance in 5- to 7-yr-old children of low birthweight. *Med Sci Sports Exerc* 32: 278–283.

113. O'Beirne C, Larkin D, Cable T (1994) Coordination problems and anaerobic performance in children. *Adapt Phys Act Quart* 11: 141–149.

114. Parker DF, Carriere L, Hebestreit H, Salsberg A, Bar-Or O (1993) Muscle performance and gross motor function of children with spastic cerebral palsy. *Dev Med Child Neurol* 35: 17–23.

115. van den Berg-Emons RJ, van Baak MA, Speth L, Saris WH (1998) Physical training of school children with spastic cerebral palsy: effects on daily activity, fat mass and fitness. *Int J Rehabil Res* 21: 179–194.

116. Chia M (2000) Assessing young people's exercise using anaerobic performance tests. *Eur J Phys Ed* 5: 231–258.

117. Verschuren O, Takken T, Ketelaar M, Gorter JW, Helders PJ (2007) Reliability for running tests for measuring agility and anaerobic muscle power in children and adolescents with cerebral palsy. *Pediatr Phys Ther* 19: 108–115.

118. Zatsiorsky VM, Gregor RJ (2000) Mechanical power and work in human movement. In: Sparrow WA, editor. *Energetics of Human Movement.* Champaign, IL: Human Kinetics, pp. 195–227.

119. Verschuren O, Ketelaar M, Gorter JW, Helders PJ, Takken T (2009) Relation between physical fitness and gross motor capacity in children and adolescents with cerebral palsy. *Dev Med Child Neurol* 51: 866–871.

120. Verschuren O, Ketelaar M, Gorter JW, Helders PJ, Uiterwaal CS, Takken T (2007) Exercise training program in children and adolescents with cerebral palsy: a randomized controlled trial. *Arch Pediatr Adolesc Med* 161: 1075–1081.

121. Leger L (1996) Aerobic performance. In: Docherty D, editor. *Measurement in Pediatric Exercise Science.* Champaign, IL: Human Kinetics, pp. 183–223.

122. Paridon SM, Alpert BS, Boas SR, et al (2006) Clinical stress testing in the pediatric age group: a statement from the American Heart Association Council on Cardiovascular Disease in the Young, Committee on Atherosclerosis, Hypertension, and Obesity in Youth. *Circ J* 113: 1905–1920.

123. Midgley AW, Bentley DJ, Luttikholt H, McNaughton LR, Millet GP (2008) Challenging a dogma of exercise physiology: does an incremental exercise test for valid VO 2 max determination really need to last between 8 and 12 minutes? *Sports Med* 38: 441–447.

124. Rowland T (2005) The importance of body size. In: *Children's Exercise Physiology.* Champaign, IL: Human Kinetics, pp. 1–20.

125. Sheehan JM, Rowland TW, Burke EJ (1987) A comparison of four treadmill protocols for determination of maximum oxygen uptake in 10- to 12-year-old boys. *Int J Sports Med* 8: 31–34.

126. Zeimetz G, McNeil J, Moss R (1985) Quantifiable changes in oxygen uptake, heart rate, and time to target heart rate when hand support is allowed during treadmill exercise. *J Cardpulm Rehabil* 5: 525–530.

127. Rowland T (1999) Crusading for the Balke protocol. *Pediatr Exerc Sci* 11: 189–192.

128. Fernhall B, Pitetti K, Stubbs N, Stadler L (1996) Validity and reliability of the 1/2-mile run–walk as an indicator of aerobic fitness in children with mental retardation. *Pediatr Exerc Sci* 8: 130–142.

129. Fernhall B, Pitetti K, Vukovich D, et al (1998) Validation of cardiovascular fitness field tests in children with mental retardation. *Am J Ment Retard* 102: 602–612.

130. Hoofwijk M, Unnithan V, Bar-Or O (1995) Maximal treadmill performance of children with cerebral palsy. *Pediatr Exerc Sci* 7: 305–313.

131. Maltais DB, Pierrynowski MR, Galea VA, Bar-Or O (2005) Physical activity level is associated with the O_2 cost of walking in cerebral palsy. *Med Sci Sports Exerc* 37: 347–353.

132. Verschuren O, Takken T, Ketelaar M, Gorter JW, Helders PJ (2006) Reliability and validity of data for 2 newly developed shuttle run tests in children with cerebral palsy. *Phys Ther* 86: 1107–1117.

133. Verschuren O, Bloemen M, Kruitwagen C, Takken T (2010) Reference values for aerobic fitness in children, adolescents, and young adults who have cerebral palsy and are ambulatory. *Phys Ther* 90: 1148–1156.

134. Wu SK, Lin HH, Li YC, Tsai CL, Cairney J (2010) Cardiopulmonary fitness and endurance in children with developmental coordination disorder. *Res Dev Disabil* 31: 345–349.

135. Pivarnik JM, Dwyer MC, Lauderdale MA (1996) The reliability of aerobic capacity (VO2max) testing in adolescent girls. *Res Quart Exerc Sport* 67: 345–348.

136. Verschuren O, Takken T (2010) Aerobic capacity in children and adolescents with cerebral palsy. *Res Dev Disabil* 31: 1352–1357.

137. Leger LA, Mercier D, Gadoury C, Lambert J (1988) The multistage 20 metre shuttle run test for aerobic fitness. *J Sports Sci* 6: 93–101.

138. Meredith MD, Welk GJ (2010) *Fitnessgram & Activitygram Test Administration Manual.* Champaign, IL: Human Kinetics.

139. Castro-Pinero J, Artero EG, Espana-Romero V, et al (2010) Criterion-related validity of field-based fitness tests in youth: a systematic review. *Br J Sports Med* 44: 934–943.

140. Robergs RA, Landwehr R (2002) The surprising history of the 'HRmax=220-age' equation. *J Exerc Physiol* 5: 1–10.

141. van MW, Hlobil H, Kemper HC (1986) Validation of two running tests as estimates of maximal aerobic power in children. *Eur J Appl Physiol Occup Physiol* 55: 503–506.

142. Cairney J, Hay J, Veldhuizen S, Faught B (2010) Comparison of VO2 maximum obtained from 20 m shuttle run and cycle ergometer in children with and without developmental coordination disorder. *Res Dev Disabil* 31: 1332–1339.

143. Cairney J, Hay JA, Faught BE, Flouris A, Klentrou P (2007) Developmental coordination disorder and cardiorespiratory fitness in children. *Pediatr Exerc Sci* 19: 20–28.

144. Burns YR, Danks M, O'Callaghan MJ, et al (2009) Motor coordination difficulties and physical fitness of extremely-low-birthweight children. *Dev Med Child Neurol* 51: 136–142.

145. Smith LJ, van Asperen PP, McKay KO, Selvadurai H, Fitzgerald DA (2008) Reduced exercise capacity in children born very preterm. *Pediatrics* 122: e287–e293.

146. Bar-Or O, Rowland TW (2004) Procedures for exercising testing in children. In: *Pediatric Exercise Medicine: From Physiologic Principles to Health Care Application.* Champaign, IL: Human Kinetics, pp. 343–366.

147. Franklin BA (1985) Exercise testing, training and arm ergometry. *Sports Med* 2: 100–119.

148. Bar-Or O, Inbar O, Spira R (1976) Physiological effects of a sports rehabilitation program on cerebral palsied and post-poliomyelitic adolescents. *Med Sci Sports* 8: 157–161.

149. Franklin BA (1989) Aerobic exercise training programs for the upper body. *Med Sci Sports Exerc* 21: S141–S148.

150. Unnithan VB, Katsimanis G, Evangelinou C, Kosmas C, Kandrali I, Kellis E (2007) Effect of strength and aerobic training in children with cerebral palsy. *Med Sci Sports Exerc* 39: 1902–1909.

151. Bar-Or O, Zwiren LD (1975) Maximal oxygen consumption test during arm exercise – reliability and validity. *J Appl Physiol* 38: 424–426.

152. Noonan V, Dean E (2000) Submaximal exercise testing: clinical application and interpretation. *Phys Ther* 80: 782–807.

153. Frost G, Bar-Or O, Dowling J, Dyson K (2002) Explaining differences in the metabolic cost and efficiency of treadmill locomotion in children. *J Sports Sci* 20: 451–461.

154. Unnithan VB, Dowling JJ, Frost G, Bar-Or O (1999) Role of mechanical power estimates in the O_2 cost of walking in children with cerebral palsy. *Med Sci Sports Exerc* 31: 1703–1708.

155. Bar-Or O (1983) *Pediatric Sports Medicine for the Practitioner: From Physiologic Principals to Clinic Applications*. New York: Springer Verlag.

156. Dahlback GO, Norlin R (1985) The effect of corrective surgery on energy expenditure during ambulation in children with cerebral palsy. *Eur J Appl Physiol* 54: 67–70.

157. Jeng SF, Holt KG, Fetters L, Certo C (1996) Self-optimization in nondisabled children and children with cerebral palsy. *J Mot Behav* 28: 15–27.

158. Berling J, Foster C, Gibson M, Doberstein S, Porcari J (2006) The effect of handrail support on oxygen uptake during steady-state treadmill exercise. *J Cardpulm Rehabil* 26: 391–394.

159. Unnithan VB, Dowling JJ, Frost G, Bar-Or O (1996) Role of co-contraction in the O_2 cost of walking in children with cerebral palsy. *Med Sci Sports Exerc* 28: 1498–1504.

160. Plasschaert F, Jones K, Forward M (2009) Energy cost of walking: solving the paradox of steady state in the presence of variable walking speed. *Gait Post* 29: 311–316.

161. Butler P, Engelbrecht M, Major RE, Tait JH, Stallard J, Patrick JH (1984) Physiological cost index of walking for normal children and its use as an indicator of physical handicap. *Dev Med Child Neurol* 26: 607–612.

162. Rose J, Gamble JG, Burgos A, Medeiros J, Haskell WL (1990) Energy expenditure index of walking for normal children and for children with cerebral palsy. *Dev Med Child Neurol* 32: 333–340.

163. Brehm MA, Becher J, Harlaar J (2007) Reproducibility evaluation of gross and net walking efficiency in children with cerebral palsy. *Dev Med Child Neurol* 49: 45–48.

164. Morgan DW, Tseh W, Caputo JL, et al (2004) Longitudinal stratification of gait economy in young boys and girls: the locomotion energy and growth study. *Eur J Appl Physiol* 91: 30–34.

165. Nene AV (1993) Physiological cost index of walking in able-bodied adolescents and adults. *Clin Rehabil* 7: 319–326.

166. Tseh W, Caputo JL, Craig IS, Keefer DJ, Martin PE, Morgan DW (2000) Metabolic accommodation of young children to treadmill walking. *Gait Post* 12: 139–142.

167. Maltais D, Bar-Or O, Pierrynowski M, Galea V (2003) Repeated treadmill walks affect physiologic responses in children with cerebral palsy. *Med Sci Sports Exerc* 35: 1653–1661.

168. Thomas SS, Buckon CE, Schwartz MH, Russman BS, Sussman MD, Aiona MD (2009) Variability and minimum detectable change for walking energy efficiency variables in children with cerebral palsy. *Dev Med Child Neurol* 51: 615–621.

169. Wiart L, Darrah J (1999) Test–retest reliability of the energy expenditure index in adolescents with cerebral palsy. *Dev Med Child Neurol* 41: 716–718.

170. De Groot JF, Takken T, Schoenmakers MA, Tummers L, Vanhees L, Helders PJ (2010) Reproducibility of energy cost of locomotion in ambulatory children with spina bifida. *Gait Post* 31: 159–163.

171. Brehm MA, Knol DL, Harlaar J (2007) Methodological consideration for improving the reproducibility of walking efficiency outcomes in clinical gait studies. *Gait Post* 27: 196–201.

172. Keefer DJ, Tseh W, Caputo JL, Apperson K, McGreal S, Morgan DW (2005) Within- and between-day stability of treadmill walking VO_2 in children with hemiplegic cerebral palsy, stability of walking VO_2 in children with CP. *Gait Post* 21: 80–84.

173. Rose J, Gamble JG, Medeiros J, Burgos A, Haskell WL (1989) Energy cost of walking in normal children and in those with cerebral palsy: comparison of heart rate and oxygen uptake. *J Pediatr Orthop* 9: 276–279.

174. Livingstone MB, Coward WA, Prentice AM, et al (1992) Daily energy expenditure in free-living children: comparison of heart-rate monitoring with the doubly labeled water ($2H_2(18)O$) method. *Am J Clin Nutr* 56: 343–352.

175. Keefer DJ, Tseh W, Caputo JL, Apperson K, McGreal S, Morgan DW (2004) Comparison of direct and indirect measures of walking energy expenditure in children with hemiplegic cerebral palsy. *Dev Med Child Neurol* 46: 320–324.

176. Ijzerman MJ, Nene AV (2002) Feasibility of the physiological cost index as an outcome measure for the assessment of energy expenditure during walking. *Arch Phys Med Rehabil* 83: 1777–1782.

177. Keefer DJ, Tseh W, Caputo JL, et al (2004) Interrelationships among thigh muscle co-contraction, quadriceps muscle strength and the aerobic demand of walking in children with cerebral palsy. *Electromyogr Clin Neurophysiol* 44: 103–110.

178. Johnston TE, Moore SE, Quinn LT, Smith BT (2004) Energy cost of walking in children with cerebral palsy: relation to the Gross Motor Function Classification System. *Dev Med Child Neurol* 46: 34–38.

179. Oeffinger DJ, Tylkowski CM, Rayens MK, et al (2004) Gross Motor Function Classification System and outcome tools for assessing ambulatory cerebral palsy: a multicenter study. *Dev Med Child Neurol* 46: 311–319.

180. Chia LC, Guelfi KJ, Licari MK (2010) A comparison of the oxygen cost of locomotion in children with and without developmental coordination disorder. *Dev Med Child Neurol* 52: 251–255.

181. Oeffinger D, Gorton G, Bagley A, et al (2007) Outcome assessments in children with cerebral palsy, part I: descriptive characteristics of GMFCS Levels I to III. *Dev Med Child Neurol* 49: 172–180.

182. Oeffinger D, Bagley A, Rogers S, et al (2008) Outcome tools used for ambulatory children with cerebral palsy: responsiveness and minimum clinically important differences. *Dev Med Child Neurol* 50: 918–925.

183. Thomas SS, Buckon CE, Piatt JH, Aiona MD, Sussman MD (2004) A 2-year follow-up of outcomes following orthopedic surgery or selective dorsal rhizotomy in children with spastic diplegia. *J Pediatr Orthop B* 13: 358–366.

184. Mossberg KA, Linton KA, Friske K (1990) Ankle–foot orthoses: effect on energy expenditure of gait in spastic diplegic children. *Arch Phys Med Rehabil* 71: 490–494.

185. Liao HF, Liu YC, Liu WY, Lin YT (2007) Effectiveness of loaded sit-to-stand resistance exercise for children with mild spastic diplegia: a randomized clinical trial. *Arch Phys Med Rehabil* 88: 25–31.

186. ATS Committee on Proficiency Standards for Clinical Pulmonary Function Laboratories (2002) ATS statement: guidelines for the six-minute walk test. *Am J Respir Crit Care Med* 166: 111–117.

187. Thompson P, Beath T, Bell J, et al (2008) Test–retest reliability of the 10-metre fast walk test and 6-minute walk test in ambulatory school-aged children with cerebral palsy. *Dev Med Child Neurol* 50: 370–376.

188. Maher CA, Williams MT, Olds TS (2008) The six-minute walk test for children with cerebral palsy. *Int J Rehabil Res* 31: 185–188.

189. Ben SH, Prefaut C, Missaoui R, Mohamed IH, Tabka Z, Hayot M (2009) Reference equation for 6-min walk distance in healthy North African children 6–16 years old. *Pediatr Pulmonol* 44: 316–324.

190. Geiger R, Strasak A, Treml B, et al (2007) Six-minute walk test in children and adolescents. *J Pediatr* 150: 395–399.

191. Li AM, Yin J, Au JT, et al (2007) Standard reference for the six-minute-walk test in healthy children aged 7 to 16 years. *Am J Resp Crit Care Med* 176: 174–180.

192. Hassan MM (2001) Validity and reliability for the Bruininks–Oseretsky Test of Motor Proficiency-Short Form as applied in the United Arab Emirates culture. *Percept Mot Skills* 92: 157–166.

193. Li AM, Yin J, Yu CC, et al (2005) The six-minute walk test in healthy children: reliability and validity. *Eur Respir J* 25: 1057–1060.

194. Lesser DJ, Fleming MM, Maher CA, Kim SB, Woo MS, Keens TG (2010) Does the 6-min walk test correlate with the exercise stress test in children? *Pediatr Pulmonol* 45: 135–140.

195. Limsuwan A, Wongwandee R, Khowsathit P (2010) Correlation between 6-min walk test and exercise stress test in healthy children. *Acta Paediatr* 99: 438–441.

196. Limsuwan A (2010) Correlation between the 6-min walk test and exercise stress test. *Acta Paediatr* 99: 958–959.

197. Takken T (2010) Six-minute walk test is a poor predictor of maximum oxygen uptake in children. *Acta Paediatr* 99: 958.

198. Andersson C, Grooten W, Hellsten M, Kaping K, Mattsson E (2003) Adults with cerebral palsy: walking ability after progressive strength training. *Dev Med Child Neurol* 45: 220–228.

199. Meyer-Heim A, Ammann-Reiffer C, Schmartz A, et al (2009) Improvement of walking abilities after robotic-assisted locomotion training in children with cerebral palsy. *Arch Dis Child* 94: 615–620.

200. Wade DT, Wood VA, Heller A, Maggs J, Langton HR (1987) Walking after stroke. Measurement and recovery over the first 3 months. *Scand J Rehabil Med* 19: 25–30.

201. Watson MJ (2002) Refining the ten-metre walking test for use with neurologically impaired people. *Physiotherapy* 88: 386–397.

202. Ruck J, Chabot G, Rauch F (2010) Vibration treatment in cerebral palsy: A randomized controlled pilot study. *J Musuloskel Neuronal Interact* 10: 77–83.

203. Leemrijse C, Meijer OG, Vermeer A, Lambregts B, Ader HJ (1999) Detecting individual change in children with mild to moderate motor impairment: the standard error of measurement of the Movement ABC. *Clin Rehabil* 13: 420–429.

204. Brown T, Lalor A (2009) The Movement Assessment Battery for Children – Second Edition (MABC-2): a review and critique. *Phys Occup Ther Pediatr* 29: 86–103.

205. Peens A, Pienaar AE, Nienaber AW (2008) The effect of different intervention programmes on the self-concept and motor proficiency of 7- to 9-year-old children with DCD. *Child Care Health Dev* 34: 316–328.

206. Schoemaker MM, Smits-Engelsman BC, Jongmans MJ (2003) Psychometric properties of the Movement Assessment Battery for Children – checklist as a screening instrument for children with a developmental coordination disorder. *Br J Educ Psychol* 73: 3–41.

207. Smits-Engelsman BC, Fiers MJ, Henderson SE, Henderson L (2008) Interrater reliability of the Movement Assessment Battery for Children. *Phys Ther* 88: 286–294.

208. Livesey D, Coleman R, Piek J (2007) Performance on the Movement Assessment Battery for Children by Australian 3- to 5-year-old children. *Child Care Health Dev* 33: 713–719.

209. Van WH, Peersman W, Lenoir M, Engelsman BC (2007) Convergent validity between two motor tests: movement-ABC and PDMS-2. *Adapt Phys Act Quart* 24: 59–69.

210. Watter P (2006) Movement Assessment Battery for Children (Movement ABC). *Aust J Physiother* 52: 68.

211. Chow SM, Henderson SE (2003) Interrater and test–retest reliability of the Movement Assessment Battery for Chinese preschool children. *Am J Occup Ther* 57: 574–577.

212. Croce RV, Horvat M, McCarthy E (2001) Reliability and concurrent validity of the movement assessment battery for children. *Percept Mot Skill* 93: 275–280.

213. Hiller S, Mcintyre A, Plummer L (2010) Aquatic physical therapy for children with developmental coordination disorder: A pilot randomized controlled trial. *Phys Occup Ther Pediatr* 30: 111–124.

214. Gard L, Rosblad B (2009) The qualitative motor observations in Movement ABC: aspects of reliability and validity. *Adv Physiother* 11: 51–57.

215. Civetta LR, Hillier SL (2008) The developmental coordination disorder questionnaire and Movement Assessment Battery for Children as a diagnostic method in Australian children. *Pediatr Phys Ther* 20: 39–46.

216. Crawford SG, Wilson BN, Dewey D (2001) Identifying developmental coordination disorder: consistency between tests. *Phys Occup Ther Pediatr* 20: 29–50.

217. Yoon DY, Scott K, Hill MN, Levitt NS, Lambert EV (2006) Review of three tests of motor proficiency in children. *Percept Mot Skill* 102: 543–551.

218. Watemberg N, Waiserberg N, Zuk L, Lerman-Sagie T (2007) Developmental coordination disorder in children with attention-deficit–hyperactivity disorder and physical therapy intervention. *Dev Med Child Neurol* 49: 920–925.

219. Sugden DA, Chambers ME (2003) Intervention in children with developmental coordination disorder: the role of parents and teachers. *Br J Educ Psychol* 73: 4–61.

220. Niemeijer AS, Smits-Engelsman BC, Schoemaker MM (2007) Neuromotor task training for children with developmental coordination disorder: a controlled trial. *Dev Med Child Neurol* 49: 406–411.

221. Ziviani J, Poylsen A (2007) Neuromotor task training for children with developmental coordination disorder. *Dev Med Child Neurol* 49: 404.

222. Mercuri E, Jongmans M, Bouza H, et al (1999) Congenital hemiplegia in children at school age: assessment of hand function in the non-hemiplegic hand and correlation with MRI. *Neuropediatrics* 30: 8–13.

223. Ulrich DA (2000) *Test of Gross Motor Development*. Austin, TX: Pro-Ed.

224. Harvey WJ, Reid G, Bloom GA, et al (2009) Physical activity experiences of boys with and without ADHD. *Adapt Phys Act Quart* 26: 131–150.

225. Apache RR (2005) Activity-based intervention in motor skill development. *Percept Mot Skills* 100: 1011–1020

226. Franjoine MR, Gunther JS, Taylor MJ (2003) Pediatric Balance Scale: A modified version of the Berg Balance Scale for the school-age child with mild to moderate motor impairment. *Pediatr Phys Ther* 15: 114–128.

227. Liao HF, Mao PJ, Hwang AW (2001) Test–retest reliability of balance tests in children with cerebral palsy. *Dev Med Child Neurol* 43: 180–186.

228. Zaino CA, Marchese VG, Westcott SL (2004) Times Up and Down Stairs Test: Preliminary reliability and validity of a new measure of functional mobility. *Pediatr Phys Ther* 16: 90–98.

229. Gorter H, Holty L, Rameckers EE, Elvers HJ, Oostendorp RA (2009) Changes in endurance and walking ability through

functional physical training in children with cerebral palsy. *Pediatr Phys Ther* 21: 31–37.

230. Podsiadlo D, Richardson S (1991) The timed 'Up & Go': a test of basic functional mobility for frail elderly persons. *J Am Geriatr Soc* 39: 142–148.

231. Gan SM, Tung LC, Tang YH, Wang CH (2008) Psychometric properties of functional balance assessment in children with cerebral palsy. *Neurorehabil Neural Repair* 22: 745–753.

232. Williams EN, Carroll SG, Reddihough DS, Phillips BA, Galea MP (2005) Investigation of the timed 'up & go' test in children. *Dev Med Child Neurol* 47: 518–524.

233. Salem Y, Godwin EM (2009) Effects of task-oriented training on mobility function in children with cerebral palsy. *Neurorehabil* 24: 307–313.

234. Katz-Leurer M, Rotem H, Keren O, Meyer S (2009) The effects of a 'home-based' task-oriented exercise programme on motor and balance performance in children with spastic cerebral palsy and severe traumatic brain injury. *Clin Rehabil* 23: 714–724.

235. Berg K, Wood-Dauphinee S, Williams JI (1990) Measuring balance in the elderly: Preliminary development of an instrument. *Physiother Can* 41: 304–311.

236. Kembhavi G, Darrah J, Magill-Evans J, Loomis J (2002) Using the Berg Balance Scale to distinguish balance abilities in children with cerebral palsy. *Pediatr Phys Ther* 14: 92–99.

237. Niznik TM, Turner D, Worrell TW (1996) Functional reach as a measurement of balance for children with lower extremity spasticity. *Phys Occup Ther Pediatr* 15: 1–16.

238. Bartlett D, Birmingham T (2003) Validity and reliability of a pediatric reach test. *Pediatr Phys Ther* 15: 84–92.

239. Boyce WF, Gowland C, Hardy S, et al (1991) Development of a quality-of-movement measure for children with cerebral palsy. *Phys Ther* 71: 820–832.

240. Ketelaar M, Vermeer A, Helders PJ (1998) Functional motor abilities of children with cerebral palsy: a systematic literature review of assessment measures. *Clin Rehabil* 12: 369–380.

241. Boyce WF, Gowland C, Russell D, et al (1993) Consensus methodology in the development and content validation of a gross motor performance measure. *Physiother Can* 45: 94–100.

242. Sorsdahl AB, Moe-Nilssen R, Strand LI (2008) Observer reliability of the Gross Motor Performance Measure and the Quality of Upper Extremity Skills Test, based on video recordings. *Dev Med Child Neurol* 50: 146–151.

243. Boyce WF, Gowland C, Rosenbaum P, et al (1998) *Gross Motor Performance Manual*. Kingston: Queens University, School of Rehabilitation Therapy.

244. Gowland C, Boyce WF, Wright V, Russell DJ, Goldsmith CH, Rosenbaum PL (1995) Reliability of the Gross Motor Performance Measure. *Phys Ther* 75: 597–602.

245. Sienko Thomas S, Buckon CE, Phillips DS, Aiona MD, Sussman MD (2001) Interobserver reliability of the Gross Motor Performance Measure: Preliminary results. *Dev Med Child Neurol* 43: 97–102.

246. Boyce WF, Gowland C, Rosenbaum PL, et al (1995) The Gross Motor Performance Measure: validity and responsiveness of a measure of quality of movement. *Phys Ther* 75: 603–613.

247. Buckon CE, Thomas SS, Piatt JH Jr, Aiona MD, Sussman MD (2004) Selective dorsal rhizotomy versus orthopedic surgery:

a multidimensional assessment of outcome efficacy. *Arch Phys Med Rehabil* 85: 457–465.

248. Buckon CE, Thomas SS, Jakobson-Huston S, Moor M, Sussman M, Aiona M (2004) Comparison of three ankle–foot orthosis configurations for children with spastic diplegia. *Dev Med Child Neurol* 46: 590–598.

249. Mathiowetz V, Federman S, Wiemer D (1985) Box and Block Test of manual dexterity: norms for 6 to 19 year olds. *Can J Occup Ther* 52: 241–245.

250. Cromwell FS (1976) *Occupational Therapist's Manual for Basic Skill Assessment: Primary Prevocational Evaluation.* Altadena, CA: Fair Oaks Printing.

251. Platz T, Pinkowski C, van WF, Kim IH, di BP, Johnson G (2005) Reliability and validity of arm function assessment with standardized guidelines for the Fugl–Meyer Test, Action Research Arm Test and Box and Block Test: a multicentre study. *Clin Rehabil* 19: 404–411.

252. Kellor M, Frost J, Silberberg N, Iversen I, Cummings R (1971) Hand strength and dexterity. *Am J Occup Ther* 25: 7–83.

253. Smith YA, Hong E, Presson C (2000) Normative and validation studies of the Nine-hole Peg Test with children. *Percept Mot Skills* 90: 823–843.

254. Poole JL, Burtner PA, Torres TA, et al (2005) Measuring dexterity in children using the Nine-hole Peg Test. *J Hand Ther* 18: 348–351.

255. Yim SY, Cho JR, Lee IY (2003) Normative data and developmental characteristics of hand function for elementary school children in Suwon area of Korea: grip, pinch and dexterity study. *J Korean Med Sci* 18: 552–558.

256. Tiffin J, Asher EJ (1968) The Purdue Pegboard: norms and studies of reliability and validity. *J Appl Psychol* 32: 234–247.

257. Siegel M, Hirschorn B (1958) Adolescent norms for the Purdue Pegboard Tests. *Pers Guid J* 36: 563–565.

258. Gardner RA, Broman M (1979) The Purdue Pegboard: Normative data on 1334 school children. *J Clin Child Psychol* 1: 156–162.

259. Mathiowetz V, Rogers SL, Dowe-Keval M, Donahoe L, Rennells C (1986) The Purdue Pegboard: norms for 14- to 19-year-olds. *Am J Occup Ther* 40: 174–179.

260. Wilson BC, Iacoviello JM, Wilson JJ, Risucci D (1982) Purdue Pegboard performance of normal preschool children. *J Clin Child Psychol* 4: 19–26.

261. DeMatteo C, Law M, Russell D, Pollock N, Rosenbaum P, Walter S (1993) The reliability and validity of Quality of Upper Extremity Skills Test. *Phys Occup Ther Pediatr* 13: 1–18.

262. Haga N, van der Heijden-Maessen HC, van Hoorn JF, Boonstra AM, Hadders-Algra M (2007) Test–retest and inter and intra reliability of the Quality of Upper Extremity Skills Test in preschool children with cerebral palsy. *Arch Phys Med Rehabil* 88: 1686–1689.

263. Klingels K, De CP, Desloovere K, et al (2008) Comparison of the Melbourne Assessment of Unilateral Upper Limb Function and the Quality of Upper Extremity Skills Test in hemiplegic CP. *Dev Med Child Neurol* 50: 904–909.

264. Beery KE, Beery NA (2006) *The Beery–Buktenica Developmental Test of Visual Motor Integration*. San Antonio, TX: Pearson.

SECTION III GLOBAL DEVELOPMENTAL FUNCTIONING – BODY FUNCTIONS, ACTIVITIES AND PARTICIPATION (NOT CLASSIFIED)

17
SCREENING FOR DEVELOPMENTAL AND BEHAVIOURAL PROBLEMS

Frances Page Glascoe and Kevin P. Marks

Overview

Early detection of developmental disabilities is greatly facilitated when quality instruments are deployed. This chapter provides a rationale for evidence-based early detection approaches, describes how to identify accurate measures and presents standards for screening tests. Included is a table delineating accurate tools for primary care, typically those relying on information from parents (e.g. Ages and Stages Questionnaire, third edition, Parent's Evaluation of Developmental Status, Parent's Evaluation of Developmental Status: Developmental Milestones, Ages and Stages Questionnaire, social-emotional, Patient Study Calendar, Modified Checklist for Autism in Toddlers plus its follow-up interview) as well as measures that are useful in settings where providers have more time and skill at eliciting behaviours from children (e.g. Brigance Screens, Bayley Infant Neurodevelopmental Screener). Also discussed are issues in the implementation of screening measures in primary care settings, how to explain results to families, where to find supporting materials for patient education and how to locate referral resources.

Rationale for developmental screening

The challenges inherent in the early detection of developmental problems are many. Although healthcare providers have abundant contact with young children and their families, well-child visits have competing demands, including physical examinations, immunizations, obesity prevention, home safety and numerous other anticipatory guidance topics. Thus, there is little time to devote to screening for developmental behavioural problems. Other primary care barriers to early detection include poor reimbursement, lack of awareness of available referral resources, misconceptions that problems are likely to be obvious without measurement, a sense that many children will simply outgrow their delays and a reluctance to give

parents difficult news. For these reasons, healthcare providers tend to use problematic approaches to early detection, including dependence on clinical observation rather than measurement, deployment of informal milestone checklists that lack validation and distinct cut-offs or use of screening tests with out-of-date, non-diverse norming samples and/or limited accuracy.[1,2] As a consequence, only about 30% of children with developmental disabilities are identified before entering school, at which point all opportunities for early intervention are lost.[3–5] In contrast, when professionals use quality instruments, early identification rates soar and, in a single administration, can detect 70% to 80% of children with disabilities.[3,6]

Because accurate screening tools, rather than informal methods, carry the burden of proof, the first critical questions are 'How can we identify a good measure?' and 'Are there tools that are feasible in busy medical settings?'. What is available for those professionals with more time to devote to the process and who may need different types of information on children (e.g. for programme evaluation, progress tracking)?

Early intervention programmes (meaning nurse home visitation, parenting education/support groups, high-quality preschool programmes, special education services, speech–language therapy, occupational therapy or physical therapy) have a known positive impact on children's development, behaviour and subsequent school performance.[7–17] As a consequence, the American Academy of Pediatrics (AAP) has published multiple policy statements on the early detection of developmental behavioural problems that promulgate standardized universal postpartum maternal depression/mood disorder screening in the first year, general (broad-band) developmental screening at 9, 18, 24 or 30 months, autism-specific screening at 18 and 24 months, socioemotional screening whenever a general developmental or autism-specific screen is abnormal, 'kindergarten-readiness' screening at 4 years and mental health/psychosocial function screening at 5 years and every well-visit until 18 years of age.[18–20] The AAP and multiple other professional organizations are clear about the need for healthcare providers to screen 'routinely and repeatedly'.[21] Why is it necessary to repeatedly rescreen patients? There are two essential reasons, as follows.

DEVELOPMENT IS PLIANT, PARTICULARLY IN THE EARLIEST YEARS

Academic, language, social and other developmental skills are readily influenced in positive directions by environments that promote and encourage learning. When parents engage children's interests, respond by talking, listening and modelling, implement positive parenting rather than punishment as an approach to teaching and have few risk factors, their children tend to perform in the average to above-average range on measures of intelligence, which is a strong predictor of school success.[22,23] In contrast, when parents' interaction style is characterized largely by commands, or limited verbal expansions on child-initiated topics of conversation, children fare less well. Four or more of these and other risk factors, including substance abuse, mental health problems, limited social support, single parent status, more than three children in the home, numerous stressful events (such as job loss, deaths in the family, physical illness, ethnic minority and low occupational status), place children at 24 times the risk of having an intelligence quotient below 85 (well below the point at which typical classroom instruction is effective).[22]

Young children with risk factors tend to demonstrate at least mild developmental delays by the age of 2 years, particularly in the area of language, which is also a strong predictor of school success. Such weakened acquisition of developmental skills creates risks for subsequent school failure. Problematic school performance is associated with in-grade retention, dropping out of secondary school, teen pregnancy, unemployment and adjudication.[14] Despite the bleakness of this picture, early risk factors can change during childhood (e.g. because of divorce or marriage, acquisition or loss of employment, fluctuations in mental health status, addition of new siblings, involvement in early intervention). Thus, developmental progress can be changed, for better or for worse. This helps to explain why single-point screening in a community setting has been shown to be problematic.[24] Therefore, to accurately monitor changes in developmental status, repeated screening is necessary.

DEVELOPMENT DEVELOPS – DEVELOPMENTAL PROBLEMS DEVELOP TOO

We cannot know, for example, that a typically developing 9-month-old infant will remain on a normal or typical developmental trajectory. What if he or she is not using words by 18 months or two-word utterances by 24 months? Even if language emerges well and progresses adequately, we cannot know whether he or she will be a successful reader at age 5 years until the child reaches the age when most children have some facility with letter and word recognition. The term 'age-related developmental manifestations'[25] captures the emerging nature of development and developmental problems. This phenomenon results in an increasing risk of disabilities across the life span. Public school special education programmes serve almost 12% of the school-age population, a figure considered quite low by epidemiologists who generally find rates of 16% to 18% for developmental disabilities alone.[26,27] When mental health problems are also included, the combined prevalence is 22%, which is quite similar to high school drop-out rates in the USA.[28] Over time, measurable delays, disorders or disabilities become more apparent at different ages; the most common (and least well identified) condition is speech–language impairment (17.5% at 30–36mo).[29,30] Prevalence varies by age, but this is followed in frequency by socioemotional disorders (9.5–14.2%),[31] attention-deficit–hyperactivity disorder (7.8%),[32] specific learning disabilities (6.5%),[33] developmental coordination disorder (1.7% at 7y to 6% at 5–11y),[34,35] cognitive disabilities (1.2% overall)[36] and autism spectrum disorder (0.66–1.1% overall).[37–39] Less common (meaning <1%) conditions include cerebral palsy (0.23%),[36] hearing impairment (0.12%),[36] vision impairment (0.08%)[36] and other forms of health or physical impairment (e.g. Down syndrome, fragile X syndrome, traumatic brain injury, metabolic disorders).

General factors to consider when measuring this domain

Owing to development's pliability and age-related manifestations, there is a clear need for screening. Detection rates are problematic when using informal methods such as checklists and clinical observation; therefore, there is a need for formal screening using quality instruments and screening repeatedly. So, what are the most accurate screens? Which ones are suitable for busy primary care clinics? Which ones are more appropriate for early intervention programmes and other settings where professionals have time to work with children directly? While there are many published tests, it is important to recognize that their publication is not regulated, particularly in the USA. In contrast, the Canadian Psychological Association (CPA) requires the publisher to report specific indicators of accuracy and avoid misleading findings such as overall hit rates.[40] Even so, the CPA guidelines regulate only reporting requirements and do not deter inaccurate measures from being marketed. Thus, professionals involved in testing should become knowledgeable about the basics of test psychometry so they can select measures that are well constructed and accurate.

Screening test technical standards and related terms are defined below. These were drawn from several sources including *Standards for Educational and Psychological Tests* published by the American Psychological Association (1999) and from the recommendations of researchers in screening.[41–44]

Screening is a brief method of distinguishing those who probably have problems from those who probably do not. Screening measures are meant to be employed universally and are especially important for those with subclinical difficulties. The group with probable problems is typically referred for diagnostic work-ups and, if diagnosed, culturally appropriate family-centred treatment is provided. It is worth noting that often a specific diagnosis is not necessary for young children to enter early intervention. Rather, the presence of quantifiable delays serves as eligibility criteria for services and complete diagnostic evaluations are typically provided later.

Screens may be *broad-band* (meaning that they tap all or most developmental domains) or *narrow-band*, meaning that they focus on a single domain of development such as motor skills or on a specific condition such as autism spectrum disorder or attention-deficit–hyperactivity disorder. The focus of this discussion is on broad-band screens, although the psychometric precepts underlying their construction also apply to narrow-band tools.

Developmental screens, even the most accurate ones, are not error free. This is not surprising given the moving target that is development itself. Developmental behavioural screening tools seek to categorize conditions which typically exist upon a spectrum, and in this regard are different from many other screens in medicine which seek to identify a strictly positive or negative condition (e.g. cystic fibrosis, sickle cell anaemia, congenital hypothyroidism, phenylketonuria). Nevertheless, developmental behavioural screens should be as accurate as possible in order to minimize the many expenses associated with both over-referrals and underdetection. The components of screening accuracy (concurrent criterion-related validity) include the following.

SENSITIVITY

Sensitivity is the percentage of children with a developmental-behavioural condition correctly detected by a screening test. Sensitivity is computed by administering diagnostic tests to a randomly selected group of children. Some will be found to have the condition of interest. If

screening tests are then given to the same group, researchers can look at the numbers correctly detected (e.g. by obtaining failing, abnormal or positive results). Standards for sensitivity are the identification of at least 70% to 80% of children with a given developmental behavioural condition at a single administration.

SPECIFICITY

Specificity is the percentage of children without a developmental behavioural condition correctly identified by a screening test. In the above example in which diagnostic tests were given to a group of children, most would be found to have typical development. If a screening test is then administered, it should identify the typically developing children as such (e.g. by passing typical or negative findings on screening). Because there are many more children with typical development than without, specificity should be approximately 80% or above, so as to minimize over-referrals.

POSITIVE PREDICTIVE VALUE

Positive predictive value is the percentage of children with failing scores on screening tests who are found to have the condition of interest. When a child does poorly on a screening test, the results means that he or she *probably* has the condition. Still, there is always a chance that the screening test is in error. How much of a chance? Put another way, what is the predictive value of a failing (or positive) test score in reflecting an actual problem? For example, if four out of five children with failing scores on screening tests are found to have developmental diagnoses, the test's positive predictive value is four-fifths, or 80%, meaning that for any screening test failure there would be an 80% risk that the child actually has a disability. In application, however, the positive predictive value is rarely so high and values of 30% to 50% are typical (meaning that for every two to three children referred, only one would result in a diagnosis). While this may seem troubling, what is interesting is the nature of false positives. Research shows that children who fail screening tests but are not found to have a developmental diagnosis are children with numerous psychosocial risk factors and below-average performance in the better predictors of school success: academics and pre-academics, language and intelligence.[45] These are children who require help. Although they will not qualify for special education, they benefit enormously from programmes such as Head Start, high-quality daycare/preschool, parent training, social services and summer school. These findings indicate that screening tests followed by additional assessments (which are usually available through early intervention programmes) are helpful in identifying the at-risk child as well as those with undetected disabilities. For this reason, there is no agreed-upon standard for positive predictive value.

OTHER CHARACTERISTICS OF QUALITY SCREENING TESTS

Screening tests must first embody the same psychometric properties as all other tests. This means that screens should be standardized on a large national and current sample whose characteristics reflect those of the country in which they are deployed (e.g. inclusion of ethnic minorities in proportion to their prevalence in the population, correct proportions of parents with varying levels of education, correct percentage of children with disabilities in relation to the population as a whole). Typically, census information is used to determine current population parameters and thus the optimal standardization sample. The representativeness of this sample is critical because it is their performance from which normative information on test performance is derived to construct the test's scores such as centiles, quotients and age equivalents. Standardization must be current, and recommendations from the American Psychological Association call for a restandardization of measures every 10 years at a minimum.[42] This is wise because population sociodemographics change and test stimuli become out of date (e.g. images of a rotary dial telephone no longer have meaning for most young children). Ideally, the standardization sample should also be naturalistically acquired (e.g. consecutive children seeking well-child care). In contrast, including groups with and without known disabilities will probably exclude those with subtle problems with a concomitant loss of gradations in developmental status in the range between atypical and typical. The result is that tests perform less than optimally in real-life applications.

Reliability

Screening tests must also include proof of reliability. Reliability of ≥90% is recommended for diagnostic decisions; 80% to 89% is adequate for screening decisions.[46] When applied to a primary care setting, a truly standardized administration method, identical to that reported in the screening test manual, is important to achieving a screen's reported reliability. There are many types including test–retest (retesting the same child by the same examiner a few weeks apart) and inter-rater reliability (retesting the same child by a different examiner). A high level of consistency shows that the directions are clear, that the items tap relatively enduring developmental behaviours and that different examiners can confidently use the test norms to compare children's performance. Internal consistency is another type of reliability and shows that items

cluster as expected into domains. If, for example, motor items and language items have a great deal of overlap, test users cannot be confident that they are measuring each domain adequately (e.g. a child with a language delay but excellent motor skills might do poorly on the latter simply because the directions were too complicated).

Validity

Validity studies should be high volume and include concurrent validity (high correlations between the screen and a broad range of diagnostic measures of language, intelligence, motor, social and self-help skills) to be sure that all developmental skills are measured well. There should also be proof of discriminant validity in which various types of disabilities are shown to have unique performance patterns (e.g. children with probable autism spectrum disorder are shown to have weaknesses [and perhaps strengths] that distinguish them from children with other disabilities such as cerebral palsy). This type of research ultimately helps practitioners to better hone referrals and better highlights the strengths and weaknesses of screens. Occasionally screening tests are also studied for their predictive validity, meaning that the screening results are compared, typically 1 to 2 years later, with diagnostic or achievement measures. High correlations, after adjusting for intervention(s), illustrate that the screen is measuring meaningful and stable aspects of development. Nevertheless, such research is fraught with thorny problems given the gaps of time during which rapid developmental changes occur where multiple confounding variables are at play (e.g. changes in the home environment, severe illness).[47] For these reasons, there are no agreed-upon standards for predictive validity.

Utility and feasibility

Utility and feasibility are terms used to describe other features of screens that are practical in nature. Ideally, peer-reviewed studies should demonstrate an instrument's effectiveness and feasibility within a busy primary care setting[48–50] where screening test psychometric properties may vary under 'real-world' constraints,[24] where less than ideal screening test return rates may exist[48] and where clinician judgement tends to haphazardly override the results of a concerning screen.[49,51] Utility features for developmental screening tools include (1) materials that are interesting to children but sufficiently minimal in number that examiners can find them easily in the test kit; (2) easy to find and read directions for items; (3) clear scoring procedures of sufficient simplicity that computation errors are minimized; (4) clear information about the amount of training required and videos and/or training exercises included with the manual; (5) directions for interpreting test results to families (e.g. examiners should be encouraged not to use diagnostic labels), to present the information and service referrals in a positive and practical way (e.g. give parents telephone numbers) and to offer ongoing support to families struggling with difficult news; (6) guidance should be given for the types of referrals that may be needed based on unique pattern performance profiles (e.g. failing scores on motor domains but average performance in other areas) and should indicate a referral to a neurologist and/or physical therapist; (7) alternative methods for administering items if needed to circumvent behavioural non-compliance, limited English proficiency or limited knowledge of the child's development on the part of the caretaker accompanying the child during screening – strategies to address these challenges may include having foreign-language translations or parent-reporting options alongside directly administered items; (8) screening toolkits should ideally include well-crafted developmental promotion tools such as developmental activity sheets or parent-centred handouts; (9) electronic/online capabilities to improve feasibility that accurately utilize the corrected age for children born preterm and automatically score the results before the beginning of a well-child visit so that results can be promptly interpreted in the context of ongoing surveillance and so potential referrals can be discussed with caregivers face to face; and (10) estimated costs that are not a barrier to implementation and sustainability as recommended by the AAP. The cost of screening is primarily a function of time and staff are required to implement a given tool using a resource-based relative valuation.[52] Total administrative costs (for normal and abnormal screens) have been found to be lower for parent-report screening tools and higher for practitioner-administered tools.[52,53] To estimate clinic costs per screen, refer to a modifiable model by Dobrez et al.[52] A final issue is that screening or assessment test forms must be periodically restocked in clinic work areas. For measures that are not available in the public domain, clinics or practitioners must be registered with the supplier and screening or assessment test forms need to be periodically reordered.

Overview of recommended measures

Appendix 17.1 provides information on the best available screening tests.

Implementation issues

It is generally insufficient to select a quality measure and then expect that it will be routinely deployed unless the primary care office is adequately prepared. Providers need to carefully consider implementation and evoke the enthusiasm of office staff. A helpful implementation resource is www.developmentalscreening.org, a website developed

by Harvard University. Providers need to be familiar with parenting information resources because many parental concerns focus on discipline, toileting or other specific developmental or behavioural milestones or tasks (see www.kidshealth.com). Providers also need skills in explaining screening results to parents. The manuals of most quality screening tools offer helpful guidance. Explaining results is easiest when parents' concerns are first elicited because affirmation is an effective springboard to discussions about referrals.

Ultimately, one of the biggest challenges for primary care providers is knowledge of referral resources (see www.pedstest.com for links to services in the USA). Providers tend to refer only to those services they know well, and they know services best when they offer prompt confirmation that referrals are received, provide copies of test results and engage providers in collaborative decision-making about needed services.[57] Thus, all service providers need to develop and maintain close communication. Finally, all providers need professional life-long learning resources. One helpful source is the AAP's section on developmental and behavioural paediatrics website (www.dbpeds.org), which provides information on disabilities and challenging cases. Another resource is the early detection discussion list hosted on www.pedstest.com, where clinicians can ask peers for ideas on training, translation issues and other related topics.

Insuring a Medical Home

Once children are identified as having special needs, the primary care provider often has the challenging role of making sure that medical care is not fragmented from the vital services of primary care (e.g. ensuring that children with special needs are immunized). Ideally, the child's primary healthcare provider should be viewed by all as the central figure in the process of coordinating referrals. The AAP's Medical Home model (www.medicalhomeinfo.org) offers helpful guidance on how primary care practices can best maintain the organization and communication needed to ensure continuity of care and to best meet the needs of children with disabilities and their families.

Summary

The administration of psychometrically sound screens is only one step in the process of caring for the developmental and behavioural needs of children. Skill in delivering difficult news to families, access to patient education materials, awareness of referral resources and locating support for care coordination are also critical. Periodic screening should be combined with a flexible longitudinal continuous and cumulative process of surveillance that includes the following:

1 eliciting and attending to parents' (and other caregiver) concerns;

2 maintaining a developmental behavioural history (milestone/skill monitoring);

3 identifying the presence of developmental behavioural (biological and environmental) risk and protective factors;

4 making accurate and informed observations about the child and the parent–child interactions;

5 promoting developmental behavioural wellness (e.g. literacy promotion/Reach Out and Read, strength-based or positive parenting counselling);

6 when indicated, responding to concerning screens with supplemental screens and/or medical tests;

7 thoughtfully interpreting screening test results;

8 referring promptly to community services;

9 documenting the process and findings;

10 reliably providing care coordination for referrals and/or office follow-up plans;

11 reviewing referral reports and recommendations and monitoring the child's early intervention/early childhood special education eligibility status and progress longitudinally over time; and

12 re-assessing a child's response to interventions when faced with a child who has chronic health conditions, and advising non-medical service providers as needed.

Developmental behavioural surveillance and screening also should adhere to the Institute of Medicine's quality aims.[56] Processes should (1) not harm patients/parents with a preterm diagnosis and yet emphasize safety by not delaying interventions for those who need them; (2) provide more equitable and effective care via less reliance on subjective clinician impressions; (3) offer timely services that are family and patient centred; and (4) provide efficient services. All of these aims can be enhanced via screening with accurate parent-report tools.[56–58]

REFERENCES

1. Sices L (2004) How do primary care physicians manage children with possible developmental delays? *Pediatrics* 113: 274–282.
2. Rydz D, Shevell MI, Majnemer A, et al (2005) Developmental screening. *Child Neurol* 20: 4–21.
3. Silverstein M, Sand N, Glascoe FP, et al (2005) Pediatricians' reported practices regarding developmental screening: do guidelines work? And do they help? *Pediatrics* 116: 174–179.
4. King T, Glascoe F (2003) Developmental surveillance of infants and young children in pediatric primary care. *Curr Opin Pediatr* 15: 624–629.
5. Halfon N, Regalado M, Sareen H, et al (2004) Assessing development in the paediatric office. *Pediatrics* 113(Suppl): 1926–1933.
6. Palfrey JS, Singer JD, Walker DK, et al (1987) Early identification of children's needs: a study of five metropolitan communities. *J Pediatr* 111: 651–659.
7. Ramey CT, Landesman Ramey S (1992) Effective early intervention. *Ment Retard* 30: 337–345.
8. Brooks-Gunn J, McCartoon CM, Casey PH, et al (1994) Early intervention in low-birth premature infants: results through age 5 years from the Infant Health and Development Program. *JAMA* 272: 1257–1262.
9. Capute AJ, Accardo PJ (1996) A neurodevelopmental perspective on the continuum of developmental disabilities. In: Capute AJ, Accardo PJ, editors. *Developmental Disabilities in Infancy and Childhood*, 2nd edition, Vol. 1. Baltimore, MD: Paul H Brookes, pp. 1–22.
10. McCarton CM, Brooks-Gunn J, Wallace IF, et al (1997) Results at age 8 years of early intervention for low-birth-weight premature infants. The Infant Health and Development Program. *JAMA* 227: 126–132.
11. Olds DL, Eckenrode J, Henderson CR Jr, et al (1997) Long-term effects of home visitation on maternal life course and child abuse and neglect: Fifteen-year follow-up of a randomized trial. *JAMA* 278: 637–643.
12. Old D, Henderson CR Jr, Cole R, et al (1998) Long-term effects of nurse home visitation on children's criminal and antisocial behavior: 15-year follow-up of a randomized controlled trial. *JAMA* 280: 1238–1244.
13. Eckenrode J, Ganzel B, Henderson CR Jr, et al (2000) Preventing child abuse and neglect with a program of nurse home visitation: the limiting effects of domestic violence. *JAMA* 284: 1385–1391.
14. Reynolds AJ, Temple JA, Robertson DL, et al (2001) Long-term effects of an early childhood intervention on educational achievement and juvenile arrest: a 15-year follow-up of low-income children in public schools. *Arch Pediatr Adolesc Med* 285: 2339–2346.
15. Reynolds AJ, Temple JA, Ou SR, et al (2007) Effects of a school-based, early childhood intervention on adult health and well-being: a 19-year follow-up of low-income families. *Arch Pediatr Adolesc Med* 161: 730–739.
16. Shonkoff JP (2003) From neurons to neighbourhoods; old and new challenges for developmental and behavioral pediatrics. *J Dev Behav Pediatr* 24: 70–76.
17. McCormick MC, Brooks-Gunn J, Buka SL, et al (2006) Early intervention in low birth weight premature infants: results at 18 years of age for the Infant Health and Development Program. *Pediatrics* 117: 771–780.
18. American Academy of Pediatrics Council on Children with Disabilities, Section on Developmental Behavioral Pediatrics, Bright Futures Steering Committee, Medical Home Initiatives for Children with Special Needs Project Advisory Committee (2006) Identifying infants and young children with developmental disorders in the medical home: an algorithm for developmental surveillance and screening. *Pediatrics* 118: 405–420 (http://aappolicy.aappublications.org/).
19. Johnson CP, Myers SM, the Council on Children with Disabilities (2007) Identification and evaluation of children with autism spectrum disorders. American Academy of Pediatrics Policy Statement. *Paediatrics* 120: 1183–1215.
20. American Academy of Pediatrics Task Force on Mental Health (2010) Enhancing pediatric mental health care: strategies for preparing a primary care practice. *Pediatrics* 125(Suppl 3): S87–S108.

21. American Academy of Pediatrics, Committee on Children with Disabilities (2001) Developmental surveillance and screening of infants and young children. *Pediatrics* 108, 192–196 (http://aappolicy.aappublications.org/).

22. Sameroff AJ, Seifer R, Barocas R, et al (1987) Intelligence quotient scores of 4-year-old children: social–environmental risk factors. *Paediatrics* 79: 343–350.

23. Aylward GP (1990) Environmental influences on the developmental outcome of children at risk. *Infants and Young Children* 2: 1–9.

24. Rydz D, Srour M, Oskoui M, Marget N, et al (2006) Screening for developmental delay in the setting of a community pediatric clinic: a prospective assessment of parent-report questionnaires. *Pediatrics* 118: e1178–e1186.

25. Bell RQ (1986) Age-specific manifestations in changing psychosocial risk. In: Farran DC, McKinney JC, editors. *Risk in Intellectual and Psychosocial Development*. Orlando, FL: Academic Press, Inc.

26. Yeargin-Allsopp M, Murphy CC, Oakley GP, Sikes RK (1992) A multiple-source method for studying the prevalence of developmental disabilities in children: The Metropolitan Atlanta Developmental Disabilities Study. *Pediatrics* 89: 624–630.

27. Newacheck, PW, Strickland B, Shonkoff, JP, et al (1998) An epidemiologic profile of children with special health care needs. *Pediatrics* 102: 117–123.

28. Lavigne JV, Binns JH, Christoffel KK, et al, the Pediatric Practice Research Group (1993) Behavioral and emotional problems among preschool children in pediatric primary care: prevalence and pediatricians' recognition. *Paediatrics* 91: 649–655.

29. Horwitz SM, Irvin JR, Briggs-Gowan MJ, Bosson Heenan JM, Mendoza J, Carter AS (2003) Language delay in a community cohort of young children. *J Am Acad Child Adolesc Psychiatry* 42: 932–940.

30. Tomblin JB, Records NL, Buckwalter P, Zhang X, Smith E, O'Brien M (1997) Prevalence of specific language impairment in kindergarten children. *J Speech Lang Hear Res* 40: 1245–1260.

31. Boydell Brauner C, Bowers Stephens C (2006) Estimating the prevalence of early childhood serious emotional/behavioral disorders: challenges and recommendations. *Public Health Rep* 121: 303–310.

32. Centers for Disease Control and Prevention (2003) *Mental Health in the United States: Prevalence of Diagnosis and Medication Treatment for Attention Deficit/Hyperactivity Disorder*. Available at: www.cdc.gov/mmwr/preview/mmwrhtml/mm5434a2.htm (accessed 1 February 2011).

33. Boyle CA, Decoufle P, Yeargin-Allsopp M (1994) Prevalence and health impact of developmental disabilities in US children. *Pediatrics* 93: 399–403.

34. Lingam R, Hunt L, Golding J, Jongmans M, Emond A (2009) Prevalence of developmental coordination disorder using the DSM-IV at 7 years of age: a UK population-based study. *Pediatrics* 123: e693–e700.

35. American Psychiatric Association (2000) *Diagnostic and Statistical Manual of Mental Disorders,* 4th edition, text revision. Washington, DC: American Psychiatric Association.

36. Barnes KE (1982) *Preschool Screening: The Measurement and Prediction of Children at Risk*. Springfield, IL: Charles C. Thomas.

37. Boyle CA, Yeargin-Allsopp M (1991) Prevalence of selected developmental disabilities in children 3–10 years of age: the metropolitan Atlanta developmental disabilities surveillance program. *MMWR Surveill Summ* 45(SS-2): 1–14. Available at: www.cdc.gov/mmwr/preview/mmwrhtml/00040928.htm (accessed 1 February 2011).

38. Bertrand JM, Boyle C, Bove F, Yeargin-Allsopp M, Decoufle P (2001) Prevalence of autism in a United States population: the Brick Township, New Jersey, investigation. *Pediatrics* 108: 1155–1161.

39. Autism and Developmental Disabilities Monitoring Network Surveillance Year 2002, Principal Investigators; Centers for Disease Control and Prevention (2007) Prevalence of autism spectrum disorders – autism and developmental disabilities monitoring network, 14 sites, United States, 2002. *MMWR Surveill Summ* 56: 12–28.

40. Kogan MD, Blumberg SJ, Schieve LA, et al (2009) Prevalence of parent-reported diagnosis of autism spectrum disorder among children in the US, 2007. *Pediatrics* 124: 1395–1403.

41. Canadian Psychological Association (1996) *Guidelines for Advertising Preschool Screening Tests*. Ottawa, ON: Canadian Psychological Association. Available at: www.cpa.ca/guide11.html (accessed 1 February 2011).

42. American Educational Research Association, American Psychological Association, National Council on Measurement in Education (NCME) (1999) *Standards for Educational and Psychological Test,* 2nd edition. Washington, DC: American Psychological Association.

43. Squires J, Nickel RE, Eisert D (1996) Early detection of developmental problems: strategies for monitoring young children in the practice setting. *JDBP* 17: 420–427.

44. Lichtenstein R, Ireton H (1984) *Preschool Screening: Identifying Young Children with Developmental and Educational Problems*. Orlando, FL: Grune & Stratton.

45. Glascoe FG (2001) Are overreferrals on developmental screening tests really a problem? *Arch Pediatr Adolesc Med* 155: 54–59.

46. Alfonso VC, Flanagan DP (2008) Assessment of preschool children: a framework for evaluating the adequacy of the technical characteristics of norm-referenced instruments. In: Mowder B, Rubinson F, Yasik A, editors. *Evidence Based Practice in Infant and Early Childhood Psychology*. New York: Wiley & Sons, pp. 3–44.

47. Marks K, Glascoe FP, Aylward G, Shevell MI, Lipkin PH, Squires JK (2008) The thorny nature of predictive validity studies on screening tests for developmental-behavioral problems. *Pediatrics* 122: 866–868.

48. Hix-Small H, Marks K, Squires J, Nickel R (2007) Impact of developmental screening at 12 and 24 months in a pediatric practice. *Pediatrics* 120: 381–389.

49. Schonwald A, Huntington N, Chan E, Risko W, Bridgemohan C (2009) Routine developmental screening implemented in urban primary care settings: more evidence of feasibility and effectiveness. *Pediatrics* 123: 660–668.

50. Marks K, Hix-Small H, Clark K, Newman J (2009) Lowering developmental screening thresholds and raising quality improvement for preterm children. *Pediatrics* 123: 1516–1523.

51. King TM, Tandon D, Macias MM, et al (2010) Implementing developmental screening and referrals: lessons learned from a national project. *Pediatrics* 125: 350–360.

52. Dobrez D, Lo Sasso AL, Holl J, Shalowitz M, Leon S, Budetti P (2001) Estimating the cost of developmental and behavioral screening of preschool children in general pediatric practice. *Pediatrics* 108: 913–922.

53. Glascoe FP, Foster MF, Wolraich ML (1997) An economic analysis of developmental detection methods. *Pediatrics* 99: 830–837.

54. Glascoe FP, Byrne KE, Chang B, Strickland B, Ashford L, Johnson K (1992) The accuracy of the Denver-II in developmental screening. *Pediatrics* 89: 1221–1225.

55. Kube DA. Wilson WM. Petersen MC. Palmer FB (2000) CAT/CLAMS: its use in detecting early childhood cognitive impairment. *Pediatr Neurol* 23: 208–215.

56. Hoon AH Jr. Pulsifer MB. Gopalan R. Palmer FB. Capute AJ (1993) Clinical Adaptive Test/Clinical Linguistic Auditory Milestone Scale in early cognitive assessment. *J Pediatr* 123: S1–S8.

57. Forrest CB. Nutting PA. Starfield B. von Schrader S (2002) Family physicians' referral decisions: results from the ASPN referral study. *J Fam Pract* 51: 215–222.

58. Institute of Medicine Committee on Quality of Health Care in America (2001) *Crossing the Quality Chasm: A New Health System for the 21st Century*. Washington, DC: National Academy Press.

APPENDIX 17.1

DEVELOPMENTAL, MENTAL HEALTH/BEHAVIOURAL AND ACADEMIC SCREENS

This appendix was compiled by Frances Page Glascoe, PhD, Professor of Pediatrics, Vanderbilt University (Nashville, TN), with assistance from other screening test authors and screening test researchers whose works are described below.

The following chart is a list of measures that meet standards for screening test accuracy, meaning that they correctly identify, at all ages, at least 70% of children with disabilities while also correctly identifying at least 70% of children without disabilities. All included measures were standardized on nationally representative samples in the USA, are proven to be reliable (i.e. inter-rater, test–retest and internal consistency of ≥0.85) and are validated against a range of diagnostic measures (and shown to have significantly high correlations). Details on the psychometric support for each tool along with research findings on discriminant validity can be found on each publisher's website (or within the manual for each test).

Measures are sorted into those that are most feasible in health care versus early childhood or other programmes (where there may be more time, skill and, for educational programming purposes, a greater need to observe and directly test children during the process of screening).

General or broad-band screens are presented first. These cover the broad domains of development (i.e. cognitive/academic, language, motor, self-help). Some broad-band screens also cover socioemotional/behavioural/mental health.

Because providers are often charged with detecting autism spectrum disorder and mental health problems (and because not all broad-band screens address such problems), a list of condition-specific or narrow-band tools follow. These measures should be administered only after problematic performance on a general screen and thus focus on only a few domains. Narrow-band tools can help determine the need for simultaneous referrals to specialty clinics focused on the diagnosis of autism and mental health. Not included are narrow-band tools that screen language or motor disorders in greater depth. Such tools are best administered by specialists such as speech–language pathologists or developmental behavioural

paediatricians. For primary care, broad-band screens are sufficient to make a decision about whether a referral is needed.

The first column in the chart provides publication information, the cost of purchasing a specimen set and the training options available. The 'Description' column provides information on alternative ways, if available, to administer measures (e.g. waiting rooms). The 'Accuracy' column shows the percentage of patients with and without problems identified correctly. The 'Time frame/costs' column shows the costs of materials per visit along with the costs of professional time (using an average salary of US$60 per hour) needed to administer and interpret each measure. Time/cost estimates do not include expenses associated with referring. For parent-report tools, administration time reflects not only scoring of test results, but also the relationship between each test's reading level and the average percentage of parents with less than a high school education (who may or may not be able to complete measures in waiting rooms owing to literacy problems and thus will need more time-consuming interview administrations). Measures in each table are arranged according to the time required to administer them by interview or directly to children, from least to most.

Information about electronic options is included at the end of the chart. Electronic applications save time, reduce human scoring errors, automate scoring, generate referral letters and aggregate results, which is helpful for programme evaluation and quality improvement initiatives. While somewhat more costly than print, electronic options offer time savings that offset the costs of hand-scoring, writing referral letters, and so on.

Note that measures such as the Denver-II, Developmental Indicators for the Assessment of Learning-III, Early Screening Profile (ESP), Early Learning Accomplishment Profile (E-LAP), Nippising are not included because they fail to meet the key technical standards for screening test construction (problematic standardization samples, out-of-date norming procedures, absent validation and limited to no proof of accuracy) and measures such as the Cognitive Adaptive Test/Clinical Linguistic and Auditory Milestone Scale, because they were standardized on referred (preterm or very low birth-weight) and not on general populations.

Also not included are diagnostic measures such as the Vanderbilt Diagnostic ADHD Scale, because such tools should only be used after a broad-band screening test indicates the need (e.g. Pediatric Symptom Checklist). The rationale is that, for example, conditions that present as ADHD can actually be symptoms of other problems such as academic deficits, depression, anxiety, and so on.

In settings where there are healthcare providers, such professionals can and should carefully document both medical history and physical examination to determine whether organic conditions are contributory; a list of exam foci are described in the footnote.[a]

When screening test results are problematic, referrals should begin with local services. This allows intervention to commence even while children typically need to wait for medical specialty exams, autism-focused clinics, etc. For medical professionals it may seem odd to refer for treatment before a diagnosis is finalized, but with young children (those who benefit most from early intervention), eligibility criteria are generally only a percentage of delay and do not require specific nosology.

---

[a] Medical history and physical examination for primary care.

Healthcare providers should conduct, along with developmental behavioural screening tests, a thorough physical examination at targeted well-visits: take note of such potentially teratogenic exposures as radiation or medications, infectious illnesses, fever, addictive substances or trauma, and review results of neonatal screens including phenylketonuria, hypothyroidism and other metabolic conditions. Your review should also consider the perinatal history, including birthweight, gestational age, Apgar scores and any medical complications. Postnatal medical factors should be considered, such as chronic respiratory or allergic illness, recurrent otitis, head trauma and sleep problems including symptoms of obstructive sleep apnoea. Family risk factors should be discussed (or captured via the Family Psychosocial Screen) and noted in the child's chart. These should include parental history of depression or anxiety, family history of developmental disabilities and substance abuse including smoking, etc

The physical examination should include attention to growth parameters, head shape and circumference, facial and other body dysmorphology, eye findings (e.g. cataracts in various inborn errors of metabolism), vascular markings and signs of neurocutaneous disorders (e.g. café-au-lait spots in neurofibromatosis, hypopigmented macules in tuberous sclerosis), muscle strength and tone, presence of abnormal reflexes and disturbance of movement. For guidance in conducting a paediatric neurodevelopmental examination, the following online video is helpful: http://library.med.utah.edu/pedineurologicexam/html/home_exam.html. Vision and hearing screening are essential. Lead screening should be provided whenever developmental problems arise, but preferably for all children, and repeated at several points during the 0- to 6-year age range.

---

1. Screens for primary care (all rely on information from parents owing to enhanced efficiency under time constraints. All cover developmental domains. Some also cover socioemotional, behavioural and mental health issues. Some can be administered by interview while others depend on parents, and optionally clinicians, to elicit skills). All also cover at least some degree of compliance with the American Academy of Pediatrics' 2006 statement on developmental behavioural screening and surveillance

Behavioural and/or developmental screens relying on information from parents	Age range	Description	Scoring	Accuracy	Time frame/costs. *Note:* publisher pricing and salary costs often change
Parents' Evaluations of Developmental Status (PEDS) (2009) www.PEDS*Test*.com (US$36) **Electronic offerings:** See below **Training options:** offers through its website self-training/train-the-trainer support via downloadable slide shows with notes, case examples, pre-/post-test questions, participant handouts, FAQs, website discussion list (covering all screens), short videos, with some live training available	Birth –8y	10 questions eliciting parents' concerns in English, Spanish, Vietnamese and many other languages. Written at the 5th-grade level. Screening/surveillance of development incuding social-emotional skills via parents' concerns. Longitudinal Score and Interpretation Forms assign risk levels, track decision-making and offer specific guidance on how to address concerns. Provides screening, longitudinal surveillance and triage for developmental as well as behavioural/social/emotional/mental health problems. PEDS can be used in conjunction with the PEDS:DM (below) for compliance with AAP policy on screening as well as surveillance, i.e. eliciting and addressing parents' concerns and monitoring milstones	Identifies when to refer and what types of referrals are needed; advise parents; monitor vigilantly; screen further (or refer for screening); or reassure	**By age** Sensitivity: 74–79% Specificity: 70–80% **By disabilities** i.e. learning, intellectual, language, mental health and autism spectrum disorders Sensitivity: 71–87%	Scoring time: 1 min Scoring cost: $1.20 Materials: $0.39 **Total (self-report): $1.59** Interview time: 2 min Interview cost: $2.40 Scoring/materials: $1.59 **Total (interview): $3.99**

Behavioural and/or developmental screens relying on information from parents	Age range	Description	Scoring	Accuracy	Time frame/costs. *Note*: publisher pricing and salary costs often change
PEDS: Developmental Milestones (PEDS-DM, screening version) www.PEDS*Test*.com ($275) **Electronic offerings:** see below **Training options:** Offers through its website self-training/train-the-trainer support via downloadable slide shows with notes, case examples, pre-/post-test questions, participant handouts, FAQs, website discussion list (covering all screens), short videos, with some live training available. The PEDS:DM manual includes extensive suggestions for training medical students, residents and nurses	0–8y	Screening and surveillance of developmental and social-emotional milestones. PEDS-DM consists of 6–8 items at each age level. Each item taps a different domain (fine/gross motor, self-help, academics, expressive/receptive language, socio-emotional). The PEDS:DM provides screening, triage and surveillance via a longitudinal score form for tracking milestones progress. Written at the 2nd to 3rd grade level, and can be completed by self-report, interview or administered directly to children. Forms are laminated and completed with a dry erase marker. Supplemental measures focused on AAP policy include the M-CHAT, Family Psychosocial Screen, Pictorial PSC-17, the SWILS, the Vanderbilt ADHD scale and the Brigance Parent–Child Interactions Scale. When combined with PEDS it ensures full compliance with AAP policy. In English, Spanish, Portuguese and Taiwanese with other languages in progress.	Pass/fail cut-offs tied to performance above and below the 16th centile for each item and its domain	**By age** Sensitivity: 70–94%; Specificity: 77–93% **By developmental domain** Sensitivity: 75–87% Specificity: 71–88%	Scoring time: 1 min Scoring cost: $1.20 Materials: $0.02 **Total (self-report): $1.22** Interview time: 3 min Interview cost: $3.00 Direct administration time: 4 min Direct administration cost: $4.00 Scoring/materials: $1.22 **Total (interview): $3.82** **Total (direct admin): $6.10**
Ages and Stages Questionnaire, Third Edition (ASQ-3) (2009) Paul H. Brookes Publishing, Inc. www.agesandstages.com ($199.95 each for English or Spanish) **Electronic offerings:** see below **Training options:** DVDs for purchase, case examples and live training	1–66 mo	Parents indicate children's developmental skills on 30 or so items plus overall concerns. The ASQ has a different form (5–8 pages) for each age interval. Written at the 4th–6th-grade level. Can be used in mass mail-outs for child-find programmes. Manual contains detailed instructions for organizing child-find programmes and includes activity handouts for parents. The ASQ-3 is available in English and Spanish, with the ASQ-2 also available in French and Korean with additional translations under way	Cut-off scores set at 2 standard deviations below the mean, in five developmental domains: indicate need for referral or monitoring	**By age** Sensitivity: 82–89% Specificity: 77–92% **By domain** Sensitivity: 83% Specificity: 91% **By disabilities,** i.e. cerebral palsy, visual and hearing impairment Sensitivity: 87% Specificity: 82%	Scoring time: 2 min Scoring cost: $2.40 Materials: $~0.36–$0.48 **Total (self-report): $2.76–$2.88** Interview time: 12 min Interview cost: $14.40 Scoring/materials: $2.76–$2.88 **Total (interview): $17.28**

AAP, American Academy of Pediatrics; ADHD, attention-deficit–hyperactivity disorder; M-CHAT, Modified Checklist for Autism in Toddlers; PSC, Pediatric Symptom Checklist; SWILS, Safety Word Inventory Literacy Screen.

2. Narrow-band screens for young children (for mental health, psychosocial risk and autism spectrum disorder. These are valuable adjuncts in primary care and elsewhere but should *not* be used as the sole measure of developmental behavioural status)

Developmental behavioural screens relying on information from parents	Age range	Description	Scoring	Accuracy	Time frame/costs. *Note*: publisher pricing and salary costs often change
Modified Checklist for Autism in Toddlers (M-CHAT) (1999) Free download at: www.mchatscreen.com Included in the PEDS:DM (www.pedstest.com). **Electronic offerings:** see below **Training options:** none	18–60mo	Parent report of 23 yes–no questions and written at 4th–6th-grade reading level. Screens for autism spectrum disorder (ASD). Downloadable scoring template and .xls files for automated scoring. Available in multiple languages. If M-CHAT is failed, then the M-CHAT Follow-Up Interview is strongly recommended by its authors. This is because 6–10% of children fail the M-CHAT at the 18- and 24-month well-visits, which leads to a high over-referral rate for an expensive, comprehensive ASD evaluation	Pass/fail scores based on failing at least two critical items, or three or more non-critical items	**By age and by disability** i.e. autism spectrum disorders Sensitivity: 90% Specificity: 99%	Scoring time: 2min Scoring costs: $2.40 Materials: $0.06 **Total (self-report): $2.46** Interview time: 5min (excluding follow-up on any failed items) Interview cost: $6.00 Scoring/materials: $2.46 **Total (interview): $8.46**
Brief Infant–Toddler Social-Emotional Assessment (BITSEA) Harcourt Assessment, Inc. http://pearsonassess.com/ ($105) **Electronic offerings:** none **Training options:** none	12–36mo	42-item parent-report measure for identifying socioemotional/behavioural problems and delays in competence. Items were drawn from the assessment-level measure, the ITSEA. Written at the 4th–6th-grade level. Available in Spanish, French, Dutch, Hebrew	Cut-off points based on child age and sex show presence/ absence of problems and competence	**By age and disability** i.e. internalizing, externalizing and ASD Sensitivity: 80–95% Specificity: 80%	Scoring time: 3min Scoring costs: $3.60 Materials: $1.56 **Total (self-report): $5.16** Interview time: 6 min Interview costs: $7.20 Scoring/materials: $5.16 **Total (interview): $12.36**
Eyberg Child Behavior Inventory/Sutter–Eyberg Student Behavior Inventory (ECBI/SESBI) Psychological Assessment Resources www.parinc.com/ ($120) **Electronic offerings:** not yet available **Training options:** e-mail support, live training (cost unknown)	2–16y	The ECBI/SESBI consists of 36–38 short statements of common behaviour problems, along with parents' perceptions of problem intensity, i.e. a probe about the degree to which a specific issue is challenging for parents. The ECBI uses parent report while the SESBI is used for teacher report. Written at the 1st to 2nd-grade level, the measure functions as a problems checklist for planning interventions. Can be used as a longitudinal indicator of progress. In print in English and licensed in Spanish and nine other languages	Single refer/ non-refer score for externalizing problems, conduct, aggression, etc. plus an intensity score per item	**By age and by disability** i.e. conduct disorders Sensitivity: 80% Specificity: 86%	Scoring time: 5 min Scoring costs: $5.00 Material costs: $1.52 **Total (self-report): $6.52** Interview time: 5 min Interview costs: $5.00 Scoring/materials: $6.52 **Total (interview): $11.52**

Developmental behavioural screens relying on information from parents	Age range	Description	Scoring	Accuracy	Time frame/costs. *Note*: publisher pricing and salary costs often change
Infant–Toddler Checklist for Language and Communication (1998) Paul H. Brookes Publishing, Inc. www.pbrookes.com ($109.95) **Electronic offerings:** Scoring CD-ROM **Training options:** live training (cost unknown)	6–24mo	Parents complete the checklist's 24 multiple-choice questions. Focuses on screening for language, social communication. Examiners are encouraged to observe child to verify parents' answers via brief observation. Reading level is ~3rd grade. Can serve as an entry point into the assessment-level, CSBS and also as a monitoring tool. Does not screen for motor milestones. In English, Spanish, Slovenian, Chinese and German	Cut-off scores for each domain: social, speech and symbolic	**By age and by disability** i.e. developmental disabilities Sensitivity: 78% Specificity: 84%	Scoring time: ~10min (by hand), ~3min with CD-ROM Observation time: ~5 min Scoring costs: $3–10.00 Observation costs: $5.00 Material costs: $0.12 **Total (self-report ±observation)=$3.12–15.12** Interview time: 8 min Interview costs: $8.00 Scoring/materials+observation: $3.12–15.12 **Total interview costs: $11.12–23.12**
Ages & Stages Questionnaires: Social-Emotional (ASQ:SE) Paul H. Brookes, Publishers www.pbrookes.com/ ($149) **Electronic offerings:** see below **Training options:** email support, training videos, live training (cost unknown)	3–66mo	Socioemotional/'broad-band behavioural' parent-report tool that is a companion measure to ASQ-3. The ASQ:SE consists of eight age-specific forms (each form is 4–6 pages long) with 19–33 items. Items focus on self-regulation, compliance, communication, adaptive functioning, autonomy, affect and interaction with people. Readability is 5–6th grade. Includes activities sheets for families. In English and Spanish	Single cut-off score indicating when a referral is needed	**By age and disability** i.e. socioemotional delays/problems Sensitivity: 71–85% Specificity: 90–98%	Scoring time: 2 min Scoring cost: $2.40 Material costs: $0.24–0.36 **Total (self-report): $2.64–$2.76** Interview time: 10min Interview cost: $12.00 Scoring/materials: $2.64–$2.76 **Total (interview): $14.64–$14.76**
Family Psychosocial Screening (FPS) Kemper KJ, Kelleher KJ. Family psychosocial screening: instruments and techniques. Included in PEDS:DM and downloadable at www.pedstest.com **Electronic offerings:** none **Training options:** none	Parents of all ages	A two-page clinic measure of psychosocial risk factors associated with developmental problems, often used for clinic intake. More than four risk factors are associated with developmental delays. The FPS also includes (1) a four-item screen for parental history of physical abuse as a child; (2) a six-item measure of parental substance abuse; (3) a four-item screen for domestic violence; and (4) a three item measure of maternal depression. Can be used along with the Brigance Parent–Child Interaction Scale to view parenting risk and resilience. More than four psychosocial risk factors are associated with developmental delays. Readability is 4th grade. In English and Spanish	Refer/no refer scores for each risk factor. Also has guides to referring and resource lists	**By condition** i.e. parental depression, substance abuse, etc. Sensitivity: >90% Specificity: >90%	Scoring time: 3 min Scoring cost: $3.60 Material costs: $0.00 (laminated)/$0.12 (photocopied) **Total (self-report): $3.60–$3.72** Interview time: 15min Interview cost: $18.00 Scoring/materials $.3.60–3.72 **Total (interview): $19.60–19.72**

CSBS, Communication and Symbolic Behavior Scales; PEDS-DM, Pediatric Emotional Distress Scale: Developmental Milestones.

3. Developmental screens relying on eliciting skills directly from children: these tools are recommended for early childhood, neonatal intensive care unit follow-up, referral clinic triage, etc. All require more time and skill than is typically available in primary care, although clinics with nurse practitioners (who generally have lots of assessment skills and who typically administer screens to a subset of general paediatric patients) may find any of the below helpful as a second-stage screen

Developmental behavioural screens relying on information from parents	Age range	Description	Scoring	Accuracy	Time frame/costs. *Note*: publisher pricing and salary costs often change
Bayley Infant Neurodevelopmental Screen (BINS) (1995) The Psychological Corporation www.pearsonassessments.com ($195) **Electronic offerings:** none **Training options:** none	3–24mo	Uses 10–13 directly elicited items per 3–6mo age range to assess neurological processes (reflexes, and tone); neurodevelopmental skills (movement and symmetry); and developmental accomplishments (object permanence, imitation and language). Standardized on a low birthweight, not general, sample	Categorizes performance into low, moderate or high risk via cut-off scores. Provides subtest cut-off scores for each domain	**By age and disability** i.e. cognitive delay and neurological/ motor impairment Sensitivity: 75–86% Specificity: 75–86%	Administration/ scoring time: 10min Administration/ scoring costs: $12.00 Materials $1.88 **Total: $13.88**
Brigance Screens-II (2005) Curriculum Associates, Inc., www.curriculumassociates.com/ ($737.00) **Electronic offerings:** see below **Training options:** live workshops (cost unknown), e-mail support, webcasts, videos, listserve	0–90mo	Nine separate forms, one for each 12mo age range. Taps speech–language, motor, readiness and general knowledge at younger ages and also reading and maths at older ages. Uses a combination of direct elicitation and observation. In the 0–2y age range, can be administered by parent interview. Includes longitudinal tracking, progress indicators plus separate psychosocial risk cut-offs for children in head start-type programmes who need 'the gift of time' before referral decisions are made. In English, with Spanish and other language directions	Cut-off, quotients, centiles, age-equivalent scores in various domains and overall	**By age and disabilities** i.e. language impairment, specific learning disabilities, mental retardation,[a] physical impairment, ASD) Sensitivity: 73–100% Specificity: 72–94% **By age, giftedness/ academic talent** Sensitivity: 81–100% Specificity: 70–94%	Administration/ scoring time: 10–15min Administration/ scoring costs: $12.00–18.00 Materials: $~1.25 **Total: ~$13.25–~19.25**
PEDS: Developmental Milestones (assessment version) (PEDS:DM) www.PEDS*Test*.com ($275) **Electronic offerings:** see below **Training options:** training is freely offered via downloadable slide shows with notes, case examples and handouts, website discussion list (covering all screens), training modules, short videos, e-mail/phone consultation with research/ training staff	0–8y	PEDS:DM assessment version uses the same items as the screening version but presents more at once in each domain (about 35 in total, depending on age) for fine motor, gross motor, self-help, academics, expressive language, receptive language and socioemotional. Items are administered by parents or professionals. Written at the 2nd-grade level. The assessment level booklet is reusable with each child and includes a longitudinal score form to track progress. Toolkit includes many supplemental measures that measure mental health/psychosocial function, risk of ASD, parent–child interactions, academic readiness and family psychosocial risk. In English and Spanish	Age-equivalent scores, percentage of delay/progress along with the same cut-offs, sensitivity/ specificity as the PEDS:DM screening version	**By age and disabilities** i.e. significant deficits in each domain of development on diagnostic measures Sensitivity: 75–94% Specificity: 71–93%	Scoring time: 5 min Scoring costs: $6.00 Materials $3.00 **Total (self-report): $9.00** Direct administration time: 10min Direct admin costs: $12.00 Scoring/materials: $9.00 **Total (direct admin): $21.00**

Developmental behavioural screens relying on information from parents	Age range	Description	Scoring	Accuracy	Time frame/costs. *Note*: publisher pricing and salary costs often change
Battelle Developmental Inventory Screening Test – II (BDIST-2) (2006) Riverside Publishing Company www.riversidepublishing.com ($311 with materials kit, $185 without materials) **Electronic offerings:** see below **Training options:** live workshops, webcasts	0–95mo	Items (at least six are needed per domain) use a combination of direct assessment, observation and parental interview to provide separate scores in adaptive behaviour, personal–social, communication, motor and cognitive domains. Used only to decide if the full BDI-2 is needed. Includes links to the Hawaii curriculum and to the BDI-2 curriculum. In English and Spanish	Age equivalents and cut-offs at 1.0, 1.5 and 2.0 standard deviations below the mean in each of five domains	**By age** Not available **By disability** i.e. to problematic performance on the full BDI-2, and only computed on a select sample with 50% of children qualifying for special services, making the following figures likely to be inflated when compared with other tools Sensitivity: 72–93% Specificity: 79–88%	Administration/ scoring time: 10–30min Admin/scoring costs: $12.00–36.00 Materials: $1.94 **Total: $13.94–37.94**

a UK usage: intellectual disability.

4. Screens for older children (these screens focus on academic skills and mental health, including attention-deficit– hyperactivity disorder [ADHD] screening. The shorter ones, such as the SWILS and PSC, are suitable for primary care)

Developmental behavioural screens relying on information from parents	Age range	Description	Scoring	Accuracy	Time frame/costs. *Note*: publisher pricing and salary costs often change
Safety Word Inventory and Literacy Screener (SWILS) PEDS*Test*.com, LLC items courtesy of Curriculum Associates, Inc The SWILS is included (laminated) in PEDS: Developmental Milestones (www.PEDS*Test*.com) **Electronic offerings:** none **Training options:** slide shows, email consultation at www.PEDS*Test*.com	6–14y	Children are asked (by parents or professionals) to read 29 common safety words (e.g. high voltage, wait, poison) aloud. The number of correctly read words is compared with a cut-off score. Results predict performance in maths, written language and a range of reading skills. Test content may serve as a springboard to injury prevention counselling and can be used to screen for parental literacy. Because even non-English speakers living in the USA need to read safety words in English, the measure is available only in English	Single cut-off score indicating the need for a referral	**By age/ academic deficits** Sensitivity: 73–88% Specificity: 77–88%	Scoring time: 1min Scoring costs: $1.20 Materials: $0.06 **Total (self report): $1.26** Admin time: ~7 min Admin/scoring costs: ~$8.40 Materials/scoring: $1.26 **Total (direct admin): ~$9.66**

Developmental behavioural screens relying on information from parents	Age range	Description	Scoring	Accuracy	Time frame/costs. *Note*: publisher pricing and salary costs often change
Pediatric Symptom Checklist (PSC) http://psc.partners.org/ The Pictorial PSC (PPSC) is useful with low-income Spanish-speaking families in its 17-item factorial version, which facilitates screening for ADHD, internalizing and externalizing disorders. The PSC is included (laminated) in the PEDS:DM (www.PEDS*Test*.com) **Electronic offerings:** none **Training options:** slide shows, email consultation at www.PEDS*Test*.com	4–16y (but 3–18y per the PSC authors)	Broad-band mental health tool that uses parent-report or adolescent self-report. 35 vs 17 short statements of problem behaviours including both externalizing (conduct) and internalizing (depression, anxiety, adjustment, etc.). The PSC/PPSC in their 17-item versions produce cut-offs for attentional, internalizing and externalizing problems. Readability is ~2nd grade and completion time is ~7 min. In English, Spanish, Portuguese, Chinese, Dutch, Filipino, French, Somali and several other languages. Standardized in 1998 (>10y ago) on national and diverse populations in the USA and Chile. There are numerous studies demonstrating its feasibility in multiple countries, socioeconomic groups and primary care settings	Single refer/ no refer score. Cut-off scores also available for attention, internalizing and externalizing problems. No questionable category	**PSC/PPSC by disability** i.e. mental health disorders of any kind, across numerous studies Sensitivity: 80–95%; Specificity: 68–100% **PSC-17/PPSC-17 by specific disability** i.e. ADHD Sensitivity: 58% Specificity: 91% **Internalizing disorders** Sensitivity: 52–73% Specificity: 74% **Externalizing disorders** Sensitivity: 62% Specificity: 89%	Scoring time: 3min Scoring cost: $3.60 Materials: laminated $0.00/photocopy ~$0.06 **Total (self-report): $3.66** Interview time: 3min Interview cost: $3.60 Materials/scoring: $3.66 **Total (interview): $7.26**
Strengths & Difficulties Questionnaire (SDQ) www.sdqinfo.com/ The SDQ is freely available in the public domain for print and online use	3–16y	Broad-band mental health tool that uses parent- and/or self-report. 25–35 questions about the child's emotions, conduct, hyperactivity, inattention and prosocial behaviours, but can include an 'impact' supplement to measure level of impairment. The four cut-off categories include 'close to average' vs 'slightly raised' vs 'high' vs 'very high'. Readability is <5th grade and completion time is ~7 min. Available in ~70 languages. www.sdqinfo.com/py/doc/b0.py. Standardized in 2001 (10y ago) on national and diverse populations in Britain and the USA	Single refer/no refer score; however, results yield four cut-off score categories	Sensitivity: 63.3% for parent-, teacher- and self-report Specificity: 94.6% for parent-, teacher- and self-report	Scoring time: 5min Scoring cost: $6.00 Materials: $0.12 **Total (self-report): $6.12** Interview time: 5min Admin/interview costs: $6.00 **Total (direct admin): $12.12**

PEDS, Parents' Evaluation of Developmental Status.

5. Electronic records options for screening with quality tools (including online and other digital approaches to administration and scoring)

Company	Training/support options	Description and pricing
CHADIS (www.chadis.com/) PEDS, ASQ, M-CHAT and other measures online for touch-screen, tablet PCs, keyboards and parent portal methods). Spanish-language version coming soon	Downloadable guides, live training at exhibits and other training services on request	CHADIS also includes decision support for a large range of other measures, both diagnostic and parent/family focused, such as the Vanderbilt ADHD Diagnostic Rating Scale, and various parental depression inventories. CHADIS offers integration with existing electronic health records. Works with a range of equipment/applications, and automatically generates reports. Pricing is ~$2.00 per use

Company	Training/support options	Description and pricing
PEDS*Test*.com LLC (www. PEDS*Test*.com/online) PEDS, M-CHAT, PEDS:DM online for keyboard and parent portal (PEDS:DM in Spanish and other translations coming soon)	Slide shows, website FAQs, email support, online videos, discussion list	This site offers PEDS, PEDS:DM and the M-CHAT for applications for keyboards (including i-Pad) allowing for actual comments from parents). Offers a parent portal (wherein families do not see the results), etc. Scoring is automated as are summary reports for parents, referral letters when needed and ICD-9/procedure codes. HL-7 integration with electronic records is available as are data export and aggregate views of records. $2.00–2.75 per use (depending on volume)
Brookes Publishing (www.agesandstages.com/) (ASQ/ASQ:SE via CD-ROM installed on keyboard computers, along with web-based scoring service)	Live training, online training, purchasable training videos, email listserv	ASQ on a CD-ROM enables users to click answers and receive an automated score. The software offers aggregation of results, report writing templates and progress tracking
Curriculum Associates (www.cainc.com) (Brigance Screens-II online for keyboards. English only but with Spanish-language score/administration forms)	Live training, online training, email and phone support, customer suggestion box	This service, web-based or via CD-ROM, provides clickable data sheets which automatically calculate scores including age equivalents, quotients, progress indicators, at-risk cut-off scores, quotients, etc. Aggregated reports are available through the online service. $3.00–5.00 per use, depending on volume
Riverside Publishing (www.riverpub.com) For Battelle Developmental Inventory along with the screening version (BDIST-II) online via keyboards and/or CD-ROM	Website FAQs, email support, live workshops, webcasts/webinars	Scoring services include report writing, all via web-based services. The website indicate a version for Personal Digital Assistants, but this will be phased out shortly. In English and Spanish. Pricing ~ $765 per year
Patient Tools (www.patienttools.com) (PEDS, M-CHAT, ASQ, ASQ:SE and others measures online for tablet PCs) Coming soon	Webcasts/webinars, live support by phone, email	Patient tools plans to offer the ASQ, ASQ:SE, M-CHAT, the Vanderbilt ADHD Scales and a wide range of behavioural/mental health measures for adolescents and adults. A parent portal approach is available via Survey Tablets. Equipment including docking stations is rented, lease-purchased, or purchased ($74.00–1320.00) after which $58.00 per month is the ongoing cost of hosting, data storage, telephone technical and installation support

Essential definitions are: keyboards, users can type in text-based answers to questions; touch-screens applications, hopefully self-explanatory but these often allow parents to also listen to questions and response options, thus reducing literacy demands; online, meaning an internet connection, preferably high speed, is needed; CD-ROM, offline but still electronic, and requiring installation on the user's computer; parent portal, applications (typically web-based and thus online) where parents can complete measures but do not see results. Rather, these are sent to a different office computer for inclusion in the medical record/sharing results; webcasts/webinars, either live or constantly available on publishers' websites. LiveWebcasts are generally translated into Webinars (a few days after a live webcast) and thus become videos/audios, usually freely available on demand. PEDS, Parents' Evaluation of Developmental Status; ASQ, Ages and Stages Questionnaire; M-CHAT, Modified Checklist for Autism in Toddlers; ADHD, attention-deficit–hyperactivity disorder; PEDS:DM, Parents' Evaluation of Developmental Status: Developmental Milestones; FAQ, frequently asked questions; ICD, International Classification of Diseases; HL-7, Health Level 7 International.

Disclosure: This table was compiled and vetted in collaboration with many researchers, clinicians and test authors, without regard to authors' potential financial interests in products mentioned.

18
GLOBAL DEVELOPMENTAL ASSESSMENTS

Barbara Mazer, Annette Majnemer, Noemi Dahan-Oliel and Irene Sebestyen

What is the construct?

Child development is the progressive ascertainment of new skills over time and is reflective of the integrity of the central nervous system.[1] Formal standardized measures of overall developmental ability are typically designed to quantify the degree of developmental progress in a range of domains, including gross and fine motor, cognition, speech and language, socioemotional and behavioural. These measures are composed of test items which assess skills thought to be indicative of those acquired within the context of typical development for age level.[2] These evaluation tools are usually tester-administered by a trained examiner who measures a child's responses to a structured set of tasks or activities, and are designed to compare a child's skills with the level of development found in the 'normal' or typically developing population. Standardized developmental tests are often viewed as the criterion standard for outcome assessment,[3] providing an objective, valid and reliable evaluation of a child's development in comparison to the norm, and typically provides standardized scores that can be used to classify developmental level.[3] Through the use of standardized administration and scoring criteria, measurement error is reduced, providing an objective, accurate evaluation of a child's abilities in various developmental domains.

Developmental assessments provide detailed information regarding skill attainment and are designed to accurately discriminate abnormality (deviance from the 'norm') and quantify the extent of developmental difficulty. In addition, they provide results of developmental progress within specific developmental domains, offering an indication of the child's areas of strength and weakness. For tests with discriminant validity, results from these assessments may be used for the early identification of children at risk for difficulties, to describe a child's skill acquisition compared with peers, to determine eligibility for services and to assess a child's specific needs for intervention.[2] Owing to the standardized administration and scoring procedures, they are also appropriate to be used on a large scale, such as in routine follow-up programmes and in research. While several tools suggest that they may be used to periodically monitor developmental progress over time, most tools have not evaluated responsiveness to change and caution should be used when interpreting scores over time.

Delays in the emergence of particular body functions (e.g. motor, speech, cognitive) are characterized clinically as developmental delays. Global developmental delay often refers to a delay (typically two standard deviations [SD] below the normative mean) in two or more domains of development.[4] The International Classification of Functioning, Disability and Health for Children and Youth (ICF-CY) interprets 'developmental delay' very broadly to include lags or delays in body functions and structures, and activities and participation.[5] Most standardized developmental assessment tools measure the child's capacity (what an individual can do), determining this by observing the child's ability to perform on a series of predetermined tasks. They provide a snapshot of a child's behaviour observed in a novel standardized situation and often within a new setting and should be considered as only one approach to gathering information regarding a child's abilities. These tests, for the most part, are not meant to provide an assessment of what the child does do in the real-life context as is the case with activities and participation measures. For this reason, we would suggest that most standardized measures of global development fit best within the body functions component.

General factors to consider when measuring this domain

A number of factors are highlighted below that can influence the use and interpretation of developmental assessments. These include administration, training, normative data, age and applicability to children with disabilities.

ADMINISTRATION

Tests of overall development are usually scored through the direct observation of child performance. While measures of a child's ability may accept proxy report of the child's ability, from a parent, caregiver or service provider, the standardized procedures of tests of overall development may not allow for proxy report. Credit for performance is provided only when each item is administered according to the prescribed guidelines and the child successfully completes the item according to preset criteria. Difficulties in obtaining an accurate measure of a child's abilities may arise when the child is tired, shy or otherwise uncooperative, reducing the validity of the resultant score. Clearly, if the purpose of the testing is to obtain standardized scores in order to compare the developmental level of an individual or group with the norm, the test must be administered in the prescribed standardized manner. When evaluating a child's abilities with the intent of obtaining a qualitative profile of development, the test may be adapted, but standardized scores should not be used.[3]

TRAINING

Developmental evaluations are administrated by a trained qualified examiner who must adhere to the stringent administration and scoring procedures. Evaluator training is imperative, as the objectivity and validity of the results are dependent upon the strict adherence to the standardized procedures. Requirements for training can include formal instruction, but typically entail reading the manual, familiarizing oneself with the detailed procedures, practising the administration of the test items and learning the scoring criteria. Evaluators are expected to have knowledge and clinical expertise related to child development.

NORMATIVE DATA

The attainment of developmental skills changes over time, suggesting that the use of norms from older tests may no longer be valid. Indeed, it has been shown that there is an upward drift in standardized scores over time,[3,6] and when older norms are used, the developmental level may be overestimated.[7] Newer tests are more likely to contain test items that are based on recent ecologically valid empirical studies and methods of assessing development, ensuring that individuals are assessed and compared with current normative standards. It is always critical to examine the make-up of the normative sample in order to determine whether the norms are applicable to the population of interest.[8]

AGE

While developmental assessments aim to evaluate the developmental level of a child in a variety of domains, the resultant scores may be influenced by several factors. The naturally occurring variations in the rate and intensity of development between the domains (e.g. at 18mo there are many more motor items than language items to test) present a barrier to the construction of a multidimensional measure with sufficient content validity across all areas.[8] If the test has a small sample of items within a specific age, it has a weak test 'floor' or 'ceiling' and may not have adequate validity for those age ranges. In those cases, test results may be variable and can lack validity owing to the large influence of a few items.[8] When assessing the development of children born preterm, it is imperative to account for delays in development due to the early birth. It is recommended to correct for the number of weeks born preterm for children born <32 weeks' gestation until at least 2 years of age.[3]

CHILDREN WITH DISABILITIES

While developmental assessments are meant to be used with atypically developing children, they are rarely standardized on children with disabilities, and it is often a challenge to administer these tools using the prescribed standardized procedures. In many cases, when testing children with disabilities, the tool cannot be adapted and the normative data and standardized scores cannot be used. It is important to note that the various facets of development are often interdependent and, therefore, to successfully complete items in a specific developmental domain may require additional skills in other domains. For example, test items in the domain of cognition may also require motor skills in order to complete the test items. Several tests offer suggested methods of adapting the items for children with disabilities. For example, it is recommended that tests that provide separate scores for verbal and non-verbal subtests be used for children with hearing and/or language impairment.

Overview of recommended measures

Several measures of overall child development have been created over the past few decades. This review will focus on seven commonly used measures that have been reported and described in the literature. These include the following:

- Battelle Developmental Inventory, second edition (BDI-2)
- Bayley Scales of Infant and Toddler Development, third edition (Bayley-III)
- Griffiths Mental Development Scales – revised (GMDS-R)
- McCarthy Scales of Children's Abilities (MSCA)

TABLE 18.1

Overview of domains assessed for the seven developmental assessments

Developmental assessment	Age range	Gross motor, fine motor	Cognition	Speech and language	Socioemotional, behavioural	Adaptive, self-care
BDI-II (Battelle)	0–7y	Yes	Yes	Yes	Yes	Yes
Bayley-III	1–42mo	Yes	Yes	Yes	Yes	Yes
GMDS-R (Griffiths)	0–8y	Yes	Yes	Yes	Yes	No
MSCA (McCarthy)	2y 6mo–8y 6mo	Yes	Yes	Yes	No	No
MPSD-R (Merrill–Palmer)	1mo–6y 6mo	Yes	Yes	Yes	Yes	Yes
MAP (Miller)	33–68mo	Yes	Yes	Yes	No	No
MSEL (Mullen)	0–5y 8mo	Yes	No	Yes	No	No

BDI-II, Batelle Developmental Inventory; GMDS-R, Griffiths Mental Development Scales, revised; MAP, Miller Assessment for Preschoolers; MPSD-R, Merrill–Palmer Scales of Development; MSCA, McCarthy Scales of Children's Abilities; MSEL, Mullen Scales of Early Learning.

- Merrill–Palmer Scales of Development – Revised (MPSD-R)
- Miller Assessment for Preschoolers (MAP)
- Mullen Scales of Early Learning (MSEL)

Table 18.1 summarizes the ages and domains evaluated by each of these measures. Furthermore, a detailed overview of the purpose, administration and scoring procedures is described for each of these measures, and their psychometric properties are summarized. Individually, charts display the key features for those measures that cover development more globally and have acceptable psychometric properties.

Other published tools which are in use but have not yet been extensively evaluated (e.g. psychometric properties) in the literature include the Developmental Assessment of Young Children (DAYC),[9] Developmental Profile 3 (DP-3),[10] Early Learning Accomplishment Profile (ELAP),[11] Infant–Toddler Developmental Assessment (ITDA)[12] and Parents' Evaluation of Developmental Status: Developmental Milestones (PEDS:DM).[13] All of these assessment tools evaluate development within a range of domains, including motor, cognitive, language and socioemotional, among others. Both the ELAP and ITDA assess the development of young children until age 3 years, the DAYC to age 5 years, the PEDS:DM to age 8 years, and the DP-3 provides information on development from 0 to 12 years. Typically, these measures use flexible administration procedures, including a combination of direct observation and caregiver interview. The DAYC also comprises a teacher-administered language screening tool for a classroom setting.[14]

BATTELLE DEVELOPMENTAL INVENTORY (BDI), SECOND EDITION

Overview and purpose
The BDI has a well-established tradition dating back to 1973, when the USA Office of Education initiated a project to evaluate the effectiveness of the Handicapped Children's Early Education Program. The BDI was completed in 1984, and revised in 2005. This recent version combines many of the important features of the earlier edition with important improvements in psychometric properties, is based on changes in life experiences of children and includes new user-friendly materials and technology.

The BDI-2 is an individually administered standardized tool that is designed and constructed as an assessment of a child's development. It may be used to identify and describe developmental delay, as well as typical or advanced development, from birth to 7 years of age. It is not intended as an instrument for diagnosing specific disabilities. The BDI-2 may be used with children with disabilities and can assist in planning intervention and evaluating programmes servicing children.

Administration and scoring
The BDI-2 uses a combination of three administration formats – structured task, interview and observation. It requires 1 to 2 hours to administer. Testing may occur over several days if necessary, but should be completed within a 2-week period.

The BDI-2 includes 450 items assessing five domains of development, including adaptive, personal–social, communication, cognitive and motor. The *adaptive domain* measures the child's ability to use the information and skills acquired in the other domains. It is divided into two subdomains: *self-care* and *personal responsibility*. The self-care subdomain assesses the child's ability to perform tasks associated with daily routines with increasing independence. Personal responsibility assesses the ability to assume responsibility for performing simple chores. The *personal–social domain* evaluates abilities and characteristics that allow a child to engage in meaningful social interactions with adults and peers and to develop his or her own self-concept and sense of social role. The behaviours measured in this domain are divided into three subdomains: *adult interaction*, *peer interaction* and *self-concept and social role*. The first two subdomains measure the quality and frequency of a child's interaction with adults and children (of similar age). The self-concept and social role subdomain evaluates a child's development with respect to self-awareness, personal knowledge, self-worth and pride, moral development, sensitivity to others' needs and feelings, and coping skills. The *communication domain* measures how effectively a child receives and expresses ideas through verbal and non-verbal means. The *receptive* subdomain looks at the ability to discriminate, recognize and understand sounds, words and information received through gestures and other non-verbal means. The *expressive* subdomain assesses the child's production and use of sounds, words or gestures to relate information, the knowledge and ability to use simple grammatical rules to produce phrases and sentences and the child's use of language as a tool for social contact. The *motor domain* evaluates the child's ability to control large and small muscle groups. The *gross motor* subdomain reflects the development of the large muscle systems used in locomotion skills and the *fine motor* subdomain assesses the development of fine muscle control, particularly the small muscles in the arms and hands. The *perceptual motor* subdomain measures the ability to integrate fine motor and perceptual skills for various tasks. Finally, the *cognitive domain* measures the skills and abilities commonly thought of as 'mental' or 'intellectual', with the exception of language and communication. The *attention and memory* subdomain includes the ability to visually and auditorally attend to environmental stimuli and to retrieve information when given relevant clues, both in the short and long term. The *reasoning and academic skills* subdomain assesses the critical thinking skills that a child needs to perceive, identify and solve problems, analyse and appraise the elements of situations, identify missing components, contradictions and inconsistencies, and judge and evaluate ideas, processes and products. The final subdomain, *perception and concepts*, assesses an infant's active sensorimotor interaction with the immediate environment

and the older child's ability to conceptualize and discriminate object features.

The BDI-2 test kit includes five item test books, one for each of the BDI-2 domains. Each test book contains the test items, administration procedures, scoring information and a list of toys and/or materials required to administer each item. The kit also includes a package of record forms, student workbooks, a set of presentation cards, stimulus book, an examiner's manual, a complete set of the BDI-2 screening test materials and a carrying case. Optional computer software components (for scoring) and objects that can be handled (toys and other materials necessary for test administration) are also available, but sold separately.

The BDI-2 domains may be administered in any order. It is recommended that the examiner administer all the subdomains within a specific domain and in the order that they appear on the score sheet. A script for the examiner to follow is provided in each of the item booklets, and the method options that may be used to administer each item are listed on the score sheet. Modifications are provided to facilitate administration for children with health conditions.

Starting points are generally determined by the child's chronological age and on known information about the child. Basal and ceiling levels must be attained. The basal level is attained by a score of 2 on three consecutive items. The ceiling is obtained by a score of 0 on three consecutive items. Each item is scored on a three-point scale, with a score of 2 indicating that the child's response meets the specified criteria, 1 that the child attempted the item but did not meet all the criteria and 0 when the response is incorrect or there is no response or opportunity to respond. Raw scores for each subdomain may be converted into subdomain scaled scores, centile ranks and age equivalents. Scaled scores for each subdomain are added together to obtain the domain scaled score, and the domain scaled scores are then added to provide the BDI-2 total score. These are converted into developmental quotients and centile ranks. The scoring of this tool makes it possible to profile domain and subdomain scores and compare weaknesses and strengths in various areas. These profiles can be used to help determine whether a child's deficit is due to weakness in all areas of development or in specific areas.[15] Scoring may be done by hand or by using the optional scoring software.

The BDI-2 screening test is another available format of the test, and was designed as a method of determining whether a child warranted further and more in-depth evaluation. It consists of the same domains and subdomains measured by the full BDI-2, but with only two to three items per age range for each subdomain.[16]

BATTELLE DEVELOPMENTAL INVENTORY, SECOND EDITION (BDI-2)	
Purpose	To measure the developmental abilities of young children in multiple domains and to identify disability or developmental delay. It can be used to measure developmental progress, and is useful for developing and implementing individualized education programmes and individualized family service plans
Population	Young children aged 0–7y; may be used with children with disabilities
Description of domains (subscales)	450 test items divided into five domains: Motor: gross motor, fine motor, perceptual motor Adaptive: self-care, personal responsibilities Communication: receptive, expressive Cognitive: attention and memory, reasoning and academic Personal–social: adult and peer interaction, self-concept and social growth
Administration and test format	Time to complete: 1–2h to administer, 30min to score Testing format: combination of structured administration, observation and interview. Modifications are provided to facilitate administration for children with various health conditions. Includes a shorter, efficient, comprehensive screening test (consists of 100 of the 450 items) Scoring: three-point scoring system: 2, response meets specified criteria; 1, attempted item but did not meet all the criteria; 0, incorrect/no response/no opportunity to respond. Subdomain raw scores are converted into scale scores, centile ranks and age equivalents. Developmental quotients and centile ranks are derived for each of the five developmental domains as well as for overall development. The BDI-2 can be scored by hand or with optional scoring software (BDI-2 data manager software) Training: no formal training is necessary. May be administered by healthcare professionals, infant intervention specialists, preschool and primary school educators and assessment specialists. Evaluators must learn and be comfortable with evaluation components
Psychometric properties	Normative sample: 2500 children in the USA, nationally represented *Reliability* Internal consistency (subdomains: r=0.85–0.95; domain developmental quotients: r=0.90–0.96; BDI-2 total score: r=0.99) Inter-rater reliability: r=0.97–0.99 Test–retest reliability (subdomains: r=0.74–0.92; domains: r=0.87–0.92; total BDI-2: r=0.94) *Validity* Criterion validity: correlations between BDI-2 and original BDI (r=0.64–0.76 for domains and r=0.78 for developmental quotients); Bayley Scales of Infant Development II (r=0.61–0.75); Denver Developmental Screening Test, second edition (r=0.83–0.90); Preschool Language Scale (r=0.63–0.73) Construct validity: subdomain scores highly correlated with total domain score, and domain scores highly correlated with the total score, except for motor domain (r=0.49)
How to order	Purchase from www.assess.nelson.com in Canada or www.riverpub.com in the USA Cost: CAD$1460; US$985 (includes full kit and manipulatives); additional cost for data manager software
Key reference	Newburg J (2005) *Battelle Developmental Inventory*, 2nd edition. Itasca, IL: Riverside Publishing Company.

The BDI-2 can be used by infant interventionists, pre-school and primary school teachers and special educators, as well as healthcare professionals. Formal training is not mandatory. A thorough understanding of the BDI-2, familiarity with child development, and appropriate training and experience working with children are prerequisites for testing.

Psychometric properties

The standardization of the BDI-2 was based on a nationally representative sample of 2500 children, from birth to 7 years 11 months. The sample was matched to the percentages of age, sex, ethnicity, geographic region and socioeconomic levels specified by the US Census Bureau (2001).

The reliability of the BDI-2 meets or exceeds traditional standards for excellence at the subdomain, domain and full test composite levels.[17] Internal consistency for the 13 subdomains ranged from $r=0.85$ to $r=0.95$. The coefficients for the domain developmental quotients ranged from $r=0.90$ to $r=0.96$ and were quite consistent across age groups. High test–retest correlations support the reliability of the BDI-2 ($r=0.74–0.92$ for subdomains; $r=0.87–0.92$ for domains; $r=0.94$ for total BDI-2). Inter-rater reliability is high with correlations of $r=0.97$ to 0.99.

Criterion validity[16] was determined when evaluating the correlation of the BDI-2 with the original BDI,[18] Bayley-II,[19] Denver Developmental Screening Test-2 ($r=0.83–0.90$),[20] Preschool Language Scales, fourth edition ($r=0.63–0.73$),[21] Vineland Social–Emotional Childhood Scales[22] and Wechsler Preschool and Primary Scale of Intelligence, third edition.[23] Correlations between the BDI-2 and the original BDI domain scores ranged from $r=0.64$ to $r=0.76$, with the total development quotient scores correlating at $r=0.78$. Correlations between the BDI-2 and the Bayley-II were reported for the cognitive ($r=0.61$), communication ($r=0.75$) and motor ($r=0.64$) domains. Correlations between the BDI-2 and these measures of development were within the moderate to high range ($r=0.63–0.90$). Construct validity was measured through age trends, intercorrelations of the total domain and subdomain scores, and factor analysis. All provided strong evidence of good construct validity, except for the correlation between the total score and the motor domain score ($r=0.49$).

BAYLEY SCALES OF INFANT AND TODDLER DEVELOPMENT, THIRD EDITION

Overview and purpose

The Bayley-III is recognized internationally as one of the most comprehensive tools to assess the development of young children. The first edition was developed in 1969 and is known as the Bayley Scales of Infant Development (BSID).[24] The need for revisions and updated normative data prompted the development of the second edition of the BSID (BSID-II), which was introduced in 1993. In 2006, the Bayley-III[25] was published and the most significant revision in this latest version was the development of five distinct scales.[26]

The original intent of this tool was to measure the developmental abilities of infants and toddlers between the ages of 1 and 42 months. It includes growth scores to monitor the child's progress over time, although responsiveness has not yet been demonstrated. Other specific purposes of the Bayley-III are to identify possible developmental delay, inform professionals about specific areas of strength or weakness when planning a comprehensive intervention and provide a method of monitoring a child's developmental progress.[26] Similar to the previous editions, the Bayley-III can also be used for individuals who are severely delayed and are outside the age range for which the test was standardized. It maintains the same types of tasks and promotes task involvement through play-based activities for individuals with limited ability, and therefore can provide detailed information on developmental ability even from non-verbal children. However, its utility as an instrument to assess individuals with severe delay has not yet been fully examined.

Administration and scoring

The Bayley-III consists of a series of developmental play tasks divided into five scales. It takes approximately 45 to 60 minutes (up to 90min for children aged ≥13mo) to administer.

The *cognitive* scale comprises 91 items, with some new items and some items taken from the mental scale of the BSID-II. The *language* scale consists of *receptive* (49 items) and *expressive* (48 items) communication subtests. The *motor* scale consists of the *fine motor* (66 items) and *gross motor* (72 items) subtests. The examiner begins by administering the cognitive, language and motor scales at a starting point corresponding to the child's chronological age (adjusted for preterm birth, if necessary, up to 24mo) and is designated by the letters A to Q. First, the examiner must establish the child's basal level, which is achieved when the first three items administered are successfully completed. If this is not established, the examiner goes to the previous starting point and continues administration until the child does not achieve five consecutive items (this criterion corresponds to the ceiling level). The examiner should start at the original age-determined starting letter for subsequent scales. Items should be administered only once

BAYLEY SCALES OF INFANT AND TODDLER DEVELOPMENT, THIRD EDITION	
Purpose	To measure the developmental functioning of infants and toddlers. May be used to identify possible developmental delay, inform professionals about specific areas of strength or weakness when planning a comprehensive intervention and monitor a child's developmental progress over time
Population	Infants and toddlers aged 1–42mo
Description of domains (subscales)	Test items divided into five domains: Cognitive Motor: fine motor, gross motor Language: expressive, receptive Socioemotional Adaptive behaviour (Adaptive Behaviour Assessment System, second edition, ABAS-II)
Administration and test format	Time to complete: 45–60min to administer for children aged ≤12mo, up to 90min for children aged ≥13mo Testing format: cognitive, motor and language scales are administered by the examiner to the child. Socioemotional and adaptive behaviour scales are conducted through parent questionnaires Scoring: items on the cognitive, motor and language scales are scored 0 (no credit) or 1 (credit). Socioemotional and adaptive behaviour scales are scored 0 to 5 ('cannot tell' to 'all the time'), and 0 to 3 ('is not able to' to 'always when needed'), respectively. Raw scores are converted into scale scores and composite scores Training: may be administered by occupational therapists, speech pathologists, psychologists or educators with expertise. Evaluators must learn and be comfortable with evaluation components
Psychometric properties	Normative sample: 1700 children in the USA, representative for parent education, race or ethnicity and geographic region *Reliability* Internal consistency was high on average using Fisher's z transformation for cognitive, language and motor scales (0.91–0.93). Test–retest reliability for these three scales was $r=0.67$–0.94 *Validity* Criterion validity: correlations between the Bayley-III cognitive and language scales and Wechsler Intelligence Scale for Children, third edition ($r=0.72$–0.79 and $r=0.71$–0.83, respectively); Bayley-III motor scale and Peabody Developmental Motor Scales, second edition ($r=0.49$–0.57); Bayley-III adaptive behaviour scale and Vineland Adaptive Behaviour Scale –interview edition ($r=0.58$–0.70)
How to order	Purchase from www.pearsonpsychcorp.com Cost: US$2509.80 (kit)
Key references	Bayley N (2006) *Bayley Scales of Infant and Toddler Development, Third Edition: Administration Manual.* San Antonio, TX: Harcourt Assessment. Bayley N (2006) *Bayley Scales of Infant and Toddler Development, Third Edition: Technical Manual.* San Antonio, TX: Harcourt Assessment.

during the course of the testing session. Every item is scored 1 (credit) or 0 (no credit). For each scale (cognitive, language and motor), raw scores of successfully completed items are converted to scale scores (mean=10; SD=3) and additionally to composite scores (mean=100; SD=15). These scores are used to determine the child's performance compared with norms from typically developing children. The *socioemotional* scale is to be completed by the child's caregiver. Each of the 35 items measures emotional development and related behaviours and is scored on a six-point scale ranging from 0 (cannot tell) to 5 (all of the time). The *adaptive behaviour* scale evaluates practical everyday skills that children require to function and meet environmental demands effectively and independently. This scale is also completed by the caregiver and indicates the extent to which the child is performing the adaptive skills when needed. This scale is scored from 0 (is not able to) to 3 (always when needed).

The Bayley-III includes a test kit that contains stimulus items and manuals; however, examiners must provide additional materials for test administration. Standard administration and scoring procedures must be followed. Three of the five scales – cognitive, motor and language – are administered by the examiner with child interaction. The two other scales – socioemotional and adaptive behaviour – are conducted with parent questionnaires. Subtests in one or more domains may be administered individually.

The Bayley-III can be administered by certified psychologists, occupational therapists, speech pathologists, or other health or education professionals who have the appropriate training and expertise in developmental assessment and interpretation. The Bayley-III may be administered in the home, but the examiner must maintain standard administration procedures and keep distractions to a minimum. The child's caregiver is encouraged to remain in the testing room; however, he or she should not interfere with the testing procedures.

Psychometric properties
The standardization sample for the cognitive, language and motor scales included 1700 US children aged 1 to 42 months and is reported to be representative in terms of parent education level, race or ethnicity and geographic region. Children with mental, physical and behavioural difficulties were later added to the sample and represent 10% of the total sample. The standardization sample for the socioemotional scale included 456 children and appears to be relatively representative of the US population. The standardization sample for the adaptive behaviour scale included 1350 children and was developed independently of the Bayley-III standardization process; norms were truncated in terms of age to represent the Bayley-III's age limit. Although the Bayley scales were standardized on US children, they have been used in studies crossculturally, including on Dutch, Indian, Kenyan and Australian infants.[7]

The psychometric properties of the BSID and the BSID-II have been extensively studied and provide support for their reliability and validity. For the Bayley-III, high average internal consistency coefficients for the cognitive, language and motor scales are reported (Fisher's z-transformation: 0.91–0.93). Test–retest reliability for these three scales ranged from $r=0.67$ to $r=0.94$ across the age span of 2 to 42 months. Moderate to high correlations were found for the Bayley-III cognitive ($r=0.72–0.79$) and language ($r=0.71–0.83$) scales when it was compared with the Wechsler Intelligence Scale for Children, third edition,[23] the motor scale with the Peabody Developmental Motor Scales, second edition ($r=0.49–0.57$),[27] and the adaptive behaviour scale with the Vineland Adaptive Behaviour Scale, interview edition ($r=0.58–0.70$).[28] Studies examining the Bayley-III administered to children with various conditions (e.g. Down syndrome, cerebral palsy, prenatal alcohol exposure, preterm infants) are also included in the technical manual.[29]

GRIFFITHS MENTAL DEVELOPMENT SCALES, REVISED

Overview and purpose
The Griffiths Mental Development Scales (GMDS) were originally designed by Dr Ruth Griffiths in the UK to assess the mental development of infants and young children aged between 0 and 2 years. They were developed by observing children in their natural environments while engaged in everyday activities. The GMDS were originally published in 1954 and were the first published scales designed to assess mental development in children <2 years of age. In 1996, a revision of the Griffiths 0–2 Scales was undertaken, in which a complete restandardization was conducted, new items were added and a revised record form was introduced.[30] During the 1960s, the Griffiths Scales were extended to cover birth to 8 years, and a sixth scale (practical reasoning) was added. The first edition for 2- to 8-year-old children was published in 1970 and revised in 1984; the third and most current edition for 2- to 8-year-old children was recently published.[31] It has also been used for a more detailed evaluation of children with developmental delays. A further use of these scales has been to evaluate the outcome of interventions by regularly repeating the assessment.[32] However, the responsiveness of the GMDS-R has yet to be determined. The GMDS-R were designed to be equal in difficulty at each month of age so that discrepancies in development for a particular child may be identified.

Administration and scoring
The GMDS-R takes 50 to 60 minutes to administer. The 0 to 2 year version includes the first five areas of

GRIFFITHS MENTAL DEVELOPMENT SCALES, REVISED (GMDS-R)	
How to order	Purchase from www.hogrefe.co.uk/?/test/show/35/
	Cost: £390 (birth–2y kit) and £699 (2–8y comprehensive starter pack)
Key references	Huntley M (1996) *The Griffiths Mental Development Scales: From Birth to 2 Years.* Amersham: ARICD.
	Luiz DM, Kotras N, Barnard A, Knoesen N (2004) *Technical Manual of the Griffiths Mental Development Scales – Extended Revised (GMDS-ER)*. Amersham: ARICD.

development listed below. The *locomotor* scale assesses gross motor skills and items include age-appropriate activities such as kicking and rolling, walking up and down stairs, running and jumping. The *personal–social* scale measures the developing abilities that contribute to independence and social development. The *hearing and language* scale assesses hearing, receptive language and expressive language. The *eye and hand coordination* scale focuses on fine motor skills, manual dexterity and visual monitoring skills. The *performance* scale measures the ability to reason through performance tests and visuospatial skills, including speed of working and precision. The *practical reasoning* scale (children 3–8y) assesses the ability to solve practical problems, understanding of basic mathematical concepts and understanding of moral issues.

The test kit includes most of the standardized equipment required to administer the items on the GMDS-R. Necessary material also includes a few sheets of white drawing paper and crayons. The GMDS-R is an evaluator-administered assessment tool, although a caregiver report may be used to assess and score certain items. It is available in English, German, Portuguese and Italian.

Raw scores for each individual subscale are computed by adding the total number of items passed and then adding these to obtain a total raw score. Raw scores can be converted into age equivalents, subquotients, general quotients and centile equivalents. A mental age can be calculated for each of the six scales, and the average score across scales defines the child's overall mental age. A general quotient may be obtained by dividing the overall mental age by the child's chronological age. Several authors have found discrepancies between the mental ages obtained on the GMDS and those from other frequently used instruments. A study by McLean and colleagues[33] found that the age equivalents obtained on the GMDS were considerably higher than those from the BSID[24] and the BDI,[18] indicating a need for the GMDS to be restandardized on a culturally diverse sample. Evaluators must therefore keep in mind that the age equivalents of the GMDS may overestimate developmental levels in infants.

Clinical use of the GMDS-R is restricted to psychologists and developmental paediatricians, although therapists may administer the measure under the supervision of a qualified evaluator. Training courses are offered through the Association for Research in Infant and Child Development.

Psychometric properties
The initial version of the GMDS was standardized on 604 infants from London during the late 1940s and early 1950s.[33] Research on the GMDS has included children from the UK, USA, Brazil and South Africa.[34] Inter-rater reliability of the earlier versions of the GMDS was assessed and was found to have greater consistency between raters on the eye–hand coordination and the performance and practical reasoning scales than on the locomotor scale, personal–social scale and the hearing–speech scale.[32] Children in mainstream educational settings had higher GMDS scores than those in special schools for children with emotional or behavioural problems,[35] supporting the discriminative ability of the GMDS in identifying children with special education needs. Crosscultural validation was established by Luiz and colleagues[36] by comparing the correlation coefficients for four South African groups (i.e. white, mixed race, Asian and black) with the British standardization sample of the GMDS. The findings suggest that the scales measure a construct which is similar across cultures. However, a recent study detected differences in performance between the South African sample and the 1996 normative group, which may be attributed to cultural differences.[34] Psychometric properties of the latest version, the GMDS-R, are not readily available.

McCARTHY SCALES OF CHILDREN'S ABILITIES

Overview and purpose
The McCarthy Scales of Children's Abilities (MSCA) was designed by Dorothea McCarthy in 1972 to facilitate the measurement of general intellectual level in children aged 2 years 6 months to 8 years 6 months. It is a meticulously developed and standardized assessment

McCarthy Scales of Children's Abilities (MSCA)	
How to order	Purchase from www.pearson.com Cost: US$669 (kit)
Key references	McCarthy D (1972) *The McCarthy Scales of Children's Abilities*. New York: Psychological Corporation.

tool, with the purpose of providing information about a child's strengths and weaknesses in important abilities that can be used to prescribe remedial programmes. It detects abilities and limitations across several skill areas, including cognitive and motor. It is suitable for use with typically developing children and those with specific learning disabilities. The MSCA is used as a means of assessing children for clinical, educational and research purposes.[37]

Administration and scoring

The MSCA is an individually administered test which takes approximately 45 to 60 minutes to administer. The MSCA consists of 18 subtests/tasks which are combined into five scales that separately evaluate verbal, perceptual, quantitative, memory and motor abilities. The *verbal* scale (five subtests) assesses comprehension and use of language. The *quantitative* scale (three subtests) measures mathematical abilities, while the *perceptual-performance* scale (seven subtests) evaluates the child's ability to conceptualize and reason without language. The *memory* scale (four subtests) tests short-term recall of words, numbers, pictures and tonal sequences. The *motor* scale (five subtests) assesses both gross and fine motor coordination. The first three scales – verbal, quantitative and perceptual-performance – are distinct, and together yield a General Cognitive Index (GCI). The GCI is a measure of overall cognitive functioning. The memory and motor scales are composed of some tests in common with the other four scales.

The MSCA is administered directly to the child using a wide range of puzzles, toys and game-like activities designed to make the evaluation interesting and enjoyable. All materials, including the necessary manuals, record forms and toys, are contained in a test kit for ease of administration.

Composite raw scores are converted to scale indices according to tables that represent 3-month age spans. All five scales have a mean of 50 (SD=10). The child's score is measured against the standard mean of children close to his or her own age. The mean of the GCI is 100 (SD=16). Children who score ≥130 are classified as very superior, 120 to 129 as superior, 110 to 119 as

bright normal, 90 to 109 as average, 80 to 89 as dull normal, 70 to 79 as borderline and ≤69 as mentally challenged. No formal training is required to administer the test; however, it is recommended that the evaluator be trained by a person with expertise in the use of this instrument.

Psychometric properties

The MSCA was standardized by testing 1032 children from a stratified sample in accordance with estimates from the US census data. Stratification variables included age, sex, colour, geographic location and father's occupation. The same sample included 'normal children' and children with suspected intellectual impairment who lived at home. Children with severe emotional or behavioural problems or who had obvious physical defects were excluded.[38]

The internal consistency coefficients for the GCI averaged $r=0.93$ across 10 age groups between 2 years 6 months and 8 years 6 months. Mean reliability coefficients for the other five index scales ranged from $r=0.79$ to $r=0.88$. The MSCA has also been shown to be relatively stable over a 3- to 6-week test–retest period (GCI: $r=0.80$; index scales: $r=0.69–0.89$)[39] as well as over a 1-year period.[40] The MSCA was found to be predictive of school performance in children at risk for developmental delay[41] and of reading readiness and achievement in first grade.[42]

This tool has not been revised or renormed since its original testing in the 1970s and the normative values are probably out of date.

MERRILL–PALMER SCALES OF DEVELOPMENT, REVISED

Overview and purpose

The Merrill–Palmer Scales of Development (MPSD) were first developed in 1931[43] with a revised version, the MPSD-R, published in 2004.[44] The items on the MPSD-R follow the natural progression of activities for children from the age of 1 month to 6 years 6 months and assess visual motor, learning and problem-solving abilities in English- and Spanish-speaking children. The MPSD-R

MERRILL–PALMER SCALES OF DEVELOPMENT, REVISED (MPSD-R)	
Purpose	To evaluate overall child development
Population	Infants and children aged 1mo to 6y 6mo; may be used with children who have with limited language skills, such as those with autism

Description of domains (subscales)	466 test items divided into five domains:
	
	  Cognitive: verbal and non-verbal reasoning, memory, visual motor, speed of processing
	  Language/communication: receptive, expressive
	  Motor: gross motor, fine motor
	  Socioemotional behaviour
	  Self-help/adaptability

Administration and test format	Time to complete: 40–50min Testing format: evaluator administered Scoring: normative standard scores, centiles, age equivalents and criterion-referenced change-sensitive 'growth scores' are derived for each of the five domains Training: a training DVD is available at an additional cost. Workshops on the administration, scoring and interpretation of the MPSD-R are available and suggested. May be administered by psychologists, counsellors or individuals in related fields with experience in test administration and scoring
Psychometric properties	Normative sample: 1400 children representative of 2000 US population *Reliability* Internal consistency: developmental index (intraclass correlation coefficient=0.97–0.98). Test–retest reliability: ranges from $r=0.84$ to $r=0.90$, excluding the expressive language subtest *Validity* Criterion validity: developmental index correlates with Bayley-II mental scale ($r=0.82$), although the scores on the MPSD-R were consistently and significantly higher
How to order	Purchase from Western Psychological Services at https://portal.wpspublish.com; PAR, Inc. at www3.parinc.com; and Stoelting at https://www.stoeltingco.com Cost: ranges from US$925 to US$995
Key references	Roid GH, Sampers J (2004) *Merrill–Palmer-R Scales of Development*. Wood Dale, IL: Stoelting.

assesses both the quality of performance as well as the achievement of developmental milestones.

The MPSD-R is useful for the early identification of developmental delays or disabilities in infants and children and for assessing the development of children with hearing impairments or deafness, autism[45] or other disabilities with limited language skills. Guidelines are provided to adapt the administration of test items for children with impairments. The MPSD-R has been described as sensitive in detecting changes in development over time, although this has not been demonstrated in reported studies. It has been used to assess children born preterm.

Administration and scoring

The MPSD-R takes approximately 40 to 50 minutes to complete. The tool provides an evaluation of overall development (466 items) as well as separate scores for the following domains: *cognitive* (111 items) – verbal and non-verbal reasoning, memory, visual motor speed of processing; *language/communication* (140 items) – receptive and expressive language, evaluated by examiner and parent; *motor* – gross motor (75 items) and fine motor (59 items); *socioemotional behaviour* (37 items) – developmental scale and clinical data, rated by examiner and parent; and *self-help/adaptability* (44 items) – developmental and global examiner and parent rating scales.

The MPSD-R is an evaluator-administered tool and can include parent report. The test kit includes the administration and scoring manual, forms, test toys and materials. Parent-report forms are also available in Spanish.

The results obtained on the MPSD-R provide normative standard scores, centiles, age equivalents and criterion-referenced change-sensitive 'growth scores' for each of the five domains. The Growth Score Profile enables the examiner to plot the scores for individual developmental index domains and identify specific areas of deficit. The results can then be used to develop an educational plan which targets those deficits.

The MPSD-R may be administered by psychologists, counsellors and professionals from related fields with experience in test administration and scoring and those with professional training in psychological measurement. A training DVD is available at extra cost, and workshops on the administration, scoring and interpretation of the MPSD-R are recommended.

Psychometric properties

The MPSD-R provides norms based on 1400 cases (including 250 atypical) representative of the 2000 US census for sex, ethnicity, socioeconomic level and geographic region. Internal consistency for the developmental index is reported as high (intraclass correlation coefficient=0.97–0.98), and test–retest reliability coefficients ranged from $r=0.84$ to $r=0.90$ (3-week retest interval) excluding the expressive language subtest. There are data on content-related and criterion-related validity, and the items indicate a good fit to the Rasch model. One study found that the developmental index correlates highly with the Bayley-II mental scale ($r=0.82$),[46] although the scores on the MPSD-R were consistently and significantly higher. The authors suggest that this difference may be because these two tools emphasize different skills. The MPSD focuses more on visuospatial tasks, whereas the Bayley-II includes items involving perspective taking and social responsivity.

MILLER ASSESSMENT FOR PRESCHOOLERS

Overview and purpose

The Miller Assessment for Preschoolers (MAP) was published in 1982, in response to the US federal mandate, Public Law 94–142, that all states must develop and implement policies that assure a free appropriate public education to all children with disabilities. It is a short, comprehensive preschool assessment designed to predict school-related problems. It is based on the assumption that the maturity of the brain is indicative of future abilities relating to school performance.[47] Its primary purpose is to identify children aged 2 years 9 months to 5 years 8 months who exhibit mild, moderate and severe pre-academic problems and who may be at risk of future learning difficulties. The MAP can indicate that a developmental problem may exist and that further evaluation is justified.[48] It is not intended to establish a diagnosis or identify children who are precocious in their development.

Administration and scoring

The MAP is administered in a playful yet structured environment and takes approximately 25 to 40 minutes to complete the 27 core items. The MAP assesses five areas of performance, providing five indices. The structure of the tasks within each index offers a comprehensive profile of the child in terms of the underlying sensory, motor and cognitive components implicated in movement and task performance.[49] The *foundation* index assesses the child's abilities involving basic motor tasks and awareness of sensations, skills fundamental to more complex activities. The *coordination* index assesses more complex motor (gross, fine, oral) tasks, combining sensory and motor components. These two indices together assess the child's sensory and motor abilities. The *verbal* index focuses on memory, sequencing, expression, comprehension and association within a verbal context. The *non-verbal* index assesses memory, sequencing, visualization and mental manipulation within a non-verbal context. The verbal and non-verbal indices together assess the child's cognitive abilities. The *complex tasks* index focuses on sensorimotor abilities in conjunction with cognitive abilities that require interpretation of visuospatial information, and thus assesses a combination of the sensory, motor and cognitive areas.

The MAP test kit includes a well-organized box containing all the necessary test items: a clearly written and illustrated manual, individual cue sheets for each item and colour-coded record sheets for each of six age groups, each one spanning 5 months. When scoring the MAP, raw scores are converted to centile scores for the total score, the subtests and each of the five indices, providing a broad overview of the child's developmental status relative to other children of the same age. Colour-coded record forms reflect the centile ranges and facilitate interpretation of the scores. Red indicates that the child's performance is within the 0 to 5th centile range, suggesting that a problem may exist and that the child needs to be referred for further evaluation. Yellow indicates that a child falls within the 6th to 24th centile, suggesting that the child needs to be followed carefully. Finally, a score that falls in the green category, above the 24th centile, indicates that the child is within normal limits.

MILLER ASSESSMENT FOR PRESCHOOLERS (MAP)

Purpose	To identify young children with mild to moderate developmental delay. May be used to detect children who are demonstrating difficulties in pre-academic abilities and who may be at risk of future school-related problems
Population	Preschool children aged 2y 9mo–5y 8mo
Description of domains (subscales)	27 test items divided into five domains: Foundation: motor tasks, awareness of sensations Coordination: gross, fine and oromotor skill Verbal: memory, sequencing, semantic associations Non-verbal: mental manipulations not requiring spoken language Complex tasks: integration of sensory, motor and cognitive skills requiring interpretation of visuospatial information
Administration and test format	Time to complete: 25–40min to administer Testing format: 27 game-like items administered through interaction between examiner and child. A MAP screening, MAP extended and MAP research format are each available within the kit Scoring: age-specific information for 6mo age categories (separate administration sheet and item score sheet for each age level). Raw scores are converted to centiles for each of the five indices and for the total score. A colour-coded record form indicates age-appropriate performance for each item. Cut-off scores for performance within normal limits and requiring further evaluation are provided Training: attendance at a MAP seminar is recommended, but not mandatory. The MAP extended format can be administered by any healthcare or educational professional. MAP screening may be administered by school personnel, educational and therapy aides, and even parent volunteers
Psychometric properties	Normative sample: 1204 children without disabilities; 90 children with disabilities *Reliability* Internal consistency: r=0.79–0.89 Test–retest reliability: established (r=0.81; range 0.72–0.94) Inter-rater reliability: r=0.98 (range 0.84–0.99) *Validity* Content validity: correlates with Weschler Intelligence Scale for Children, revised (r=0.45–0.50) and Woodcock–Johnson math, reading and language subtests (r=0.35–0.38) Construct validity: distinguishes between groups at risk and not at risk Sensitivity and specificity: MAP 25% cut-off point indicates sensitivity and specificity (>0.7) in predicting children who later had difficulty in kindergarten Predictive validity: accurate prediction of academic performance
How to order	Can be purchased by a healthcare or educational professional from www.pearsonassess.org and www.wpspublish.com Cost: US$799 (kit)
Key reference	Miller LJ (1988) *The Miller Assessment for Preschoolers*. San Antonio, TX: Psychological Corporation.

A MAP screening format is available and may be administered by school personnel, educational and therapy aides, and even parent volunteers. The MAP can be used by a variety of clinical and educational personnel and formal training is not mandatory. However, it is strongly recommended that users of this instrument attend a MAP seminar for training and obtain the most up-to-date normative information. The highly organized collection of test materials makes it fairly easy even for new examiners to learn test administration.[49]

Psychometric properties
Standardization of the MAP involved a randomly selected, nationally representative sample of children, based on the 1970 US census. The sample was stratified according to region, age, sex, race and size of residential community and included 1204 'normal' children and 90 'at risk' children. The MAP demonstrates excellent internal consistency and inter-rater reliability (*r*=0.79–0.89; *r*=0.98, respectively).[49] Test–retest reliability indicates that the MAP total score is quite stable over time (*r*=0.81; ranging from 0.72 for the coordination index to *r*=0.94 for the non-verbal index).[49]

Various studies have been conducted to determine the validity of the MAP. MAP scores distinguished between groups at risk and not at risk in their first year in school, measured according to teachers' ratings.[50] Lemerand[51] found that the classification, according to the MAP's 25% cut-off point, resulted in moderate sensitivity and specificity rates (>0.7) in predicting children who had difficulty in kindergarten 1 year later.[51] The MAP, when administered to preschoolers, adequately predicted intelligence and academic performance 4 years later.[52] These results were validated in a subsequent study,[53] suggesting that the MAP is a screening tool capable of predicting performance of school-age children over a substantial period of time (7 years) and is accurate in predicting academic performance.

Studies have a found that there is a moderate significant correlation between the MAP and the Wechsler Intelligence Scale for Children, revised (*r*=0.45–0.50)[49] and the Woodcock–Johnson maths, reading and language subtests (*r*=0.35–0.38).[54]

MULLEN SCALES OF EARLY LEARNING

Overview and purpose
The Mullen Scales of Early Learning (MSEL) is a standardized test assessing five domains of development in children aged 0 to 5 years 8 months (gross motor scale: 0–33mo). It permits early targeted educational intervention by providing a measure of early information processing skills in the areas of motor, cognitive and language development. The MSEL pinpoints the child's strengths and weaknesses and is ideal for assessing school readiness, providing separate standard verbal and non-verbal summaries.

Administration and scoring
The MSEL is individually administered and takes between 15 and 60 minutes to complete, with younger children requiring less administration time. It consists of five subscales: *gross motor* (skills from head control to walking), *fine motor* (bilateral and unilateral manipulation), *visual reception* (visual perception), *receptive language* (ability to decode verbal input) and *expressive language* (spontaneous language, vocal or verbal responses to questions and high-level concepts).

Included with the MSEL are the toy kit, the examiner manual, the administration manual and the stimulus book. Items are scored through direct testing, although several may be scored through parental interview.

Each scale is scored separately and provides a T-score (mean=100; SD=15), centile and age-equivalent score. An early-learning composite score is derived from the visual receptive, fine motor, receptive language and expressive language scales and provides a summary measure of general functioning. The age-equivalent scores appear to be more appropriate for children with autism spectrum disorders (ASD) than the T-scores, as children with ASD may have scores below the minimum T-score of 20, representing a score three or more SDs below the mean or an IQ of approximately 55.[55] Computer scoring from the publishers is also available at an additional cost.

The MSEL has been used mainly in research studies involving children with autism, with children with ASD scoring significantly less than typically developing children,[55,56] as well as with children with Down syndrome.[57]

The MSEL may be administered by a variety of clinical and educational personnel with a background in developmental assessment, though formal training is not required. A video is available to train examiners in the administration of the tool.

MULLEN SCALES OF EARLY LEARNING (MSEL)	
How to order	Purchase from www.pearsonassessments.com or www.wpspublish.com
	Cost: US$770–785 (complete kit)
Key reference	Mullen EM (1995) *Mullen Scales of Early Learning*. Circle Pines, MN: American Guidance Service Inc.

Psychometric properties

The MSEL was standardized on 1849 children without physical or cognitive impairment. The sample was representative of the 1990 US census according to sex, father's occupation, race/ethnicity and urban/rural residence. Internal consistency of the five subdomains ranges from $r=0.75$ to $r=0.83$; evidence that the subscales measure distinct abilities. Test–retest reliability within a 2-week interval ranged from $r=0.83$ to $r=0.98$, while inter-rater reliability was $r=0.99$.[58] This instrument has demonstrated strong concurrent validity with other well-known developmental tests of language, motor and cognitive development.[58,59] High correlations have been found between the MSEL, the BSID, the Preschool Language Assessment and the Peabody Developmental Motor Scales.[59]

REFERENCES

1. Lipkin PH, Allen MC (2005) Introduction: developmental assessment of the young child. *Ment Retard Dev Disabil Res Rev* 11: 171–172.
2. Long CE, Blackman JA, Farrell WJ, Smolkin ME, Conaway MR (2005) A comparison of developmental versus functional assessment in the rehabilitation of young children. *Pediatr Rehabil* 8: 156–161.
3. Johnson S, Marlow N (2006) Developmental screen or developmental testing? *Early Hum Dev* 82: 173–183.
4. Shevell MI (2010) Present conceptualization of early childhood neurodevelopmental disabilities. *J Child Neurol* 25: 120–126.
5. World Health Organization (2007) *International Classification of Functioning, Disability and Health – Child and Youth Version*. Geneva: WHO Press.
6. Flynn J (1999) Searching for justice. The discovery of IQ gains over time. *Am Psychol* 54: 5–20.
7. Gagnon SG, Nagle RJ (2000) Comparison of the revised and original versions of the Bayley Scales of Infant Development. *Sch Psychol Int* 21: 293–305.
8. Kenny TJ, Holden EW, Santilli L (1991) The meaning of measures: pitfalls in behavioral and developmental research. *J Dev Behav Pediatr* 12: 355–360.
9. Voress JK, Maddox T (1998) *Developmental Assessment of Young Children: Examiner's Manual*. Austin, TX: Pro-Ed.
10. Alpern GD, Boll T, Shearer J (2007) *Developmental Profile 3 (DP-3)*. Los Angeles, CA: Western Psychological Services.
11. Hardin BJ, Peisner-Feinberg ES (2001) *The Early Learning Accomplishment Profile (Early LAP) Examiner's Manual and Reliability and Validity Technical Report*. Lewisville, NC: Kaplan Press.
12. Provence S, Erikson J, Vater S, Palmeri S (1995) *Infant–Toddler Developmental Assessment (IDA)*. Rolling Meadows, IL: Riverside Publishing.
13. Glascoe FP, Robertshaw NS (2006) *Parents' Evaluation of Developmental Status: Developmental Milestones Measurements for Children*. Nashville, TN: Ellsworth and Vandermeer Press.
14. Andersson L (2006) Use of the communication development subtest of the DAYC as a teacher-administered language-screening instrument. *Commun Dis Quar* 27: 206–212.
15. Berls AT, McEwen IR (1999) Battelle Developmental Inventory. *Phys Ther* 79: 8–16.
16. Bliss SL (2007) Test Reviews: Battelle Developmental Inventory Second Edition. *J Psychoeduc Assess* 25: 409–414.
17. Newborg J (2005) *Battelle Developmental Inventory*, 2nd edition. Itasca, IL: Riverside Publishing Company.
18. Newborg J, Stock JR, Wnek I, Guidubaldi J, Svinicki J (1984) *Battelle Developmental Inventory*. Rolling Meadows, IL: Riverside Publishing.
19. Bayley N (1993) *Bayley Scales of Infant Development*, 2nd edition. San Antonio, TX: Psychological Corporation.
20. Frankenburg WK, Dodds JB (1986) *Denver Developmental Screening Test*. Denver, CO: Denver Developmental Materials.
21. Zimmerman IL, Steiner VG, Pond RE (2002) *Preschool Language Scale*, 4th edition. San Antonio, TX: Psychological Corporation.
22. Sparrow SS, Balla DA, Cicchetti DV (1998) *Vineland Social–Emotional Early Childhood Scales*. Circle Pines, MN: AGS.
23. Wechsler D (2002) *Wechsler Intelligence Scales for Children*, 3rd edition. San Antonio, TX: Psychological Corporation.
24. Bayley N (1969) *Bayley Scales of Infant Development*. San Antonio, TX: The Psychological Corporation.
25. Bayley N (2006) *Bayley Scales of Infant and Toddler Development*, 3rd edition. Administration Manual. San Antonio, TX: Harcourt Assessment.
26. Albers CA, Grieve AJ (2007) Test review: Bayley N (2006) Bayley Scales of Infant and Toddler Development, 3rd edition. *J Psychoeduc Assess* 25: 180–190.
27. Folio MR, Fewell RR (2000) *Peabody Developmental Motor Scales*, 2nd edition. Austin, TX: Pro-Ed.
28. Sparrow SS, Balla DA, Cicchetti DV (1984) *Vineland Adaptive Behavior Scales*. Circles Pines, MN: American Guidance Service, Inc.
29. Bayley N (2006) *Bayley Scales of Infant and Toddler Development, Third Edition: Administration Manual*. San Antonio, TX: Harcourt Assessment.
30. Huntley M (1996) *The Griffiths Mental Development Scales: From Birth to 2 Years*. Amersham: ARICD.
31. Luiz DM, Kotras N, Barnard A, Knoesen N (2004) *Technical Manual of the Griffiths Mental Development Scales – Extended Revised (GMDS-ER)*. Amersham: ARICD.
32. Aldridge Smith J, Bidder RT, Gardner SM, Gray OP (1980) Griffiths Scales of mental development and different users. *Child Care Health Dev* 6: 11–16.
33. McLean ME, McCormick K, Baird SM (1991) Concurrent validity of the Griffith's Mental Developmental Scales with a population of children under 24 months. *J Early Interv* 15: 338–344.
34. Amod Z, Cockcroft K, Soellaart B (2007) Use of the 1996 Griffiths Mental Developmental Scales for infants: a pilot study with a Black, South African sample. *J Child Adolesc Ment Health* 19: 123–130.
35. Conn P (1993) The relation between Griffiths scales assessments in the pre-school period and educational outcomes at 7+ years. *Child Care Health Dev* 19: 275–289.
36. Luiz DM, Foxcroft CD, Stewart R (2001) The construct validity of the Griffiths Scales of Mental Development. *Child Care Health Dev* 27: 73–83.
37. McCarthy D (1972) *The McCarthy Scales of Children's Abilities*. New York: Psychological Corporation.
38. Hayes JS (1981) The McCarthy Scales of Children's Abilities: their usefulness in developmental assessment. *Pediatr Nurs* 7: 35–37.
39. Bryant CK, Roffe MW (1978) A reliability study of the McCarthy Scales of Children's Abilities. *J Clin Psychol* 34: 401–406.

40. Davis EE, Slettedahl RW (1976) Stability of the McCarthy Scale over a year. *J Clin Psychol* 32: 798–800.

41. Funk SG, Sturner RA, Green JA (1986) Preschool prediction of early school performance. *J Sch Psychol* 24: 181–194.

42. Massoth NA, Levinson RL (1982) The McCarthy Scales of Children's Abilities as a predictor of reading readiness and reading achievement. *Psychol Sch* 19: 293–296.

43. Stutsman R (1931) Guide for administering the Merrill–Palmer Scale of Mental Tests. In: Terman L, editor. *Mental Measurement of Preschool Children*. New York: Harcourt, Brace & World, pp. 139–262.

44. Roid GH, Sampers J (2004) *Merrill–Palmer-R Scales of Development*. Wood Dale, IL: Stoelting.

45. Lord C, Schopler E (1989) Stability of assessment results of autistic and non-autistic language-impaired children from preschool years to early school age. *J Child Psychol Psychiatry* 30: 575–590.

46. Magiati I, Howlin P (2001) Monitoring the progress of preschool children with autism enrolled in early intervention programmes: problems in cognitive assessment. *Autism* 5: 399–406.

47. Miller L, Sprong T (1987) A comparison of the Miller Assessment for Preschoolers and developmental indicators for the assessment of learning-revised. *Phys Occup Ther Pediatr* 7: 57–69.

48. Banus B (1983) Miller Assessment for Preschoolers (MAP): an introduction and review. *Am J Occup Ther* 37: 333–340.

49. Miller LJ (1988) *The Miller Assessment for Preschoolers*. San Antonio, TX: Psychological Corporation.

50. Cohn SH (1986) *An analysis of the predictive validity of the Miller Assessment for Preschoolers in a suburban public school district* [unpublished doctoral dissertation]. Denver, CO: University of Denver Colorado.

51. Lemerand P (1988) Predictive validity of the Miller Assessment for Preschoolers (MAP). *Sensory Integration News* 16: 1–8.

52. Miller L, Lemerand P, Cohn S (1987) A summary of three predictive studies with the MAP. *Occup Ther J Res* 7: 378–381.

53. Parush S, Winokur M, Goldstand S, Miller LJ (2002) The prediction of school performance using the Miller Assessment for Preschoolers (MAP): a validity study. *Am J Occup Ther* 56: 547–555.

54. Woodcock RW, Johnson MB (1977) *The Woodcock–Johnson Psycho-educational Battery*. Hingham, PA: Teaching Resources.

55. Akshoomoff N (2006) Use of the Mullen Scales of Early Learning for the assessment of young children with autism spectrum disorders. *Child Neuropsychol* 12: 269–277.

56. Landa R, Garrett-Mayer E (2006) Development in infants with autism spectrum disorders: a prospective study. *J Child Psychol Psychiatry* 47: 629–638.

57. Fidler DJ, Hepburn S, Rogers S (2006) Early learning and adaptive behaviour in toddlers with Down syndrome: evidence for an emerging behavioural phenotype? *Downs Syndr Res Pract* 9: 37–44.

58. Schraeder BD (1993) Assessment of measures to detect preschool academic risk in very-low-birth-weight children. *Nurs Res* 42: 17–21.

59. Mullen EM (1995) *Mullen Scales of Early Learning*. Circle Pines, MN: American Guidance Service Inc.

SECTION IV ACTIVITIES AND PARTICIPATION

19

ACTIVITIES AND PARTICIPATION: AN OVERVIEW OF GENERIC MEASURES

Christopher Morris and Annette Majnemer

What is the construct?

The World Health Organization (WHO) first published the International Classification of Functioning, Disability and Health (ICF) as a generic framework[1] and then later published a specific version for children and youth (ICF-CY).[2] Replacing the International Classification of Impairments, Disability and Handicap, the ICF moved away from a conceptual model of 'consequences of disease' towards a framework for 'components of health'. The ICF distinguishes the health concepts of 'body functions and structures' from 'activities and participation' and classifies all these as 'functioning' in its broadest sense.

In the ICF, 'activities' is defined as the *execution of tasks or actions* and 'participation' is *involvement in life situations*. However, the distinction between activities and participation is not well defined and, rather confusingly, the domains of 'activities and participation' are provided in the ICF as a single list. The activities and participation domains for children include learning and applying knowledge, general tasks and demands, communication, mobility, self-care, domestic life (including housing and acquiring goods), school life, social life, interpersonal relationships, and leisure and recreation (Tables 19.1 and 19.2). A full listing of the subdomains and components can be accessed through the online version (www.who.int/classifications/icfbrowser and selecting the Children and Youth version).

Activities and participation are relevant and the same for all children whether or not they have a disability. Importantly, activities and participation are objective verifiable phenomena, and therefore conceptually distinct from 'quality of life', which is defined as a person's subjective perception of their well-being.[3] The ICF advocates the qualifiers 'capacity' and 'performance' for activities and participation. 'Capacity' describes the best that a person can achieve in a standardized environment, whereas 'performance' describes what a person actually does in their lived environment. Inconsistencies between capacity and performance are proposed to be due to mediating contextual factors, labelled as 'environmental' or 'personal'. Environmental factors are classified as (1) products and technology, (2) natural environment and human-made changes to environment, (3) support and relationships, (4) attitudes and (5) services, systems and policies. Personal factors are not classified in the ICF, but include sex, race, age, culture, lifestyle, habits and coping styles among others.

The term 'social inclusion' is commonly used as a goal in health and social care policy, and is variously defined. Nevertheless, most definitions of social exclusion emphasize 'lack of participation in social activities as the core characteristic'.[4] Therefore, social inclusion appears to be conceptually synonymous with many aspects of participation.

Factors to consider when measuring this domain

The ICF has been an important conceptual development in childhood disability and health research. However, several major issues and difficulties emerge when one tries to conduct applied measurement of the construct.[5] Important considerations include moving from construct definitions to the content validity of instruments, age appropriateness, whether to measure capacity or performance or 'capability', how to scale 'execution' (for activities) and 'involvement' (for participation), and who should report a child's activities and participation. When selecting instruments for measuring activities and participation, the usual criteria for appraising such instruments should include appropriateness, reliability, validity, responsiveness, precision, interpretability, acceptability and feasibility.[6]

CONSTRUCT DEFINITIONS TO CONTENT VALIDITY

Having separate definitions for activities and participation but then combining them in a single list makes it

TABLE 19.1

Chapter titles of the key domains for activities and participation in the International Classification of Functioning, Disability and Health

Major domains of activities and participation
Learning and applying knowledge
General tasks and demands
Communication
Mobility
Self-care
Domestic life
Interpersonal interactions and relationships
Major life areas
Community, social and civic life

TABLE 19.2

Sublevels of item d510 'washing oneself' in the chapter on 'self care' as an example of the hierarchical structure of the International Classification of Functioning, Disability and Health

Chapter 5 Self-care	
+ *d510*	*Washing oneself*
d5100	Washing body parts
d5101	Washing whole body
d5102	Drying oneself
d5108	Washing oneself, other specified
d5109	Washing oneself, unspecified

difficult to distinguish between what in life constitutes tasks (for activities) and life situations (for participation). McConachie et al[7] characterized four primary types of life situations as (1) essential for survival, (2) those that are supportive of child development, (3) education related and (4) discretionary roles. Coster and Khetani[8] reviewed the measurement of participation in some detail and pointed out that clarity in the construct definition is fundamental to the validity of any measurement. Badley[9] proposed that activities and participation could be recategorized in three domains (1) acts, (2) tasks and (3) societal participation. She does this with reference to the construct of the component, individual effects (role of cognitive and volition) and contextual influences, including scene setters, facilitators and cultural variants. Badley's approach has merit to distinguish acts without context, tasks which are coordinated acts and are broadly consistent with 'activities of daily living', and socially inclusive pursuits defined by social roles.[9]

While many elements of activities and participation are generic wherever in the world a child lives, some aspects of participation are country- or culture-specific. An issue that is particularly relevant for young children,

but also to all young people, is that many aspects of life are nested within a family context. Therefore codependence must be recognized when assessing activities and participation in the realms titled 'domestic life' and 'interpersonal interactions and relationships'.[7,8]

The instruments included in this chapter are relevant to 'activities and participation'; however, none is entirely consistent with, or provides comprehensive coverage of, the items classified in the ICF simply because the ICF has been so recently developed.[10] Coster and Khetani[8] acknowledged that, until consensus emerges on these difficult but crucial issues, the fact that existing instruments measure subtly, or substantially different, constructs precludes any effective synthesis and interpretation of results across studies.

AGE APPROPRIATENESS

The social context of children's lives varies at different stages of development; hence, depending on the purpose of measurement, the content may need to be adjusted for different age groupings. Fifteen-year-old adolescents obviously participate in different life situations than 5-year-olds, although it is often also desirable to measure change over time and between age groups. Therefore, a balance must be struck between focusing on age-specific roles (thus ensuring internal validity) and including broader content that will be generalizable to a wider age range (external validity).

CAPACITY AND PERFORMANCE, OR CAPABILITY?

The ICF qualifiers of 'capacity' (can do, at best) and 'performance' (does do) are useful but may not capture the whole picture when measuring functioning. Aside from environment, whether a child performs, particularly in discretionary situations, is to a large degree mediated by them having the opportunity (capability), and then choosing to do so. Having the 'opportunity' is consistent with the intention that activities and participation should be framed within a rights agenda alongside the UN Conventions on the Rights of the Child.[11] The 'capability approach'[12] (and for application to disability see references 13–15) offers a corollary framework to the ICF to enable consideration of the *opportunity* and *choice* elements to be incorporated in measuring activities and participation.[16]

SCALING 'EXECUTION' AND 'INVOLVEMENT'

Coster and Khetani,[8] and also Bedell et al,[17] reflect upon what constitutes 'involvement' in the situations and roles of life and how this can be scaled for measurement. It remains unclear whether involvement requires active versus passive engagement in a situation or task; whether a child who requires some level of assistance, either human or assistive technology, to perform is participating to a lesser extent; or how frequency or intensity of performance can be incorporated into assessment. Such issues are important as they influence whether children with physical or learning disabilities can achieve higher levels of participation and social inclusion, or whether their level of performance is always penalized by their impairments or need for help.

WHO SHOULD REPORT?

Relevant questionnaires have, to date, typically been administered with parents or carers as part of semi-structured interviews or in postal surveys; however, it is increasingly recognized that children should be engaged in self-reporting their health.[18] The chapters and categories in the ICF are descriptive but not necessarily operationalized in language that can be readily understood by, and perceived as meaningful for, children. Questionnaires evaluating children's activities and participation should be based on pertinent child-orientated situations that ask about how things are, typically, in everyday life. Any questions that are to be administered directly to children

must incorporate age-appropriate words and phrases. Multiple respondents could be considered; for instance, Sakzewski et al[19] recommended three instruments to gain a complete profile of a child's participation, requiring input from the child, parent and teacher. Such variety could be viewed either as a strength of the approach or a psychometric weakness, as each reporter brings a different perspective.

Primary global generic measures of activity and participation

Six tools commonly used in practice and research are described in detail below, with key attributes tabulated at the end of each section.

FUNCTIONAL INDEPENDENCE MEASURE FOR CHILDREN

Overview and purpose

Functional status measures were first developed in the 1960s for adult populations in order to quantify activity limitations and level of functional independence in individuals with disabilities. One of the most widely used measures for adults is the Functional Independence Measure. Wide utility in rehabilitation settings prompted development of a paediatric version called the WeeFIM (Functional Independent Measure for Children), which began in 1987.[20,21] The original intent of this tool was for use with an inpatient paediatric rehabilitation population; however, it has much wider clinical applicability to include use in hospital settings, home care and community-based services. The WeeFIM II® system includes the instrument, the 0 to 3 years module (recently developed for young infants and undergoing psychometric validation) and software that enables the generation of reports (www.udsmr.org). Institutions may subscribe to this system package, which includes comprehensive training workshops and ongoing services and supports. For example, institutional data may be compared with population-based data.

The purpose of the WeeFIM is to evaluate and monitor performance in functional (daily living) skills in infants and young children with congenital or acquired disabilities between 6 months and 7 years of age. It may also be used in older children (7–18y) who are functioning at <7 years of age. It has been used in research on children with a wide range of physical limitations and global developmental disabilities (e.g. spinal cord and traumatic brain injury, musculoskeletal disorders, cerebral palsy, developmental delay). This assessment tool provides a measure of severity of disability in terms of how much assistance is required beyond what would be considered age appropriate. This tool provides an appreciation of

FUNCTIONAL INDEPENDENCE MEASURE FOR CHILDREN (WeeFIM)®	
Purpose	To measure and monitor performance in functional (daily living) skills in infants and young children or older children with activity limitations. An indicator of severity of disability with reference to level of assistance required to perform routine everyday tasks. May be used as an outcome measure of medical and rehabilitation interventions. May be helpful in identifying social and economic supports and assistance required to complete daily tasks
Population	6mo–7y, or older children who are functioning at <7y
Description of domains (subscales)	Adapted from the adult FIM™ instrument. Six domains/three subscales: self-care, sphincter control, transfers, locomotion, communication, social cognition; self-care (eight items), motor (five items), cognition (five items)
Administration and test format	Time to complete: 10–20min to administer Testing format: 18 items; interview with primary caregiver and/or by observation Scoring: seven-point ordinal scale, criterion-referenced. Independent (7) or modified independent with devices (6), modified dependence (3–5), complete dependence (1–2) Training: available with credentialing of institutions
Psychometric properties	Normative sample: >500 children without disabilities; >700 children with disabilities *Reliability* Inter-rater and test–retest reliability established (intraclass correlation coefficient range: 0.73–0.98) Equivalence reliability for telephone compared with face-to-face interview *Validity* Experts involved in establishing content validity. Developmentally sensitive with progressive sequence of items associated with increasing age (construct validity). Correlates with (1) Vineland Adaptive Behaviour Scale, (2) Battelle Developmental Inventory, (3) Pediatric Evaluation of Disability Inventory: rho between 0.53 and 0.96 but >0.88 for similar subscale associations (concurrent validity). Differentiates between children with and without disabilities (construct validity) *Responsiveness* Measures change in children with disabilities over a 1-year period
How to order	Institutions can become accredited with users trained in the administration and scoring of the tool. Requires an annual subscription fee Available at: www.udsmr.org
Key references	Deutsch A, Braun A, Granger C (1996) The Functional Independence Measure (FIMSM Instrument) and the Functional Independence Measure (WeeFIM® Instrument): ten years of development. *Crit Rev Phys Rehabil Med* 8: 267–281. Ottenbacher KJ, Msall ME, Lyons NR, Duffy LC, Granger CV, Braun S (1997) Interrater agreement and stability of the Functional Independence Measure for Children (WeeFIM TM): use in children with developmental disabilities. *Arch Phys Med Rehabil* 78: 1309–1315. Ottenbacher KJ, Msall ME, Lyons N, et al (2000) The WeeFIM instrument: its utility in detecting change in children with developmental disabilities. *Arch Phys Med Rehabil* 81: 1317–1326.

the physical, social, economic and technological burden experienced by the families and as such identifies resource needs.[20,22] The WeeFIM is meant to be a minimal data set and is used to track outcomes following rehabilitation interventions.[21,23] It should be emphasized that it is not meant to replace a more detailed and comprehensive assessment of activity limitations across the spectrum of functioning. Furthermore, it does not evaluate why children are experiencing activity limitations, therefore it is not a diagnostic tool but rather an evaluative tool that measures change over time. It is part of a 'uniform data set' (for medical rehabilitation) which collects additional demographic and medical information.[20,21,23]

Administration and scoring

The WeeFIM can be used across disciplines by any health professional who is trained in its use. It is typically administered by interview and/or direct observation, together with a primary caregiver who is very familiar with the child's functional abilities. It takes approximately 20 minutes to administer and includes 18 items classified into three domains. The self-care domain includes eating, grooming, bathing, dressing the upper and lower body, and sphincter control. The motor domain includes transfers and locomotion, whereas cognition includes items related to communication (expression and comprehension) and social cognition (social interaction, problem solving, memory).[20,22] The items include activities routinely performed as part of daily activities, and scoring of these items is on 'actual' performance. In other words, it is possible that the child has the capacity to do the activity, but in everyday-life experience the child does not actually perform the task. This may be for a number of reasons, and would need to be investigated in order to maximize functional independence.

Each item is scored on a seven-point ordinal scale. A high score indicates complete (7) or modified (6; with a device) independence. Modified dependence would include the need for supervision to complete the task (5), minimal assistance (4) or moderate assistance (3). Complete dependence occurs when there is the need for maximal assistance (2) or total assistance (1). Scores per domain and total score can be compared with normative data and can be converted to quotients. Quotients between 50 and 75 indicate moderate disability, whereas those below 50 imply severe disability.[22]

Psychometric properties

Development of this tool involved pilot testing on children both with and without disabilities. More than 500 typically developing children were evaluated using the WeeFIM instrument, which was helpful in refining administration, developing normative data, evaluating the effects of age and comparing scores with those of children with disabilities.[21,23] Rasch models were used to calculate normative data in 4-month intervals.[20] Rasch analyses were also used to verify the clustering of items and distinct dimensions of this tool.[23,24] Changes in functional status with increasing age were also confirmed, with a high coefficient of determination (r^2=0.83), contributing to

construct validity. Discriminant validity was determined by comparing children with and without disabilities.[20,21,23] There was a high level of correlation (>0.88) between the more detailed Pediatric Evaluation of Disability Inventory (PEDI) and the WeeFIM, thus confirming concurrent validity.[25] Similar strong correlations were obtained with the Vineland Adaptive Behavior Scale (VABS) and the Battelle Developmental Inventory.[26] Test–retest and inter-rater reliability were very good to excellent, with an intra-class correlation coefficient (ICC) ranging from 0.73 to 0.98, with total score reliabilities of 0.96 (different rater) and 0.98 (same rater). Furthermore, equivalence reliability (telephone vs face-to-face interviews) has also been established, with no significant differences in scores for the two administration formats.[22,27] Furthermore, the five indices of responsiveness all demonstrated significant changes over time (over a 1-year period) in children with disabilities.[28] Cross-cultural testing to include establishment of normative data and small adjustments to items has been pursued in Chinese, Japanese, Thai and Turkish children.[29–32]

PEDIATRIC EVALUATION OF DISABILITY INVENTORY

Overview and purpose

The PEDI may be used to assess abilities for a variety of functional activities as well as the level of caregiver assistance required in order to do functional tasks. A range of functional activities that are typically performed in children between 6 months and 7 years 6 months of age are evaluated. The purpose of the PEDI is to detect whether there are limitations in functional activities (discriminative) and to monitor change over time (evaluative). It is often used in the clinical setting for programme evaluation, and particular components of the measure may be completed by professionals from different health disciplines. This assessment may be carried out on children with a variety of disabilities, both congenital and acquired. The PEDI provides a more detailed and comprehensive assessment of activity limitations across the spectrum of functioning than the WeeFIM.[33,34]

Administration and scoring

The PEDI can be used by any health professional who has expertise in standardized assessment and in functional activities and is trained in its use. It can be administered by direct observation by one or more health professionals who are familiar with the child's functional performance. However, it is typically administered by structured interview (with a recommended questioning strategy) with the primary caregiver who is most familiar with the child's level of independence in functional activities. It takes

PEDIATRIC EVALUATION OF DISABILITY INVENTORY (PEDI)	
Purpose	To evaluate a wide range of functional capabilities of children with disabilities and to monitor progress in functional performance over time. It is an indicator of the level of caregiver assistance required to perform routine everyday tasks. It may be used to evaluate programmes. It provides quantification of modifications made to the environment and equipment needed in order to execute functional activities
Population	6mo–7y 6mo, or older children who are functioning at <7y
Description of domains (subscales)	1. Functional skills scale – 197 items (with scores for self-care, mobility, social functions) 2. Caregiver assistance scale – 20 items (with scores for self-care, mobility, social functions) 3. Modifications scale – 20 items
Administration and test format	Time to complete: typically 45–60min to administer, depending on functional level Testing format: direct observation by health professional and/or structured interview with primary caregiver most familiar with the child's typical performance. Computer adaptive testing (CAT) version – computer selects optimal items based on previous responses, greatly reducing the number of items Scoring: 0 (unable, limited) or 1 (capable in most situations) scored for each item. Normative standard scores (adjusted for age, mean: 50; standard deviation: 10) or scaled score (not age-adjusted, 0–100 from easy to difficult) Training: guidelines are described in the manual
Psychometric properties	Normative sample: 412 children without disabilities, 14 age groups *Reliability (with trained interviewers)* Inter-rater reliability established (intraclass correlation coefficient range: 0.74–0.95). Inter-rater reliability excellent for sample with typically developing children (0.95–0.99) *Validity* Experts involved in establishing content validity. Developmentally sensitive with progressive sequence of items associated with increasing age (construct validity). Correlates with (1) Battelle Developmental Inventory and (2) WeeFIM (correlations >0.70) (concurrent validity). Differentiates children with/without disabilities (construct validity). Validation studies conducted on Dutch-, Spanish-, Swedish- and Turkish-language versions *Responsiveness* Measures change in children with disabilities over a 6-month period
How to order	Manual, forms and software may be purchased from Harcourt Assessment Inc. (http://harcourtassessment.com/pedi) Cost: approximately US$425 (manual, forms, software)
Key references	Berg M, Jahnsen R, Froslie KF, Hussain A (2004) Reliability of the Pediatric Evaluation of Disability Inventory (PEDI). *Phys Occup Ther Paediatr* 24: 61–77. Coster WJ, Haley SM, Ni P, Dumas HM, Fragala-Pinkham MA (2008) Assessing self-care and social function using a computer adaptive testing version of the Pediatric Evaluation of Disability Inventory. *Arch Phys Med Rehabil* 89: 622–629. Haley SM, Coster WJ, Ludlow LH, Haltiwanger JT, Andrellos PJ (1992) *Pediatric Evaluation of Disability Inventory (PEDI). Version 1.0: Development, Standardization and Administration Manual.* Boston, MA: New England Medical Center Hospitals Inc.

approximately 20 minutes to 1 hour to administer, depending on the age of the child and level of capability. There are three sections to the tool: (1) the functional skills scale (197 items), which includes performance in self-care, mobility and social functions; (2) the caregiver assistance scale (20 items), which quantifies level of caregiver assistance needed to perform each task; and (3) the modifications scale (20 items), which records the environmental modifications and equipment required. Each scale can be used separately. The tool includes the manual, score forms and software to generate scores and profiles.[33]

There are three domains (self-care, mobility, social functions) for which individual scale scores may be obtained within the functional skills and for caregiver assistance. The self-care domain includes capabilities within eating, grooming, dressing and toileting. Mobility includes transfer skills (e.g. getting in and out of the bathtub, chair, car, bed) as well as body transport activities (e.g. floor mobility, locomotion, stairs, outdoor surfaces, manipulating objects during locomotion). Social functions are diverse and include expression and comprehension, peer interactions, play, problem solving, household chores and orientating to self and time.[33] Each item is scored as either zero (unable or limited capability) or one (capable of performing the task in most situations). Summary scores are derived, which include (1) normative standard scores (mean: 50, standard deviation: 10) for each of the three functional skill domains and each of the three caregiver assistance domains, and (2) scaled scores from 0 to 100 (easy to difficult). The scaled scores are not age adjusted, whereas the normative standard scores are adjusted for age expectations based on the normative sample (n=412; 14 age groups). Children without disabilities were recruited from the north-east region of the USA using a stratified quota sampling strategy. There are explicit scoring criteria for each item in the manual. The modifications scale counts the type and extent of environmental modifications and equipment needed to perform functional activities.[33]

Psychometric properties
Development of the content of the tool was initially developed from the literature, previous tests and clinical expertise. An initial version was then field tested on children with disabilities. The item pool was narrowed, and reliability and internal consistency were estimated. Further validation was done involving a panel of 31 experts (content validity), to ensure that the measure was comprehensive and representative of functional activities. The final standardization version has undergone further psychometric testing (see below). Rasch models were applied for scale construction.

Internal consistency using Cronbach's coefficient alpha for the six scales (three for functional scale, three for caregiver assistance) is excellent (0.95–0.99). Inter-interviewer reliability (i.e. two individuals scoring the same interview) for the normative sample is also excellent (ICC 0.96–0.99). Inter-rater reliability ICC ranges from 0.74 to 0.96, with the modifications scale being somewhat less reliable. Inter-rater and intrarater reliability (trained interviewers) on a sample of Norwegian children without disability was excellent (ICC 0.95–0.99). Discrepancy between parents and teachers (inter-respondent reliability) was highest (ICC 0.64–0.99).[35] Construct validity is supported as the scores are associated with age. Furthermore, the PEDI discriminates between children with and without disabilities. Concurrent validity with the Battelle Developmental Inventory (0.70–0.73) and the WeeFIM (0.80–0.97) is acceptable.[25,33] Preliminary data demonstrated that the PEDI is responsive to changes over a 6-month period.[33] Responsiveness to change in motor ability was shown (effects size and standardized response mean values >0.8) in children with cerebral palsy, with greater responsiveness in children <4 years of age.[36] In one study, minimally clinically important change, as determined by clinicians, was associated with PEDI change scores of approximately 11%.[37] Content and concurrent and discriminant validity were demonstrated with the Spanish language version;[38,39] reliability and construct validity has been shown for the Turkish version;[40] content validity has been established for the Swedish version;[41] and discriminative validity and reliability were evident in the Dutch version.[42,43]

Recently, a computer adaptive testing (CAT) version (short form) of the functional skills subscales of the PEDI has been developed. This uses an interface that selects the most optimal items based on previous responses, and thus reduces the total number of items. The score estimates from this short computerized version are comparable to those of the long version, but substantially decrease administration time.[44,45] Multidimensional CAT applications have greater precision and efficiency.[46] The CAT is able to detect functional changes over time; however, this is with reduced sensitivity (greater variability in score estimates) when compared with the full-length version.[47]

VINELAND ADAPTIVE BEHAVIOR SCALE, SECOND EDITION

Overview and purpose
The VABS-II is a self-administered questionnaire that measures adaptive behaviour and is appropriate for all age groups from birth to adulthood (0–90y). Domains evaluated include communication, daily living skills, socialization and motor skills (0–6y only for motor) as well as maladaptive behaviour (problem behaviours). This new edition has been expanded to include more items for the 0- to 3-year age group, items for adults and items that are

VINELAND ADAPTIVE BEHAVIOUR SCALE, SECOND EDITION (VABS-II)	
Purpose	To measure adaptive behaviour across functional domains in an individual across the lifespan. To determine strengths and limitations in daily functioning and to ascertain the need for referral for special services. To assist with differential diagnosis and programme planning. To monitor progress in functioning
Population	Birth to age 90y; 0–6y for motor skills domain
Description of domains (subscales)	Four domains to yield an adaptive behaviour composite score (three domains if age >6y): communication (receptive, expressive, written); daily living skills (personal, domestic, community); socialization (interpersonal relationships, play and leisure time, coping skills); and motor skills (gross, fine)
	Optional: maladaptive behaviour domain (a composite of undesirable behaviours that may limit functioning) for individuals aged >3y
Administration and test format	Time to complete: 20min–1h to administer, depending on age or developmental level; 15–30min required for scoring
	Testing format: interview with primary caregiver and/or by self-report
	Scoring: for each item/activity – habitually performed (2), performed sometimes or partially without help (1), never/rarely performed (0), no opportunity (NO), do not know (DK). Standard scores and centile ranks may be derived
	Training: the manual contains detailed directions for the administration of the tool
Psychometric properties	Normative sample: >3600 individuals
	Psychometric properties for Survey Interview Form domains are summarized below (Parent Rating Form properties are described in the manual)
	Reliability
	Internal consistency: median split-half coefficients range from 0.86 to 0.98
	Inter-rater: intraclass correlation coefficients (ICCs) range from 0.68 to 0.80 and test–retest reliability has been established (most ICCs >0.85, range 0.75–0.96)
	Validity
	Experts involved in establishing content validity. Developmentally sensitive with progressive sequence of items associated with increasing age (construct validity). Correlates strongly with Vineland Adaptive Behaviour Scale, first edition. Differentiates between children with and without disabilities (construct validity). Correlations with the Weschler Intelligence Scale for Children are low, but were highest for the communication domain (0.30–0.36)
How to order	Computer software is available to generate scores and reports. It can be ordered from http://psychcorp.pearsonassessments.com/HAIWEB/Cultures/en-us/Productdetail. htm?Pid=Vineland-II
	Cost: approximately US$160 for starter kit, US$430 with software
Key reference	Sparrow SS, Cicchetti DV, Balla DA (2005) *Vineland Adaptive Behaviour Scales, Second Edition. Survey Forms Manual*. Minneapolis, MN: NCS Pearson Inc.

more culturally appropriate. The purpose of the VABS-II is to provide an overview of an individual's daily life functioning and may be applied to children and young people with a range of conditions and developmental disabilities. More specifically, this instrument measures adaptive behaviour (i.e. performance necessary for personal and social sufficiency) and integrates four principles as follows: (1) there are age-related changes in functioning, characterized by increasing complexity, (2) it is defined by the expectations and the standards of others, (3) it is potentially modifiable and (4) it is a measure of performance (does do), not capacity (can do).[48]

Administration and scoring

Administration format is flexible and can include face-to-face semi-structured interviews (survey interview form) as a preferred format but can also be administered by proxy self-report (parent/caregiver rating form) approaches. Expanded interview and teacher rating forms are also available. The respondent should be an adult who is very familiar with the daily functioning of the individual being evaluated, and is typically a parent. More than one respondent may be used for separate domains. Explicit instructions are provided in the manual to guide the interview format. The interview can take 20 minutes to 1 hour to complete, depending on the functional level of the child. The interview may be administered in other languages by a bilingual interviewer. The tool includes the manual and score sheets, and software can be purchased as well. Each item represents an activity and is scored as either habitually performed (2), sometimes/partially performed (1) or rarely/not performed (0). A score of 'no opportunity' or 'do not know' can also be provided. Detailed information is provided in the manual to differentiate these scores. Basal and ceiling scores are established. Subdomain raw scores are computed and then converted to derived scores for each of the domains and the adaptive behaviour composite score. Normative scores include standard scores, age equivalents, centile ranks and stanines.[48]

Psychometric properties

The new items on the revised VABS were generated from a large pool of items that were reviewed by an expert panel and accordingly retained or excluded. Items were subsequently reviewed for relevance and bias by 12 clinicians from the USA who routinely evaluate individuals with developmental disabilities from diverse ethnic backgrounds. The revised instrument was then field tested on a random sampling of 1843 individuals (0–77y) from a pool of over 5800 people and a clinical sample of 392 individuals with developmental disabilities was also tested. A Rasch model was applied for item fit. Exploratory factor analyses and a split-half procedure supported internal consistency. Normative data and psychometric testing were determined from samples across 20 age group categories. The normative sample included 3695 individuals randomly selected from a large pool, matching for demographic characteristics by age group. Representation was sought across ethnicity, socioeconomic status, sex and geographic region. Internal consistency, test–retest and inter-rater reliability are very good to excellent overall (see chart below).[48] Telephone versus face-to-face equivalence reliability has been established for the VABS first edition.[49]

Content validity is supported with respect to representativeness of content by domains (item-scale structure supported) and relationship to increasing age. Confirmatory factor analysis supports the theoretical structure of the VABS-II. The instrument differentiates children with global delays, pervasive developmental disorders and other disabilities with the reference sample, supporting discriminative validity. When comparing the VABS first and second edition, VABS-II scores are somewhat higher, especially for daily living skills, although the scores across the two editions are highly correlated overall (most correlation coefficients: 0.80s and 0.90s). Correlations with the Wechsler Intelligence Scale for Children, third edition, are low, supporting that these two instruments measure different constructs.

ASSESSMENT OF LIFE HABITS

Overview and purpose

The Assessment of Life Habits (LIFE-H) was developed to measure involvement in life situations as the 'social participation' domain of the Disability Creation Process (DCP).[50] The DCP and ICF share many similarities, as the developers of the DCP were involved in the construction of the ICF; however, there are also substantive differences in their concepts and categories.[51] The LIFE-H was initially developed for assessing adults; the children's version for children aged 5 to 13 years was created by modifying the adult instrument.

The LIFE-H was initially administered to parents of children with cerebral palsy; these children experienced the most disruption to situations involving recreation, community, personal care, education, mobility, housing and nutrition.[52,53] Further work has explored the use of the instrument for children with other conditions.[54] The LIFE-H was administered as part of a large European study examining factors affecting participation of children with cerebral palsy across several countries.[55]

Administration and scoring

There are short (64 items) and long (197 items) versions that are administered to parents as an interview. Item responses are scored by difficulty and assistance required, with the final item score calculated as a composite of the two elements (0–9). Items are grouped into 11 domains for nutrition, fitness, personal care, communication, housing, mobility, responsibilities, interpersonal relationships, community life, education and recreation. Domain scores are expressed as a percentage (0–100%), where higher scores represent greater disruption to life habits.

ASSESSMENT OF LIFE HABITS (LIFE-H)

Purpose	To measure social participation consistent with the Disability Creation Process
Population	Children aged 5–13y; a version has also been produced for infants aged 0–4y but is not evaluated here
Description of domains (subscales)	Domains for nutrition, fitness, personal care, communication, housing, mobility, responsibilities, interpersonal relationships, community life, education and recreation
Administration and test format	Time to complete: typically 45–60min to administer Testing format: structured questionnaire-based interview with primary caregiver Scoring: item scores are a composite of accomplishment (five levels) and assistance required (four levels) to perform roles; domain scores are expressed as a percentage (0–100%), where higher scores represent greater disruption to life habits Training: guidelines described in the manual and courses also available
Psychometric properties	*Reliability* Intra-observer reliability: intraclass correlation coefficient (ICC) >0.78 for 10 domains, ICC=0.58 for the 'interpersonal relationship' domain Inter-observer reliability: ICC >0.78 for 10 domains, ICC=0.63 for the 'interpersonal relationship' domain *Validity* Content validity supported by expert panel. Appropriate convergent correlations with Pediatric Evaluation of Disability Inventory and Functional Independence Measure for Children scales *Responsiveness* No evidence of responsiveness is available
How to order	Related documents can be ordered through the International Network on the Disability Creation Process (www.ripph.qc.ca)
Key references	Fougeyrollas P, Noreau L, Bergeron H, Cloutier R, Dion SA, St-Michel G (1998) Social consequences of long term impairments and disabilities: conceptual approach and assessment of handicap. *Int J Rehabil Res* 21: 127–141. Lepage C, Noreau L, Bernard P-M, Fougeyrollas P (1998) Profile of handicap situations in children with cerebral palsy. *Scand J Rehabil Med* 30: 263–272. Noreau L, Lepage C, Boissiere L, et al (2007) Measuring participation in children with disabilities using the Assessment of Life Habits. *Dev Med Child Neurol* 49: 666–671.

Psychometric properties

Content validity was supported by an expert panel that included parents, clinicians and researchers. The intra-observer and interobserver reliability (ICC) for 10 domains exceeded 0.78; reliability was slightly lower (ICC=0.58) for 'interpersonal relationships'. Construct validity was supported by appropriate convergent and divergent correlations with scores from the PEDI functional skills and caregiver assistance scales and WeeFIM domains. No evidence of responsiveness is available from longitudinal studies.[54]

ACTIVITIES SCALE FOR KIDS

Overview and purpose

The Activities Scale for Kids (ASK) was developed as a self-report instrument to measure physical functioning in children aged 5 to 15 years. Two versions are available which are constructed to assess capability (ASKc) and performance (ASKp). The performance version measures what a child usually does in his or her life, whereas the capability version measures what the child thinks he or she could have done without taking his or her environment into account.[56] The ASK was initially developed for children affected by musculoskeletal problems, but has since been used to assess physical functioning in children with cerebral palsy and a range of disabling conditions.[57–59]

Administration and scoring
The questionnaire can be completed by children themselves or be completed by a proxy such as a parent. A non-scoring question asks how much help children had in completing the questionnaire. The items cover a range of activities including personal care, dressing, eating and drinking, play and mobility. The initial version of the ASK that was tested had 30 items; however, a 38-item version is proposed to improve precision. Five response options are scaled as the frequency at which the activity was performed (performance version) or difficulty (capability version). Items are scored (0–4) and a single summary percentage score (0–100%) is calculated, with higher scores indicating better functioning.

Psychometric properties
The content validity of the ASK is supported by the fact that children were involved in generating and ranking the items. Test–retest reliability was high (ICC=0.97), and reliability between children and parents was also high (ICC=0.94).[56] Rasch analysis demonstrated that the 30-item version measured a unidimensional construct. Construct validity was supported by appropriate convergence and divergence with scores from the Child Health Questionnaire and Health Utilities Index (HUI3) domains.[60] Good responsiveness was demonstrated in children predicted to experience clinically important change over time.[60]

ACTIVITIES SCALE FOR KIDS (ASK)	
Purpose	To measure physical functioning. There are separate versions for assessing capacity (could do) and performance (frequency)
Population	Children aged 5–15y
Description of domains (subscales)	Single summary scores for either 'capacity' and/or 'performance' in physical functioning – personal care, dressing, eating and drinking, mobility, play, stairs, standing skills
Administration and test format	Time to complete: 10–30min
	Testing format: questionnaire self-completed by child or primary caregiver
	Scoring: items are scored 0–4 and summary score is expressed as a percentage (0–100%); higher scores represent better physical functioning and activity performance
	Training: guidelines are described in the manual
Psychometric properties	*Reliability*
	Child test–retest intraclass correlation coefficient (ICC)=0.97, child and parent agreement ICC=0.96. Internal consistency (Cronbach's alpha) of 0.99
	Validity
	Initially developed with input from children with musculoskeletal problems. Convergent correlation with Childhood Health Questionnaire (0.82) and mobility item from Health Utilities Index, third edition (HUI-3) (0.74) and moderate correlation with Child Health Questionnaire 'physical function' scale. Divergent correlation with HUI-3 classification of emotion (0.15) and speech (0.09)
	Responsiveness
	Sensitivity to change over time has been demonstrated
How to order	Contact the developers. See www.activitiesscaleforkids.com
Key references	Plint AC, Gaboury I, Owen J, Young N (2003) Activities Scale for Kids: an analysis of normals. *J Pediatr Orthop* 23: 788–790.
	Young NL, Williams JI, Yoshida KK, Bombardier C, Wright JG (1996) The context of measuring disability. Does it matter whether capability or performance is measured? *J Clin Epidemiol* 49: 1097–1101.
	Young NL, Williams JI, Yoshida KK, Wright JG (2000) Measurement properties of the Activities Scale for Kids. *J Clin Epidemiol* 53: 125–137.

Overview and purpose

The Lifestyle Assessment Questionnaire (LAQ-CP) was developed as a discriminative parent-assessed measure of the 'impact of disability' on children with cerebral palsy aged 3 to 10 years and their families.[61] A generic version of the instrument evolved from the cerebral palsy-specific instrument. The generic measure (LAQ-G) was developed with children with a variety of medical conditions and unimpaired children aged 5 to 7 years.[62] The LAQ-G has six domains: communication, mobility, self-care, domestic life, interpersonal interactions and relationships, and community and social life.

Administration and scoring

The LAQs are intended to be completed by a parent and are usually administered by mail. Items have varying levels of response options (between two and five) but are all scored on a 0 to 4 scale. Domain scores are percentage scores (0–100%), which are weighted in the case of the LAQ-CP based upon perceived relative importance to clinicians and parents, but not weighted for the LAQ-G; higher scores represent greater impact of disability.

Psychometric properties

The content of the cerebral palsy-specific version was generated by clinicians; reliability was reported to be satisfactory.[61] The LAQ-G built on the LAQ-CP by taking account of surveys with children and families, a literature

LIFESTYLE ASSESSMENT QUESTIONNAIRE (LAQ-CP AND LAQ-G)	
Purpose	To measure 'impact of disability' on child and family life
Population	LAQ-CP children aged 3–10y; LAQ-G children aged 5–7y
Description of domains (subscales)	LAQ-CP domain scores for mobility, physical independence, clinical burden, economic burden, schooling and social integration
	LAQ-G domains for communication, mobility, self-care, domestic life, interpersonal interactions and relationships, community and social life
Administration and test format	Time to complete: typically 15–20min to complete
	Testing format: questionnaire completed by primary caregiver
	Scoring: items scored 0–4 and percentage domain scores scored 0–100%, where a higher score represents a greater impact of disability
	Training: guidelines are described in the manuals
Psychometric properties	*Reliability*
	Test–retest for same assessor: intraclass correlation coefficient (ICC) ranged from 0.64 to 0.96
	Interobserver between different assessors: ICC ranged from 0.62 to 0.91
	Internal consistency (Cronbach's alpha) ranged from 0.73 to <0.90, except interpersonal relationships (0.40)
	Validity
	Content validity assessed by expert panel. Convergent correlation with scores from the Central Motor Deficit Form ($r=0.76$; $p<0.0001$)
	Responsiveness
	No evidence of responsiveness
How to order	Contact the developers. See http://research.ncl.ac.uk/cargo-ne/contents.html
Key references	Jessen EC, Colver AF, Mackie PC, Jarvis SN (2003) Development and validation of a tool to measure the impact of childhood disabilities on the lives of children and their families. *Child Care Health Dev* 29: 21–34.
	Mackie PC, Jessen EC, Jarvis SN (1998) The Lifestyle Assessment Questionnaire: an instrument to measure the impact of disability on the lives of children with cerebral palsy and their families. *Child Care Health Dev* 24: 473–486.

review and consultation with a range of professionals.[62] Internal consistency (Cronbach's alpha) for the LAQ-G domains ranged from 0.66 to 0.91. Test–retest analyses were satisfactory for the LAQ-G, but were reported only at the item level rather than by correlating domain scores. Construct validity for the LAQ-G was demonstrated by the items discriminating between children with and without disability.

Summary

The WeeFIM and PEDI are measures of severity of disability (level of independence in functional skills) and are limited by a ceiling effect when measuring children who are higher functioning, with minimal activity limitations.

Therefore, these tools are more appropriate for children with physical limitations that impede the capability to perform a variety of everyday activities. The LIFE-H and the ASK were also primarily developed for children with physical disabilities, whereas the VABS and the LAQ may be used more broadly for children with a range of developmental disabilities. The VABS is unique in its applicability across all age groups, whereas the other measures have specific age requirements for application. None of these tools covers the entire spectrum of activity and participation domains, as defined by the ICF. Indeed, there is an urgent need for measures that accurately capture the activity and participation domains, as conceptualized by the ICF classification framework.

REFERENCES

1. World Health Organization (2001) *International Classification of Functioning, Disability and Health.* Geneva: WHO.
2. World Health Organization (2007) *International Classification of Functioning, Disability and Health Version for Children and Youth.* Geneva: WHO.
3. World Health Organization (1998) Quality of Life Instruments Assessment Group Development and general psychometric properties. *Soc Sci Med* 46: 1569–1585.
4. Morgan C, Burns T, Fitzpatrick R, Pinfold V, Priebe S (2007) Social exclusion and mental health: a conceptual and methodological review. *Br J Psychiatry* 191: 477–483.
5. Morris C (2007) Measuring children's participation. *Dev Med Child Neurol* 49: 645.
6. Fitzpatrick R, Davey C, Buxton MJ, Jones DR (1998) Evaluating patient-based outcome measures for use in clinical trials. *Health Technol Assess* 2: 1–74.
7. McConachie H, Colver AF, Forsyth RJ, Jarvis SN, Parkinson KN (2006) Participation of disabled children: how should it be characterized and measured? *Disabil Rehabil* 28: 1157–1164.
8. Coster W, Khetani MA (2008) Measuring participation of children with disabilities: issues and challenges. *Disabil Rehabil* 30: 639–648.
9. Badley EM (2008) Enhancing the conceptual clarity of the activity and participation components of the International Classification of Functioning, Disability and Health. *Soc Sci Med* 66: 2335–2345.
10. Morris C, Kurinczuk JJ, Fitzpatrick R (2005) Child or family assessed measures of activity performance and participation for children with cerebral palsy: a structured review. *Child Care Health Dev* 31: 397–407.
11. Simeonsson RJ, Leonardi M, Lollar D, Bjorck-Akesson E, Hollenweger J, Martinuzzi A (2003) Applying the International Classification of Functioning, Disability and Health (ICF) to measure childhood disability. *Disabil Rehabil* 25: 602–610.
12. Sen A (1992) *Inequality Re-examined.* Oxford: Oxford University Press.
13. Terzi L (2005) A capability perspective on impairment, disability and special needs. *Theory Res Edu* 3: 197–223.
14. Robeyns I (2005) The capability approach: a theoretical survey. *J Hum Dev* 6: 93–114.
15. Mitra S (2006) The capability approach and disability. *J Dis Pol Stud* 16: 236–247.
16. Morris C (2009) Measuring participation in childhood disability: how does the capability approach improve our understanding? *Dev Med Child Neurol* 51: 92–94.
17. Bedell G, Coster W (2008) Measuring participation of school-aged children with traumatic brain injuries: considerations and approaches. *J Head Trauma Rehabil* 23: 220–229.
18. United Nations (1989) *Convention on the Rights of the Child.* Available at: www.unicef.org/crc.
19. Sakzewski L, Boyd R, Ziviani J (2007) Clinimetric properties of participation measures for 5- to 13-year-old children with cerebral palsy: a systematic review. *Dev Med Child Neurol* 49: 232–240.
20. Deutsch A, Braun A, Granger C (1996) The Functional Independence Measure (FIM™ Instrument) and the Functional Independence Measure (WeeFIM® Instrument): ten years of development. *Crit Rev Phys Rehabil Med* 8: 267–281.
21. Msall ME, DiGaudio K, Rogers BT, et al (1994) The Functional Independence Measure for Children (WeeFIM): conceptual basis and pilot use in children with developmental disabilities. *Clin Pediatr* 35: 421–430.
22. Ottenbacher KJ, Msall ME, Lyons NR, Duffy LC, Granger CV, Braun S (1997) Interrater agreement and stability of the Functional Independence Measure for Children (WeeFIM™): use in children with developmental disabilities. *Arch Phys Med Rehabil* 78: 1309–1315.
23. Msall ME, DiGaudio K, Duffy LC, LaForest S, Braun S, Granger CV (1994) WeeFIM: normative sample of an instrument for tracking functional independence in children. *Clin Pediatr* 35: 431–438.
24. Chen CC, Bode RK, Granger C, Heinemann AW (2005) Psychometric properties and developmental differences in children's ADL item hierarchy: a study of the WeeFIM® Instrument. *Am J Phys Med* 84: 671–679.
25. Ziviani J, Ottenbacher KJ, Shephard K, Foreman S, Astbury W, Ireland P (2001) Concurrent validity of the Functional Independence Measure for Children (WeeFIM™) and the Pediatric Evaluation of Disabilities Inventory in children with developmental disabilities and acquired brain injuries. *Phys Occup Ther Pediatr* 21: 91–101.
26. Newborg J (2005) *Battelle Developmental Inventory*, 2nd edition. Itasca, IL: Riverside Publishing Company.
27. Ottenbacher KJ, Taylor ET, Msall ME, et al (1996) The stability and equivalence reliability of the WeeFIM® instrument. *Dev Med Child Neurol* 38: 907–916.
28. Ottenbacher KJ, Msall ME, Lyons N, et al (2000) The WeeFIM instrument: its utility in detecting change in children with developmental disabilities. *Arch Phys Med Rehabil* 81: 1317–1326.

29. Aybay C, Erkin G, Elhan AH, Sirzai H, Ozel S (2007) ADL assessment of nondisabled Turkish children with the WeeFIM instrument. *Am J Phys Med Rehabil* 86: 176–182.

30. Jongjit J, Komsopapong L, Saikaew T, et al (2006) Reliability of the Functional Independence Measure for Children in normal Thai children. *Pediatr Int* 48: 132–137.

31. Tsuji T, Liu M, Toikawa H, Hanayama K, Sonoda S, Chino N (1999) ADL structure for nondisabled Japanese children based on the functional independence measure for children (WeeFIM™). *Am J Phys Med* 78: 208–212.

32. Wong V, Wong S, Chan K, Wong W (2002) Functional independence measure (WeeFIM) for Chinese children: Hong Kong cohort. *Pediatrics* 109: e-36.

33. Haley SM, Coster WJ, Ludlow LH, Haltiwanger JT, Andrellos PJ (1992) *Pediatric Evaluation of Disability Inventory (PEDI). Version 1.0: Development, Standardization and Administration Manual.* Boston, MA: New England Medical Center Hospitals Inc.

34. Ostensjo S, Bjorbaekmo W, Carlberg EB, Vollestad NK (2006) Assessment of everyday functioning in young children with disabilities: an ICF-based analysis of concepts and content of the Pediatric Evaluation of Disability Inventory (PEDI). *Disabil Rehabil* 28: 489–504.

35. Berg M, Jahnsen R, Froslie KF, Hussain A (2004) Reliability of the Pediatric Evaluation of Disability Inventory (PEDI). *Phys Occup Ther Pediatr* 24: 61–77.

36. Vos-Vromans, DC, Ketelaar M, Gorter JW (2005) Responsiveness of evaluative measures for children with cerebral palsy: the Gross Motor Function Measure and the Pediatric Evaluation of Disability Inventory. *Disabil Rehabil* 27: 1245–1252.

37. Iyer LV, Haley SM, Watkins MP, Dumas HM (2003) Establishing minimal clinically important differences for scores on the Pediatric Evaluation of Disability Inventory for inpatient rehabilitation. *Phys Ther* 83: 888–898.

38. Gannotti ME, Cruz C (2001) Content and construct validity of a Spanish translation of the Pediatric Evaluation of Disability Inventory for children living in Puerto Rico. *Phys Occup Ther Pediatr* 20: 7–24.

39. Wren TAL, Sheng, M, Bowen, RE, et al (2008) Concurrent and discriminant validity of Spanish language instruments for measuring functional health status. *J Pediatr Orthop* 28: 199–212.

40. Erkin G, Elhan AH, Aybay C, Sirzai H, Ozel S (2007) Validity and reliability of the Turkish translation of the Paediatric Evaluation of Disability Inventory (PEDI). *Disabil Rehabil* 29: 1271–1279.

41. Normark E, Orban K, Hagglund G, Jarnlo GB (1999) The American Pediatric Evaluation of Disability Inventory (PEDI). Applicability of PEDI in Sweden for children aged 2.0–6.9 years. *Scand J Rehabil Med* 31: 95–100.

42. Custers JW, van der Net J, Hoijtink H, Wassenberg-Severijnen JE, Vermeer A, Helders PJ (2002) Discriminative validity of the Dutch Pediatric Evaluation of Disability Inventory. *Arch Phys Med Rehabil* 83: 1437–1441.

43. Wassenberg-Severijnen JE, Custers JW, Hox JJ, Vermeer A, Helders PJ (2003) Reliability of the Dutch Pediatric Evaluation of Disability Inventory (PEDI). *Clin Rehabil* 17: 457–462.

44. Coster WJ, Haley SM, Ni P, Dumas HM, Fragala-Pinkham MA (2008) Assessing self-care and social function using a computer adaptive testing version of the pediatric evaluation of disability inventory. *Arch Phys Med Rehabil* 89: 622–629.

45. Mulcahey MJ, Haley SM, Duffy T, Pengsheng N, Betz RR (2008) Measuring physical functioning in children with spinal impairments with computerized adaptive testing. *J Pediatr Orthop* 28: 330–335.

46. Haley SM, Ni P, Ludlow LH, Fragala-Pinkham MA (2006) Measurement precision and efficiency of multidimensional computer adaptive testing of physical functioning using the Pediatric Evaluation of Disability Inventory. *Arch Phys Med Rehabil* 87: 1223–1229.

47. Haley SM, Fragala-Pinkham MA, Ni P (2006) Sensitivity of a computer adaptive assessment for measuring functional mobility changes in children enrolled in a community fitness programme. *Clin Rehabil* 20: 616–622.

48. Sparrow SS, Cicchetti DV, Balla DA (2005) *Vineland Adaptive Behavior Scales*, 2nd edition. Survey Forms Manual. Minneapolis, MN: NCS Pearson Inc.

49. Limperopoulos C, Majnemer A, Steinbach CL, Shevell MI (2006) Equivalence reliability of the Vineland Adaptive Behavior Scale between in-person and telephone administration. *Phys Occup Ther Pediatr* 26: 115–127.

50. Fougeyrollas P, Noreau L, Bergeron H, Cloutier R, Dion SA, St-Michel G (1998) Social consequences of long term impairments and disabilities: conceptual approach and assessment of handicap. *Int J Rehabil Res* 21: 127–141.

51. Levasseur M, Desrosiers J, Tribble D (2007) Comparing the Disability Creation Process and International Classification of Functioning, Disability and Health Models. *Can J Occup Ther* 74: 233–242.

52. Lepage C, Noreau L, Bernard PM (1998) Association between characteristics of locomotion and accomplishment of life habits in children with cerebral palsy. *Phys Ther* 78: 458–469.

53. Lepage C, Noreau L, Bernard PM, Fougeyrollas P (1998) Profile of handicap situations in children with cerebral palsy. *Scand J Rehabil Med* 30: 263–272.

54. Noreau L, Lepage C, Boissiere L, et al (2007) Measuring participation in children with disabilities using the Assessment of Life Habits. *Dev Med Child Neurol* 49: 666–671.

55. Fauconnier J, Dickinson HO, Beckung E, et al (2009) Participation in life situations of 8–12 year old children with cerebral palsy: cross sectional European study. *BMJ* 338: b1458.

56. Young NL, Williams JI, Yoshida KK, Bombardier C, Wright JG (1996) The context of measuring disability. Does it matter whether capability or performance is measured? *J Clin Epidemiol* 49: 1097–1101.

57. Law M, Finkelman S, Hurley P, et al (2004) Participation of children with physical disabilities: relationships with diagnosis, physical function, and demographic variables. *Scand J Occup Ther* 11: 156–162.

58. Morris C, Kurinczuk JJ, Fitzpatrick R, Rosenbaum P (2006) Do children's abilities explain their activities and participation? *Dev Med Child Neurol* 48: 954–961.

59. Palisano RJ, Copeland WP, Galuppi BE (2007) Performance of physical activities by adolescents with cerebral palsy. *Phys Ther* 87: 77–87.

60. Young NL, Williams JI, Yoshida KK, Wright JG (2000) Measurement properties of the Activities Scale for Kids. *J Clin Epidemiol* 53: 125–137.

61. Mackie PC, Jessen EC, Jarvis SN (1998) The Lifestyle Assessment Questionnaire: an instrument to measure the impact of disability on the lives of children with cerebral palsy and their families. *Child Care Health Dev* 24: 473–486.

62. Jessen EC, Colver AF, Mackie PC, Jarvis SN (2003) Development and validation of a tool to measure the impact of childhood disabilities on the lives of children and their families. *Child Care Health Dev* 29: 21–34.

20
LEARNING AND APPLYING KNOWLEDGE (D110–D179)

Kirsten M. Ellingsen, Andrea R. Burch and Andy V. Pham

What is the construct?

Learning is an essential activity for children. The ability to acquire new information from experience, practice or instruction and subsequently apply this knowledge enables children to develop increasing independence and successfully participate in expected social roles. One of the major roles for children in many societies is to be a student who performs successfully in a school environment. Progress from one level or grade to another depends on successful demonstration of academic skills and application of knowledge. Yet, learning difficulties have been proposed as the most common childhood disability or disorder.[1] Therefore, it is important to reliably identify children who demonstrate problems with learning academic material, starting with those who have significant difficulty learning how to read, write or calculate so that early instruction and intervention can promote future educational success.

Appropriately identifying and addressing learning problems is not a simple process. Learning is influenced by capabilities and functioning across developmental domains, as well as by individual experiences, instructional opportunities and environmental resources. Culture and language also play a significant role in learning and acquiring knowledge. Language is the primary resource that teachers have and use for mediating learning in schools. Culture and language shape a child's academic and social experiences by offering opportunities to learn new concepts and ways of understanding the world. Measuring learning problems appropriately requires an understanding that a child's ability to learn and engage as a student can be influenced by a range of factors, from neighbourhood events to neuropsychological functioning. Varying experiences and resources available in early childhood have been differentially related to children's preparedness for school entry at kindergarten and subsequent academic achievement in later grades.

In addition, children may be predisposed to problems with learning for different aetiological reasons, including perinatal injury, having a specific neurological or medical condition (e.g. lead poisoning, fetal alcohol syndrome, fragile X syndrome), or impairment in auditory processing, visual perception, attention, memory or language processing.[1] Thus, measuring learning outcomes necessitates a multidimensional and bio-ecological perspective so that the information gathered is sufficient and meaningful.

Assessment methods should take into account general health and functioning as well as environmental variables to understand where, how and why problems exist so that appropriate treatment and interventions can be designed and implemented. Specific information taught to children and expectations regarding how to demonstrate knowledge or skills may vary within different educational systems, curricula, cultures or political environments. Despite these differences, there has been international agreement about important skills and abilities for children, as evident in the global adoption of the World Health Organization's International Classification of Functioning, Disability and Health for Children and Youth (ICF-CY). The learning skills and behaviours outlined in the ICF-CY are represented under the 'Learning and applying knowledge' chapter in the activities and participation domain; select codes are shown in Table 20.1.

Using this framework, a comprehensive evaluation of learning difficulties would require measuring dimensions of functioning at the ICF-CY body, person and environment level. This perspective also facilitates identification of early modifiable predictors of problems. Specific learning disabilities or problems are often conceptualized, labelled, defined and assessed differently across countries; however, identified concerns in many countries typically involve lower performance in the academic areas of reading, writing and mathematics.[1]

TABLE 20.1
**Select International Classification of Functioning, Disability and Health for Children
and Youth Chapter 1 'Learning and applying knowledge' codes**

Purposeful sensory experiences (d110–d129)

d110	Watching
d115	Listening
d120	Other purposeful sensing

Basic learning (d130–d159)

d130	Copying
d131	Learning through actions with objects
d132	Acquiring information
d133	Acquiring language
d135	Rehearsing
d137	Acquiring concepts
d140	Learning to read
d145	Learning to write
d150	Learning to calculate
d155	Acquiring skills

Applying knowledge (d160–d179)

d160	Focusing attention
d163	Thinking
d166	Reading
d170	Writing
d172	Calculating
d175	Solving problems
d177	Making decisions

Because the ICF-CY is a globally endorsed, crosscultural classification system of child functioning, the focus of this chapter will be on measurement techniques and tools that align with select academic and pre-academic codes shown in Table 20.2.

A review of issues to consider when measuring learning outcomes is presented, followed by an overview of three general accepted methods that guide the assessment of academic problems and diagnosis of problems such as a specific learning disability. Specific instruments and curriculum-based measures used to assess dimensions of academic learning are described next and are accompanied by charts of the standardized measures that describe the instrument purpose, administration and psychometric properties, as well as ordering information. The measures and general practices outlined for assessing learning problems are primarily focused on those used in the USA; however, the areas assessed are linked to the ICF-CY at the end of the chapter.

LEARNING AS A PROCESS
The learning process and methods employed by children to acquire new knowledge change over the course of the first two decades of life. Various theories about the developmental process of learning have been hypothesized and tested over the past several decades. Jean Piaget's work remains highly influential in the present understanding of changes in the process of childhood learning and reasoning (for more information see *The Learning Theory of Piaget & Inhelder*[2] and *The Psychology of the Child*[3]). Piaget's research and theory provide a framework for expected behaviours during different ages or developmental stages. According to Piaget's theory, learning is subordinate to development, so acquiring knowledge from experience or instruction is dependent upon maturation and cognitive development.

The expected sequence of behaviours used by young children to learn about their social and physical worlds is a dynamic process observable in the sensory exploration of infants, purposeful communication of

TABLE 20.2
Measures of pre-academic and academic skills

Measures of school readiness/pre-academic skills

Bracken Basic Concept Scale, revised, or Bracken School Readiness Assessment, third edition (BSRA-3)

Kaufman Survey of Early Academic and Language Skills (K-SEALS)

Achievement tests

Woodcock–Johnson Tests of Achievement, third edition (WJ-III)

Wechsler Individual Achievement Test, third edition (WIAT-III)

Kaufman Test of Educational Achievement, second edition (KTEA-II)

Monitoring Basic Skills Progress (MBSP) (curriculum based)

Reading

Dynamic Indicators of Basic Early Literacy Skills (DIBELS)

Gray Oral Reading Test, fourth edition (GORT-4)

Test of Reading Comprehension, fourth edition (TORC-4)

Mathematics

KeyMaths Revised, Test of Early Mathematics Ability, third edition

Writing

The Oral and Written Language Scales (OWLS) or Test of Written Language, fourth edition (TOWL)

toddlers and imaginative play of preschoolers. Learning strategies employed by children are inextricably linked to the attainment of major cognitive, motor, language and socioemotional developmental milestones. Strategies employed to acquire information become increasingly purposeful, sophisticated and distal. Early sensory exploration and repeated social interactions provide a foundation for academic learning. Learning proceeds as children discover more about themselves and their environment from direct actions to symbolically representing objects in words and pictures. Learning strategies continue to change with the increased use of effective verbal and written communication during childhood and the ability to engage in abstract thinking during adolescence.

In many countries, demonstrating success as a learner involves progressing as a student through a formal education system, starting at around the age of 5 years and continuing until late adolescence. The outcomes of learning can be viewed broadly as passing academic classes or graduating to a new grade level. Efforts to identify problems in learning and find effective remediation techniques become essential when children fail to meet educational expectations. The ability to read, express ideas with written language and perform mathematics accurately facilitates the attainment of increasingly complex and specific academic knowledge. In the USA, the process to assess learning and qualify preschool or elementary children for

special education services typically follows one of three general approaches.

IDENTIFYING LEARNING PROBLEMS AND ESTABLISHING A DIAGNOSIS OF LEARNING DISABILITY

Identifying problems in learning academic material is an important topic in medical and educational settings. However, different classification systems are used to guide evaluations and establish when problems constitute a disability. According to research conducted by the National Institutes of Health, 20% of the US school-age population, or one in five US students, has a learning disability (www.ldworldwide.org/parents/parent-articles/357). However, there is no global consensus regarding how to conceptualize, define or identify a specific learning disability.[4] In the USA, students must meet specific eligibility criteria mandated by federal legislation to obtain special education support. According to the Individuals with Disabilities Education Act (IDEA) of 2004, children can qualify as having a specific learning disability if they express difficulties in one of the following areas: oral expression, listening comprehension, written expression, basic reading skill, reading fluency skills, reading comprehension, mathematics calculation and mathematics problem solving. The specific learning disability special education classification has been considered to be the 'most controversial' special education disability category in the USA, and is the only category with diagnostic criteria in federal legislation.[5] Learning difficulties must not be due to poor instruction or lack of experience. However, the criteria for 'quality' instruction and necessary early experiences remains unclear.[6] Excluding experience and instruction has been widely criticized as difficult to untangle diagnostically. Disagreement exists about the origin of learning difficulties and the role of experience, and experts debate classifying problems as information processing differences, neurological impairment or lack of relevant educational experiences, and exposure to early academic concepts (see reference 7 for a review of these issues).

Factors to consider when measuring this domain
Recent conceptualizations and proposed strategies to measure problems in learning or applying knowledge reflect a broader philosophical shift in viewing child disability as no longer existing exclusively within the child, but rather as a manifestation of ongoing dynamic interactions between a child and his or her environment. There are three common models used to identify learning problems: an aptitude-achievement discrepancy, intra-individual differences or lack of response to intervention (RTI). The types of measures selected under each model vary. A discrepancy model would require standardized measures of IQ and achievement tests in different academic domains; an intra-individual model involves cognitive or neuropsychological tests; a model that uses RTI would rely on curriculum-based measurement (CBM). Each model is described next.

THE TRADITIONAL DISCREPANCY MODEL
Traditionally, the presence or absence of a specific learning disability was determined by examining the degree of discrepancy between a child's overall cognitive abilities and academic skills as measured by standardized tests. This 'discrepancy model' has been the predominant model in the USA. Children determined to be achieving significantly below expectation qualified for specialized educational services to address the content areas indicated (e.g. reading, maths calculations, written expression). The discrepancy model has been referred to as the 'wait-to-fail' method because the testing is often insensitive to subtle developmental differences in cognitive abilities and academic skills, making early identification of specific learning disabilities unlikely. Other problems include inconsistency in application across schools, districts and states, overidentification of students from diverse backgrounds and little guidance on which 'IQ' score should be used for comparison with achievement scores.[8]

Individual diagnostic tests can assess a student's strengths and weaknesses so that educators can develop appropriate interventions in order to remediate weaknesses. Diagnostic tests can also be given to determine whether a student qualifies for educational services, with the student's performance compared with scores of other same-aged peers. However, individual diagnostic tests are not considered appropriate to evaluate the effectiveness of instruction or important gains made by individual students. Group survey tests are generally used to evaluate instructional effectiveness for large groups of students or classrooms. Disagreement regarding the usefulness of the traditional ability–achievement discrepancy model to inform intervention or measure individual gains resulted in a process-orientated RTI approach to determine eligibility for special education.

RESPONSE TO INTERVENTION AS A MEANS OF IDENTIFICATION OF SPECIFIC LEARNING DISABILITIES
RTI is a comprehensive tiered framework that integrates assessment and intervention. It requires the delivery of high-quality, differentiated instruction to all students. The reauthorization of the IDEA in 2004 states that response to 'scientific, research-based intervention' can be used as part of the process of determining whether a child has a specific learning disability (20 U.S.C. §1414 [b][6]).[9] RTI represents a major paradigm shift in viewing and approaching children with learning difficulties. RTI is a relatively new term, but it represents the culmination of many practices used in schools (e.g. individualized help for struggling students, problem-solving approaches, monitoring student progress).[10]

A key component of RTI is universal screening, a process by which all students are assessed for academic risk. Data are usually collected three or four times per year. The collected data are compared with a set of predetermined benchmarks. Based on data collected from a universal screening process, children are assigned to one of the intervention tiers according to their needs. Students who do not demonstrate benchmark-level performance are monitored on a regular basis in order to evaluate the effectiveness of subsequent instruction and intervention.[11] A unique characteristic of RTI as an assessment model is the manner in which norms are used to compare performance.[12]

Common principles of RTI models include the following: multiple tiers of increasingly intensive services, research-based interventions, high-quality instruction and ongoing monitoring.[13] Multiple tiers or levels of intervention are implemented, with the first for children who demonstrate appropriate progress through the regular education curriculum. Tiers two and three are more specialized and offer more intensive support. The secondary level often comprises students who are at risk for learning difficulties and participate in group-based supplementary instruction as a preventative measure.[13] The third tier is for students who require targeted intensive interventions. 'Evidence-based' interventions must be used (i.e. those with documented success at improvement in at least one experiment or quasi-experiment with a student or group of students). Evidence-based interventions can be located in journals or websites that provide analyses of the intervention effectiveness (www.rti4success.org/).[14]

Identifying and monitoring the progress of students who are at risk for learning difficulties is not sufficient. Instruction delivered to all students should be of high quality. Not only do individualized interventions require empirical evidence of their effectiveness, but instructional practices should also be backed by research. Examples of evidence-based instructional practices found to be effective with tier-one students include co-operative learning, inquiry learning and universal design for learning.[15] Although there is some evidence that all students can benefit from these instructional practices, students with support needs will probably require more structured and individualized support and accommodations (e.g. response prompting, use of objects and visuals for conceptual understanding, organizational strategies for retention of information, peer tutoring strategies, scaffolding, explicit skill modelling, organization and explicit practice).[16,17] The aim of implementing an empirically validated curriculum that is aligned with state standards across and within grade levels is to ensure that all students acquire the necessary skills and knowledge that they are expected to learn.

The RTI framework provides an alternative to the use of the traditional discrepancy model alone to diagnose learning disabilities. Although RTI has deep theoretical roots in applied behavioural analysis and ecological perspectives, it developed largely out of movements in the field of education and psychology towards problem-solving approaches, data-based decision-making, evidence-based practice and preventative measures. The problem-solving aspects of the RTI framework make it possible to evaluate and adjust instructional practices for students who are not making appropriate academic progress. Using assessment data, teachers can determine which students may be in need of differentiated learning activities in order to gain access to the instructional programme. Traditional standardized tests require comparison with a nationally representative normative group in order to judge a student's progress in one or several domains. RTI procedures involve the comparison of a specific child's performance to level of mastery and rate of learning of a local normative group (other students in the school or district). Therefore, students are expected to reach a series of goals at a rate commensurate to their peers. Under the RTI model, a child's progress can only be appropriately monitored if the child's functioning is assessed over time. CBMs are commonly used as screening tools and progress-monitoring instruments.

RTI AND SPECIFIC LEARNING DISABILITY IDENTIFICATION

Using RTI data to identify students with specific learning disabilities would require the use of a 'dual discrepancy' approach.[18] Students who exhibit a dual discrepancy demonstrate not only a severe educational need, but also a lack of response to research-based interventions implemented with fidelity. Practitioners warn against the use of 'failure to respond' alone because it has not been empirically validated at this time. The current research and support for RTI is largely focused on reading development in the elementary grades; support for methods used at the secondary level and across content areas is yet to be established.

INTEGRATED MODELS

An international comparison of specific learning disability classification and school-based practices in Australia, Belgium, the USA and Zimbabwe led to the development of an integrated and comprehensive method proposed to assess it.[1] Methods to identify specific learning disabilities examined similar academic constructs. For the comparison, specific learning disability was commonly defined as underachievement in one of the following areas: reading, maths, written expression or oral language. The proposed model includes the following steps: screening for a specific learning disability, assessing achievement, diagnosing nature of problem and monitoring intervention effects. Screening may include teacher-created, norm or criterion-referenced measures. The second step involves assessing achievement with norm-referenced tests in reading, maths, and written and oral language to identify children performing below peers or below their assumed academic aptitude. In the third stage, additional tests are recommended to examine individual intelligence, psychological processes such as memory and comorbid conditions (e.g. attention-deficit–hyperactivity disorder, depression). These measures should have high reliability and validity and be administered and interpreted by trained professionals. The authors also recommend monitoring the intended specific areas of skill development.

This proposed method is similar to the stepwise model advocated by school psychologists and specific learning disability experts in the USA. Specifically, a 'hybrid' model that incorporates RTI, norm-referenced measures, and assessment of contextual factors and potential other conditions has been proposed.[6] Essential to this approach is that specific learning disabilities are not determined based on a single assessment and the child must have had adequate instruction and opportunity to learn. Progress monitoring occurs by multiple administration of normed tests, or CBMs. Research also supports positive outcomes for students in reading, spelling and maths when teachers use CBM data to guide instruction.[6] Moreover, these integrative models align with the ICF-CY framework.

Overview of recommended measures

In the following section, the assessment of pre-academic, academic, reading, maths and written expression are described. The measures that are included are linked to specific ICF-CY codes as shown in Table 20.3. To address the different models of assessment used to measure learning problems, an overview of the construct is presented followed by standardized measures and then CBMs.

PRE-ACADEMIC FUNCTIONING/SCHOOL-READINESS ASSESSMENT

Children enter formal education systems with differences in background and early experiences that have been linked to education outcomes. In the USA, kindergarten children are expected to be able to learn to work independently, follow a daily time schedule and acquire basic literacy and maths skills.[19] Children who are not successful in meeting these expectations struggle academically and socially. The following five domains of development were identified by the National Education Goals Panel's Technical Planning Group on School Readiness as important to a child's preparation for school: physical well-being and motor development; social and emotional development; approaches to learning; language usage; and cognition and general knowledge identified.[20] (For a review of national data on early experience and school readiness see National Center for Education Statistics reports for the National Household Education Study [NHES], the Early Childhood Longitudinal Study birth cohort [ECLS-B] and ECLS kindergarten cohort [ECLS-K] at http://nces.ed.gov/pubsearch/).

Lower academic achievement has been associated with inequalities in knowledge and skills at the start of school.[21] High-quality childcare and early intervention services provided to children who were at risk for underachievement has significantly improved the educational success of children (e.g. Abcedarian study and Perry Preschool Program). Because early language and literacy were found to be connected to preparedness for school, these areas were initially emphasized. Less research has been conducted on early social and emotional

development and its prediction to later academic outcomes and school adjustment relative to early literacy and numeracy skills.[19] School readiness indicators have been defined as 'individual characteristics and observable behaviors that children show while taking part in learning activities' and includes persistence, emotion regulation, attentiveness, flexibility and organization.[22]

In a nationally representative longitudinal study (ECLS-K), teachers reported that being physically healthy, rested and well nourished, able to communicate and being enthusiastic and curious in approaching new activities were the most essential qualities for children to be ready for kindergarten.[19]

The mastery of the advanced and complex academic skills necessary for reading and mathematical competency is built on simple skills that start in early childhood. For reading, simple skills include becoming familiar with the conventions of print (e.g. reading from left to right and from top to bottom), recognizing letters by name, associating sounds with letters and understanding the meaning of spoken words and phrases, as cited by Zill and West.[20,23] For arithmetic, simple skills include rote counting, one-to-one correspondences, recognizing written numerals and understanding greater, lesser and equal relationships.[20] Executive functioning skills (e.g. planning, attending, self-control and emotion regulation) have also been correlated with academic outcomes.[21] Problems with spatial representation, visual reasoning, working memory and self-regulation in early childhood have been connected to discrepancies in mathematical competence in higher grades.[21]

Consequently, children are screened for school-readiness skills upon entry into kindergarten with standardized measures. Standardized measures of the presumed basic concepts and knowledge may be administered, with the same test given at the beginning and end of the academic year to determine progress. Additionally, these measures can be used in conjunction with cognitive measures for intervention recommendations or as part of an evaluation during special education eligibility decisions. The Bracken School Readiness Assessment, third edition (BSRA-3) and the Kaufman Survey of Early Academic and Language Skills (K-SEALS) are two popular standardized measures for academic readiness. Both are briefly described below. These are followed by a description of comprehensive academic achievement measures and then specific measures for reading, maths and written expression.

Bracken School Readiness Assessment, third edition
The BSRA-3 is an individually administered measure of a child's exposure to concepts necessary for learning at

TABLE 20.3

International Classification of Functioning, Disability and Health codes under pre-academic and early academic domains

Activities and participation: ICF-CY learning codes

School readiness/pre-academic skills

d132	Acquiring information
d137	Acquiring concepts
d140	Learning to read
d145	Learning to write
d150	Learning to calculate

Activities and participation: applying knowledge codes

Academic Achievement

d160	Reading
d1660	Using general skills and strategies of the reading process
d1661	Comprehending written language
d172	Calculating
d1720	Using simple skills and strategies of the calculation process
d1721	Using complex skills and strategies of the calculation process
d170	Writing
d1700	Using general skills and strategies of the writing process
d1701	Using grammatical and mechanical conventions in written compositions

school. The BSRA-3 is a standardized instrument that evaluates the child's knowledge of concepts of colours, letters, numbers/counting, sizes, comparisons and shapes for children between the ages of 3 years and 6 years 11 months. These academic markers are foundational terms and concepts that have traditionally been considered as important to know before participation in formal education.

Kaufman Survey of Early Academic and Language Skills

The K-SEALS is described by the authors as a measure of language, pre-articulation and articulation skills of young children. It is individually administered to children between the ages of 3 years and 6 years 11 months. The K-SEALS is marketed as a brief measure that consists of the following three separate subtests: vocabulary subtest, numbers, letters and words subtest and articulation survey.

GENERAL ACADEMIC ACHIEVEMENT MEASURES

Diagnostic achievement tests are the most frequently used tests in educational settings. These tests evaluate knowledge and understanding in several curricular areas, such as reading or maths. Most achievement tests are norm-referenced, although some are criterion-referenced or performance measures. Individually administered tests allow examiners the opportunity to observe students working

and solving problems so they can note valuable qualitative information in addition to the qualitative information that the scores provide. Below are some of the most commonly used academic achievement measures used in educational settings.

The Woodcock–Johnson, Normative Update, Tests of Achievement, third edition

The Woodcock–Johnson, Normative Update, Tests of Achievement, third edition (WJ-III-Ach) is an individually administered test of achievement designed to assess various academic skills (e.g. reading, maths and written expression) in children, adolescents and adults. It allows the examiner to administer a single subtest or any combination of subtests to assess achievement in one or more domains. These tests are often used in conjunction with the WJ-III Tests of Cognitive Abilities to assess an individual's abilities on many specific cognitive clusters. The norms for the cognitive and achievement tests are based on data from the same sample of individuals, which allows direct comparisons among and within an individual's scores that have a degree of accuracy that is not possible when comparing scores from separately normed tests. In addition to providing ability–achievement discrepancies, examiners can evaluate domain-specific achievement skills and the cognitive abilities related to those skills.[24]

KAUFMAN SURVEY OF EARLY ACADEMIC AND LANGUAGE SKILLS (K-SEALS)	
Purpose	A brief measure designed to evaluate pre-academic concept development, language, pre-articulation and articulation skills
Population	Ages 3y 0mo to 6y 11mo
Description of domains (subscales)	The K-SEALS is a brief measure of children's receptive and expressive language, pre-academic skills (i.e. number skills, letter skills, word skills) and articulation skills
Administration and test format	Time to complete: 15–25min to administer
	Testing format: 100 items in five categories, individually administered direct assessment. The test uses a flip-easel format for ease of administration. Colourful pictures are used to engage young children
	Scoring: yields a survey, early academic and language skills composite score, as well as language scales (expressive skills and receptive skills), early academic scales, number skills, letter skills and word skills. Standard scores with a mean of 100 (standard deviation=15), centiles, descriptive categories and age equivalents. Articulation survey subtest can be interpreted using descriptive categories or item error analysis procedures
Psychometric properties	Normative sample: 1000 children representative of the US population by age, sex, race/ethnicity, geographic region and parent education level. Many of the individuals did not attend preschool or school programmes
	Reliability
	Test–retest stability was found to be good to excellent for subtests, scales and composite scores (0.88–0.94). Internal consistency for scales, subtests and composites was also strong, ranging from 0.81 to 0.94
	Validity
	The K-SEALS composite scores correlate with the Kaufman Assessment Battery for Children and Stanford–Binet, at approximately 0.80. The K-SEALS composite score also correlates moderately with teacher ratings of ability, approximately $r=0.60$
How to order	Online: www.pearsonassessment.com; email: Clinicalcustomersupport@Pearson.com
	International orders: www.pearsonassessments.com/pai/ca/IO/international.htm
Key references	Ackerman PL (1995) [Review of the Kaufman Survey of Early Academic & Language Skills]. In: Conoley JC, Impara JC, editors. *The Twelfth Mental Measurements Yearbook*. Lincoln, NE: Buros Institute of Mental Measurements.
	Ford L (1995) [Review of the Kaufman Survey of Early Academic & Language Skills]. In: Conoley JC, Impara JC, editors. *The Twelfth Mental Measurements Yearbook*. Lincoln, NE: Buros Institute of Mental Measurements.
	Kaufman Survey of Early Academic and Language Skills (1995) *The Twelfth Mental Measurements Yearbook*. Available from: http://buros.unl.edu/buros/

Kaufman Test of Educational Achievement, second edition

The Kaufman Test of Educational Achievement, second edition (KTEA-II) is an individually administered measure of academic achievement for ages 4 years 6 months to 25 years. The test is available in two versions: the brief form, which assesses achievement in reading, maths and written expression; and the comprehensive form, which includes a wider range of achievement domains and provides an error analysis. It was developed from a clinical model of assessment in order to provide more than a profile of norm-referenced scores. Curriculum experts helped to define the specific skills measured by each subtest and the different types of errors students are likely to make on each subtest, which can prove useful for developing instructional interventions.[25]

WOODCOCK JOHNSON TESTS OF ACHIEVEMENT, THIRD EDITION (NORMATIVE UPDATE) (WJ-III-ACH [NU])

Purpose	To document and assess academic skills in children and adolescents. To help determine needs for special support services for specific academic domains and examine existence/ severity of a specific learning disability when used in a comprehensive student evaluation. Information can also be used to determine areas of academic skill strengths and weaknesses or reveal deficits in areas of knowledge
Population	Ages 2–90+y
Description of domains (subscales)	The WJ-III-Ach has 22 tests measuring five academic areas (reading, mathematics, written language, oral language and academic knowledge) that are typical of curricular areas emphasized in the school setting. There are two forms, A and B, and two batteries – standard (12 subtests) and extended (10 additional subtests); one or both can be administered. Several cluster scores and individual subtest scores can be obtained, including oral expression, listening comprehension, written expression, basic reading skills, reading comprehension, reading fluency, maths calculation skills, maths reasoning
Administration and test format	Time to complete: time to administer varies depending on the number of subtests given. Approximately 5min per subtest.
	Testing format: direct assessment with children individually administered
	Scoring: scores are age- and grade-based standard scores (mean=100; standard deviation=15), centile ranks, norm curve equivalence (for title 1) stanines, age and grade equivalents. Hand scoring and computer scoring are available. Specific scoring criteria set for each test in the examiner's manual.
	Training: graduate-level training in educational assessment and a background in diagnostic decision-making are recommended. Knowledge of exact scoring and administration procedures as delineated in the examiner's manual
Psychometric properties	Normative sample: the WJ-III-Ach was normed to represent the US population from ages 24mo to 90+y in a sample of 8818 individuals from 100 geographically diverse communities
	Reliability
	Most of the WJ-III-Ach subtests show strong reliabilities of 0.80 or higher; several are 0.90 or higher. The WJ-III-NU interpretive plan is based on cluster interpretation, which shows strong reliabilities, most at 0.90 or higher
	Validity
	The WJ-III-Ach's two batteries were conormed, which means that the normative data are based on a single sample. Normative data from the USA were obtained by stratified sampling of 8818 individuals selected to represent the general population
	Responsiveness
	Two parallel forms to monitor individuals' progress over time
How to order	Online: www.riverpub.com/products/wjIIIAchievement/pricing.html
	US orders: email RPC_Customer_Service@hmhpub.com; Canadian orders: email inquire@nelson.com; international orders: email rpinternational@hmhpub.com
Key references	Ford L, Swart S, Negreiros J, Lacroix S, McGrew KS (2010) *Use of the Woodcock– Johnson III NU Tests of Cognitive Abilities and Tests of Achievement with Canadian Populations (Woodcock- Johnson III Assessment Service Bulletin No. 12)*. Rolling Meadows, IL: Riverside Publishing.
	Fletcher J, Lyon GR, Fuchs LS, Barnes MA (2007) *Learning Disabilities From Identification to Intervention*. New York: The Guilford Press.
	McGrew KS, Woodcock RW (2001) *Woodcock–Johnson III: Technical Manual*. Itasca, IL: Riverside Publishing.

Mather N, Jaffe L (2001) *Woodcock–Johnson III Reports, Recommendations, and Strategies*. New York: John Wiley and Sons.

Woodcock RW, Schrank FA, Miller DC, Wendling BJ (2001) *Essentials of WJ-III Cognitive Abilities Assessment*. New York: John Wiley and Sons.

Woodcock RW, Mather N, Wendling B (2001) *Essentials of WJ-III Tests of Achievement Assessment. Volume 7 of Essentials of Psychological Assessment Series 'Assessment Made Simple' (S145)*. New York: Wiley.

KAUFMAN TEST OF EDUCATIONAL ACHIEVEMENT, SECOND EDITION (KTEA-II)

Purpose	Academic achievement test that provides composite scores for first grade and older students in reading, maths, written language and oral language. Also yields a comprehensive achievement composite
Population	Ages 4y 6mo–25y for the comprehensive form. Ages 4y 6mo–90+y for the brief form
Description of domains (subscales)	The KTEA-II comprehensive subtests and composites include reading composite (letter and word recognition, reading comprehension) reading-related subtests (phonological awareness, nonsense word decoding, word recognition fluency, decoding fluency, associated fluency, naming facility); maths composite (maths concepts and applications, maths computation); written language composite (written expression, spelling); oral language composite (listening comprehension, oral expression); comprehensive achievement composite
	The KTEA-II brief form includes three subtests: reading (word recognition and reading comprehension), maths (computation and application problems) and written expression (written language and spelling)
Administration and test format	Time to complete: administration prekindergarten=30min, grades 1–2=50min, grades 3+=80min; the brief form for ages 4y 6mo–90y=15–45min
	Testing format: 18 items; interview with primary caregiver
	Scoring: age- and grade-based standard scores (mean=100, standard deviation=15), age and grade equivalents, centile ranks, normal curve equivalents and stanines
	Training: training videos are available to order (www.pearsonassessments.com)
Psychometric properties	A nationally representative age-normed sample of 3000 individuals and a nationally represented grade-norm sample of 2400 students in grades K through 12 were tested across 39 states and the District of Columbia
	Reliability
	Inter-rater reliabilities are all very high (0.90s), except for associational fluency and oral expression. Internal consistency reliabilities are all within the upper 0.90s for every composite except oral and language, and oral fluency, which are within the mid to upper 0.80s
	Validity
	Subtests within most achievement domains correlate highly, between 0.46 and 0.80. Correlations with the WJ-III-Ach were >0.80, except for oral language composite and listening comprehension
	Responsiveness
	Two parallel forms to monitor the individual's progress over time
How to order	Online: www.pearsonassessment.com; e-mail: ClincalCustomerSupport@Pearson.com
	International orders: www.pearsonassessments.com/pai/ca/IO/International.htm
Key reference	Kaufman AS, Kaufman NL (2004) *Kaufman Test of Educational Achievement*, 2nd edition. Circle Pines, MN: AGS Publishing.

Wechsler Individual Achievement Test, third edition

The Wechsler Individual Achievement Test, third edition (WIAT-III) is an individually administered diagnostic achievement test designed for students in grades prekindergarten through 12, or ages 4 years 0 months through 19 years 11 months, with adult norms from ages 20 to 50 years. The WIAT-III is a revision of the WIAT-II, and includes 16 subtests designed to measure listening, speaking, reading, writing and maths skills.[26] The WIAT-III was standardized on a national sample of 2775 students and features comprehensive normative information.

ASSESSMENT OF READING

Reading proficiency requires decoding, word recognition, vocabulary, reading fluency and comprehension.[27] Many research studies looking at reading development have

WECHSLER INDIVIDUAL ACHIEVEMENT TEST, THIRD EDITION (WIAT-III)	
Purpose	To measure the academic strengths and weaknesses of an individual child, inform decisions regarding special support services eligibility and diagnosis of a learning disability and provide information about skills in specific academic areas, for instruction or intervention. This measure of academic achievement can be used in clinical, educational and research settings
Population	Ages 4y–19y 11mo (adult norms for ages 20–50y have been available since mid-2010)
Description of domains (subscales)	There are 16 subtests to measure the eight areas of achievement specified by US federal legislation to identify and classify specific learning disabilities
	Subtests: listening comprehension, oral expression, early reading skills, word reading, pseudoword decoding, reading comprehension, oral reading fluency, alphabet writing fluency, spelling, sentence composition, essay composition, maths problem solving, numerical operations, maths fluency – addition, maths fluency – subtraction, maths fluency – multiplication
	Composites: oral language total reading basic reading, reading comprehension and fluency, written expression, mathematics, maths fluency, total achievement
Administration and test format	Time to complete: varies by grade and number of subtests administered
	Testing format: direct assessment with individual child
	Training: knowledge of exact scoring and administration procedures as delineated in the examiner's manual
	Scoring: Scoring Assistant software or hand scoring, criteria set for each test; scores are age- and grade-based standard scores (mean=100; standard deviation=15), centile ranks, normal curve equivalents, stanines, age and grade equivalents
Psychometric properties	Normative sample: nationally standardized in the USA on 2775 students
	Reliability
	Internal consistency reliabilities are over 0.80, except for listening comprehension and sentence completion (0.75 and 0.79, respectively)
	Validity
	Intercorrelations range from 0.46 to 0.93 among the oral language, total reading, basic reading, reading comprehension and fluency, written expression, mathematics and maths fluency composites. Stronger correlations among reading composites, and weaker correlations between the maths fluency composite and other composites
How to order	Online: www.pearsonassessment.com; email: ClinicalCustomerSupport@Pearson.com
	International orders: www.pearsonassessments.com/pai/ca/IO/International.htm
Key references	Fletcher J, Lyon GR, Fuchs LS, Barnes MA (2007) *Learning Disabilities From Identification to Intervention*. New York: The Guilford Press.
	Lichtenberger EO, Breaux KC (2010) *Essentials of WIAT-III and KTEA-II Assessment*. New York: John Wiley & Sons Inc.

suggested that children at various developmental stages use different reading components and processes to meet their reading goals.[28] For example, beginner readers who are learning how to read use basic skills and strategies to recognize or decode words correctly. Advanced readers, on the other hand, are reading to learn by comprehending and accumulating knowledge from the text. Their basic literacy skills are fully developed and becoming automatic; thus, children are reading more fluently and spending more of their cognitive resources for reading comprehension.

Decoding or word analysis skills are those used to derive the pronunciation of a word through phonetic and structural analysis or contextual cues. Phonetic analysis allows the reader to use letter–sound correspondence and blending to identify words. Structural analysis, on the other hand, allows the reader to segment the word into meaningful parts. Because lack of decoding skills may be an indication of reading difficulties, basic reading assessments can be used to analyse decoding skills, including letter–sound identification, blending phonemes or sound-deletion tasks (elision tasks). One commonly used decoding assessment is to provide a child a list of nonsense words or unfamiliar words and then ask the child to read them aloud. The child must use decoding strategies to ascertain what the words are and how they can be pronounced.

Tasks which assess word recognition skills allow the examiner to determine the child's identification and accuracy of 'sight words'. If the student reads and is exposed to a word repeatedly and becomes more familiar with it, then eventually he or she may be able to recognize the word automatically without having to decode it. Thus, a child who attains proficient sight word recognition does not necessarily utilize their decoding skills. Word recognition tasks are principal measures on diagnostic reading assessments. The examiner provides the child with a list of familiar sight words, either in isolation or in context, to determine whether the child is able to identify them.

Reading fluency broadly refers to the ability to read words in connected text effortlessly, accurately and with prosody. Therefore, when assessing oral reading fluency, two variables are measured: reading rate and reading accuracy. Both rate and accuracy are equally important indicators, because fluency as an index of speed without accuracy may not provide an accurate profile of the child's reading. For example, a child who reads 80 words per minute with 20 errors is a different reader from another child who reads 80 words in the same passage for 5 minutes without any errors. Fluent readers can maintain reading performance for long periods of time and can generalize across texts. Oral reading fluency is commonly assessed

by allowing the child to read several paragraphs aloud as the examiner notes reading errors and behaviours. Silent reading fluency can also be evaluated, but it may be harder to observe reading errors if they are not heard aloud.

In addition, specific conditions in early childhood should warrant closer monitoring for learning difficulties when children reach school age. A preschool diagnosis of language impairment has been determined to be a risk factor for later reading difficulty as well as written expression disorders.[27] Reading comprehension is considered the ultimate goal of reading. Reading comprehension broadly refers to the process of extracting and constructing meaning through the reciprocal interaction of ideas between the reader and the message of a particular text. Within this reader–text dyad, the reader possesses the basic skills in phonemic awareness, accuracy and fluency and vocabulary, as well as prior knowledge and inference-making abilities. The text provides the discourse, genre and print or linguistic structure, which the reader must readily interpret. When many factors are not matched with the reader's skills, previous knowledge and learning experiences, the text becomes too difficult for optimal comprehension to occur. Therefore, reading comprehension requires active and deliberate cognitive processes that readers must engage in while they interact with the text.

One informal method of assessing reading comprehension is to give readers access to material and have them retell or paraphrase what they have just read.[29] Retold passages may be scored on the basis of the number of words or phrases recalled. Retelling may be conducted in an oral or written format. Another method of assessing reading comprehension is to ask students questions about what they have just read. Questions can address main ideas, important relationships, specific characters, conflicts/events and other relevant details. Often, answers to questions are open ended in order to assess their recall of details; however, if a child has difficulty responding to a question, an alternative method is to provide multiple choices to determine whether the child recognizes the correct answer.

Below are two standardized measures of reading that are commonly used to assess reading fluency and comprehension: the Gray Oral Reading Test, fourth edition (GORT-4) and the Test of Reading Comprehension, fourth edition (TORC-4).

Gray Oral Reading Test, fourth edition
The GORT-4 is an individually administered norm-referenced measure of oral reading fluency, accuracy and comprehension that is used to assess individuals from 6 to 18 years of age. Individuals are required to read paragraphs of increasing complexity orally and respond

GRAY ORAL READING TEST, FOURTH EDITION (GORT-4)

Purpose	The GORT-4 provides an efficient and objective measure of growth in oral reading fluency and comprehension and aids in the diagnosis of oral reading difficulties
Population	Ages 6y–18y 11mo
Description of domains (subscales)	Five scores are reported on a student's oral reading skills in terms of: Rate – the amount of time in seconds to read a passage Accuracy – the number of deviations from print made in the passage Fluency – the student's rate and accuracy scores combined Comprehension – the number of questions answered correctly from each passage Overall reading ability – the fluency (i.e. rate and accuracy) and comprehension scores combined
Administration and test format	Time to complete: 20–30min to administer Testing format: direct child assessment, individually administered Scoring: age- and grade-based standard scores (mean=100, standard deviation [SD]=15), grade and age equivalents. (Subtests yield scale scores mean=10, SD=3 and grade and age equivalents)
Psychometric properties	Normative sample: 1600 students *Reliability* Internal consistency reliabilities are 0.90 or above. Test–retest reliability ranges from 0.78 to 0.95, suggesting moderate to excellent reliability *Validity* Criterion prediction validity with other measures of reading ranged from 0.45 to 0.74. Inter-correlations between subtests ranged from 0.39 to 0.85 *Responsiveness* Two parallel forms to monitor the individual's progress over time
How to order	Online: www.pearsonassessment.com; e-mail: ClinicalCustomerSupport@Pearson.com International orders: www.pearsonassessments.com/pai/ca/IO/International.htm
Key reference	Wiederholt JL, Bryant BR (2001) *Gray Oral Reading Test*, 4th edition. Austin, TX: Pro-Ed.

to five comprehension multiple-choice questions for each passage. Multiple scores are derived from the child's reading (rate, accuracy and rate plus accuracy) and a single score is derived for comprehension. A composite score can be calculated, which is derived from the fluency and comprehension scores.

Dynamic Indicators of Basic Early Literacy Skills

The Dynamic Indicators of Early Literacy Skills (DIBELS; http://dibels.org/dibels.html) are a specific type of curriculum-based measure (CBM) designed to assess the acquisition of early literacy skills in kindergarten through to sixth grade. Like most CBMs, DIBELS are quick and efficient indicators of a child's acquisition of early literacy skill; each measure can be administered in one minute. Specifically, DIBELS are composed of seven measures designed to assess the five essential skill areas in reading as identified by the national reading panel (i.e. phonemic awareness; alphabetic principle; accuracy and fluency; vocabulary; and comprehension). DIBELS benchmark measures can be used to identify students who may be at risk for reading difficulties. DIBELS progress monitoring probes allow for the monitoring of students who receive interventional or additional instructional support to ensure that they are making adequate progress.

Test of Reading Comprehension, fourth edition

The TORC-4 is a multidimensional measure of silent reading comprehension given to students from grades 2 to 12 (ages 7–18y). The TORC-4 is used to identify students who need to improve reading proficiency. It is also useful in documenting the effectiveness of remedial efforts in reading comprehension.

DYNAMIC INDICATORS OF BASIC EARLY LITERACY SKILLS (DIBELS)	
Purpose	Designed to measure the acquisition and mastery of early reading skills in elementary school children. Measures are brief and easily administered; materials are available for collecting benchmark data and for monitoring individual student progress
Population	Kindergarten to sixth grade
Description of domains (subscales)	DIBELS were designed to measure the five big ideas of early literacy, developed by the national reading panel: phonological awareness, alphabetic principle, fluency with connected text, vocabulary and comprehension
	Measures of phonological awareness: Initial Sounds Fluency– assesses a child's skill at identifying and producing the initial sound of a given word; Phonemic Segmentation Fluency – assesses a child's skill at producing the individual sounds within a given word
	Measure of alphabetic principle and phonics: Nonsense Word Fluency – assesses a child's knowledge of letter–sound correspondences as well as his or her ability to blend letters together to form unfamiliar 'nonsense' (e.g. ut, fik, lig, etc.) words; Oral Reading Fluency – if accuracy is <95%
	Measure of accuracy and fluency with connected text: Oral Reading Fluency – assesses a child's skill at reading connected text in grade-level materials.
	Measure of comprehension: Oral Reading Fluency and Retell Fluency – assesses a child's understanding of verbally read connected text
	Measure of vocabulary and oral language: Word Use Fluency – assesses a child's ability to accurately use a provided word in the context of a sentence
Administration and test format	Administration and scoring procedures are available for download along with the test materials. Measures are designed to be administered as one minute probes
Psychometric properties	See www.dibels.org/papers/DIBELSNextTechAdequacySupplement.pdf
How to order	Many materials are free and available for download at https://dibels.uoregon.edu/dibels Subscription to the DIBELS data system is also available for purchase
Key reference	Puranik CS, Petscher Y, Otaiba SI, Catts HW, Lonigahn CJ (2008) Development of oral reading fluency in children with speech or language impairments a growth curve analysis. *J Learning Dis* 41: 545–560.

CURRICULUM-BASED MEASURES

Another approach to measuring learning is the use of CBMs. CBMs are a fast and effective means of assessment and progress monitoring within the RTI framework. CBMs were developed by Stanley Deno and colleagues in the late 1970s and early 1980s. They are derived directly from the classroom curriculum. A favourable alternative to traditional standardized assessments, the outcomes assessed by CBMs are more directly related to what the student is required to learn in the classroom.[12] CBMs directly measure academic skills using elements of the curriculum. These skills include reading fluency (speed and accuracy), reading comprehension, spelling, written expression (mechanics and grammar), maths problem solving, maths computation and maths fluency. CBMs gained recognition in the literature of the early 1980s,

and have since been widely accepted as useful progress-monitoring tools and means for assessment of instructional level. More recently, CBMs have been employed for screening and eligibility determination.[30] There is also emerging evidence that reading and maths CBM data correlate moderately and positively with state-wide achievement tests and other widely used norm-referenced achievement tests.[31]

ASSESSMENT OF MATHEMATICS

Like reading, diagnostic testing in mathematics is used to identify strengths and weaknesses within the subject area. It is intended to provide detailed information to determine eligibility and placement decisions, or to develop interventions for remediation. There are relatively fewer maths assessments than reading assessments, but maths skills

TEST OF READING COMPREHENSION, FOURTH EDITION (TORC-4)	
Purpose	Assesses silent reading comprehension that can be used to (1) identify children and adolescents who score significantly below their peers and who therefore might need help in improving their reading proficiency and comprehension, (2) document student progress in remedial programmes and (3) serve as a research tool in studies investigating reading problems in children and adolescents. Studies in the TORC-4 manual indicate that the test has high reliability and strong validity, especially criterion prediction validity
Population	Ages 7y–17y 11mo (grades 2–12)
Description of domains (subscales)	The test has five subtests, all of which measure word identification and contextual meaning: Relational vocabulary Sentence completion Paragraph construction Text comprehension Contextual fluency
Administration and test format	Time to complete: 45min Testing format: direct child assessment, individually administered Scoring: age- and grade-based standard scores (mean=100, standard deviation [SD]=15), grade and age equivalents. Subtests yield scale scores mean=10, SD=3 and grade and age equivalents
Psychometric properties	Normative sample: 1942 students *Reliability* Internal consistency reliabilities are ≥0.90 *Validity* Studies cited in the examiner's manual indicate strong validity, including criterion prediction validity
How to order	Online: www.pearsonassessment.com; e-mail: ClinicalCustomerSupport@Pearson.com International orders: www.pearsonassessments.com/pai/ca/IO/International.htm
Key reference	Brown VL, Hammill DD, Wiederholt JL (2008) *Test of Reading Comprehension*, 4th edition. Austin, TX: Pro-Ed.

are generally more straightforward to assess than reading skills. Specifically, mathematical operations often depend on successful performance in another (e.g. multiplication often depends on addition), and therefore it is easier to sequence the skill development and assessment of maths than reading. Maths assessments typically sample various skills such as maths concepts and operations, as well as applications and reasoning.

The academic subject of mathematics requires at least four different domain-specific components of knowledge and skills, including conceptual knowledge, procedural knowledge and skills, fictional knowledge and problem-solving skills. Children who have demonstrated difficulty with learning maths have also been found to have weaknesses related to basic cognitive functions such as working

memory, verbal and visuospatial short-term memory, processing speed and inhibitory control.[32]

KeyMath-3 Diagnostic Assessment
One standardized measure of maths is the KeyMath-3 Diagnostic Assessment, which is a comprehensive norm-referenced measure of essential mathematical concepts and skills. It can be used with individuals aged between 4 years 6 months and 21 years. Items are grouped into 10 subtests that represent three general maths content areas: basic concepts (conceptual knowledge), operations (computation skills) and applications (problem solving). The content covers the full spectrum of maths concepts and skills, ranging from early experiences with rote and rational counting through experiences with algebraic and linear equations.

KEYMATH-3 DIAGNOSTIC ASSESSMENT (KEYMATH-3-DA)	
Purpose	To assess and provide information to improve maths skills of students. This measure is designed to evaluate the student's understanding and application of essential maths concepts and skills (e.g. counting through algebra)
Population	4y 6mo–21y 11mo (grades K–12)
Description of domains (subscales)	Three areas, 10 subtests: basic concepts (numeration, algebra, geometry, measurement, and data analysis and probability); operations (mental computation and estimation, written computation: addition and subtraction, written computation: multiplication and division); and applications (foundations of problem solving, applied problem solving)
Administration and test format	Time to complete: 30–90min to administer Testing format: direct child assessment, individually administered Scoring: computer scoring software is available (KeyMaths-3-DA ASSIST). Age- and grade-based standard scores (mean=100; standard deviation [SD]=15), grade and age equivalents, and growth scale values. Subtests yield scale scores mean=10, SD=3, and grade and age equivalents Training: comprehensive system includes new KeyMaths-3 essential resources instructional program. Web seminars are also available
Psychometric properties	Normative sample: 3630 participants representative of US population by sex, race, socioeconomic status, region and disability groups *Reliability* Most of the internal consistency reliabilities are in the upper 0.80s or 0.90s. Test–retest reliability is 0.86 for younger examiners and 0.88 for older examiners. All area score reliabilities are in the mid-0.90s *Validity* All three area scores generally correlate in the 0.80s with one another, and their correlations with the total test scores generally surpass 0.90. Correlations with the KeyMath-R/NU subtests lie within the range of 0.50 and 0.75. Correlations between the total test scores for the two editions are 0.91 for kindergarten through Grade 5, and 0.91 for Grades 6 through 12 *Responsiveness* Two parallel forms to monitor the individual's progress over time
How to order	Online: www.pearsonassessment.com; e-mail: ClinicalCustomerSupport@Pearson.com International orders: www.pearsonassessments.com/pai/ca/IO/International.htm
Key reference	Connolly AJ (2007) *Key Maths 3*. Upper Saddle River, NJ: Pearson Assessment

Curriculum-based maths measures

In the area of mathematics, CBMs typically assess computation skills or concept development and application of mathematical problem-solving skills. CBMs for computation skills can be organized in sets of single-skill measures (e.g. only single-digit addition) or mixed-skill measures (e.g. single-digit addition, double-digit addition and double-digit addition with regrouping). Commonly used scoring procedures for computation CBMs involve counting the number of digits correct in the final answer of each problem and using the total number of digits correct in the given time period to represent the student's performance on the probe.

Curriculum-based measures of maths concepts and applications are designed to assess the mastery of particular concepts and application of mathematical skills for a particular grade level. These can include, but are not limited to, counting, number concepts, number naming, understanding charts and graphs, using money, understanding fractions and solving word problems. Students typically receive points for each part of the problem answered correctly and the total number of points is

MONITORING BASIC SKILLS PROGRESS (MBSP)	
Purpose	To measure a student's progress in computational skills and application of mathematical concepts and problem-solving skills over the course of a school year
Population	Basic Maths Computation: grades 1–6 Basic maths concepts and applications: grades 2–6
Description of domains (subscales)	Basic maths computation: addition, subtraction, multiplication and division of whole numbers, fractions and decimals Basic maths concepts and application: number concepts, names of numbers and vocabulary, measurement, charts and graphs, grid reading, areas and perimeters, fractions, decimals and word problems
Administration and test format	Brief probes are administered for the specified time period according to grade level Time limit for computation tests: 2–6min, depending on grade level Time limit for concepts and application tests: 6–8min, depending on grade level Standard administration instructions are available in the manual
Psychometric properties	Basic maths computation: test–retest reliability for computation measures ranges from 0.73 (moderate) to 0.92 (excellent). Content validity was judged as adequate and criterion validity established through correlation with other curriculum-based measures and standardized assessments Basic maths concepts and application: reliability and validity for these data are adequate with reliability (internal consistency) >0.90
How to order	Online: www.proedinc.com; e-mail: info@proedinc.com
Key reference	Fuchs FS, Fuchs D, Hamlett CL, et al (1994) Technical features of a mathematical concepts and application curriculum based measurement system. *Diagnostic* 19: 23–49.

recorded as a measure of the student's progress. Maths CBMs are typically administered for longer than 1 minute, and the length of time for administration can differ depending upon the complexity of the problems. Shapiro[12] suggests 3 minutes for probes involving addition and subtraction and 5 minutes for those measuring multiplication and division skills. There are several computerized and web-based programs that can generate maths probes:

- Mathematics Worksheet Factory by School House Technologies: www.schoolhousetech.com
- Aplus Math: www.aplusmath.com
- Maths Worksheet Generator: http://interventioncentral.org

The Monitoring Basic Skills Progress
The Monitoring Basic Skills Progress (MBSP) was created in order to allow teachers to monitor student's progress in mathematics over the course of a school year using commercially prepared CBMs. The MBSP includes two programmes: basic maths computation (addition, subtraction, multiplication and division of whole numbers, fractions and decimals) and basic maths concepts and applications (number concepts, names of numbers and vocabulary, measurement, charts and graphs, grid reading, areas and perimeters, fractions, decimals and word problems). There are 30 tests in every skill domain for each grade level. Each test is designed with the same level of difficulty; a higher score on subsequent sets would reflect improvement in the student's ability to solve the maths problems at that grade level in the curriculum. Directions for administering and scoring the tests are available in the manual; answer keys are located in the appendix. Blackline master copies of the tests are provided in separate books.

Consistent with the CBM model of assessment, standard scores are not available. Maths computation tests can be scored in terms of the number of correct problems or number of correct digits. According to the test manual, concepts and applications tests are scored by totalling the number of parts answered correctly

TEST OF WRITTEN LANGUAGE, FOURTH EDITION (TOWL-4)	
Purpose	Designed to identify students who are poor writers and may require intervention; determine strengths and weaknesses in various writing abilities; and document progress following writing intervention programmes
Population	9y–17y 11mo
Description of domains (subscales)	Seven subtests designed to assess the conventional, linguistic and conceptual aspects of a student's writing as well as contrived and spontaneous writing
Administration and test format	Time to complete: 60–90min to administer. The TOWL-4 contains seven subtests; subtests 1–5 use contrived formats and subtests 6 and 7 use a spontaneously written story to assess important aspects of written language 1. Vocabulary: sentence writing that incorporates a stimulus word 2. Spelling: sentence writing from dictation, making proper use of spelling rules 3. Punctuation: sentence writing from dictation, making proper use of punctuation and capitalization rules 4. Logical sentences: editing an illogical sentence so that it makes better sense 5. Sentence combining: integrating the meaning of several short sentences into one grammatically correct written sentence 6. Contextual conventions: story writing in response to a stimulus picture, with points earned for satisfying arbitrary requirements relative to orthographic and grammatical conventions 7. Story composition: story evaluation relative to the quality of its composition
Psychometric properties	The TOWL-4 was normed on a sample of 2205 individuals *Reliability* Internal consistency and test–retest reliabilities exceeded 0.80 *Validity* Correlations with other criterion-based measures are primarily between 0.50 and 0.75 *Responsiveness* Two parallel forms to monitor an individual's progress over time
How to order	Online: www.pearsonassessment.com; e-mail: Clinicalcustomersupport@Pearson.com International orders: www.pearsonassessments.com/pai/ca/IO/international.htm
Key reference	Hammill DD, Larsen SC (2009) *Test of Written Language*, 4th edition. Austin, TX: Pro-Ed.

for each problem. These measures were developed on 14 cohorts of students over 20 years. Included were students with mild to moderate disabilities as well as typically developing children. Test–retest reliability for basic maths computation measures ranges from 0.73 (moderate) to 0.92 (excellent). Content validity was judged by having regular education and special education teachers and curriculum supervisors evaluate the content of the tests for each grade level. The content validity was judged to be adequate. Criterion validity was established through moderate to strong correlations with three different measures: the Maths Computation Test and two subtests of the Stanford Achievement Test. For basic maths concepts and applications, internal consistency was established by computing a student's average score across all even-numbered assessments and all odd-numbered assessments. Correlations between these averages were at the 0.90 level and higher. Concurrent validity coefficients were calculated between the basic maths concepts and applications and basics maths computation scores. Correlations ranged from moderate to excellent.

ASSESSMENT OF WRITING

Writing is a critical skill that is important for academic achievement in schools. It is a fundamental way to communicate and express ideas. Writing combines many skills and relies on development in many areas. Written expression integrates fine motor, visuospatial, executive functioning, working memory, cognitive processing and critical thinking skills. Successful writing is a complicated process as it involves mastering both physical and cognitive skills and is associated with oral language and reading skill acquisition.[33] Research has found children's writing development to be a sociocultural, generative and developmental process.[34] Moreover, specific neurological and cognitive processes have been associated with difficulties in writing. Improvements in non-writing specific skills can facilitate the process of writing, and associated underlying cognitive processes that influence writing are important as educators work to support academic success and competency for all children in their classes (www.pbs.org/wgbh/misunderstoodminds/writingdiffs.html). Promoting writing development begins in early childhood with print awareness and oral language acquisition. The writing process may continue throughout adult life, with mastery of new genres of writing and refinement of various forms of writing for different audiences. Categories of knowledge that readers and writers use include meta-knowledge (pragmatics), domain knowledge about substance and content (previous knowledge, content knowledge gained while reading and writing), knowledge about universal text attributes and procedural knowledge and skill to negotiate reading and writing.[33] Two approaches to measurement of written language are presented below. Other standardized measures of handwriting performance are described in detail in Chapter 23.

Test of Written Language, Fourth Edition

The Test of Written Language, Fourth Edition, is a norm-referenced individually administered assessment of written expression. Its seven subtests represent three writing components (conventional, linguistic and conceptual) and the two writing assessment formats (contrived and spontaneous). It is designed for individuals aged 9 years to 17 years 11 months. The assessment can be used to (1) identify students who write poorly and therefore need special help, (2) determine students' particular strengths and weaknesses in their writing abilities, (3) document student progress in special writing programmes or interventions and (4) serve as measurement tools in writing research.

Curriculum-based measures of written expression

Mastery of writing skills can be more difficult to measure, as many schools have not developed a set of curricular objectives as they have for reading and maths. Writing CBMs are administered in order to obtain an understanding of a student's skill development using a more general technique across grade levels. Evidence supporting writing CBM has shown that having students write a story for 3 minutes, given an age-appropriate story starter, is a reliable and valid general outcome measure of general written expression.[35] General procedures described by Shapiro[12] suggest developing a number of narrative 'story starters' to give the student an idea to write about; he also suggests allowing the child to think about the 'story starter' for 1 minute before asking the child to respond to the prompt. Suggested scoring procedures include totalling the number of words written correctly per minute (recognizable and legible), ignoring capitalization, spelling and punctuation. Other scoring methods involve counting correct word sequences, where credit is received if the word sequence contains correct spelling, punctuation, grammar and syntax.[36] Written expression probes can be generated online at Aimsweb (http://interventioncentral.org).[37] This system includes written expression probes.

Curriculum-based measures of spelling

Assessment materials for spelling can easily be derived from the curriculum as many schools have a spelling series in early grades. Spelling CBM probes typically consist of 20 words; these words are dictated to the student at a rate of about one word per every 10 seconds for first or second graders and one word per every 7 seconds for children in the third grade and higher.[12] Words are scored in terms of 'correct letter sequences'. Aimsweb provides graded spelling lists of equal difficulty comprising the most frequently used words from seven different spelling series and reading word lists.[37] The following websites have CBM materials available for purchase: www.aimsweb.com; www.easycbm.com; www.edcheckup.com; and www.isteep.com.

Conclusion

Given the diagnostic and conceptual variability within the educational, psychological and medical fields for assessing learning difficulties, a universal standard classification system would be helpful to facilitate communication and provide a common framework. This is possible through the application of the ICF-CY as the first universal taxonomy of child health and disability. For example, Table 20.4 demonstrates how ICF-CY codes link to the standardized school readiness academic measures reviewed in this chapter. Common expectations about the general academic skills that allow a child to successfully participate as a student within formalized educational settings

TABLE 20.4

International Classification of Functioning, Disability and Health: learning and applying knowledge

---

Construct school readiness

Bracken Basic Concept Scale, revised, or Bracken School Readiness Assessment, third edition (BSRA-3), Kaufman Survey of Early Academic and Language Skills (K-SEALS)

ICF-CY	**d140** Learning to read
	d150 Learning to calculate
	d145 Learning to write
	d132 Acquiring information
	d137 Acquiring concepts

Academic achievement standardized measures

Woodcock–Johnson Tests of Achievement, third edition (WJ-III-Ach), Wechsler Individual Achievement Test, second edition (WIAT-III); Kaufman Test of Educational Achievement, second edition (KTEA-II); Monitoring Basic Skills Progress (MBSP) (curriculum based)

Reading

Dynamic Indicators of Basic Early Literacy Skills (DIBELS)

Gray Oral Reading Test, fourth edition (GORT-4)

Test of Reading Comprehension, fourth edition (TORC-4)

WJ-III, WIAT-III, KTEA-II subtests

ICF-CY	**d140** Learning to read
	d160 Reading
	d1660 Using general skills and strategies of the reading process
	d1661 Comprehending written language

Maths

KeyMath 3 Diagnostic Assessment

Test of Early Mathematics Ability, third edition

WJ-III, WIAT-III, KTEA-II subtests

ICF-CY	**d150** Learning to calculate
	d172 Calculating
	d1720 Using simple skills and strategies of the calculation process
	d1721 Using complex skills and strategies of the calculation process

Writing

The Oral and Written Language Scales (OWLS)

Test of Written Language, fourth edition (TOWL)

WJ-III, WIAT-III, KTEA-II subtests

ICF-CY	**d145** Learning to write
	d170 Writing
	d1700 Using general skills and strategies of the writing process
	d1701 Using grammatical and mechanical conventions in written compositions

---

are available for the first time with the recent introduction of the ICF-CY. Included at the person level of functioning, under the activities and participation domain of the ICF-CY, is a chapter that delineates areas of learning and applying knowledge for children from birth to the age of 17 years. Thus, the specific items included in the ICF-CY represent early behaviours and prerequisite abilities starting in infancy as well as pre-academic early childhood skills.

Measuring academic learning has widely come to mean assessing academic areas for a disability in learning where a child is performing at an unexpected level given his or her cognitive ability (assessed with a standardized intelligence test). Typically a child's academic knowledge is evaluated and compared with same-aged peers. While understanding that the child's general cognitive ability can inform classroom expectations, measuring what they learn and determining how to best promote learning is central. Most standardized measures only identify where a difference exists; understanding the cause of problems would require administering and interpreting measures of cognitive, socioemotional and physical functioning to inform instructional and intervention efforts. However, targeting skills or gaps in knowledge seems to be a priority in designing relevant individualized interventions for a child in maths, reading or writing. With recent legislative support, a new model of RTI would align with classroom- and skill-specific individualized 'curriculum-based assessments' for children who are not performing as expected in a particular academic area.

RTI was proposed as an alternative model for making decisions about the presence or absence of a specific learning disability. Reflecting more of a functional assessment of learning difficulties, the RTI method identifies students based on problems with academic performance over time rather than reflecting one time point where performance on standardized measures are compared. While RTI conceptualization appears to better align with a bio-ecological framework of functioning, it does not readily seek to understand if and how neuropsychological processes are compromised and need to be addressed until a child has failed to respond to intervention. With some fundamental issues related to RTI unresolved, a better strategy may be to more rigorously implement existing identification criteria (e.g. discrepancy and psychological processing deficits) or an integrative model and use a structured psychometric framework.[4]

The bidirectional ecological framework presented in the ICF-CY supports the inclusion of environmental factors in the documentation of learning problems. The ICF-CY classification system applied to learning concerns would provide a profile of child functioning, reflecting the degree of difficulty in performing specific behaviours or activities under the learning and applying knowledge codes. In addition, environmental facilitators and barriers and problems at the body structure/body functions level would be included. Although the following areas are specified as important functional components of child learning and application of knowledge, these specific codes are always considered along with the present level of functioning at the body and system level. An ability to read, express ideas with written language and perform mathematics accurately facilitates the attainment of increasingly complex and specific academic knowledge.

Establishing a common definition of a specific learning disability would require consensus about areas or academic knowledge and skills that need to be measured. Further, a universal definition would reflect agreement about the level at which deficits or problems in these areas would indicate a disability. The methods and approach to diagnose a specific learning disability would examine functioning and capability in these identified areas using reliable and valid instruments for standardized comparisons to the established criteria. Alternatively, assessing academic learning at an individual level may be more meaningful when performance in current learning environments is examined, with the purpose of determining obstacles to understanding and retaining or applying information. This type of approach would include examining situational factors, personal factors, cultural, and environmental factors that might facilitate or impede the learning process. For example, when problems exist, consideration about previous knowledge and experiences, instructional match and classroom environment would be examined as well as problems in foundational cognitive processes (e.g. attention, memory, visuospatial processing) or socioemotional functioning that might hinder learning. The intent of the assessment might be viewed as a problem-solving process to determine the cause of difficulties and lead to the identification of areas to target for treatment or intervention.

The method of measuring child learning within the ICF-CY framework would then produce a profile of functioning as well as a picture of environmental and relational factors that would promote or hinder optimal functioning rather than yield a 'yes' or 'no' response for whether a disability exists. Integrating information about potential environmental, instructional, experiential, physical, neurobiological or psychological factors that contribute to successful learning and performance in an educational setting is essential to establishing appropriate interventions. The evaluation of learning problems would include measures of important factors in each of these areas. The ICF-CY provides both a framework and detailed taxonomy that would capture functioning across these areas when learning and applying knowledge measures are combined with reliable measures across the body, person and environment levels.

Additional resources

Learning Disabilities Association of America: www.ldaamerica.org/about/position/rti.asp
National Association of School Psychologists: www.nasponline.org/about_nasp/positionpapers/StudentsLearningDisabilities.pdf
National Center for Learning Disabilities: www.rtinetwork.org/
National Joint Committee on Learning Disabilities: www.ldonline.org/about/partners/njcld#reports

REFERENCES

1. Oakland T, Mpofu E, Gregoire J, Faulkner M (2007) An exploration of learning disabilities in four countries: implications for test development and use in developing countries. *Int J Test* 7: 53–70.

2. McCarthy J, Reid DK (2002) *The Learning Theory of Piaget & Inhelder*. Lincoln, NE: Brooks/Cole Publishing Company.

3. Piaget J, Inhelder B (1969) *The Psychology of the Child*. New York: Basic Books.

4. Kavale K (2005) Identifying specific learning disability. Is responsiveness to intervention the answer? *J Learn Disabil* 38: 553–562.

5. Speece DL (2008) Learning disabilities in the US: operationalizing a construct. In: Florian L, McLaughlin MJ, editors. *Disability Classification in Education: Issues and Perspectives*. Thousand Oaks, CA: Corwin Press, pp. 227–239.

6. Weiss IR, Pasley JD, Smith PS, Bainlower ER, Heck DJ (2003) *Looking Inside the Classroom: A Study of K-12 Mathematics and Science Education in the United States*. Chapel Hill, NC: Horizon Research. Available from: www.horizonresearch.com/insidetheclassroom/reports/looking/

7. Fletcher JM, Lyon GR, Fuchs LS, Barnes MA (2007) *Learning Disabilities: From Identification to Intervention*. New York: Guilford Press.

8. Hale J, Alfonso V, Berninger V, et al (2010) Critical issues in response to intervention, comprehensive evaluation, and specific learning disability identification and intervention: an expert white paper consensus. *Learn Disabil Q* 33: 223–236.

9. Individuals with Disabilities Education Act (2008) 20 U.S.C. § et seq.

10. Brown-Chidsey R, Steege M (2010) *Response to Intervention: Principles and Strategies for Effective Practice*, 2nd edition. New York: Guilford Press.

11. Deno SD, Reschly AL, Lembke ES, et al (2009) Developing a school-wide progress monitoring system. *Psychol Sch* 46: 44–55.

12. Shapiro ES (2004) *Academic Skills Problems*, 3rd edition. New York: Guilford Press.

13. Glover TA, DiPerna JC (2007) Service delivery models for response to intervention: core components and directions for future research. *Sch Psychol Rev* 36: 526–640.

14. National Center on Response to Intervention. Available from: www.rti4success.org (accessed 10 December 2010).

15. Copeland SR, Crosbey J (2008) Making progress in the general curriculum: rethinking effective instructional practices. *Res Pract Persons Severe Disabil* 33: 214–227.

16. Maccini P, Gagnon JC (2006) Mathematics instructional practices and assessment accommodations by general and special educators. *Except Child* 72: 217–234.

17. Swanson HL, Hoskyn M (2001) Instructing adolescents with learning disabilities: a component and composite analysis. *Learn Disabil Res Pract* 16: 109–119.

18. Shinn MR (2007) Identifying students at risk, monitoring performance, and determining eligibility within response to intervention: research on educational need and benefit from academic intervention. *Sch Psychol Rev* 36: 601–617.

19. Hair E, Halle T, Terry-Humen E, Lavelle B, Calkins J (2006) Children's school readiness in the ECLS-K: predictions to academic, health, and social outcomes in first grade. *Early Child Res Q* 21: 431–454.

20. Zill N, West J (2001) *Entering Kindergarten: A Portrait of American Children When They Begin School: Findings From the Condition of Education 2000*. Washington, DC: US Department of Education, National Center for Education Statistics NCES, pp. 2001–2035.

21. Clark CA, Pritchard VE, Woodward LJ (2010) Preschool executive functioning abilities predict early mathematics achievement. *Dev Psychol* 46: 1176–1191.

22. Li-Grining CP, Votruba-Drzal E, Maldonado-Carreno C, Haas K (2010) Children's early approaches to learning and academic trajectories through fifth grade. *Dev Psychol* 46: 1062–1077.

23. Snow C, Burns S, Griffin P (1998) *Preventing Reading Difficulties in Young Children*. Washington, DC: National Academy Press.

24. McGrew KS, Woodcock RW (2000) *Technical Manual. Woodcock–Johnson III*. Itasca, IL: Riverside Publishing.

25. Kaufman AS, Kaufman NL (2004) *Kaufman Test of Educational Achievement, Second Edition (KTEA-II)*. Circle Pines, MN: American Guidance Service.

26. Pearson Assessment Support. New York: Pearson. Available from: www.pearsonassessmentsupport.com/ (accessed 6 June 2010).

27. Puranik CS, Petscher Y, Otaiba SA, Catts HW, Lonigan CJ (2008) Development of oral reading fluency in children with speech or language impairments. *J Learn Disabil* 41: 545–560.

28. Shaywitz SE, Morris R, Shaywitz BA (2008) The education of dyslexic children from childhood to young adulthood. *Annu Rev Psychol* 58: 451–475.

29. Salvia J, Ysseldyke J (2004) *Assessment in Special and Inclusive Education*, 9th edition. New York: Houghton-Mifflin.

30. Fuchs LS, Fuchs D, Hamlett CL, Thompson A, Roberts PH (1994) Technical features of a mathematical concepts and application curriculum based measurement system. *Diagnosis* 19: 23–49.

31. Keller-Margulis MA, Shapiro ES, Hintze JM (2008) Long-term diagnostic accuracy of curriculum-based measures in reading and mathematics. *Sch Psychol Rev* 37: 374–389.

32. Andersson U (2010) Skill development in different components of arithmetic and basic cognitive functions: findings from a 3-year longitudinal study of children with different types of learning difficulties. *J Educ Psychol* 2: 115–134.

33. Fitzgerald J, Shanahan T (2000) Reading and writing relations and their development. *Educ Psychol* 35: 39–50.

34. Lu MY (2000) *Writing Development. ERIC D159*. Bloomington (IN): ERIC Clearinghouse on Reading English and Communication. Available from: www.ericdigests.org/2001–3/development.htm (accessed 1 December 2010)

35. Deno SL, Marston D, Mirkin P (1982) Valid measurement procedures for continuous evaluation of written expression. *Except Child* 48: 368–371.

36. Espin CA, Skare S, Shin J, Deno SL, Robinson S, Brenner B (2000) Identifying indicators of growth in written expression for middle-school students. *J Spec Educ* 34: 140–153.

37. Aimsweb: Assessment and Data Management for RTI (2010) New York: Pearson. Available from: www.aimsweb.com (accessed 6 July 2010).

21
GENERAL TASKS AND DEMANDS OF CHILDREN (D210–250)

Susana Castro, Shannon Lewis and Rune J. Simeonsson

What is the construct?

The International Classification of Functioning, Disability and Health for Children and Youth (ICF-CY)[1] describes the term 'activity' as 'the execution of a task' and 'participation' as 'involvement in life situations'. The activities and participation component of the ICF and ICF-CY has been the object of many studies where the focus has been to clarify the conceptual distinction between the two terms – activities and participation – in spite of the fact that they are included within the same section of the classification (e.g. references 2–4).

In line with this focus, Badley[2] suggested a new way of categorizing functioning, based on the ICF components. In this proposal, the activities and participation component of the ICF could be divided into *acts*, *tasks* and *societal involvement*. Contextual influences, in the form of environmental factors in the ICF-CY, are seen as scene-setters, facilitating or creating barriers for the execution of acts, tasks and societal involvement. In this conceptualization of activities and participation, the acts component would consist of the general things a person is able to do independent of context or purpose and in an automatic way. Tasks are seen as the purposeful things people do in daily life in a specific context; often they also are automatic, but have a specific objective defined. Acts and tasks (corresponding to the current notion of activity) form a continuum, along with the societal involvement (corresponding to the current notion of participation).

According to Badley,[2] isolated acts form the execution of purposeful tasks, which is illustrated in the 'general tasks and demands' chapter. Therefore, the ICF-CY chapter regarding general tasks and demands of an individual can be positioned in this continuum. In fact, the categories embraced within this chapter – undertaking purposeful tasks, managing routines, handling stress and managing behaviour – are presented in a developmental sequence in which the first ones (such as 'undertaking a single task')

are close to the notion of activity, and the last and more complex ones (such as managing behaviour) are closer to participation, as they imply a certain level of societal involvement. This chapter first classifies the ability to execute tasks, which could be seen as acts (first isolated and then simultaneous acts), and then presents more purposeful and orientated behaviours such as carrying out daily routines. The following categories refer to how the child behaves in those daily activities: how he or she handles stress and other psychological demands and how he or she manages his or her own behaviour. The chapter is, then, organized in a continuum from the simple execution of isolated tasks to purposeful, orientated tasks, but without addressing societal involvement in a specific context.

In order to fully understand how the child is able to perform tasks in his or her daily routines, the assessment of behaviour must be conducted within children's natural environments. Routines are naturally occurring activities that happen with some regularity, and they include both caregiving events and leisure times. The study and understanding of children's daily routines and the management of their daily demands warrant the need for further understanding on the level of engagement of children in those activities.[5] This notion of engagement is similar to the ICF notion of participation in regards to 'involvement in life situations'. Thus, the complete understanding of children's life situations requires the assessment of their level of participation. Also, this definition of engagement includes the interactions that are established between the child and their surrounding environments,[6] which fits with the notion of the environmental factors as scene-setters for the performance of daily routines and behavioural demands of children in their natural environments. This notion of engagement, which considers the surrounding environment, is also close to the idea of goodness of fit, which proposes that when the characteristics of a child fit with the demands and expectations of the environment, adaptive outcomes will result.[7] This further validates the need to measure the child's ability to manage his or her daily life, and behaviour and psychological demands that might appear in that process.

The Goodness of Fit Model and the concept of a child's engagement with the environment within his or her daily routines can be seen to be consistent with the conceptual framework of the ICF-CY, which is known as a biopsychosocial model of functioning.[1]

In line with these theoretical assumptions, this chapter will focus on describing measurements that were developed to assess aspects of the general tasks and demands that children face in their daily lives. To pursue this aim, the understanding of the children's routines in a comprehensive way is of foremost relevance. We suggest that the Routines-based Interview (RBI)[8] is a good measure of children's and families' daily experiences, as well as of how children deal with the challenges presented in those routines. Among the various challenges that daily life might present to children, complex demands such as managing feelings of stress and controlling their own behaviours are of large relevance. In order to assess the general performance of the child in task execution, we suggest using the Performance Skills Questionnaire (PSQ).[9] To assess children's management of stress and use of effective coping skills, two measures were selected: the Early Coping Inventory (ECI)[10] and the Stress Impact Scale.[11] To assess the ability to self-control and the behavioural style of children in daily lives, we selected two measures: the Child Self-control Rating Scale (CSCRS)[12] and the Behavioral Style Questionnaire.[13] Table 21.1 lists the selected measures.

UNDERTAKING SINGLE AND MULTIPLE TASKS AND CARRYING OUT A DAILY ROUTINE
The focus of this chapter is on tasks defined in terms of activities performed by children in their daily life routines. This approach takes a broad view of the assessment of undertaking tasks, as most of the tasks performed by

children imply a specific setting and are related to their daily routines.[5] General performance on task execution might then be observed by assessing the child's management of routines defined by codes in the ICF-CY component of activities and participation. However, the capacity of the child to execute independent and/or simultaneous tasks might also be assessed through measurements of executive function, which is classified in the body functions component of the ICF-CY. Routines are defined as activities that are repeated on a day-to-day basis. Common routines include morning, mealtime, departure and bedtime routines, and each of these has specific subtasks, executed repeatedly every day. Routines are reported to be critical in the establishment of a child's sense of predictability and feelings of security. In toddlers, routines are believed to foster smooth transitions between different activities and to be related to the development of independence, trust and security,[14] which is why it is developmentally appropriate that a child gradually becomes more and more able to predict and manage his or her routines independently.

Among older children, a substantial proportion of routines involve learning tasks in academic settings. Among preschool and elementary children, routines often involve behaviour and are thought to moderate impulsivity and overactivity, while aiding in the development of self-control,[14] which is why the ICF-CY domains of carrying out daily routines, handling psychological demands and managing one's own behaviour are interrelated and integrated under the umbrella of 'general tasks and demands'. Coping strategies in dealing with stress and other demands, as well as self-control and behaviour management, are essential aspects to carry out more basic-level activities such as daily routines or simple tasks. In fact, several studies demonstrate this relationship between behavioural-oppositional problems in children and a lack of predictability in daily routines.[14] Also, it is widely recognized in the scientific literature on early childhood intervention that the best outcomes are obtained when the process of assessment and intervention is conducted in an embedded way, within a child's daily routines.[5] However, some measures were developed specifically for the purpose of assessing the children's abilities on the performance of tasks, and some of them are conceptually framed by the ICF-CY model of functioning and use the ICF-CY taxonomy that describes the task performance substeps. In this scope, the Occupational Therapy Practice Framework suggests that the child's underlying capacities are contributors to functional performance, and that the child's capacities by themselves cannot fully explain participation. Thus, a more detailed terminology is developed in which three

TABLE 21.1
Selected measures for the assessment of general tasks and demands of children

Measurements
Performance Skills Questionnaire[9]
Routines-based Interview[8]
Early Coping Inventory[10]
Stress Impact Scale[11]
Child Self-control Rating Scale[12]
Behavioral Style Questionnaire[13]

components are considered: (1) client factors (capacities); (2) performance patterns (routines, habits and roles); and (3) performance skills. According to this framework, performance skills are elements of functional performance and contribute to the effective execution of any activity or occupation, and include motor skills, process skills and communication skills.[9]

HANDLING STRESS AND OTHER PSYCHOLOGICAL DEMANDS

There is growing evidence that children's experience of stress affects their health and adjustment. Effective coping skills in children potentially may distinguish those who eventually learn to manage stress appropriately from those who do not possess the ability to do so, or succumb to the stress effects by developing psychiatric or psychosomatic symptoms.[15] The assessment of individual coping skills and strategies has been addressed in the life stress literature,[15,16] based on the recognition that health consequences of stress are influenced by coping and the amount of stress an individual is exposed to.[16]

Stress is linked with both physical and psychological factors, and might be explained through homeostatic system functioning in which life changes upset the homeostasis, requiring that adjustments be made. Therefore, children's health is affected by both personal and environmental factors. In this context, some risk factors that might affect their health and well-being are troubled families, specific life events (such as loss of a family member, illness, moving, parental divorce), internal factors such as attributions and locus of control, temperament, self-esteem and coping styles.[17]

Much of what is known about stress in children comes from parental reports as measurements of stress from the child's perspective are still rare. Some of the indicators of stress in children are body language, deviations from their regular behaviour, specific emotional responses and physiological reactions.[17] Stress can be defined as an imbalance between an individual's perceptions of demands and his or her perceptions of capabilities available to meet those demands.[15]

According to Ptrezlik and Sylva,[18] Lazarus refers to 'distress' as a reaction to stress with emotional overtones and defines 'coping' as 'constantly changing cognitive and behavioral efforts to manage the specific external and/or internal demands that are appraised as taxing or exceeding the resources of the person' (p. 141). Thus, from Lazarus' perspective, distress is an emotional reaction, whereas coping always involves efforts to deal with the stress. The coping strategies that are used by an individual vary across types of stressors and over time. Therefore, coping is the process of making adjustments to fit both

personal needs and the demands of the environment, and is a process that is influenced by such factors as a child's developmental skills, temperament, physical health, previous experience and social support. Over time, each child develops a unique coping style that grows in complexity and reflects his or her own way of handling the opportunities, challenges and frustrations in their daily lives.[19]

MANAGING ONE'S OWN BEHAVIOUR

The definition of self-control involves two components: cognitive and behavioural.[20] From the cognitive point of view, self-control implies deliberation, problem solving, planning and evaluation in a given situation where it is required. On the other hand, the behavioural component comprises the ability to execute the behaviour that was chosen after deliberation and inhibition of the disregarded behaviours. This conceptualization of self-control also allows us to conclude that a non-impulsive child is a self-controlled child.

Self-control or self-management skills have been frequently cited as necessary competences for children's successful school and life adjustment. The concept of locus of control has been recognized by self-management theorists as being related to the attainment of self-controlling skills.[21] An internal locus of control orientation has been associated with more adequate levels of self-control,[12] whereas a child with an external locus of control manifests an orientation more likely to attribute success or failure to external factors.

Self-control in children has also been studied in relation to disruptive behaviours as well as hyperactive behaviours that are expressed by many children. Both behaviours have been related with poor self-control management.[20]

General factors to consider when measuring this domain

The assessment of task performance and level of participation in task performance is of immense importance when planning for interventions for children. In fact, the ultimate goal of any intervention programme is to ensure that the child is able to perform the necessary activities and to become actively engaged in their daily routines. Within the natural process of development, young children are expected to learn how to perform certain acts, reunite them in the performance of activities that grow in complexity over time and, finally, they are also expected to face their own psychological demands, such us tolerating frustration in the process of learning and organize their body language and general behaviour according to the rules of the environment. Also, this learning process occurs in an embedded way, according to each child's daily living routine. The ICF-CY contemplates the ability of the child to manage his or her routines, which highlights the importance of having a complete and profound knowledge of the child's daily living when conducting an assessment. In this process of assessment of task performance in daily routines of children, attention should be given to the particularities among different age groups, cultures, family backgrounds and other relevant contextual factors that can influence general tasks. Furthermore, routines are thought to moderate impulsivity and overactivity in preschool and elementary school children, while aiding in the development of self-control. In older children, routines typically focus on chores and homework.[14]

Therefore, the constructs of coping and self-control should be assessed in light of these previous conditions: measures should be selected and administered in a way that allows enough opportunity to acquire knowledge about the particular daily living conditions of each child, without imposing a preconceived matrix of expectations for the child's behaviour and routine. The routine is defined by each family.[8] Attention should also be given to the particular features of the environment that might influence the task performance or the level of engagement that the child demonstrates in daily routines. Existing research suggests a relationship between certain factors (e.g. low socioeconomic status,

maternal depression, marital discord) and problematic child behaviours.[14]

Overview of recommended measures

PERFORMANCE SKILLS QUESTIONNAIRE

The PSQ was developed based on the Occupational Therapy Practice Framework and its items were adjusted to fit the young children's general performance in different types of activities. It has 34 items in three domains: motor skills (10 items), process skills (14 items) and communication skills (10 items). The immediate caregiver, usually the parent, should rate each item on a six-point Likert scale, where a higher score indicates better performance skills of the child. It provides information on the ability of the child to initiate, perform and end certain activities related to well-defined developmental domains, according to the parent's report. This questionnaire has recently been developed, and preliminary psychometric properties appear to be acceptable for use in clinical practice.

ROUTINES-BASED INTERVIEW

This measure consists of a semi-structured interview designed to collect systematic information about the activities that occur in the typical day of families and classrooms, identifying the child's abilities within those

PERFORMANCE SKILLS QUESTIONNAIRE (PSQ)	
Purpose	Evaluates the young children's general activity and performance
Population	Ages 4–6y
Description of domains	Motor skills, communication skills and process skills
Administration and test format	Time to complete: 10–15min
	Testing format: the 34 items of the PSQ are rated on a six-point Likert scale, where a higher score indicates better performance skills of the child
	Scoring: each item is scored on a Likert scale from 1 to 6, where a higher score indicates better performance skills
	Training: no specific training needed
Psychometric properties	Internal consistency: Cronbach's coefficient alpha of the items within motor skills, process skills and communication skills is 0.89, 0.92 and 0.84, respectively
	Inter-rater reliability: weighted kappa ranges from 0.44 to 0.89 and agreement per cent ranges from 57.5% to 95% for all 34 items. Intraclass correlation coefficients for mean scores of the three performance skill measures ranged from 0.92 to 0.96
How to order	Contact the authors
Key reference	Bart O, Rosenberg L, Ratzon NZ, Jarus T (2010) Development and initial validation of the Performance Skills Questionnaire (PSQ). *Res Dev Disabil* 31: 46–56.

ROUTINES-BASED INTERVIEW (RBI)	
Purpose	Collects systematic information about the activities that occur in the family's and the classroom's typical day, identifying a child's abilities within those contexts
Population	Children and their families
Description of domains	General daily routine
Administration and test format	Time to complete: 90–120min
	Testing format: semi-structured interview
	Scoring: data are of a qualitative nature. There is a routine rating from 1 to 5
	Training: the interview is best conducted by someone who is going to have a long-term relationship with the family and who is knowledgeable in child development and family functioning. The RBI implementation checklist and the top 10 signs of correct implementation may be downloaded from: http://ectc.nde.ne.gov/rbi/training_skill_building.htm
Psychometric properties	Not applicable. This measure consists of a qualitative interview
How to order	Protocol and instructions can be downloaded from: http://ectc.nde.ne.gov/rbi/rbi.htm
	For the Routines-based Early Intervention purchase: www.brookespublishing.com/store/books/mcwilliam-70625/index.htm
Key references	McWilliam RA (2000) It's only natural … to have early intervention in the environments where it's needed. In: Sandall S, Ostrosky M, editors. *Young Exceptional Children Monograph Series No. 2: Natural Environments and Inclusion.* Denver, CO: The Division for Early Childhood of the Council for Exceptional Children, pp. 17–26.
	McWilliam RA (2010) *Working with Families of Young Children with Special Needs.* New York: The Guilford Press.

contexts. It was developed in the scope of the Early Intervention in Natural Environments model, developed by Robin McWilliam.[5] This model comprises five components: (1) understanding the family ecology; (2) functional intervention planning; (3) integrated services; (4) effective home visits; and (5) collaborative consultation for childcare. These components illustrate the importance of understanding children's routines and their ability to manage them for effective early intervention outcomes. Each component is addressed with a specific practice for its assessment. The RBI is related to the component of 'functional intervention planning' because it highlights the importance of addressing a child's natural environment and specific routines for effective planning of interventions. According to the author, functional outcomes are those that address participation or engagement needs, independence needs and social-relationship needs. This is consistent with the ICF-CY definition of participation as 'involvement in life situations'.

EARLY COPING INVENTORY

This observation instrument generates a profile of coping behaviours of young children across three categories: sensorimotor organization, reactive behaviour and self-initiated behaviour.[19] Sensorimotor organization refers to the regulation of psychophysiological functions and the integration of sensory and motor systems. Reactive behaviour includes the behaviour used to react to demands of the physical and social environment. Items that typify this category are the ability to respond to vocal or gestural direction, to react to the feelings and moods of others, to bounce back after stressful situations, to adjust to daily routines and to accommodate to changes in the surroundings. The Self-initiated Behaviour Subscale examines a child's autonomously generated behaviours, which help individuals to interact with people and objects. Such coping behaviour is intrinsically motivated and not directly linked to environmental cues. Sample items include the child's ability to apply a previously learned behaviour to new situations, to initiate interactions with others, to demonstrate persistence during activities, to anticipate events

EARLY COPING INVENTORY (ECI)	
Purpose	To measure children's individual patterns of behaviour (coping styles), level of coping effectiveness and characteristic coping strengths and vulnerabilities
Population	Ages 4–36mo
Description of domains	Three subscales (sensorimotor organization, reactive behaviour, self-initiated behaviour) comprise a total of 48 items
Administration and test format	Time to complete: administration time varies depending on the observer's familiarity with the child
	Testing format: items on the ECI are rated using a five-point Likert scale where 1 is ineffective, 2 is minimally effective, 3 is situationally effective, 4 is effective more often than not and 5 is consistently effective
	Scoring: a mean rating of the items is computed for each of the three subscales with a global indicator of coping effectiveness, called the Adaptive Behaviour Index, representing an average of the three subscales. A list of six to eight of the most and least adaptive coping behaviours is also compiled to aid in intervention planning
	Training: no specific training is required. The assessment process can be conducted by anyone with knowledge of child development
Psychometric properties	Psychometric validation of the instrument, reported in the ECI manual (Zeitlin et al, 1988) is based on a series of studies that established its construct and content validity, inter-rater reliability, test–retest reliability and item reliability. Inter-rater reliability coefficients ranged from a low of 0.80 for sensorimotor organization to a high of 0.94 for self-initiated behaviour, with an average of 0.91. Test–retest reliability (6-week interval): Friedman's analysis of variance test was used to test for significant differences between ECI test–retest scores for each child on the coping clusters and the adaptive behavioural index. The authors reported no statistical significant shift in scoring on 11 of the 16 tests. Validity of the instrument was supported
How to order	Scholastic Testing Service, Inc.: www.ststesting.com.
	Cost: US$62.65 for the Early Coping Inventory Starter Set Observation Form (one manual and 20 forms)
Key reference	Zeitlin S, Williamson GG, Szczepanski M (1988) *Early Coping Inventory*. Bensenville, IL: Scholastic Testing Service.

and to explore objects independently using a variety of strategies.[19,22]

The ECI is primarily a clinical tool to help practitioners plan intervention services that enhance adaptive functioning. Each item identifies a specific behavioural characteristic that has been documented in the research literature or by expert clinical judgement as highly relevant to coping in young children. As coping is an integrative process, items in the inventory tap a range of domains – temperament, sensory processing, motor control, psychological functions and socio-emotional factors. The item scores, representing the target behaviours, are obtained through responses on a five-point Likert scale and are not elicited in a test situation. Instead, ratings are assigned after observations of the child in a variety of circumstances, as coping behaviour reflects the general capabilities of the child to effectively respond to the multiple demands of functional living.[19]

CHILD SELF-CONTROL RATING SCALE

The CSCRS[12] was designed to parallel the Self-control Rating Scale (SCRS),[20] which is an often-used, reliable and valid measure of children's self-control, as rated by parents. The CSCRS is a measure that consists of 33 items where children should rate their ability to control themselves in the given situations. Interventions designed to increase children's self-control have often utilized pencil-and-paper measures for ratings by parents and teachers to assess the effectiveness of the interventions. However,

CHILD SELF-CONTROL RATING SCALE (CSCRS)	
Purpose	To measure children's conduct problems and perceived ability to control one's behaviour, using self-reported ratings. The Self-control Rating Scale (SCRS) is for parent and teacher proxy rating and has the same structure and theoretical basis as the CSCRS
Population	Ages 8–11y; from third grade to fifth grade
Description of domains	No areas or domains are specified
Administration and test format	Time to complete: not specified Testing format: the scale has 33 items that are rated on a four-point Likert scale. For each item, the child is first asked to decide which kind of child is mostly like him or her and then decide if this is only sort of true or really true. In the SCRS format, the items are rated by parents or teachers on a seven-point scale Scoring: all items are summed to yield a total score, with a higher score reflecting a greater lack of self-control Training: no specific training is required. The assessment process can be conducted by anyone with knowledge of child development
Psychometric properties	Test–retest reliability: 0.88. No information on inter-rater reliability
How to order	Contact: Cynthia A Rohrbeck (rohrbeck@gwu.edu)
Key references	Kendall PC, Wilcox LE (1979) Self-control in children: development of a rating scale. *J Consult Clin Psychol* 47: 1020–1029. Rohrbeck CA, Azar ST, Wagner PE (1991) Child Self-Control Rating Scale: validation of a Child Self-Report Measure. *J Clin Child Psychol* 20: 179–183.

parents' and teachers' judgements might be biased because of the subjectivity of their own perceptions. Assessing children's perceptions of their own self-control is more likely to reflect their true behaviour across all situations, including in both home and classroom settings.[12] In the CSCRS, children have to position themselves within the behaviours and situations presented, providing us with a self-report assessment of their own self-control and behaviour management to be used along with the ratings provided by the parents and teachers using the SCRS.

BEHAVIOURAL STYLE QUESTIONNAIRE

The Behavioural Style Questionnaire (BSQ)[13] provides a means of assessing temperament through personal and social functioning observation of young children with disabilities between 3 and 7 years of age, which is often non-verbal. Assessment of temperament is of foremost importance, especially in young children with disabilities, as it can provide a profile of real or perceived personal characteristics of importance to parents and other care-givers.[23] Despite the fact that temperament is a mental function (within body functions), there is a relationship in the way it expresses a particular behaviour style and participation in task performance. In other words, this instrument can assess the way in which the child manages his or her behaviour according to temperamental features. Parents can rate the child's behaviour according to nine variables adapted from the definition of temperament by Thomas and Chess:[24] activity, rhythmicity of biological functions, initial approach–withdrawal, adaptability, intensity, mood, persistence, distractibility and sensory threshold. The ratings are made according to three levels: *easy, difficult* and *slow to warm up*. Another measure – the Middle Childhood Temperament Questionnaire – is based on the same approach as the BSQ, but it is designed for children between 8 and 12 years of age.

STRESS IMPACT SCALE

The Stress Impact Scale (SIS)[11] is a measure designed to assess the perceptions and feelings about stressful life events and occurrences potentially faced by children and adolescents between the ages of 8 and 20 years. Items on the SIS include events and situations that may occur at school, home or in the community and constitute aspects

BEHAVIOUR STYLE QUESTIONNAIRE (BSQ)

Purpose	To measure children's behavioural style and temperament
Population	Ages 3–7y; a second version for children aged between 8y and 12y is also available (the Middle Childhood Temperament Questionnaire)

Description of domains	Nine behavioural features to be rated:
	     High activity/low activity
	     Arrhythmic/rhythmic
	     Withdrawal/approach
	     Slow adaptation/very adaptive
	     Intense/mild
	     Negative mood/positive mood
	     Low persistence/high persistence
	     Low distractibility/high distractibility
	     Low threshold/high threshold

Administration and test format	Time to complete: not specified by the authors Testing format: parent's rating of children's behaviour Scoring: scoring for each item is made by choosing one of three categories: easy, difficult and slow to warm up Training: no specific training is required
Psychometric properties	Test–retest reliability was 0.89. Internal consistency measured with alpha coefficients ranged from 0.47 to 0.80 with a median of 0.70. Internal consistency for the total instrument was 0.84
How to order	Contact the authors
Key references	McDevitt SC, Carey WB (1978) Measurement of temperament in 3 to 7 year old children. *J Child Psychol Psychiatry* 19: 245–253. Carey WB, McDevitt SC, Baker D (1979) Differentiating minimal brain dysfunction and temperament. *Dev Med Child Neurol* 21: 765–772.

STRESS IMPACT SCALE (SIS)

Purpose	To assess the perceptions and feelings of children and adolescents regarding potentially stressful life events and occurrences
Population	Ages 8–20y
Description of domains	Three stress quotients: (1) Stress Occurrence Quotient (SOQ), (2) Stress Impact Quotient (SIQ) and (3) Stress Impact Differential Quotient (SID). The SOQ indicates the total number of stressful events reported by the respondent, the SIQ is a sum of the ratings for which the respondent reported that the event bothered him or her and the SID is derived by subtracting the raw SOQ from the raw SIQ and converting it into a standard score. The standard score indicates the level of stress reported when previous stressful situations are eliminated from the total SIQ
Administration and test format	Time to complete: administration time not reported Testing format: the SIS is a 70-item self-reported instrument where respondents are asked to indicate a yes or no to denote if an event occurred. If the respondent marked yes next to an event, he or she is then asked to indicate if he or she is still bothered by the event, using a Likert-type scale that ranges from none (1) to a lot (3). It can be administered to a group

	Scoring: the sum of the items stress occurrence items gives the SOQ and the sum of the stress impact domains gives the SIQ. Subtracting the raw SOQ from the raw SIQ scores and converting to a standard score results in the Stress Impact Differential quotient Training: no specific training needed
Psychometric properties	Reliability coefficients for each scale are consistently >0.85 and are reported by age, grade, race, sex, parent education level, parent occupation and national geographic area. The test–retest reliability coefficients of the stress occurrence and stress impact scales ranged from 0.83 to 0.93 across grades. The stress occurrence and stress impact scales are highly correlated (r=0.86). The norms appear to be representative across demographic groups
How to order	Contact Pro-Ed, Inc. (www.proedinc.com)
Key reference	Stress Impact Scale (1990) In: Conoley JC, Impara JC, editors. *The Supplement to the Eleventh Mental Measurements Yearbook*. Lincoln, NE: Buros Institute of Mental Measurements, pp. 238–240.

of academic performance and behaviour, social isolation and peer rejection, problems with relationships, mobility and other traumatic events. Respondents are asked to indicate 'yes' or 'no' to denote whether an event has occurred. If the respondent marked 'yes' beside an event, he or she is then asked to indicate if he or she is still bothered by the event using a scale that ranges from none (1) to a lot (3). The respondent's questions provide three stress quotients that include the stress occurrence quotient, stress impact quotient and the stress impact differential quotient.

REFERENCES

1. World Health Organization (2007) *International Classification of Functioning, Disability and Health Version for Children and Youth*. Geneva: WHO.
2. Badley E (2008) Enhancing the conceptual clarity of the activity and participation components of the International Classification of Functioning, Disability, and Health. *Soc Sci Med* 66: 2335–2345.
3. McConachie H, Colver A, Forsyth R, Jarvis S, Parkinson K (2006) Participation of disabled children: how should it be characterized and measured? *Disabil Rehabil* 28: 1157–1164.
4. Egilson S, Traustadottir R (2009) Participation of students with physical disabilities in the school environment. *Am J Occup Ther* 63: 264–272.
5. McWilliam RA (2000) It's only natural… to have early intervention in the environments where it's needed. In: Sandall S, Ostrosky M, editors. *Young Exceptional Children Monograph Series No. 2: Natural Environments and Inclusion*. Denver, CO: The Division for Early Childhood of the Council for Exceptional Children, pp. 17–26.
6. McWilliam RA, Bailey DB (1992) Promoting engagement and mastery. In: Bailey DB, Wolery M, editors. *Teaching Infants and Preschoolers with Disabilities*. Columbus, OH: Merrill, pp. 229–255.
7. Thomas A, Chess S (1977) *Temperament and Development*. New York: Brunner/Mazel.
8. McWilliam (2010) *Routines-Based Early Intervention: Supporting Young Children and Their Families*. Baltimore, MD: Paul H. Brookes Publishing Co.
9. Bart O, Rosenberg L, Ratzon NZ, Jarus T (2010). Development and initial validation of the Performance Skills Questionnaire (PSQ). *Res Dev Disabil* 31:46–56
10. Zeitlin S, Williamson GG, Szczepanski M (1988) *Early Coping Inventory*. Bensenville, IL: Scholastic Testing Service.
11. Hutton JB, Roberts TG (1990) *The Stress Impact Scale*. Austin, TX: Pro-Ed, Inc.
12. Rohrbeck CA, Azar ST, Wagner PE (1991) The Child Self-control Rating Scale: validation of a child self report. *J Child Psychol* 20: 179–183.
13. McDevitt SC, Carey WB (1978) Measurement of temperament in 3 to 7 year old children. *J Child Psychol Psychiatry* 19: 245–253.
14. Sytsma SE, Kelley ML, Wymer JH (2001) Development and initial validation of the Child Routines Inventory. *J Psychopathol Behav Assess* 23: 241–251.
15. Dise-Lewis JE (1988) The Life Events and Coping Inventory: an assessment of stress in children. *Psychosomat Med* 50: 484–499.
16. Tobin DL (1989) The hierarchical factor structure of the Coping Strategies Inventory. *Cogn Ther Res* 13: 343–361.
17. Romer GH (1993) Assessing stress in children: a literature review. Paper presented at the Mid-south Educational Research Association Conference, 9–12 November, New Orleans, Louisiana, pp. 1–17.
18. Pretzlik U, Sylva K (1999) Paediatric patients' distress and coping during medical treatment: a self report measure. *Arch Dis Child* 81: 525–527.
19. Zeitlin S, Williamson G (1990) Coping characteristics of disabled and nondisabled young children. *Am J Orthopsych* 60: 404–411.
20. Kendall P, Wilcox LE (1979). Self-control in children: development of a rating scale. *J Consult Clin Psychol* 47: 1020–1029.
21. Nowicki S, Strickland B (1973). A locus of control scale for children. *J Consult Clin Psychol* 40: 148–154.
22. Hughes S, Catania P, Derevensky JL, Dongier S, Boucher C (1997) The relationship between maternal psychiatric disorder and very young children's coping behaviours. *Infant Ment Health J* 18: 58–75.
23. Huntington GS, Simeonsson RJ (1987) Temperament characteristics of infants and toddlers with Down syndrome. *Child Care Health Dev* 13: 1–11.
24. Thomas A, Chess S (1977) *Temperament and Development*. New York: Brunner/Mazel.

22
COMMUNICATION (D310–D369)

Sharynne McLeod, Elspeth McCartney and Jane McCormack

What is the construct?

This chapter describes assessment of the activities and participation domain of communication (d3) as it relates to children and young people with developmental disabilities. In the International Classification of Functioning, Disability and Health for Children and Youth (ICF-CY), communication relates to 'general and specific features of communicating by language, signs and symbols…'[1] and encompasses the following: communicating – receiving (d310–d329); communicating – producing (d330–d349); and conversation and use of communication devices and techniques (d350–d369).

COMMUNICATING – RECEIVING (D310–D329)

Comprehending the messages produced by others is an essential element of successful communication. Messages may take a number of forms, both verbal and non-verbal, and successful comprehension involves being able to understand both literal and implied meanings expressed in those messages.[1] In infancy, successful comprehension is typically evaluated as an infant's ability to recognize and respond to the human voice (i.e. a spoken message) (d3100) with changes to breathing, gaze or movement. In childhood, comprehension of spoken messages is assessed as the ability to respond appropriately, with words or actions, to increasingly complex messages from basic commands or requests (d3101) through to questions and multistep instructions (d3102). As children develop, comprehension of other forms of messages (e.g. non-verbal messages, sign-language measures, written messages) may be evaluated as well.

COMMUNICATING – PRODUCING (D330–D349)

The ability to produce messages, whether in verbal or non-verbal forms, is the other essential element of communication. In infancy, the messages produced may be vocal, but may not consist of real words. Thus, children's vocalizations (pretalking) (d331) may be evaluated for communication intent (e.g. babbling when parent is close or during turn-taking activities). In childhood and adolescence, producing verbal messages may be evaluated through activities such as speaking (d330) and singing (d332), while the production of non-verbal messages may be assessed through examining the use of body language (e.g. facial gestures, body movements, postural changes) (d3350) and more formal sign language (d340), such as that used by children with hearing loss. In addition, children's production of non-verbal messages may be evaluated through examining their ability to convey meaning through activities such as producing signs and symbols (d3351) or drawings (d3352) and, for older children, producing written messages (d345).

CONVERSATION AND USE OF COMMUNICATION DEVICES AND TECHNIQUES (D350–D369)

Successful communication involves both receiving and producing messages, whether with familiar or unfamiliar people, with one person or several and in formal or informal settings. In conversation (d350), this reciprocity takes the form of an exchange of ideas, which may be evaluated through examining an individual's ability to initiate, sustain and terminate dialogue. In discussion (d355), the reciprocity takes the form of examination of matter, argument or debate. Both conversations and discussions may be carried out using verbal or non-verbal means, and both are activities that may be performed by children and young people. Other communication-based activities that may be evaluated involve the use of communication devices such as telephones (d3600), computers (d3601) and use of communication techniques (e.g. lip reading) (d3602). Some people require the use of specific assistive products and technology for communication (e1251) if they are unable to speak.[2]

When measuring the domain of communication (d3), it is important to consider both an individual's communicative *capacity* and communicative *performance*. Capacity refers to the ability to execute a task or an action and so aims to indicate 'the highest probable level of functioning that a person may reach in a given domain at a given moment'.[1,3] According to the World Health Organization (WHO), capacity is measured in a 'uniform or standard environment', and thus 'reflects the environmentally adjusted ability of the individual'.[1,3] In contrast, *performance* refers to 'what an individual does in his or her current environment...' (and) can be understood as 'involvement in a life situation'.[1,3] Evaluation of communicative performance considers children's communication skills in the context in which they live, and so also takes into account their performance with any assistive devices they typically use or personal assistance that they have.

General factors to consider when measuring this domain

ASSESSING CAPACITY VERSUS ASSESSING PERFORMANCE

The difference between a child's capacity and his or her performance reflects the difference between his or her skills in a standardized environment versus his or her everyday environment.[1] Previous researchers have described the limited availability of tools to explore the communication domain in the activities and participation component.[4] Our understanding of the capacity and performance qualifiers leads us to agree that there are few tools available to assess *performance*, but also to suggest that there are a number available to assess *capacity*. As capacity refers to a child's ability to execute an action in a standard environment, communicative capacity may be measured by standardized tools. Many standardized assessments of communication measure the functions underlying communication (e.g. voice and speech functions [b3] or specific mental functions of language [b167]), as well as the outcome of these functions: communication and conversation. Thus, the tools described in relevant body functions chapters (b167, 'Specific mental functions of language', Chapter 12 in this text; and b3, 'Voice and speech functions', Chapter 15) also apply to the assessment of communication capacity. The rules for administration of standardized tools (such as the *Clinical Evaluation of Language Fundamentals, fourth edition*[5] or the *Diagnostic Evaluation of Articulation and Phonology*[6]) are intended to limit the influence of environmental factors so as to ensure that the test context is uniform or standard, regardless of the child participating

in the assessment. Consequently, these tools enable professionals to determine a child's ability to execute activities without strategies, prompts, cues or devices to assist; that is, to determine a child's 'true ability'.[3]

The measurement of communicative capacity focuses on the skills of the individual, and, as stated, contrasts with the measurement of communicative performance, which takes into account environmental factors such as the impact of the physical, attitudinal and social world on children's communication-based activities and participation. Tools available to assess communication capacity are described elsewhere (see Chapters 12 and 15) and so will not be a focus of the current chapter, which will concentrate on the limited number of assessments that explore children's performance of communication activities in their everyday environments (see 'Overview of recommended measures', below).

The WHO[3] suggested that comparing capacity and performance 'provides a useful guide as to what can be done to the environment of the individual to improve performance'. One way to examine what can be done to improve performance is to assess a child's ability to execute an activity in a standard environment, but with assistance. For children with developmental disabilities, dynamic assessment provides one way to examine capacity with assistance. Dynamic assessment involves evaluating a child's ability to execute activities when provided with additional cues or information; that is, when the linguistic context is modified. This contrasts with static, standardized assessments, when adult input is minimized and the environment stays constant.[7] There is a range of dynamic assessment techniques (e.g. scaffolding, test–teach–retest) for children with developmental disabilities (e.g. autism, Down syndrome, language impairment)[8] as well as for children from culturally and linguistically diverse backgrounds.[9,10] It has been suggested that dynamic assessments reveal 'learning potential' rather than simply measuring skills, and provide direction about the best ways to help children achieve potential and facilitate the transfer of skills to other environments.[11]

ASSESSING COMMUNICATION ACTIVITIES VERSUS ASSESSING LIFE ACTIVITIES

It is important to recognize that successful communication encompasses many ICF-CY chapters beyond communication (d3). Other activity and participation domains should be considered simultaneously when evaluating communication in order to avoid 'ignoring the effect that a communication disability may have on all areas of life'.[12] Indeed, Eadie et al[4] stated: 'Although specific communication acts are found in the third chapter of the ICF-CY manual, communication is a construct that is pervasive and is required to fulfil other aspects of participation found in most of the other chapters (e.g. communication involved in job performance, academic performance, self-care, community roles, establishing and maintaining relationships)'. For example, activities and participation that may be difficult for children with speech impairment (b320) identified in a recent systematic review[13] include learning to read (d140), reading (d166), learning to write (d145), writing (d170), focusing attention (d160), thinking (d163), calculating (d172), mobility (d4), self-care (d5), interpersonal interactions and relationships (d7), relating with persons in authority (d7400), informal relationships with friends/peers (d7500/d7504), parent–child relationships (d7600), sibling relationships (d7602), major life areas (d8), school education (d820), and acquiring, keeping and terminating a job (d845) in addition to communication (d3).[13,14]

Holistic assessment of communication skills incorporates assessment of the full range of activities and participation domains, along with consideration of all other ICF-CY components. Researchers have identified that assessment data are most useful (in terms of determining eligibility for services, developing intervention plans and evaluating treatment effects) when information about impairments of body structures and functions are considered in association with functional abilities and limitations.[15,16]

Overview of recommended measures
Several measures to assess children's communicative performance have been created, including some which use the ICF-CY as a guiding framework. This review will focus on five recent measures. These measures have been selected for inclusion in this chapter because they rely on different communicative partners (speech–language pathologists [SLPs], parents and teachers) assessing the child's communication performance in typical everyday contexts. The perspectives of parents may well differ from the perspectives of professionals.[17,18] Additionally, the perspectives of children regarding their communication performance, areas of strength and difficulty, potential need for assistance and goals for intervention may well differ from adults.[19] Thus, in the evaluation of communicative performance, it is important to consider the range of different perspectives that may exist. Additional measures are presented in summary tables throughout this chapter. Some of the measures evaluate the communication performance of children and young people with specific communication impairments (e.g. speech impairment/speech sound disorder, voice disorder or stuttering), while other measures may be used for a range of populations.

SPEECH–LANGUAGE PATHOLOGIST – REPORT MEASURES
Speech–language pathologists are professionals specializing in the area of communication, and have traditionally focused assessment and intervention plans on functions underlying communication (e.g. body functions and structures, including voice and speech functions and mental functions of language) or communicative capacity – components which are more concrete and easier to test objectively than other components.[4,20–22] However, the success (or otherwise) of a child's communication may be judged by his or her communication performance; that is, his or her ability to engage in the full range of life activities in which he or she wishes to take part in his or her everyday environment. The Therapy Outcome Measures (TOMs) is an assessment tool developed for use by professionals as a way of evaluating communication performance. The TOMs are described in more detail below. The Focus on the Outcomes of Communication Under Six (FOCUS) is another tool that may be used by professionals to evaluate a child's ability to communicate and participate in a range of activities (see summary table), while tools such as the American Sign Language Proficiency Assessment (ASL-PA)[23] and Profile of Multiple Language Proficiencies (PMLP)[24] provide this information specifically for children with hearing loss.

Therapy outcome measures

Overview and purpose
The TOMs[25] were developed as a pre- and post-therapy measure to reflect outcomes in the WHO's ICF categories of impairment, activity and participation. In addition, they use a construct entitled 'well-being/distress', which aims to capture 'emotions, feelings, burden of upset, concern and anxiety and level of satisfaction with the condition'.[25] There are individual TOM scales for a variety of clinical conditions (including speech, language, voice and fluency), and also a core scale that may be adapted for any client. The TOMs have been adapted for use in Australian clinical practice (AusTOMs).[26]

Administration and scoring
The child's SLP assesses impairment, activity, participation and well-being/distress based on his or her knowledge of the child. Severity on each is scaled from 0 (most severe/profound) to 5 (appropriate for the child's age and culture) using the best fit from a series of illustrative descriptors. Half-way points on the 0 to 5 scale give an 11-point ordinal scale.

THERAPY OUTCOME MEASURES (TOMs)	
Purpose	Published standardized protocol
	Aims to assess outcomes in the World Health Organization International Classification of Functioning, Disability and Health categories of body function and activity and participation, and assess 'well-being/distress'. May be used as an outcome measure
Population	Any child client
Description of domains (subscales)	Domains not specified. One scale for each functional impairment, e.g. phonological disorder, dysarthria, dysfluency, dysphonia
Administration and test format	Time to complete: around 10min
	Testing format: speech–language pathologist (SLP) evaluates impairment, activity, participation and well-being/distress based on his or her knowledge of the child
	Scoring: 11-point ordinal severity scale ranging from 0 to 5, where 0 is most severe/profound and 5 is appropriate for the child's age and culture (half-way points may be used). SLP selects the best fit from the descriptors provided
	Training: designed for SLPs; training within SLP services recommended
Psychometric properties	No normative sample
	Reliability
	Inter-rater: SLPs working in the same service: Spearman's correlations for impairment 0.84–0.94; activity 0.77–0.91; participation 0.71–0.91; well-being/distress 0.70–0.93. No across-service information
	Validity
	Face validity: specialist SLPs involved in constructing the descriptors:
	Construct: TOMs Impairment Scale Spearman's correlation –0.50 with speech production scores, both computed by the same SLP
	Responsiveness
	No information retrieved
How to order	Available in Enderby et al (2006).
Key references	Enderby P, John A, Petheram B (2006) *Therapy Outcome Measures for Rehabilitation Professionals*: *Speech and Language Therapy, Physiotherapy, Occupational Therapy*, 2nd edition. Chichester: John Wiley & Sons.
	Roulstone S, John A, Hughes A, Enderby P (2004) Assessing the construct validity of the Therapy Outcome Measure for pre-school children with delayed speech and language. *Int J Speech Lang Pathol* 6: 230–236.

Psychometric properties

Reliability studies carried out by SLPs are reviewed in the manual. A total of 80 SLPs working with children in six UK national health services were included. SLPs were trained on TOMs procedures using their own clients as examples, and then rated videotapes and case history data. SLPs working for the same service showed inter-rater reliability Spearman's correlations for impairment were 0.84 to 0.94; activity 0.77 to 0.91; participation 0.71 to 0.91; and well-being/distress 0.70 to 0.93. No service descriptions are provided. Training within services to establish reliability is recommended in the manual.

Face validity was established by specialist SLPs contributing to the content of the scales' descriptors using Delphi techniques and comparing TOMs results with their own observations. Construct validity was tested by SLPs completing a TOMs scale and a range of communication measures for children under 3 years of age involved in

FOCUS ON THE OUTCOMES OF COMMUNICATION UNDER SIX (FOCUS)	
Purpose	To measure 'real world' outcomes of communication interventions (i.e. a child's ability to communicate and participate in the community)
Population	Preschool children (<6y)
Description of domains (subscales)	50 items (statements) in two parts: Part I requires respondents to identify how well items describe the child (e.g. 'My child talks a lot'). Part II requires respondents to identify the amount of cueing required by the child to complete items (e.g. 'My child will sit and listen to stories')
Administration and test format	Two versions (one for parents and one for clinicians) containing identical items FOCUS items are rated at the start and completion of intervention and a difference between the ratings indicates change Time to complete: around 10min Testing format: parent/clinician responds to written statements Scoring: seven-item Likert scales. For Part I, responses range from 'not at all like my child' to 'exactly like my child'. For Part II, responses range from 'cannot do at all' to 'can always do without help' to evaluate the level of assistance required to complete items successfully Training: no training required
Psychometric properties	Scale development sample: no normative comparisons are available owing to the nature of the measure. Testing of the measure occurred with 165 families of children (mean age 3.8y, standard deviation 0.91y, range 1.2–5.5y) attending speech and language services (and their clinicians). 72% (n=119) of participants were males, 13% (n=22) had specific medical diagnoses (including autistic spectrum disorders, cerebral palsy and Down syndrome). Most participants had developmental speech disorders (80%) or expressive language disorders (72%) *Reliability* Internal consistency: clinicians' internal consistency was high at the start of treatment (Cronbach's alpha 0.97) and completion (Cronbach's alpha 0.94). Test–retest – parents' test–retest correlation was high (r>0.95), and clinicians' test–retest correlation was acceptable (r>0.70). Rater – inter-rater reliability has been established as high (r>0.90) for both Part I and Part II of the FOCUS *Validity* Content validity: FOCUS items were derived and worded from prospective observations of change as reported by parents and clinicians of 210 preschool children. The FOCUS measure was developed and tested with parents and clinicians of an additional 165 children. Constructs used in the FOCUS measure were derived from the ICF and respondents reported that they accurately captured children's communication skills Construct validity: 22 parents also completed the Pediatric Quality of Life Inventory (PedsQL) at the start and completion of intervention. Children with higher FOCUS scores after treatment also had higher PedsQL scores (r=0.47, p=0.029) Correlation with PedsQL: psychosocial domain was particularly strong (r=0.49, p=0.013) *Responsiveness* The FOCUS is currently undergoing validity testing to establish its responsiveness to change
How to order	FOCUS items are listed in the journal article (below) describing its development. The user version of the FOCUS is available from www.hollandbloorview.ca/research/FOCUS/index.php

| Key reference | Thomas-Stonell N, Oddson B, Robertson B, Rosenbaum P (2010) Development of the FOCUS (Focus on Outcomes of Communication Under Six): a communication outcome measure for preschool children. *Dev Med Child Neurol* 52: 47–53. |

a large trial,[27] including 27 children with predominately speech difficulties. The TOMs impairment scale showed a highly significant Spearman's correlation of –0.50 with phonology error scores, although both were computed by the child's SLP. The result gives some support to the construct validity of the TOMs impairment scale for this client group. Lubinski et al[28] note, however, that SLP-gathered treatment outcomes of this type could be viewed as potentially biased and present less good evidence than even professional consensus opinion.

PARENT-REPORT MEASURES

Parents have unique knowledge of their children and can provide insights into their children's communication performance in their everyday environment. There is an increasing number of measures available to assess the perspective of parents regarding their children's communication skills. Some of these, such as the Pediatric Voice Handicap Index (pVHI)[29] (see description below), Intelligibility in Context Scale (ICS)[30] and the Parents' Evaluation of Aural/Oral Performance of Children (PEACH)[31] (see summary chart) focus solely on the perspective of parents. However, other measures, such as the FOCUS[32] (see summary chart), enable a comparison of the perspectives of parents and others. Some measures have determined the different perspectives of parents and professionals. For example, the Communication Function Classification System[33] for individuals with cerebral palsy is a validated measure of communicative function informed by the ICF-CY, and has been determined to have good professional inter-rater reliability and moderate parent–professional inter-rater reliability.[33]

Pediatric Voice Handicap Index

Overview and purpose

The adult version of the VHI[29] is a self-assessment quality of life measure for dysphonic clients, with items derived from case history interviews. The VHI assesses severity of functional, physical and emotional impacts of voice impairment. A revised and shortened adult version (VHI-10) is also available. The paediatric version (pVHI) was derived from the adult VHI as a proxy version to be completed by parents or carers of a child with voice dysfunction.[29]

Administration and scoring

The pVHI is a questionnaire for parents/carers who rate their child's overall talkativeness and then rate 23 descriptions of functional, physical and emotional aspects of voice on five-point subscales. A total score is also computed.

Psychometric properties

The adult VHI met the HSTAT 52 reliability and validity criteria,[34] and in a further study met seven of 11 criteria and was the preferred measure in relation to item information, practicality and reliability, thus supporting its clinical use.[35] The pVHI was standardized[29] on 45 parents of children aged 3 to 12 years with no history of voice dysfunction, and 33 parents/guardians of dysphonic children aged 4 to 21 years awaiting or following laryngotracheal reconstruction. Test–retest reliability was established by 10 parents of dysphonic children who received no intervening treatment, repeating the assessment within 3 weeks: Pearson's coefficients 0.95 (functional), 0.77 (physical), 0.79 (emotional), 0.82 (total).

Mean scores differentiated dysphonic from non-dysphonic children – means for dysphonic children were 13.94 (functional), 15.48 (physical), 12.15 (emotional) and 41.58 (total); means for non-dysphonic children were 1.47 (functional), 0.20 (physical), 0.18 (emotional) and 1.84 (total), suggesting little overlap in scores and therefore construct validity. Correlations between subscales ranged from 0.59 (functional and physical) to 0.86 (functional and emotional). A moderate correlation was obtained between parent report of severity on a visual analogue scale and the pVHI total score. A systematic review[36] including pVHI agreed validity and reliability criteria were met, but no responsiveness data were given. The review noted that in common with other instruments adapted from existing adult measures for paediatric use, the pVHI was constructed by eliminating items not relevant to children rather than establishing items that were specifically relevant to quality of life in childhood. The use of such instruments as outcome measures is limited by this factor.

CHILD-REPORT MEASURES

According to the United Nations Convention on the Rights of the Child, children ought to be asked about their views on issues that concern them, and their views should be given due consideration.[37] A recent book documented methodologies for listening to children and young

PARENTS' EVALUATION OF AURAL/ORAL PERFORMANCE OF CHILDREN (PEACH) SCALE	
Purpose	To evaluate the oral and aural abilities in daily life of infants and children with hearing impairment using parent observations
Population	Infants (aged 1mo) through to school-aged children
Description of domains (subscales)	11-item questionnaire for assessing functional auditory performance in everyday life Two subscales: six items examine children's auditory performance in 'quiet' situations (e.g. respond to name in quiet, respond to verbal instructions in quiet); five items examine children's auditory performance in 'noise' (e.g. respond to name in noise, respond to verbal instructions in noise)
Administration and test format	Time to complete: questionnaire is completed by parents (approximately 10min) based on child's behaviour during the previous week Testing format: if the PEACH were used to evaluate aided performance, parents are requested to check that their children use hearing devices for >50% of their waking hours, and that the use of devices does not lead to loudness discomfort. Parents then rate the frequency (never: 0%, seldom: 1–25%, sometimes: 26–50%, often: 51–75%, always: 75–100%) with which their children display behaviours in different real-life scenarios described in the questionnaire. Parents may be interviewed regarding their responses on the questionnaire. The interviewer (speech–language pathologist or audiologist) scores questionnaire items on the basis of parent reports and interviews Scoring: five-item scales (0=never, no examples of behaviour given; 1=seldom, 2=sometimes; 3=often; 4=almost always, more than six examples given or behaviour reported more than 75% of time). The PEACH scale provides an overall score, a 'quiet' and 'noise' subscale score based on subsets of items. A comparative score, on a five-point scale, is also available when the PEACH is used for comparing performance in two conditions Training: speech–language pathologist/audiologist required to interview and score PEACH
Psychometric properties	Scale Development Sample: parents of 90 children with normal hearing (mean age 13.4mo; standard deviation [SD] 11.4mo; range 0.25–46.0mo) and 90 children with hearing impairment (mean age 95.6mo; SD 64.0mo; range 4.0mo–19.8y). Hearing status of children with normal hearing was ascertained by a pass at newborn hearing screening or a pass in visual reinforcement audiometry. No children with normal hearing had any known history of ear/hearing problems. Children with hearing impairments varied in degree of hearing loss (mild to profound) and type of amplification used (seven unaided, two with unilateral hearing aids, 65 with bilateral hearing aids, 16 with hearing aid and cochlear implant in opposite ears). Children with known disabilities (in addition to hearing loss) were excluded *Reliability* Internal consistency: factor analysis revealed moderate reliability of items in the 'quiet' subscale (Cronbach's alpha 0.76) and 'noise' subscale (Cronbach's alpha 0.79). The correlation between the quiet and noise subscales was 0.85 ($p<0.001$). Test–retest: the PEACH was re-administered within 2–4 weeks to a subsample of parents (15 had children with normal hearing; 17 with hearing impairment). Test–retest correlation was high for all scales: overall: $r=0.93$; quiet: $r=0.81$; noise: $r=0.93$. Rater: inter-rater reliability has been established as high ($r=0.95$, $p<0.001$) for the overall score on the PEACH *Validity* Content validity: the PEACH focuses on aural/oral behaviours in real-life speech communication situations, as the goal of amplification is to ensure audibility for speech input. Professionals including teachers of the deaf, early intervention teachers, and audiologists contributed to the design of the items. Construct validity: functional performance in real life as measured by the PEACH was significantly correlated with auditory comprehension and expressive communication as measured by the Pre-school Language Scale (Ching et al, 2010)

	Sensitivity
	The sensitivity of the PEACH scale to differences in amplification strategies has been shown in Ching et al (2008)
How to order	The PEACH questionnaire has been modified for use with teachers (TEACH) and for children to self-report their listening function (SELF). All three questionnaires and score forms can be freely downloaded from the Australian National Acoustics Laboratory website: www.outcomes.nal.gov.au. The key references (below) also contain questionnaire items as appendices
Key references	Ching TYC, Hill M (2007) The Parents' Evaluation of Aural/Oral Performance of Children (PEACH) Scale: normative data. *J Am Acad Audiol* 18: 220–235.
	Ching TYC, Hill M, Dillon H (2008) Effect of variations in hearing aid frequency response on real-life functional performance of children with severe or profound hearing loss. *Int J Audiol* 47: 461–475.
	Ching TYC, Crowe K, Martin V, et al (2010) Language development and everyday functioning of children with hearing loss assessed at 3 years of age. *Int J Speech Lang Pathol* 12: 124–131.

PEDIATRIC VOICE HANDICAP INDEX (pVHI)

Purpose	Standardized questionnaire, derived from the adult VHI
	A quality-of-life self-assessment for dysphonic clients that aims to assess functional, physical and emotional impacts of voice disorder and provide a proxy quality of life measure via parents or carers of a child with voice dysfunction. May be used as an outcome measure
Population	Standardized on dysphonic children aged ≥3y
Description of domains (subscales)	Seven domains/five subscales: talkativeness (one item); functional (seven items); physical (nine items); emotional (seven items); and overall severity (one item)
Administration and test format	Time taken to complete: estimated 5–10min
	Testing format: questionnaire for parents/carers, who rate the child's overall talkativeness, and 23 descriptions of functional, physical and emotional impact of voice disorder
	Scoring: five- to seven-point rating scales for talkativeness, and functional, physical and emotional scales (subscale and total scores). There is a visual analogue scale for severity
	Training: none required
Psychometric properties	Normative sample: 45 parents of children aged 3–12y with no history of voice dysfunction. 33 parents/guardians of dysphonic children aged 4–21y awaiting/following laryngotracheal reconstruction
	Reliability
	Test–retest: Pearson's coefficients 0.95 (functional), 0.77 (physical), 0.79 (emotional), 0.82 (total)
	Validity
	Subscales correlated from 0.59 (functional with physical) to 0.86 (functional with emotional). Moderate correlation for total score with severity. Scores differentiated dysphonic from non-dysphonic children
	Responsiveness: no information retrieved
How to order	Information can be found in Zur KB, Cotton S, Kelchner, Baker S, Weinrich B, Lee L (2007) Paediatric Voice Handicap Index (pVHI): a new tool for evaluating paediatric dysphonia. *Int J Pediatr Otorhinolaryng* 71: 77–82.

Key references	Branski RC, Cukier-Blaj S, Pusic A, et al (2010) Measuring quality of life in dysphonic patients: a systematic review of content development in patient-reported outcomes measures. *J Voice* 24: 193–198.
	Franic DM, Bramlett RE, Bothe AC (2005) Psychometric evaluation of disease specific quality of life instruments in voice disorders. *J Voice* 19: 300–315.

people with speech, language and communication needs.[38] Although it may be difficult to establish the views of very young children when reliant solely on verbal measures, their views can be investigated using other modes. For instance, researchers have recommended that drawings can be used as a way of enabling children to express themselves and enabling others to access children's perspectives.[19,39,40] In addition, self-report measures have recently been developed for children with speech impairments (e.g. Speech Participation and Activity Assessment of Children [SPAA-C[22]]) and dysfluency (e.g. the Behavior Assessment Battery for School-age Children who Stutter[41] [BAB]) to determine their perspective regarding their communication performance. The SPAA-C will be reviewed in the next section; the dysfluency measures are described in further detail below.

Behavior Assessment Battery for School-age Children who Stutter

Overview and purpose

The BAB[41] aims to investigate the personal views of children aged 6 years and over concerning their fluency-associated emotional, disruptive, coping and attitudinal reactions. Children decide if statements about speech and fluency apply to them. There are three separate scales to offer a multidimensional view: the Speech Situation Checklist (SSC); the Behavior Checklist; and the Communication Attitude Test (CAT). Responses index activity and participation in communication, particularly conversation, interpersonal interactions and relationships, and education.

The SSC has two independent subscales: emotional reactions (ER), measuring a child's reported emotional reactions to speech situations; and speech disruption, measuring the amount of difficulty a child perceives when talking in a range of different situations. The Behavior Checklist details the child's conscious avoidance behaviours when anticipating a moment of stuttering, and so is not a measure of activity or participation. The CAT measures a child's negative and positive beliefs about his or her speech ability.

Administration and scoring

The scales are administered by the child's SLP, who reads statements for the child to evaluate, or supports older children as they read the statements themselves. Responses are true or false or semantically scaled, and are summed and compared with the mean and standard deviation for children in the standardization sample who did and did not stutter.

Psychometric properties

The standardization sample comprised 578 children aged 6 to 13 years with no history of stuttering and 139 stuttering children. Mean scores for children who stuttered were systematically and significantly lower in all subscales than those who did not, but the distributions overlap.[41]

An evaluation of instruments measuring health-related quality of life in children and adults who stuttered[42] included versions of the SSC-ER subscale and the CAT. The CAT met stringent criteria for internal consistency and test–retest reliability, but not content validity measures, as some questions did not relate to health-related quality of life. The SSC-ER addressed only mental functioning, and so failed the strict content validity criterion as a quality of life measure, and also failed strict test–retest criteria.

As the CAT differentiated children who stuttered from those who did not, the review's authors considered that its ability to differentiate stuttering from typical fluency suggested it would be responsive to major changes in a child over time, but no data were collected. Additionally, no data were available on longitudinal responsiveness. The authors recommended the 'cautious' use of the CAT scale as the best available measure for group-level decision-making for dysfluent children in the absence of a more psychometrically sound measure. Studies of children with speech difficulties other than stuttering (reviewed by Johannisson et al[43]) suggested that the CAT also differentiated among children with voice, speech and fluency disorders.

BEHAVIOR ASSESSMENT BATTERY FOR SCHOOL-AGE CHILDREN WHO STUTTER (BAB)	
Purpose	Published standardized assessment
	Aims to investigate the child's personal views concerning their fluency-associated emotional, disruptive, coping and attitudinal reactions. May be used as an outcome measure
Population	Children ≥6y who stutter
Description of domains (subscales)	Five domains/four subscales: Behaviour Checklist (BC); Communication Attitude Test (CAT); emotional reactions (ER); speech disruption (SD)
Administration and test format	Time to complete: estimated 8–9min
	Testing format: child evaluates statements read by speech–language pathologist (SLP)/child
	Scoring: True/false or semantic scale. Scores are compared with norms from stuttering (stammering) and non-stuttering children
	Training: designed for SLPs
Psychometric properties	Normative sample: 578 children aged 6–13y with no history of stuttering and 139 stuttering children
	Reliability
	CAT scales meet stringent criteria for test–retest reliability and internal consistency. ER fails strict test–retest criteria
	Validity
	Mean scores for children who stutter are lower in all subscales than for non-stuttering children, but distributions overlap. CAT scale addresses quality of life, but not all items are relevant to this construct. ER addresses only mental functioning, and so fails a strict content validity criterion as a quality of life measure.
	Responsiveness: no longitudinal data retrieved
How to order	Available in Brutten G, Vanryckeghem M (2006) *Behaviour Assessment Battery for School-age Children who Stutter*. San Diego, CA: Plural Publishing.
Key references	Franic DM, Bothe AK (2008) Psychometric evaluation of condition-specific instruments used to assess health-related quality of life, attitudes, and related constructs in stuttering. *Am J Speech Lang Pathol* 17: 60–80.

Communication Attitude Test for Pre-school and Kindergarten Children who Stutter

Overview and purpose
Stuttering frequently manifests in the preschool years. The KiddyCAT (CAT for Pre-school and Kindergarten Children who Stutter)[44] investigates the communication attitudes of children (3–6y) who stutter in relation to their communication skills. It is a downward extension of the CAT, one of the subtests in the BAB[41] (described in the preceding section).

Administration and scoring
The SLP asks the child 12 questions relating to stuttering, recording a 'yes' or 'no' answer. Responses are summed and compared with the mean and standard deviation for children in the standardization sample who did and did not stutter.

Psychometric properties
A standardization sample was composed of 63 children aged 3 to 6 years with no history of stuttering and 45 stuttering children. Mean scores for children who stuttered were systematically and significantly lower in all subscales than for those who did not, but distributions overlapped. Split-half reliability measures report Cronbach's alpha as

COMMUNICATION ATTITUDE TEST FOR PRESCHOOL AND KINDERGARTEN CHILDREN WHO STUTTER (KIDDYCAT)	
Purpose	Published standardized assessment. A downward age extension of the CAT subscale of the Behaviour Assessment Battery for School-Age Children who Stutter (BAB). Aims to assess talk-associated attitudes of preschool children. May be used as an outcome measure
Population	Children aged 3–6y who stutter
Description of domains (subscales)	Two domains/one scale (12 items)
Administration and test format	Time to complete: estimated 5–10min
	Testing format: speech–language pathologist asks the child 12 yes/no questions about talking
	Scoring: true/false. Total score is compared with norms from stuttering (stammering) and non-stuttering children
	Training: designed for use by speech–language pathologists
Psychometric properties	Normative sample: 63 children aged 3–6y with no history of stuttering and 45 stuttering children
	Reliability
	Split-half Cronbach's alpha 0.72 for non-stuttering children, 0.75 for children who stutter
	Test–retest: no information retrieved
	Validity
	Mean scores for children who stutter are lower in all subscales than for non-stuttering children, but distributions overlap. Reports criterion and construct validity measures based on studies of the CAT (above)
	Responsiveness: no longitudinal data retrieved
How to order	Available in Vanryckeghem M, Brutten G (2006) *KiddyCAT: Communication Attitude Test for Preschool and Kindergarten Children who Stutter*. San Diego, CA: Plural Publishing.
Key reference	Brutten G, Vanryckeghem M (2006) *Behaviour Assessment Battery for School-age Children who Stutter*. San Diego, CA: Plural Publishing.

0.72 for non-stuttering children and as 0.75 for children who stutter, suggesting internal consistency. Test–retest reliability measures are not given. The KiddyCAT reports criterion-related and construct validity measures based on studies of the CAT (see above).

MEASURES OF MULTIPLE PERSPECTIVES (INCLUDING CHILD-, TEACHER- AND FRIEND-REPORT)
There may be a number of 'significant others', such as a child's teacher or friends, who can also provide valuable information about their communication performance during a range of communication-based activities in everyday contexts. The perspective of teachers and friends regarding the communication performance of a child with

speech impairment may be obtained through the use of measures such as the SPAA-C[22] (described below) and ICS,[30] which both also enable comparison with parent perspectives. Other measures which provide information about the communication of children with specific difficulties include the teacher version of the PEACH,[31] the Teachers' Evaluation of Aural/Oral Performance of Children (TEACH),[45] which investigates teachers' perspectives of the communication performance of children with hearing loss, and the Peer Attitudes Toward Children who Stutter,[46] which explores the communication skills of children with fluency difficulties from the perspective of their friends.

SPEECH PARTICIPATION AND ACTIVITY OF CHILDREN: VERSION 2.0 (SPAA-C2)	
Purpose	Preliminary development of semi-structured interview protocol
	Aims to evaluate aspects of activity and participation relevant to children with speech impairments and support the planning of intervention to impact upon a child's whole life
Population	Children with speech impairment and their parents, teachers, friends, siblings and others, as appropriate
Description of domains (subscales)	Four domains/one scale: 5–27 items, according to respondent category
Administration and test format	Time to complete: interviews 10min upwards. Transcription and content analysis time not retrieved
	Testing format: semi-structured interview with the child and/or relevant others
	Scoring: scaled responses to 10 child items (and field notes)
	Training: designed for speech–language pathologists (SLPs)
Psychometric properties	Normative sample: no normative comparisons retrieved
	Reliability
	No data retrieved
	Validity
	Content validity: >200 SLPs involved in the construction of the questionnaire. Thematic analysis identified four major themes relevant to sibling experience and three major themes relevant to children with speech impairment and their parents
	Responsiveness
	No information retrieved
How to order	Provided as an appendix in McLeod S (2004) Speech pathologists' application of the ICF to children with speech impairment. *Int J Speech Lang Pathol* 6: 75–81.
Key references	Barr J, McLeod S, Daniel G (2008) Siblings of children with speech impairment: cavalry on the hill. *Lang Speech Hear Serv School* 39: 21–32.
	McCormack J, McLeod S, McAllister L, Harrison LJ (2010) My speech problem, your listening problem, and my frustration: the experience of living with childhood speech impairment. *Lang Speech Hear Serv School* 41: 379–392.

Speech Participation and Activity Assessment of Children: Version 2.0

Overview and purpose

The SPAA-C[22] is a preliminary attempt to evaluate aspects of activity and participation relevant to children with speech impairments and to plan intervention that impacts upon the child's whole life. It comprises semi-structured interview schedules for children with speech impairment and/or their friends, siblings, parents, teachers and relevant others, as appropriate. It was developed by over 200 SLPs during a conference and refined at a separate workshop. The questions derive from attendees' collected narratives about the impact of communication impairment with a focus on child speech difficulties. Activity, participation, and environmental and personal factors were considered in constructing questions. Further SLP professional critique was undertaken to derive the second version (Version 2.0).

Administration and scoring

Semi-structured interviews (lasting from 10 minutes to 1 hour) are carried out, depending upon the number of participants being interviewed at one time and the age of the interviewee – child interviews are shorter than adult interviews.[19,47] Friends, siblings and relevant others are asked five or six questions about the child, such as what they like about them, what they like doing together, what the child has trouble with and what the interviewee does if he or she does not understand the child's speech. Questions to the child's siblings and friends are broad and do not directly mention speech, in order to avoid affecting children's relationships with each other, although there is opportunity to discuss speech skills. Questions for the child with speech impairment, parents and teachers do overtly invite responses about speech and the impact of speech difficulty. The child with the speech impairment is asked up to 27 questions about his or her preferences, friends, school or preschool and talking. Included are 10 questions on how they feel about talking in a variety of contexts, scaled using cartoon 'smiley faces' indicating 'happy', 'in the middle', 'sad', 'another feeling' or 'do not know'. Parents are asked 20 questions about their child, their child's speech and the impact of the speech difficulty, including questions about exclusion, limits to

participation and responses. Teachers are asked up to 19 questions about the child's school participation and talk in class.

Psychometric properties

Over 200 SLPs were involved in constructing the SPAA-C.[22] The SPAA-C is a semi-structured interview to obtain standard descriptive information, but is not scored. It is designed to elicit qualitative information with maximum flexibility, and no information on psychometric properties has been published, although work is ongoing. Activity, participation, and environmental and personal factors are not distinguished. When the SPAA-C was used to examine the experience of preschool children with speech impairment[19] and siblings of children with speech impairment,[47] the data elicited could be coded reliably and thematic analysis could be used to identify major themes relevant to their experiences.

ACKNOWLEDGEMENT

The first author acknowledges support from the Australian Research Council Future Fellowship (FT0990588) and the third author acknowledges support from The Sir Robert Menzies Memorial Research Scholarship in the Allied Health Sciences.

REFERENCES

1. World Health Organization (2007) *International Classification of Functioning, Disability and Health – Children and Youth Version.* Geneva: WHO.
2. Raghavendra P, Bornman J, Granlund M, Björck-Åkesson E (2007) The World Health Organization's International Classification of Functioning, Disability and Health: implications for clinical and research practice in the field of augmentative and alternative communication. *Aug Alt Comm* 23: 349–361.
3. World Health Organization (2001) *International Classification of Functioning, Disability and Health.* Geneva: WHO.
4. Eadie TL, Yorkston KM, Klasner ER, et al (2006) Measuring communicative participation: a review of self-report instruments in speech–language pathology. *Am J Speech Lang Pathol* 15: 307–320.
5. Semel WA, Wiig EH, Secord WA (2003) *Clinical Evaluation of Language Fundamentals – Fourth Edition.* San Antonio, TX: The Psychological Cooperation.
6. Dodd B, Hua Z, Crosbie S, Holm A, Ozanne A (2002) *Manual of Diagnostic Evaluation of Articulation and Phonology (DEAP).* London: Psychological Corporation.
7. Donaldson AL, Olswang LB (2007) Investigating requests for information in children with autism spectrum disorders: static versus dynamic assessment. *Int J Sp Lang Pathol* 9: 297–311.
8. Law J, Camilleri B, editors (2007) Special issue: Dynamic assessment. *Int J Sp Lang Pathol* 9(4).
9. Laing SP, Kamhi A (2003) Alternative assessment of language and literacy in culturally and linguistically diverse populations. *Lang Speech Hear Serv Sch* 34: 44–55.
10. Peña E, Iglesias A, Lidz CS (2001) Reducing test bias through dynamic assessment of children's word learning ability. *Am J Speech Lang Pathol* 10: 138–154.
11. Law J, Camilleri B (2007) Dynamic assessment and its application to children with speech and language learning difficulties. *Int J Sp Lang Pathol* 9: 271–272.
12. Worrall L, Hickson L (2008) The use of the ICF in speech–language pathology research: towards a research agenda. *Int J Speech Lang Pathol* 10: 72–77.
13. McCormack J, McLeod S, McAllister L, Harrison LJ (2009) A systematic review of the association between childhood speech impairment and participation across the lifespan. *Int J Sp Lang Pathol* 11: 155–170.
14. Teverovsky EG, Bickel JO, Feldman HM (2009) Functional characteristics of children diagnosed with childhood apraxia of speech. *Dis Rehab* 31: 94–102.
15. Lollar DJ, Simeonsson RJ (2005) Diagnosis to function: classification for children and youths. *J Dev Beh Pediatr* 26: 323–330.
16. Reed GM, Lux JB, Bufka LF, et al (2005) Operationalizing the International Classification of Functioning, Disability and Health in clinical settings. *Rehab Psych* 50: 122–131.
17. McCormack J, McLeod S, Harrison LJ, McAllister L (2010) The impact of speech impairment in early childhood: investigating parents' and speech–language pathologists' perspectives using the ICF-CY. *J Comm Dis* 43: 378–396.
18. Thomas-Stonell N, Oddson B, Robertson B, Rosenbaum P (2009) Predicted and observed outcomes in preschool children following speech and language treatment: parent and clinician perspectives. *J Commun Disord* 42: 29–42.

19. McCormack J, McLeod S, McAllister L, Harrison LJ (2010) My speech problem, your listening problem, and my frustration: the experience of living with childhood speech impairment. *Lang Speech Hear Serv Sch* 41: 379–392.

20. Eadie TL, Baylor CR (2006) The effect of perceptual training on inexperienced listeners' judgments of dysphonic voice. *J Voice* 20: 527–544.

21. McCooey-O'Halloran R, Worrall L, Hickson L (2004) Evaluating the role of speech–language pathology with patients with communication disability in the acute care hospital setting using the ICF. *J Med Sp Lang Path* 12: 49–58.

22. McLeod S (2004) Speech pathologists' application of the ICF to children with speech impairment. *Int J Sp Lang Pathol* 6: 75–81.

23. Maller S, Singleton J, Supalla S, Wix T (1999) The development and psychometric properties of the American sign language proficiency assessment (ASL-PA). *J Deaf Stud Deaf Educ* 4: 249–269.

24. Goldstein G, Bebko JM (2003) The Profile of Multiple Language Proficiencies: a measure for evaluating language samples of deaf children. *J Deaf Stud Deaf Educ* 8: 452–463.

25. Enderby P, John A, Petheram B (2006) *Therapy Outcome Measures for Rehabilitation Professionals*: *Speech and Language Therapy, Physiotherapy, Occupational Therapy*, 2nd edition. Chichester: John Wiley & Sons.

26. Perry A, Skeat J (2004) *AusTOMs for Speech Pathology*. Melbourne: LaTrobe University.

27. Roulstone S, John A, Hughes A, Enderby P (2004) Assessing the construct validity of the Therapy Outcome Measure for pre-school children with delayed speech and language. *Int J Sp Lang Pathol* 6: 230–236.

28. Lubinski R, Golper LA, Frattali CM (2007) *Professional Issues in Speech–Language Pathology*, 3rd edition. Clifton Park: Thomson Delmar Learning.

29. Zur KB, Cotton S, Kelchner L, Baker S, Weinrich B, Lee L (2007) Pediatric Voice Handicap Index (pVHI): a new tool for evaluating pediatric dysphonia. *Int J Ped Otorhinolary* 71: 77–82.

30. McLeod S, Harrison LJ, McCormack J (2012) Intelligibility in Context Scale: validity and reliability of a subjective rating measure. *J Sp Lang Hear Res* 55: 648–656.

31. Ching TYC, Hill M (2007) The Parents' Evaluation of Aural/Oral Performance of Children (PEACH) Scale: normative data. *J Am Acad Audiol* 18: 220–235.

32. Thomas-Stonell NL, Oddson B, Robertson B, Rosenbaum PL (2010) Development of the FOCUS (Focus on the Outcomes of Communication Under Six): a communication outcome measure for preschool children. *Dev Med Child Neurol* 52: 47–53.

33. Hidecker MJC, Paneth N, Rosenbaum PL, et al (2011) Developing and validating the Communication Function Classification System (CFCS) for individuals with cerebral palsy. *Dev Med Child Neurol* 53: 704–710.

34. Biddle A, Watson L, Hooper C, Lohr KN, Sutton SF (2002) *Evidence/report technology assessment No. 52.* (Prepared by the University of North Carolina Evidence-based Practice Center under Contract No 290-97-0011). AHRQ Publication No. 02-E010. Rockville, MD: Agency for Healthcare Research and Quality.

35. Franic DM, Bramlett RE, Bothe AC (2005) Psychometric evaluation of disease specific quality of life instruments in voice disorders. *J Voice* 19: 300–315.

36. Branski RC, Cukier-Blaj S, Pusic A, et al (2010) Measuring quality of life in dysphonic patients: a systematic review of content development in patient-reported outcomes measures. *J Voice* 24: 193–198.

37. UNICEF (1989) *The United Nations Convention on the Rights of the Child (UNCRC)*. Available at: www2.ohchr.org/english/law/crc.htm (accessed 25 May 2009).

38. Roulstone S, McLeod S (2011) *Listening to Children and Young People with Speech, Language and Communication Needs*. London: J&R Press.

39. Einarsdottir J, Dockett S, Perry B (2009) Making meaning: children's perspectives expressed through drawings. *Early Child Dev Care* 179: 217–232.

40. Holliday EL, Harrison LJ, McLeod S (2009) Listening to children with communication impairment talking through their drawings. *J Early Child Res* 7: 244–263.

41. Brutten G, Vanryckeghem M (2006) *Behavior Assessment Battery for School-age Children who Stutter*. San Diego, CA: Plural Publishing.

42. Franic DM, Bothe AK (2008) Psychometric evaluation of condition-specific instruments used to assess health-related quality of life, attitudes, and related constructs in stuttering. *Am J Sp Lang Pathol* 17: 60–80.

43. Johannisson TB, Wennerfeldt S, Havstam C, Naeslund M, Jacobson K, Lohmander A (2009) Communication Attitude Test (CAT-S): normative values for 220 Swedish children. *Int J Lang Com Dis* 44: 813–825.

44. Vanryckeghem M, Brutten G (2006) *KiddyCAT: Communication Attitude Test for Preschool and Kindergarten Children who Stutter*. San Diego, CA: Plural Publishing.

45. Ching TYC, Hill M, Dillon H (2008) Effect of variations in hearing-aid frequency response on real-life functional performance of children with severe or profound hearing loss. *Int J Audiol* 47: 461–475.

46. Langevin M, Kleitman S, Packman A, Onslow M (2009) The Peer Attitudes Toward Children who Stutter (PATCS) scale: an evaluation of validity, reliability and the negativity of attitudes. *Int J Lang Com Dis* 44: 352–368.

47. Barr J, McLeod S, Daniel G (2008) Siblings of children with speech impairment: cavalry on the hill. *Lang Speech Hear Serv Sch* 39: 21–32.

23
MOBILITY (D410–D489)

Heidi Marie Sanders, F. Virginia Wright and Patricia A. Burtner

What is the construct?

The construct of focus in this section is chapter 4 (Mobility, d4) of the World Health Organization International Classification of Functioning, Disability and Health (ICF) activities and participation domain. Within this chapter of the ICF, multiple constructs are addressed, including changing and maintaining body position, transferring oneself, carrying, moving and handling objects, moving objects with lower extremities (e.g. kicking), fine hand use, hand and arm use, walking and moving, moving around (crawling, running, jumping), moving around in different locations and moving around using transportation. Measurement can be done either as an observational assessment by a therapist or as a child- or parent-report questionnaire.

There is some controversy as to whether specific measures of motor ability should be categorized as measures of body function or activity and participation. Indeed, several measures may have items and subscales that overlap these two domains of the ICF. The measures discussed in this review are felt by the authors to evaluate the key aspects of motor activities that relate to mobility. Future studies that link individual items of a measure to specific ICF items will be helpful to clarify the ICF chapter categorization of various motor measures.

General factors to consider when measuring this domain

Although motor skills are the primary focus of the evaluation tools presented in this section, other factors are considered that may affect the reliability and validity of the assessment. If verbal standardized instructions are required for the assessment, the child with limitations in communication may do poorly on the test, resulting in a low score. The child's scores in this instance may not reflect motor dysfunction, but rather a difficulty in understanding directions. Deficits in cognition may be related to a child's poor motor performance, especially if complex movements or advanced motor planning are required. Because somatosensory functions are closely tied to motor functions, the examiner should consider the possibility that a child's poor motor performance may be a measure of poor sensation rather than poor motor control. Such sensory deficits are especially noted in children with cerebral palsy (CP). Visual deficits often confound motor performance; when spatial orientation is distorted, movement is less precise and may appear disorganized. Sensory modulation and regulation of attention should also be considered as possible reasons for decreased or delayed motor skills. Lastly, the child's mastery motivation and psychosocial issues related to his or her environment may affect motor performance in the test situation or in the child's natural environment.

Overview of recommended measures

Using the ICF framework for measures of activities and participation, there is a well-established differentiation between *capacity* and *performance*.[1] Krumlinde-Sundholm[2] describes activity capacity as what the child *can do*, whereas activity performance is what the child *does do*. Indeed, capacity refers to the person's ability to execute a task or an action at his or her highest possible level of functioning in a standardized environment. Thus, tests in which the person is observed in their performance of motor functions such as grasping, transferring and releasing objects, or walking/running at the child's optimal level, are measures of *activity capacity*. In contrast, activity performance is used to reflect participation in life situations. Thus, *performance* measures incorporate real-life tasks or environments to observe or report on typical motor functions rather than the child's optimal performance. With this in mind, motor measures in this section are identified as *capacity* or *performance* measures.

The majority of tests discussed in the next section are not based on normative values, but rather evaluate the extent to which a child is able to do gross or fine motor tasks. The premise behind these tests is that many children with disabilities will not ever function at the age level of their peers, and their scores may fall further off the normative curve as they get older, meaning that important gains in gross and fine motor function will not be detected if plotting progress on normative curves is the only test available.

MEASURING GROSS MOTOR CAPACITY FOR ACTIVITIES AND PARTICIPATION

The Gross Motor Function Measure (GMFM) is the international standard to measure gross motor foundational skills and evaluate change, and is discussed below. While the GMFM is able to capture changes in children in Gross Motor Function Classification System (GMFCS) levels II to V, concerns have been expressed about its potential ceiling effect with school-age children in GMFCS level I. Thus, other gross motor tests that cover more advanced motor skills are also applied and are discussed below. The quality of movement companion measure to the GMFM, known as the Gross Motor Performance Measure (GMPM), was presented in Chapter 16 as it has a strong link with the balance measures and other movement quality measures presented there.

Gross Motor Function Measure

Purpose
The GMFM is an observational measure of motor capability related to five dimensions (lie/roll, sit, crawl, stand, walk/run/jump). It is used across the spectrum of motor severity for children with CP (GMFCS levels I–V, ages ≥5mo), and also with children who have developmental delay. It is accepted as the international standard to measure gross motor foundational skills and evaluate change. The GMFM has been refined by its authors to incorporate Rasch scaling measurement concepts. Specifically, it was created and first validated as an 88-item measure (GMFM-88)[3] and, through use of Rasch scaling, it was redesigned as a 66-item unidimensional interval scaled measure known as the GMFM-66.[4]

Administration and scoring
Testing with the GMFM can be done by a therapist in a clinical, home or school setting with minimal set-up and basic equipment. The only challenge with setting up outside a therapy department is that removable tape lines need to be placed on the floor for some of the walk dimension items, and space needs to be sufficient to provide

a walking/running distance >5m. The GMFM-66 and GMFM-88 are supported by a user's manual,[5] and there is a self-instructional training CD-ROM as well as Gross Motor Ability Estimator (GMAE) scoring software for the GMFM-66. There is no formal GMFM certification test; however, there is evidence that administration skill is enhanced after completion of the GMFM's self-training.

The child's best score for a maximum of three attempts per item is recorded. Each item is scored on a four-point extent of accomplishment response scale. While GMFM testing is usually done first with the child barefoot, it can also be done with walking aids and orthoses with a reduced set of items from the GMFM-88, as outlined in the GMFM manual.[5] The GMFM-88 typically requires 45 to 60 minutes to administer with a child who is fully compliant. The GMFM-66 usually takes less time as it has 22 fewer items. While the GMFM-88 can be scored manually (dimension and total percentage scores), the GMFM-66 has to be scored by GMAE software. Indeed, the GMFM-66 can be scored even if some of its 66 items are not tested, as the GMAE scoring programme is able to give a valid score estimate from the Rasch-based item hierarchy as long as at least 13 items are tested. The GMAE provides a GMFM-66 summary score as well as the standard error of measurement estimates and 95% confidence intervals associated with the child's score. The GMAE places the child's scores on an item map that can assist with the identification of the next potentially achievable gross motor skills.

Psychometric properties
There is extensive GMFM validation work in CP as well as evaluation with children with Down syndrome[3,6–9] or head injury.[5] Adaptations to its administration are advised when used with children with Down syndrome.[10] A summary of some of the key validation results is provided in the GMFM table in this chapter. In brief, internal consistency is very high (alpha 0.99), inter-rater and test–retest reliability are excellent (intraclass correlation coefficients [ICCs] from 0.75 to 0.99), strong construct validity has been established with a wide variety of impairment and activity measures (*r* from 0.50 to 0.90) (as summarized by Harvey et al[11] and Damiano et al[12]), and longitudinal validity was confirmed with children with CP over a 5-year follow-up.[13] Clinically important change has been established as 1.5 to 3 points for the GMFM-88 and GMFM-66,[5,14] with evidence of greater specificity of the GMFM-66 to change.[14] The primary limitation of the GMFM is a ceiling effect with children in GMFCS level I.[12,15] To this end, a proposed adjunct to the GMFM (known as the Challenge Module) has been developed

GROSS MOTOR FUNCTION MEASURE (GMFM-88 AND GMFM-66)	
Purpose	To evaluate gross motor capabilities in the areas of lying/rolling, sitting, crawling, standing and walking in children and young people with cerebral palsy (CP), Down syndrome and acquired brain injury. The skills evaluated are foundational gross motor skills that typically developing 5-year-old children are capable of performing
	Primary use is as an outcome measure of medical, surgical and rehabilitation interventions
	Useful for longitudinal tracking of a child's gross motor skill development from infant through to teenage years
	Assists with identification of gross motor goals using the GMFM-66 item map as a guide
Population	Children with CP, aged 5mo through teenage years. Also valid for use with children with Down syndrome and acquired brain injury
Description of domains (subscales)	GMFM-88's items are: lying/rolling (17 items); sitting (20 items); crawling (14 items); standing (13 items); walking/running/jumping (24 items)
	GMFM-66's items are: lying/rolling (four items); sitting (15 items); crawling (10 items); standing (13 items as per GMFM-88); walking/running/jumping (24 items as per GMFM-88)
Administration and test format	Time to complete: 45–60min to administer (dependent on number of dimensions tested and abilities of the child)
	Testing format: observational assessment of the child performing the items (up to three trials per item)
	Scoring: four-point scale used for both the GMFM-88 and -66: completes (3), partial completion (2), initiates (1), does not initiate (0). The GMFM-88 is an ordinal scale that is treated as interval in the scoring. GMFM-66 scores are converted by the Gross Motor Ability Estimator (GMAE) programme to an interval level summary score. GMFM-88 has a Total% score as well as five Dimension% scores. GMFM-66 requires GMAE software (provided with GMFM manual) to calculate a single total score with standard error of measurement and 95% confidence interval. An item map (by item difficulty order or by item order) is also generated and the child's scores are profiled on this map. Goal total score (for chosen dimensions) can also be calculated when the GMFM-88 is used. Can also evaluate a child's abilities with aids and orthoses (applicable primarily to the stand and walk dimensions) and calculate separate aids and orthoses GMFM stand and walk scores as described in the manual (Russell et al, 2002). May be a very pertinent score when thinking of functional abilities and changes post intervention such as orthopaedic surgery. Not suitable, though, for scoring using the GMFM-66 as the Rasch scaling for that scoring approach applies only to the barefoot testing condition
	Training: training CD-ROM available with purchase of GMFM manual – self-instruction approach – no criterion test
Psychometric properties	*Reliability*
	Internal consistency high in CP (Cronbach's alpha >0.95). Inter-rater reliability in CP (Kendall coefficient and intraclass correlation coefficient [ICC], range 0.74–0.99). Test–retest reliability in CP (Kendall coefficient and ICC range: 0.68–0.99). Inter-rater and test–retest reliability in Down syndrome (ICC range: 0.90–0.98)
	Validity
	Face and content validity: established by expert paediatric therapists for use in CP
	Construct validity related to use in CP: correlates to a moderate or strong degree with a wide variety of impairment and activity measures (r from 0.50 to 0.90 for measures such as timed walk tests, Bayley Scales of Infant Development, Berg Balance Scale, Bruininks–Oseretsky Test of Motor Proficiency, Child Health Assessment Questionnaire Disability Index, Pediatric Evaluation of Disability Inventory, Pediatric Outcomes Data Collection Instrument and judgements of change by parents/clinicians). Construct validity related to use in Down syndrome

	Discriminant validity: differentiates among children in different Gross Motor Function Classification System (GMFCS) levels, younger and older children, and those with different types of CP
	Responsiveness
	Successfully measures change in children with CP after rehabilitation, surgical or medical interventions. The greatest changes have been noted in children aged <5y who are in GMFCS levels I and II. The GMFM-66 is comparable or better than the GMFM-88 in terms of responsiveness to change. Longitudinal construct validity – similar ability to detect change after selective dorsal rhizotomy by the GMFM-88, goal total scores and GMFM-66 for long-term follow-up of children, but some advantage of the GMFM-88 and goal total scores when used in the short term, particularly with older children and those in GMFCS levels IV and V
How to order	GMFM manual (hardcover) with GMAE scoring programme can be ordered through Mac Keith Press at a cost of US$110 (www.wiley.com/WileyCDA/WileyTitle/productCd-1898683298,descCd-collegeFeatures.html) and US$75 for the self-instructional training CD (www.wiley.com/WileyCDA/WileyTitle/productCd-1898683301.html). Score sheets are downloadable for free from *CanChild*: http://motorgrowth.canchild.ca/en/GMFM/resources/GMFMscoresheet.pdf
Key references	Russell DJ, Avery LM, Rosenbaum PL, Raina PS, Walter SD, Palisano RJ (2000) Improved scaling of the Gross Motor Function Measure for children with cerebral palsy: evidence of reliability and validity. *Phys Ther* 80: 873–885.
	Russell DJ, Rosenbaum PL, Avery LM, Lane M (2002) *Gross Motor Function Measure (GMFM-66 & GMFM-88) User's Manual*. London: Mac Keith Press.
	Wang H-Y, Yang YH (2006) Evaluating the responsiveness of 2 versions of the Gross Motor Function Measure for children with cerebral palsy. *Arch Phys Med Rehabil* 87: 51–56.
	Gemus M, Palisano R, Russell D, et al (2001) Using the Gross Motor Function Measure to evaluate motor development in children with Down syndrome. *Phys Occup Ther Pediatr* 21: 69–79.

for school-aged children and young people in GMFCS level I.[16]

The GMFM often serves as a validation standard for other rehabilitation measures. It has been successfully used to measure change in effectiveness studies related to physiotherapy, other types of therapy (e.g. conductive education, hippotherapy, robotic-assisted locomotion training, random perturbation therapy), spasticity reducing interventions (e.g. botulinum toxin injections, dorsal rhizotomy, intrathecal baclofen therapy), lower limb orthopaedic surgery and comparative evaluations of orthotic and assistive devices. Typical amounts of change seen in clinical trials vary from 2 to 5 percentage points.[17–21] The GMFM-88 is used alongside the GMFM-66 in some published studies and is the proper choice when investigators want specific dimension scores, when the child is tested with shoes/orthoses (as there is no GMFM-66 scoring calculation for this) or if the child has a neuromotor diagnosis other than CP.

Work is under way to test abbreviated item-set versions of the GMFM-66 with children with CP.[22,23] The GMFM was used as the foundation for motor growth curves that help to delineate patterns of gross motor development in children and young people with CP.[24–26] The quality of movement measure known as the GMPM that is based on the GMFM was described in detail in Chapter 16.

MEASURING UPPER LIMB MOTOR CAPACITY FOR ACTIVITIES AND PARTICIPATION

Quality of movement is also an important consideration when assessing hand function. Movements to be assessed include reach, grasp, release, manipulation and postural control during activity. By assessing quality of movement, it is possible to measure changes that occur in function often before there are changes in developmental skills. Four tests are commonly used to measure quality of movement in upper limb function and to document research outcomes. Brief descriptions of each test's purpose, administration and psychometric properties are reviewed.

MELBOURNE ASSESSMENT OF UNILATERAL UPPER LIMB FUNCTION	
Purpose	Criterion-referenced test to measure quality of upper limb motor function in children with diagnosed neurological impairments Designed to measure only one limb at a time
Population	Children with neurological impairment, mild to severe, ages 5–15y
Description of domains (subscales)	Sixteen items rated for multiple areas of movement quality. Items include reaching, grasping, releasing, drawing, manipulation, pointing, pronation/supination, transferring objects and movements required for self-care
Administration and test format	Time to complete: 30min to administer, 30min to score Testing format: 16 play-based items that the child performs while being video-taped Scoring: review of videotape to score items on a three-point scale. Items are added for a total raw score. Raw score is divided by the total number of possible points (122 points) for a percentage score Training: recommendations are available for training for reliable scoring
Psychometric properties	Normative sample: criterion-referenced assessment *Reliability* Internal consistency was completed (Cronbach's alpha reliability coefficients, range 0.62–0.92). Test–retest reliability studies range from 0.69 to 0.91. Inter-rater reliability completed (intraclass correlation coefficients, range 0.87–0.96). *Validity* Content reviewed by eight experienced occupational therapists (content validity) Predictive validity: 11 children with traumatic brain injury who clinicians predicted would change rapidly were followed for three assessments. Excluding one child who regressed, data showed significant progress documented with the Melbourne ($p<0.05$). Correlation coefficients with the Quality of Upper Extremity Skills Test total score and score on hemiplegic side were 0.83 and 0.81, respectively (concurrent validity) *Responsiveness* 11 children with traumatic brain injury who clinicians predicted would change rapidly were followed for three assessments. Excluding one child who regressed, data showed significant progress documented with the Melbourne ($p<0.05$)
How to order	Contact the Occupational Therapy Department, Royal Children's Hospital, Melbourne, Australia (otdept@cryptic.rch.unimelb.edu.au)
Key references	Bourke-Taylor H (2003) Melbourne Assessment of Unilateral Upper Limb Function: Construct validity and correlation with the Paediatric Evaluation of Disability Inventory. *Dev Med Child Neurol* 45: 92–96. Cusick A, Vasquez M, Knowles L, Wallen M (2005) Effect of rater training on reliability of Melbourne Assessment of Unilateral Upper Limb Function scores. *Dev Med Child Neurol* 47: 39–45. Klingels K, De Cock P, Desloovere K, et al (2008) Comparison of the Melbourne Assessment of Unilateral Upper Limb Function and the Quality of Upper Extremity Skills Test in hemiplegic CP. *Dev Med Child Neurol* 50: 904–909. Randall M, Carlin JB, Chondros P, Reddihough D (2001) Reliability of the Melbourne Assessment of Unilateral Upper Limb Function. *Dev Med Child Neurol* 43: 761–767.

Melbourne Assessment of Unilateral Upper Limb Function

Overview and purpose

The Melbourne Assessment of Unilateral Upper Limb Function is a criterion-referenced test designed to measure quality of upper limb motor function in children between the ages of 30 months and 15 years who are diagnosed with CP or other neurological impairments.[27] Quality of unimanual movement is rated on 16 items, including reaching forward to a target, reaching forward to an elevated target position, reaching sideways to a target, grasping a crayon, releasing a crayon, grasping a pellet, releasing a pellet, manipulation of a cube with finger dexterity, pointing accuracy, reaching to brush forehead to back of neck (simulating hair brushing), palm to bottom (simulating toileting skills) pronation/supination, hand-to-hand transferring of objects, reaching to opposite shoulder (simulating dressing) and hand-to-mouth movements (simulating eating). Fluidity, target accuracy, range of motion and speed are some parameters rated in the different test items. The Melbourne Assessment provides useful information regarding changes in function after medical and/or clinical intervention and for describing quality of movement to professionals and families. Clinical utility as a descriptive/discriminative assessment as well as an evaluative tool has been established. Since the development and dissemination of the Melbourne Assessment, it has been recommended as the tool of choice as a capacity-based test of hand function for intervention studies of children with hemiplegic CP.[28]

Administration and scoring

The Melbourne Assessment is videotaped by one examiner while another examiner administers the test using standardized procedures. Performance on the 16 upper limb activity items are scored during a review of the videotape, with each item rated on quality and task achievement using a three-point scale. Total raw scores are converted to percentage scores. Training in the administration of the assessment is recommended but not required. The Melbourne Assessment requires approximately 30 minutes to administer and 30 minutes to score.

Psychometric properties

Concurrent-criterion validity was reported in a study of 21 children with hemiplegic CP tested with the Melbourne Assessment and the Quality of Upper Extremity Skills Test (QUEST). Melbourne Assessment scores and QUEST total scores and scores on the hemiplegic side were 0.83 and 0.81, respectively ($p<0.001$).[28,29] Scores on the Melbourne Assessment were also compared with four QUEST domain scores on the children's hemiplegic side, resulting in the following correlation coefficients: dissociated movements ($r=0.87$; $p<0.001$); grasp ($r=0.83$; $p<0.001$); weight bearing ($r=0.50$; $p<0.021$); and protective extension ($r=0.36$; $p<0.114$). However, the authors concluded that the Melbourne Assessment and the QUEST measure different dimensions of hand function. When the Melbourne Assessment was administered to 20 children with varying degrees of CP with videos scored by 15 occupational therapists, inter-rater reliability correlation coefficients were high, varying from 0.87 to 0.96. Test–retest reliability correlation coefficients using repeat videotaping ranged from 0.69 to 0.91.[30] The smallest detectable difference based on this sample was 8.9 points.[30]

Shriner's Hospital for Children Upper Extremity Evaluation

Overview and purpose

The Shriner's Hospital for Children Upper Extremity Evaluation (SHUEE) is a criterion-referenced test used to assess unimanual upper extremity function in children with hemiplegic CP, specifically the ability to perform grasp and release tasks.[31] The assessment focuses on spontaneous functional and dynamic positional analysis of the elbow, forearm, wrist, thumb and fingers in children aged 3 to 18 years. The SHUEE is useful as a diagnostic/discriminative measure, as well as an evaluative assessment comparing dynamic segmental alignment before and after medical or clinical intervention.

Administration and scoring

Sixteen developmentally appropriate activities of daily living, including unscrewing a cap, throwing a ball and pulling playdough are completed while the child is videotaped. Measurements of active and passive range of motion, muscle tone and a history-based assessment of performance of daily living skills are also completed. Administration of activities requires approximately 15 minutes. Upon video review, tasks are scored in three domains: spontaneous functional analysis (nine tasks on five-point scale), dynamic positional analysis (five tasks on three-point scale) and grasp and release analysis (two tasks on a three-point scale). Each domain score is reported as a percentage of the optimal score.

Psychometric properties

Eleven children with hemiplegic CP, aged 3 to 18 years, participated in reliability and validity studies, and 18

SHRINER'S HOSPITAL FOR CHILDREN UPPER EXTREMITY EVALUATION (SHUEE)	
Purpose	To assess involved upper extremity function in children with hemiplegic cerebral palsy (CP), specifically the ability to perform grasp and release tasks
	Focuses on spontaneous functional and dynamic positional analysis of elbow, forearm, wrist, thumb and fingers
	Compares dynamic, segmental alignment pre and post intervention
Population	Children with hemiplegic CP aged from 3 to 18y
Description of domains (subscales)	Through the performance of 16 developmentally age-appropriate activities of daily living, including unscrewing a cap, throwing a ball and pulling playdough apart, the following are evaluated:
	spontaneous functional analysis (SFA)
	dynamic positional analysis (DPA)
	grasp/release analysis (GRA)
	The activities are grouped together to evaluate specific joint movement. Range of motion, tone and history of activities of daily living are also evaluated
Administration and test format	Time to complete: approximately 15min to administer
	Testing format: video-based evaluation of the spontaneous use of the involved extremity and the segmental alignment of the extremity while performing tasks on demand; measurements of active and passive range of motion, tone and a history-based assessment of the performance of activities of daily living
	Scoring
	SFA: nine tasks are scored; modified House Scale of 0 to 5 (less to more spontaneous) is used; scores are expressed as a percentage of normal or optimal score
	DPA: five segments analysed; four tasks for each segment; score: 0–3 (pathological alignment to normal or optimal alignment); scores are expressed as a percentage of normal or optimal score
	GRA: two hand functions analysed in three wrist positions; score: 0–3 (pathological alignment to normal or optimal alignment); scores are expressed as a percentage of normal or optimal score
	Training: evaluator training before clinical application of the SHUEE should include:
	reading the SHUEE manual;
	viewing the key interpretation video; and
	completing the video proficiency test.
Psychometric properties	Normative sample: 11 children with hemiplegic CP aged 3–18y participated in reliability and validity studies, 18 children participated in the construct validity study
	Reliability
	Intra-observer reliability established (r=0.98–0.99)
	Interobserver reliability established (r=0.89–0.90)
	Validity
	Concurrent validity determined by the comparison of SHUEE, the Pediatric Evaluation of Disability Inventory and the Jebson–Taylor Test of Hand Function scores from the same cohort
	Responsiveness
	Construct validity determined by the analysis of SHUEE scores before and after a common orthopaedic surgical intervention designed to improve wrist alignment
How to order	Available for download at www.ejbjs.org/cgi/content/full/88/2/326/DC1

Key reference	Davids JR, Peace LC, Wagner LV, Gidewall MA, Blackhurst, DW, Roberson WM (2006) Validation of the Shriner's Hospital for Children Upper Extremity Evaluation (SHUEE) for children with hemiplegic cerebral palsy. *J Bone Jt Surg – Am* 88: 326–333.

children participated in a construct validity study. Intra-observer reliability coefficients were high (Pearson r=0.98–0.99), as were interobserver reliability coefficients (Pearson r=0.89–0.90). No studies have been completed for test–retest reliability.[31]

Concurrent validity was determined by the comparison of the SHUEE, the Pediatric Evaluation of Disability Inventory (PEDI) and the Jebson–Taylor Test of Hand Function (JTT) scores from the same cohort, with fair to moderate correlation (r=0.47 and r=0.76, respectively). Construct validity was determined by the analysis of SHUEE scores before and after a common orthopaedic surgical intervention designed to improve wrist alignment. The SHUEE wrist score improved for all 18 individuals following flexor tendon transfer with significant mean improvement (p<0.001).[31]

Jebsen–Taylor Test of Hand Function

Overview and purpose
The JTT was developed as a short, objective norm-referenced assessment of hand functions commonly used in activities of daily living.[32] The test was specifically developed for healthcare providers working with individuals needing hand restoration. Seven subtests include fine motor timed items: (1) writing/copying a 24-letter sentence, (2) turning over 3-inch × 5-inch index cards, (3) picking up small common objects such as a paper clip, bottle cap and coins, (4) simulated feeding using spoon and five kidney beans, (5) stacking checkers, (6) picking up large light objects (empty tin cans) and (7) picking up large heavy objects (full tin cans weighing approximately 0.5kg).

The JTT has been used extensively to measure hand skills of individuals with neurological, developmental and orthopaedic conditions. The test provides unimanual measurement of each hand as the child completes the seven simulated functional tasks. Normative data provide the means to compare a child's performance with peers of a similar age and sex. The JTT has often been used in research studies as a measure of changes in children's hand function pre- and post intervention.[33–36] Clinically, the JTT may be used for discriminative/descriptive as well as evaluative purposes.

Administration and scoring
Standardized instructions are followed first with testing of the non-dominant hand and then testing of the dominant hand. Children who are ≤6 years of age are not administered the writing portion of the test. Time to administer the test is approximately 30 minutes, and scoring using age norms yields z-scores for the child tested. Centile norms are also available for the Australian population.

Psychometric properties
Test–retest reliability coefficients ranged from 0.87 to 0.99 for dominant and non-dominant hands, suggesting excellent reliability. High correlations were also found between the subtests and total test score, with the exception of the handwriting subtest.[37]

MEASURING CAPACITY FOR GROSS AND FINE MOTOR DEVELOPMENT
Tests which measure motor activities in the context of developmental milestones as opposed to real-life functional activities are included in this section. These tests are typically norm-referenced and often include a combination of capacity, motor performance and motor developmental milestones and cover fine and gross motor skills within the same test. The ones reviewed are those most often cited in the literature and are also often used in clinical practice.

Peabody Developmental Motor Scales, second edition

Overview and purpose
The Peabody Developmental Motor Scales (PDMS) is a norm-referenced, standardized test designed to measure motor abilities that develop in early life (birth through 71mo) as compared with age-related peers, and also allows comparison of gross and fine motor skill levels within a child.[38] With the US mandate for educational services for children with developmental delays to include the Education of the Handicapped Act Amendments of 1986 and Individuals with Disabilities Education Act,[39] the authors of the PDMS noted the need for a norm-referenced, standardized test.[38] The 249-item PDMS-2 is divided into two scales: (1) the Gross Motor Developmental Scale, which consists of four subtests – reflexes (for children from birth through 11mo), stationary (ability to sustain control of body within its centre of gravity), locomotion (ability to move from one place to

JEBSON–TAYLOR HAND FUNCTION TEST	
Purpose	A short, objective test of hand functions used in activities of daily living
Population	Individuals with neurological or musculoskeletal conditions involving deficits in hand use. Normative data are available for individuals from age 6y through adults. There is also research published for use with clients with acquired neurological disorders, spinal cord injury and stroke
Description of domains (subscales)	Test items include fine motor, weighted and non-weighted hand function activities which are timed, including: writing (copying) a 24-letter sentence (*omitted for children aged 6–7y) turning over 3-inch × 5-inch cards picking up small common objects such as a paper clip, bottle cap and coin simulated feeding using a teaspoon and five kidney beans stacking checkers picking up large light objects (empty tin can) picking up large heavy items (full tin cans weighing approximately 0.5kg)
Administration and test format	Time to complete: approximately 15min, up to 45min for clients with slower performance Testing format: the test is conducted according to published procedures (Jebsen et al, 1969). The test is administered by the therapist. Performance of each item is timed. The non-dominant hand is tested first, then the dominant hand, for each item Scoring: the time required to complete each item is recorded during test administration. Times are then compared with normative data Training: no training is required
Psychometric properties	Normative sample: normative data are available for males and females ages 6–90y. Centile norms are also available for the Australian population *Reliability* Test–retest reliability established for children (intraclass correlation coefficient 0.83–0.99) *Validity* Content, construct and criterion validity established for adults. No studies of validity reported for use with children *Responsiveness* Less stable test–retest results have been reported in the subtest for writing and feeding
How to order	Test items can be compiled by the therapist, based upon descriptions from the original publication. Items can also be purchased from Westons Home and Medical Equipment Internet Catalogue (www.westons.com) or from Psychtest (www.psychtest.com) Cost: US$425
Key references	Hiller LB, Wade CK (1992) Upper extremity functional assessment scales in children with duchenne muscular dystrophy: a comparison. *Arch Phys Med Rehabil* 73: 527–534. Jebsen RH, Taylor N, Trieschmann RB, Trotter MJ, Howard LA (1969) An objective and standardized test of hand function. *Arch Phys Med Rehabil* 50: 311–319. Lynch KB, Bridle MJ (1989) Validity of the Jebsen–Taylor hand function test in predicting activities of daily living. *Occup Ther J Res* 9: 316–318. Rider B, Linden C (1988) Comparisons of standardized and non-standardized administration of the Jebsen Hand Function Test. *J Hand Ther* 2: 121–123. Taylor N, Sand PL, Jebsen RH (1973) Evaluation of hand function in children. *Arch Phys Med Rehabil* 54: 129–135.

another) and object manipulation (ability to manipulate balls for children aged ≥12mo); and (2) the Fine Motor Developmental Scale, which is made up of two subtests – grasping (ability to use hands) and visuomotor integration (ability to use visual perceptual skills to perform complex eye–hand coordination tasks).[38,40] As a motor developmental test, the PDMS has been used with children with developmental, neurological or orthopaedic diagnoses.

According to the authors,[38] the purposes of the test are to (1) assess motor skills in children relative to their peers, (2) identify children whose motor skills are delayed and to obtain knowledge about the child's present motor skills through thorough analysis, and (3) translate findings into individualized goals and objectives. The PDMS-2 serves best as a diagnostic/discriminative measure, but it is also used to document developmental trends in childhood populations[41] and as an evaluative assessment tool in intervention studies.[42] At the time of writing this chapter, the test kit was US$455 and could be obtained through http://portal.wpspublish.com/portal/page?_pageid=53%2C69919&_dad=portal&_schema=PORTAL. The test kit comes with an activity manual designed to assist in setting motor objectives for the child and to provide strategies for fostering the development of targeted skills.

Administration and scoring
The PDMS-2 is administered by professionals who have experience with standardized test administration. The entire test takes 45 to 60 minutes to administer. Each item is scored on a three-point scale outlined by each item in the examiner's record booklet, with a score of '2' for mastery or the child performing the item according to criteria, a score of '1' for performance of the item in clear resemblance but not fully meeting criteria for mastery and a score of '0' if the child cannot/will not attempt the item or if attempts made do not show that the skill is emerging. A basal level is established when the child scores a 2 on three items in a row, and the ceiling level is when the child scores 0 on three consecutive items on a specific subtest. Gross, fine motor and total motor composite quotient scores are generated from the subtests. These scores are presented as age equivalents, centile ranks and standard scores. In addition, there are age-stratified normative scores for 2000 children.

Psychometric properties
Updated normative data for the PDMS-2 were collected in 1998 on 2000 children from birth to age 71 months, residing in 46 states and one Canadian province with sample representation of the sex, race, ethnicity and socio-economic factors reported by the US Census Bureau for the population <5 years of age.[38] The normative sample

included children with identified physical and mental disabilities. Norms are available in monthly increments for children from birth through 23 months, and older child norms are in 2- to 5-month increments.

Reliability was established through a series of studies. Specifically, test–retest reliability of infants and children aged 2 to 11 months and 12 to 17 months was established by two tests administered within a 1-week window of time. Correlation coefficients for the gross motor composite (range: 0.73–0.94) and the fine motor composite (range: 0.73–0.94) are acceptable. Inter-rater reliability was established for the gross motor composite (coefficient: 0.97) and fine motor composite (coefficient: 0.98). When tested with children with and without motor delay (ages 4 and 5y), the inter-rater (n=18 children) and test–retest reliability (n=12 children) was excellent (r=0.84 and 0.99, respectively).[43] Reliability evaluation with 32 children with CP (ages 27–64mo) revealed strong test–retest reliability (ICCS ≥0.88).[44] However, there is also evidence that practice trials have an effect on performance in preschool-aged children, and it has been recommended that several trials for each item be allowed to ensure that scores reflect optimal performance.[45]

Internal consistency was high for subtest and composite scores, with Cronbach's alpha between 0.92 and 0.99;[38] more recent Rasch analytical work has revealed that the unidimensionality of the fine motor scale would be enhanced by the elimination of 10 items that did not appear to fit the Rasch model.[46]

Content validity of the PDMS-2 was established though a review panel of professionals who implemented motor interventions as well as item analyses.[38] Concurrent validity was fair to moderate (r from 0.13 to 0.96) for age-equivalent scores when tested against the Bayley Scales of Infant Development (BSID-II) Motor Scale,[40,47,48] moderate when compared with the Movement Assessment Battery for Children (ABC) (r=0.69)[43] and strong when tested against the Early Intervention Developmental Profile[49] and the Alberta Infant Motor Scale.[50]

An evaluation of responsiveness to change in 32 children with CP (ages 27–64mo) for the three motor composite scores over a 3-month reassessment interval demonstrated acceptable responsiveness to change (Guyatt Responsiveness Index values of 1.7–2.3).[44] While the PDMS-2 and GMFM were similar in the magnitude of change they detected over a 6-month follow-up when used with infants with CP or motor delay,[51] Palisano et al[52] noted that the PDMS was not overly responsive to change (i.e. index of responsiveness was 0.5) when used with the infants with CP who were enrolled in an early intervention programme. The PDMS-2 has been used with varying success as an outcome measure in studies with children with CP, for example constraint-induced movement therapy,[53] botulinum toxin injections[54] and use of virtual reality for children with CP.[55] Olesch et al[54] noted that the lack of responsiveness of the PDMS in their study, despite the gains in hand abilities, may suggest the need to adopt better measures of hand activity such as the Assisting Hand Assessment.

Bruininks–Oseretsky Test of Motor Proficiency, second edition

Overview and purpose
The Bruininks–Oseretsky Test of Motor Proficiency (BOTMP)[56,57] is a standardized, norm-referenced measure that was designed for use by physical and occupational therapists, physical education teachers and special education professionals. It assesses motor proficiency in advanced gross and fine motor skills of children from 4 years 6 months to 14 years 6 months of age who have motor problems.[58,59] This includes children with developmental delay, clumsiness, sensory integrative issues or developmental coordination disorder, as well as those with learning/intellectual disabilities.[60,61] The test is used as a descriptive, discriminative and supportive diagnostic measure for children with mild motor problems, and also frequently serves as an outcome measure.[60]

The second edition of the BOTMP, the BOT-2,[57] contains substantial revisions by the BOTMP's developers[56] to increase its functional relevance. New features include items that expand skill coverage and make the test more fun, improved equipment, an expanded age range to 21 years and enhanced measurement properties with children aged 4 and 5 years.[62] Its 53 items are divided into four composite scales and eight subtests: fine manual control subscale (fine motor precision and fine motor integration) subtests; manual coordination (manual dexterity, upper limb coordination); body coordination (bilateral coordination, balance); and strength and agility (running speed and agility, strength). Items for assessment of fine motor function and gross motor function are age-specific, consisting of game-like tasks.[63] Like the BOTMP, the BOT-2 has a short form which contains 14 of the measure's 53 items (six from gross motor skills subtest; six from fine motor skills subtest; two from gross and fine motor skills subtest). The short form is best suited for use in school settings[64] or as a screening measure.[59]

Administration and scoring
This assessment uses the BOTMP/BOT-2 test kit and has standardized administration instructions. Depending on the item, single or multiple trials are allowed. The time to administer is 40 to 60 minutes plus 10 minutes' set-up time for the complete BOTMP or BOT-2 and 20 minutes to score.[62] The short form requires 15 to 20 minutes to administer plus 15 minutes to set up and score. The BOT-2 comes with a training video for test administration and scoring software.

A Total Index of Motor Proficiency score is calculated from the eight subtest scores to represent the overall motor performance of the child. For each subtest, raw scores are converted to scaled scores with 90% confidence intervals and age-equivalent scores. Four composite scores are also calculated, each representing two related subtests. Age-based standard score and centile ranking are available for the four composite scores and total index score. Five-point descriptive standings (well below to well above average) are available for all subtest and composite scores.

While normative scores for the BOTMP were developed from testing an age-stratified sample of 765 typically developing children from the USA, normative scores for the BOT-2 were constructed from a random sample of 1520 US children (12 age groups). Approximately 11% of these children had a special education designation (variety of disabilities represented). Normative scores for other cultures are available, such as Greece[59] and United Arab Emirates.[64] Standard age-based scores are required for purposes of diagnosis. For evaluation of change over time, the use of raw scores has been recommended as a more sensitive approach for detecting change.[60] This is a common recommendation for tests with age-based scores as children with delays may fall behind age-related peers over time, despite small gains in motor skills.

Psychometric properties
The test developers' reliability and validity studies are reported in the BOTMP/BOT-2 test manuals.[56,57] Test–retest and inter-rater reliability are excellent (r>0.80) for subtest and composite scores, although use of Pearson r (association) rather than ICCs (agreement) reduces the interpretability of the results. Concerns have been expressed about test–retest reliability, given the large standard error of measurement (4–5 points) that indicates that true scores can fall between the fourth and 50th centiles.[65] Evidence about reliability for children with CP is limited to one test–retest study of the balance subtest.[66] High internal consistency (Cronbach's alpha >0.80) has been confirmed.[59,64] Rasch analysis with children with intellectual disability revealed that items in each composite group of the BOT-2 fit the Rasch model and had excellent reliability (range 0.90–0.97).[67] Rasch analysis has not been done for other diagnostic groups.

Discriminant validity has been demonstrated through testing of age group differentiation with typically developing children,[64,68–70] discrimination between children with

BRUININKS–OSERETSKY TEST OF MOTOR PROFICIENCY (BOTMP, AND SECOND EDITION KNOWN AS BOT-2)	
Purpose	To evaluate motor proficiency on advanced gross and fine motor skills of children and young people. Test purposes in the BOTMP/BOT-2 manual are stated as screening, clinical evaluation, research and assistance with school placement decisions
Population	Children ages 4y 6mo–14y 6mo who have motor problems not related to identified neurological disorders. This includes children with developmental delay, developmental coordination disorder, learning/intellectual disability, Down syndrome or sensory integrative issues. Also used with children with cerebral palsy (CP) in clinical trials

Description of domains (subscales)	Four composite scales and eight subtests with 53 items in total:
	  fine motor control (fine motor precision, fine motor integration) (15 items)
	  manual coordination (manual dexterity, upper limb coordination) (12 items)
	  body coordination (bilateral coordination, balance) (16 items)
	  strength and agility (strength, running speed and agility) (10 items)
	The short form has 14 items across the four composite scales

Administration and test format	Time to complete: the full test requires 40–60min to complete plus 30min to set up and score afterwards. The short form takes 15–20min to administer and 15min to set up and score afterwards Testing format: observational assessment of the child performing the items (single or multiple trials allowed, depending on the item) Scoring: scores based on prespecified timed cut-off points. For each subtest, raw scores are converted to called scores with 90% confidence interval and age-equivalent scores. Total index of motor proficiency as well as scores for the four composite scales, age-based standard score and centile ranking calculated from BOTMP's score tables. Five age-based descriptive standings also available ('well below average' to 'well above average') Training: self-training from the test-administration manual
Psychometric properties	Normative sample: normative data from a sample of US children that includes 10% with special education designation. Also available from other cultures, e.g. Greece and United Arab Emirates *Reliability* Internal consistency high (Cronbach's alpha >0.80). Inter-rater reliability established for children with mild motor problems (r >0.80). Test–retest reliability established for children with mild motor problems (r >0.80) with standard error of measurement of four to five points *Validity* Face and content validity: established by BOTMP developers and reported in manual. Construct validity: minimal BOTMP-focused work done in this area; evidence of moderate validity (r >0.60) from studies of other measures such as Movement Assessment Battery for Children where BOTMP used as a comparison standard. Discriminant validity: differentiates between typically developing children and those with motor problems, and also those with learning disabilities. May be a floor effect with children with physical disabilities, e.g. children with CP in Gross Motor Function Classification System levels I and II, i.e. measure is too difficult. Rasch analysis: good fit of data to the Rasch model with children with intellectual disability

	Responsiveness
	Use of raw scores recommended as a more sensitive approach than age-based scores to evaluating change. No specific work on responsiveness to change, although evaluation studies with children with developmental coordination disorder, CP or Down syndrome have shown postintervention changes in BOTMP scores
How to order	BOT-2 test kit with specialized equipment and test manual with standardized administration instruction and score forms can be purchased from Pearson Assessments (www.pearsonassessments.com)
	Cost: US$795.
Key references	Bruininks RH, Bruininks B (2005) *Bruininks–Oseretsky Test of Motor Proficiency*, 2nd edition. Minneapolis: NCS Pearson.
	Dietz J, Kartin D, Kopp K (2007) Review of the Bruininks–Oseretsky Test of Motor Proficiency, Second Edition (BOT-2). *Phys Occup Ther Pediatr* 27: 87–102.
	Venetsanou F, Kambas A, Aggeloussis N, Fatouros I, Taxildaris K (2009) Motor assessment of preschool aged children: a preliminary investigation of the validity of the Bruininks–Oseretsky test of motor proficiency – short form. *Hum Move Sci* 28: 543–50.
	Wilson BN, Polatajko HJ, Kaplan BJ, Faris P (2001) Use of the Bruininks–Oseretsky Test of Motor Proficiency in occupational therapy. *Percept Mot Skills* 92: 157–166.

and without motor problems[71] and differentiation between children with and without learning disabilities.[56] Construct validity has received little direct study, for example concurrent validity was demonstrated for children with learning disabilities when BOTMP scores were compared with Southern California Sensory Integration Test scores.[72] Several studies using the BOTMP to validate measures such as the Movement-ABC have revealed moderate correlation[73] or agreement.[74]

Despite criticisms about the difficulty of items for children with CP,[63] the BOTMP/BOT-2 has been used in an outcome measure set in several studies with children with CP, for example constraint-induced movement therapy, hand–arm bimanual intensive therapy, botulinum toxin injections, effectiveness of orthotic garments and predictors of hand-writing performance.[35,39,75–79] The enhanced set of items for children in the 4- to 5-year age range in the BOT-2 may result in a better fit of the measure for children with CP in GMFCS levels I and II. However, scoring issues have been noted with the BOT-2 with typically developing children aged 4 to 6 years as many of the items were still too difficult.[70]

The BOTMP/BOT-2 has been used both as a screening tool in children with developmental coordination disorder[67,80] and as an outcome measure following cognitive treatment.[81] It has also been used as the balance subtest with children with Down syndrome in whom the effectiveness of ankle orthoses was being tested,[82] following gross motor skills training in children with Down syndrome[83] and in an early intervention programme with children with Down syndrome.[84]

As the version used is not always specified, readers should confirm from the reference list of papers published after 2005 whether the BOTMP or BOT-2 was used because the tests are different in item content. Difference (change) scores and associated standard deviations from the clinical studies provide estimates of what might be expected when used with children with different diagnoses. However, test–retest reliability work is needed in each of these populations to provide the standard error of measurement and minimum detectable change, both of which are needed when interpreting change scores.

MEASURING GROSS MOTOR PERFORMANCE IN THE CONTEXT OF DAILY LIFE ACTIVITIES

The measures in this section focus on the assessment of what a child does in gross motor-related functional skills in daily life. The measures range from focused measures of functional mobility (e.g. the Functional Mobility Scale [FMS] and Gillette Functional Assessment Questionnaire [FAQ]) to a broader measurement of motor skills in the context of home, school and community activities. Measurement can also be done using a mobility subscale(s) of broad-based functional measures such as the Pediatric Outcomes Data Collection Instrument (PODCI), PEDI, Activity Scale for Kids (ASK), WeeFIM® Instrument and School Function Assessment (SFA). The FMS, FAQ, PODCI and SFA are discussed in depth in the following section, and the reader is referred to Chapter 19 for detailed reviews of the ASK, PEDI and WeeFIM.

Functional Mobility Scale

Overview and purpose

This brief parent- or clinician-report scale was designed by an orthopaedic surgery/physiotherapy/gait laboratory team to describe the functional mobility of children with CP and to evaluate change after orthopaedic surgery. This assessment of what the child does in daily life was intended to be a communication conduit between orthopaedic surgeons and other healthcare professionals. The FMS focuses on a child's mobility in three different 'real-world' environmental contexts: home, school and community (summarized as 5-, 50- and 500-m mobility distances, respectively). The targeted age for the scale is 6 years and up, fitting with the years when orthopaedic surgery is most often performed and when gait changes are no longer attributable primarily to development. The rating system uses a six-point walking ability response scale, representing progressive levels of assistive device use from the use of a wheelchair, to the use of walking aids, through to independent walking. The FMS recognizes that different methods of mobility as well as different gait devices (i.e. walker vs crutches vs cane[s]) may be employed in various environments and is more specific than the GMFCS in documenting mobility/device differences according to context and demands.

Administration and scoring

The FMS form is completed by parents or health professionals. It takes 5 to 10 minutes to do[85] and requires no special training. The six-point response scale is completed for each of 5-, 50- and 500-m walking distances. The scale is illustrated in pictorial form in the appendix by Harvey et al.[85]

Psychometric properties

The FMS demonstrated high internal consistency (Cronbach's alpha >0.95) and excellent inter-rater reliability for surgeon and research fellow rating comparisons for each of the walking distances (ICCs >0.93)[86] and when surgeon and physical therapist raters did the evaluation (weighted kappas 0.86–0.92). This was applicable to administration of the scale in person or by telephone.[87] From a validity standpoint, FMS scores decreased as the walking distance increased, and it discriminated well among children with hemiplegia, diplegia and spastic quadriplegia.[86] The FMS correlated strongly with the Child Health Questionnaire (CHQ), PODCI and a measure of 'up time'. FMS change scores demonstrated strong correlations with 6- and 12-month postoperative change scores from the CHQ, PODCI, energy expenditure and up time (0.50<*r*<0.86),[86] indicating sensitivity to change in both deterioration and improvement situations. The FMS's developers, Harvey et al[88], found substantial agreement (kappa >0.70) between the parent-report FMS and observation of the child's mobility in the three environmental contexts.

With respect to responsiveness, Harvey et al[88] noted significant changes (deterioration followed by improvement) on the FMS over a 2-year period after orthopaedic surgery (as measured every 3mo) in contrast to consistency in GMFCS level over this time, especially for children in GMFCS level III (note: the GMFCS was not designed to be a measure of change).[85] Other research groups have since verified the FMS's ability to detect change after orthopaedic surgery.[89,90] There is no mention by its creators of its potential use in other intervention contexts in children with CP. While one non-surgical study evaluated the impact of plantar flexor training in children with CP, there were no changes detected in function overall or in the FMS after training.[91] Thus, its responsiveness remains an area to be explored.

Gillette Functional Assessment Questionnaire

Overview and purpose

The FAQ is a parent-report measure that measures the functional gait of children with neuromuscular disorders (e.g. CP, spina bifida, brain injury, osteogenesis imperfecta).[92] The FAQ's first part is a 10-level walking scale that indicates the functional capability of the child. The second part consists of 22 gait-related items (skills such as running, jumping, biking and getting on/off an escalator) that are rated on ease of performance. The targeted age is not specified, although in the original validation study children aged 2 to 17 years were tested.

Administration and scoring

The entire FAQ requires approximately 10 minutes to complete. A parent or usual caregiver assigns the child an FAQ level from 0 to 10. This level is based on the type of ground covered, the distance travelled without significant problems and assistance required for walking. Level 10 denotes normal walking performance without any assistance, level 5 is consistent with household or classroom walking, while 0 indicates an inability to walk and full caregiver dependence. The 22 items of the second part are rated on a four-point degree of difficulty scale, and a 'performed as part of routine' yes/no scale. The FAQ can be accessed at www.gillettechildrens.org/fileUpload/GFAQsurveypreview2.pdf.

Psychometric properties

The FAQ's developers established inter-rater (parent vs parent and parent vs school team member) and test–retest reliability (1mo retest interval) (ICCs >0.90) for the 10-level walking scale portion of the test (part 1). Evaluation of concurrent validity compared FAQ part 1 scores with the PODCI (r=0.76), WeeFIM® Instrument (r=0.63) and oxygen uptake (r=0.46).[92] The FAQ showed moderate correlations with heart rate index and GMFCS level (r>−0.50)[93,94] and Edinburgh gait scale (r=0.51),[95] and discriminated among children in different GMFCS levels.[96] One issue noted with FAQ studies is the restriction of samples to children who score in the upper mobility range. It still requires validation with less mobile children. From the perspective of orthopaedic surgical interventions, part 1 of the FAQ detected change in children undergoing femoral osteotomy,[93] BoNT-A injections,[97] multilevel surgery for crouch gait[98] and dorsal rhizotomy.[99] Results may be different with rehabilitation interventions in which functional change is smaller in magnitude. For example, McNee et al[91] used part 1 of the FAQ as one of two measures of functional mobility in a trial on plantar flexor strength training in children with CP.[91] While strength and muscle bulk improved, there was no evidence of functional changes on the FAQ, Functional Mobility Scale or Timed Up and Go Test during follow-up (it is possible that functional change did not occur).

Novachek et al[92] noted in their FAQ validation study the absence of work on the psychometric properties of part 2 of the FAQ (the 22-question section). Initial Rasch analysis work showing its item hierarchy is promising in this regard.[100]

Pediatric Outcomes Data Collection Instrument

Overview and purpose

The PODCI is a parent and youth report questionnaire that was commissioned by the Pediatric Orthopaedic Society of North America to assess musculoskeletal health.[101] It evaluates physical function, pain and its impact on the child's participation in daily activities. Its 86-item and response scales were designed to assess the potential outcomes of orthopaedic treatment. The PODCI can be used across a wide age range (2–18y). There are four main subscales (upper extremity and physical function [eight items], transfers and basic mobility [11 items], sports/physical functioning [21 items], pain/comfort [three items]) as well as a global functioning scale that is a composite score of the four subscales. While the PODCI also has scales of satisfaction with symptoms, happiness

and treatment expectations and items regarding health, these scores are not part of the global score.

Administration and scoring

The PODCI paper questionnaire can be completed by parents and by children aged ≥11 years and takes approximately 15 minutes. Its response scales use a three- to six-point format with various anchoring terms (e.g. degree of difficulty, extent of time). Standardized scores are calculated (0–100), and normative scores are available at the PODCI website. The response option 'too young' is treated as missing data in the scoring of the parent version for children aged <11 years (version 2).[102] The PODCI (version 2) is available online at no charge from www.aaos.org/research/outcomes/outcomes_peds.asp, and includes an Excel-based scoring programme.

Psychometric properties

In the initial validation study by Daltroy et al,[101] children with CP were part of a larger orthopaedic and neurological sample. Inter-rater reliability (young people and parents) was good to excellent for the four main subscales and global score (ICC 0.76–0.87) and test–retest reliability (1–2 days) were excellent (ICC 0.83–0.97). Internal consistency was high for all subscale scores (alpha >0.80) for both parent and young person data. The PODCI also identified significant mobility differences between children with different distributions of spastic CP, although there was evidence that the mobility subscale has a floor effect.[102] While the PODCI's subscales differentiated between children in GFMCS levels I, II and III,[103,104] discriminant validity has not been studied with children in levels IV and V. PODCI scores have been established with typically developing children,[105] and Barnes et al[106] extended this work by establishing mean scores for age and GMFCS level I to III groupings.[106] With respect to construct validity, there is evidence of moderate to strong correlation of the PODCI global score, sports and transfer subscales with measures such as the Activities Scale for Kids (r=0.80)[107] and GMFM walk dimension (0.50<r<0.80).[12,102,108] In a group of children with musculoskeletal disorders, parents' and children's scores were strongly correlated with clinicians' scores.[101]

The PODCI has received considerable attention as a means of detecting change in function after orthopaedic intervention. When used with children who had orthopaedic surgery, the PODCI detected change 9 months postoperatively, was more sensitive to change than the Child Health Questionnaire[101] and correlated well with FAQ changes.[109] Another orthopaedic study determined that the PODCI's transfers and mobility and sports

PEDIATRIC OUTCOMES DATA COLLECTION INSTRUMENT (PODCI)

Purpose	To assess musculoskeletal health in the areas of physical function, pain and its impact on health and function
Population	Children with a musculoskeletal condition (acute or chronic). Includes children with a neurological diagnosis such as cerebral palsy (CP) who have associated musculoskeletal issues

Description of domains (subscales)	Four main subscales:
	
	    upper extremity and physical function (eight items)
	
	    transfers/mobility (11 items)
	
	    sports/physical functioning (21 items)
	
	    pain/comfort (three items)
	
	Separate scales to measure satisfaction with symptoms, happiness and treatment expectations, as well as health-based items

Administration and test format	Time to complete: 15min Testing format: parent-report questionnaire and child-report version for young people aged ≥11y Scoring: response scales use three- to six-point response option format with various anchoring terms (i.e. degree of difficulty, extent of time). Standardized scores can be calculated from raw scores for the global score and the four subscales. Symptoms, happiness and treatment expectation scores are not part of the global or subscale scores Training: none – parent/young person report
Psychometric properties	Standard scores: normative data were established with typically developing children and are available at the PODCI website. Mean scores also established for children with CP in Gross Motor Function Classification System (GMFCS) levels I to III to use a benchmark for clinical comparison *Reliability* Internal consistency: high for all subscale scores (alpha >0.80) for both parent and young person data. Inter-rater reliability (teenagers vs parents) – good to excellent for four main subscales and global score (intraclass correlation coefficient [ICC] 0.76–0.87). Test–retest reliability – excellent for four main subscales and global score (ICCs 0.84–0.97) *Validity* Face and content validity not reported Construct validity: evidence of moderate to strong correlation of PODCI global score, transfers/mobility subscale score with the Activities Scale for Kids (r >0.80) and Gross Motor Function Measure (GMFM) walk dimension ($0.50<r<0.80$). Strong correlation between parent/young person scores and clinicians' scores Discriminant validity: differentiates among children in GMFCS levels I to III. Not studied yet for GMFCS levels IV and V *Responsiveness* Formal testing of responsiveness has been done with children with CP receiving orthopaedic surgery, i.e. children who are more sensitive to change than the Child Health Questionnaire, and better able to detect changes in children in GMFCS level I than GMFM, and no evidence of a ceiling effect
How to order	Available at no charge from www.aaos.org/research/outcomes/outcomes_peds.asp, and includes an Excel-based scoring program

Key references	Allen DD, Gorton GE, Oeffinger DJ, Tylkowski C, Tucker CA, Haley SM (2008) Analysis of the Paediatric Outcomes Data Collection Instrument in ambulatory children with cerebral palsy using confirmatory factor analysis and item response theory methods. *J Pediatr Orthop* 28: 192–198.
	Daltroy LH, Liang MH, Fossel AH, et al (1998) The POSNA Paediatric Musculoskeletal Functional Health questionnaire: report on reliability, validity, and sensitivity to change. *J Pediatr Orthop* 18: 561–571.
	Damiano DL, Gilgannon MD, Abel MF (2005) Responsiveness and uniqueness of the Paediatric Outcomes Data Collection Instrument compared to the Gross Motor Function Measure for measuring orthopaedic and neurosurgical outcomes in cerebral palsy. *J Pediatr Orthop* 25: 641–645.
	McMulkin ML, Baird GO, Gordon AB, Caskey PM, Ferguson RL (2007) The Paediatric Outcomes Data Collection Instrument detects improvements for children with ambulatory cerebral palsy after orthopaedic intervention. *J Pediatr Orthop* 7: 1–6.

subscales were more sensitive to changes in children in GMFCS level I[103] than the GMFM, and there was no evidence of a ceiling effect. PODCI gains were in the magnitude of 4% to 5% overall postoperatively. It has also demonstrated change when used with children aged 2 to 3 months after lower limb BoNT-A injections.[110] While the PODCI detected change after muscle lengthening in children with CP (the sports and physical function scale was particularly responsive), it did not function as well as the GMFM with children after rhizotomy.[12] Factor analysis by members of the development group[111] revealed a modified three-factor structure (and different item groupings than the original PODCI) that showed greater sensitivity to change after orthopaedic intervention with children with CP.

Measuring Fine Motor Performance in the Context of Daily Life Activities

The measures in this section focus on assessment of what a child does in fine motor-related functional skills in daily life. The measures range from observational measures of hand function in play activities (e.g. the AHA), to upper limb function questionnaires (ABILHAND), to school-based function measures that include fine motor/upper limb tasks (School Assessment of Motor and Process Skills [School AMPS] and School Function Assessment [SFA]). As with gross motor skills, measurement can also be done using the self-care subscale(s) of broad-based functional measures such as the PEDI or WeeFIM Instrument. The AHA, ABILHAND, School AMPS and SFA are discussed in depth in the following section, and Chapter 19 provides detailed reviews of the PEDI and WeeFIM Instrument.

Assisting Hand Assessment

Overview and purpose
In typical bimanual activities, the two hands serve different roles. The dominant hand manipulates objects and has greater speed than the non-dominant hand, which has the stabilizing or holding role.[112] Such synchrony in hand function is often interrupted in children who experience unilateral upper limb dysfunction. The AHA was developed for use with children who have a unilateral dysfunction, such as those with hemiplegia or congenital brachial plexus injury. With the different roles of hands in bimanual hand activities in mind, the AHA measures the performance of the child's two hands during play.[113]

The stated purpose of the AHA is to describe and measure how effectively people with a unilateral dysfunction actually use the affected arm/hand with the well-functioning hand to perform tasks requiring bimanual performance.[113] The test is designed to measure usual rather than best performance and is not intended to describe underlying causes of dysfunction such as spasticity, strength or sensation. The AHA is designed for children aged 18 months to 12 years with two levels of measures: Small Kids AHA 18 months to 5 years, and School Kids AHA 6 to 12 years. Recent published reviews rate the AHA as the best performance-based measure of bimanual upper limb activity in children with hemiplegia[114] owing to the presence of strong psychometric properties, and for children with radius deficiencies owing to strong validity of the measure to the types of radial deficiency, functional hand grips and therapist's global assessment.[115] The primary purposes of the AHA are as a descriptive/discriminative measure and as an evaluative measure of a child's progress.

ASSISTING HAND ASSESSMENT (AHA)	
Purpose	To measure and describe how effectively children with a unilateral disability spontaneously use the affected hand together with the well-functioning hand in play with toys requiring bimanual performance
Population	Ages 18mo–12y with hemiplegic cerebral palsy (CP) or brachial plexus palsy Small Kids AHA: 18mo–5y School Kids AHA: 6–12y

Description of domains (subscales)	The items describe different types of object-related actions of the assisting hand under the following headings:
	    General usage, three items (timing and amount of use)
	    Arm use, three items (reaching and use of varied arm movements)
	    Grasp-release, seven items (how objects are grasped, handled and released)
	    Coordination, two items (interaction between hands)
	    Pace, three items (fluency of performance)

Administration and test format	Time to complete: play session with child approximately 15min, scoring 30–45min Testing format: a semi-structured video-recorded play session is conducted in which specific toys from the AHA test kit requiring bimanual handling are used. The scoring is performed by a review of the video Scoring: 22 items on a one- to four-point rating scale. The AHA generates a sum score (range 22–88, higher points indicates higher ability) or transformed to a percentage score (range 1–100). Through a Rasch analysis, an interval measure can be obtained in the unit logits, by contact with the developers (range –10.18 to +8.70 logits) Training: required; information available at www.ahanetwork.se
Psychometric properties	Standardization sample: developed with Rasch measurement analysis of 409 assessments of children aged 18mo–12y (88% from children with hemiplegic CP) *Reliability* Intrarater, inter-rater and test–retest reliability established (intraclass correlation coefficients range from 0.97 to 0.99 for sum scores) *Validity* Construct validity studies reported Responsiveness: person strata separated=7 Standard error of measurement=1.40, giving a smallest detectable difference of 3.89 raw scores. A change of 3.89 sum scores has a significance of p=0.046
How to order	The AHA test kit with material for children aged between 18mo and 12y can be ordered at an AHA course or during the certification procedure from Handfast AB (www.ahanetwork.se)
Key references	Holmefur M, Krumlinde-Sundholm L, Eliasson A-C (2007) Interrater and intrarater reliability of the Assisting Hand Assessment. *Am J Occup Ther* 61: 79–84. Holmefur M, Aarts P, Hoare B, Krumlinde-Sundholm L (2009) Test–retest and alternate forms reliability of the Assisting Hand Assessment. *J Rehab Med* 41: 886–891. Holmefur M, Krumlinde-Sundholm L, Bergström J, Eliasson AC (2010) Longitudinal development of hand function in children with unilateral cerebral palsy. *Dev Med Child Neurol* 52: 352–257. Krumlinde-Sundholm L, Eliasson A-C (2003) Development of the Assisting Hand Assessment: a Rasch-built measure intended for children with unilateral upper limb impairments. *Scand J Occup Ther* 10: 16–26.

Krumlinde-Sundholm L, Holmefur M, Kottorp A, Eliasson A-C (2007) The Assisting Hand Assessment: current evidence of validity, reliability and responsiveness to change. *Dev Med Child Neurol* 49: 259–264.

Administration and scoring

Training for AHA certification is required to proficiently administer and reliably score the instrument. The AHA is administered as a semi-structured video-recorded 15-minute play session in which specific toys from the AHA test kit requiring bimanual handling are used. The scoring is performed by a review of the video and takes approximately 30 to 45 minutes to complete. The 22 AHA items are scored on a one- to four-point rating scale. The items describe different types of object-related actions of the assisting hand under the following headings: general usage – three items (timing and amount of use); arm use – three items (reaching and use of varied arm movements); grasp–release – seven items (how objects are grasped, handled and released); coordination – two items (interaction between hands); and pace – three items (fluency of performance). Ratings are interpreted as follows: 4=effective; 3=somewhat effective; 2=ineffective; and 1=does not do. The manual provides descriptions of behaviours within scoring categories for each item. Examiners use the most commonly used performance (habitual performance) for scoring each item rather than the child's best performance.

A total of the item scores is computed to generate a sum score (range 22–88, higher points indicates higher ability), which may be transformed to a percentage score (range 1–100). Through a Rasch analysis, an interval measure can be obtained in the unit logits by contacting the AHA developers (range –10.18 to +8.70 logits). Information on training programmes for the AHA is available at www.ahanetwork.se.

Psychometric properties

Standardization of the AHA was completed with a sample of 409 assessments of children aged 18 months to 12 years (88% from children with hemiplegic CP). Rasch measurement analysis was used to construct the measure. Studies have been completed for intrarater reliability (ICC range=0.97–0.99 for sum scores) and inter-rater reliability between two raters (r=0.98) and 20 raters (r=0.97),[116] as well as test–retest reliability for the Small Kids AHA (r=0.97) and School Kids AHA (r=0.98).[117] Construct validity studies reported discrimination between children with different levels of hand function.[113,118] As an evaluative measure, validity was established by person separation reliability estimate (r=0.97) with 303 children aged 18 months to 12 years.[113] A standard error of measurement

(SEM) of 1.40 was established with a sample of 55 children, aged 18 months to 12 years, and the minimum detectable difference was estimated to be 3.89 points.[117] There is also evidence that the AHA score from children with unilateral CP at age 18 months can be used in discussions of future development of affected hand use.[119]

ABILHAND

Overview and purpose

ABILHAND was originally developed as a measure of *manual ability* for *adults* with *upper limb impairments*. Based on this assessment, ABILHAND-Kids[120] was developed for children aged 6 to 16 years. The scale measures a person's ability to manage *daily activities* that require the use of the upper limbs with whatever strategies are involved. Unlike other measures with scores based on observation of the child's performance, the ABILHAND-Kids applies a questionnaire format based on a Rasch model. The ABILHAND-Kids has been found to be useful in individuals at different levels, with psychometric support for its use as a discriminative/descriptive measure.

Administration and scoring

The parent-completed questionnaire includes 21 routine tasks performed by the child, with performance rated on a three-point scale ('can do with ease', 'can do with difficulty' or 'impossible'). The raw data collected on the 21 items are submitted for online analysis to www.rehabscales.org/abilhand.html, where the score is converted to a linear measure of manual ability. Online analysis of raw and percentage scores to logits is free of charge and completed in a timely manner. The administration time required is not reported by the test developers. Information on accessing the ABILHAND-Kids is available at www.rehab-scales.org/abilhand.html.

Psychometric properties

Internal consistency is reported as strong, with a person separation reliability estimate of 0.94 based upon 113 children aged 6 to 15 years with a variety of types of CP. Test–retest reliability was established with 36 children (r=0.91).[120] Support for construct validity is reflected in the relationship of the ABILHAND-Kids with the GMFCS[121] and the types of CP and school education level of the children tested.[120]

SCHOOL ASSESSMENT OF MOTOR AND PROCESS SKILLS (SCHOOL AMPS)

Purpose	To measure school-based task performance in typical classroom settings
	Standardized measure of a student's school motor skills and school process ability – performance
	Examines the relationship between the student, the school task and the environment
	Compares the quality of task performance with that of same-aged peers
Population	Age 3–12y
Description of domains (subscales)	Five categories of school tasks:
	pen/pencil writing tasks;
	drawing and colouring tasks;
	cutting and pasting tasks;
	computer writing tasks; and
	maths manipulative tasks.
	Except for the manipulative task category, which includes two tasks, each category of schoolwork tasks includes four or five specific tasks, for a total of 21 School AMPS tasks
Administration and test format	Time to complete: varies depending on task and student skills
	Testing format: observation based, conducted in the student's classroom, during his or her typical routine, while performing two school tasks assigned by the teacher; interview with the student's teacher
	Scoring: four-point rating scale is used to score each of 16 school-motor and 20 school-process skills, for each task performed
	Training: five-day training course and calibration as a reliable rater is required
Psychometric properties	Normative sample: included children with developmental disabilities, as well as a cross-cultural study of children residing in the USA and in Brazil
	Reliability
	Inter-rater reliability – five out of six raters demonstrated goodness of fit (mean squared error ≤ 1.4 and $z < 2$).
	Validity
	Construct, criterion and person response validity studies reported acceptable goodness of fit
How to order	See www.schoolamps.com for the School AMPS Manual
	Cost: US$65
Key references	Atchison BT, Fisher AG, Bryze K (1998) Rater reliability and internal scale and person response validity of the School Assessment of Motor and Process Skills. *Am J Occup Ther* 52: 843–850.
	Fingerhut P, Madill H, Darrah J, Hodge M, Warren S (2002) Classroom-based assessment: validation for the School AMPS. *Am J Occup Ther* 56: 210–213.
	Fisher AG, Bryze K, Atchison BT (2000) Naturalistic assessment of functional performance in school settings. Reliability and validity of the School AMPS. *J Outcome Measure* 4: 504–522.
	Fisher AG, Bryze K, Hume V, Griswold LA (2005) *School AMPS: School Version of the Assessment of Motor and Process Skills*. Fort Collins, CO: Three Star Press.

MEASURING GROSS AND FINE MOTOR PERFORMANCE IN THE CONTEXT OF THE SCHOOL ENVIRONMENT

There is also the opportunity to take an integrated look at fine motor or gross motor skill performance in the context of the school environment. Four well-known measures, three observational and one teacher-report, are profiled below. The first two measures look at overall school task performance, while the last two focus on handwriting skills in the classroom.

School Assessment of Motor and Process Skills

Overview and purpose

The School AMPS is a criterion- and norm-referenced test designed to measure a child's ability to perform school tasks in naturalistic classroom settings.[122,123] The School AMPS was developed from the adult measure, the Assessment of Motor and Process Skills (AMPS), to address the need for a valid, reliable and clinically useful tool to measure a child's abilities in classroom activities.[123] To measure motor and process skills, the therapist observes the child in the classroom setting, thus providing an opportunity to examine the relationship between the student, the school task and the environment. Five categories of school tasks that may be observed and later rated are pen/pencil writing tasks, drawing and colouring tasks, cutting and pasting tasks, computer writing tasks and maths manipulative tasks. Except for the manipulative task category, which includes two tasks, each of the other categories of schoolwork tasks includes four or five specific tasks, for a total of 21 School AMPS tasks.

The observed School AMPS tasks completed by the child are rated for the quality of his or her motor skills, including posture, mobility, coordination, strength and effort, and energy. The child's performance during the observed task is also rated for process skills, which include attention, using knowledge, temporal organization, using space and objects, and adaptation. The data collected are compared for quality of task performance with those of peers aged 3 to 12 years.

Administration and scoring

Before administration of the School AMPS, the therapist meets with the classroom teacher to choose two tasks (from the 21 School AMPS tasks) that provide a challenge to the child being tested. Observation by the therapist takes place in the classroom during the time that the chosen tasks are completed by the total class. The therapist takes notes of the child's skills during task completion but does not rate performance. Observation notes are later used to rate the quality of the child's performance on a four-point rating scale used to score each of 16 school

motor and 20 school process skills. The School AMPS software provides an addition criterion and normative data to assess the child's performance. Because factors supporting and hindering performance are identified, the School AMPS provides a framework for intervention strategies to use in the classroom. The time to complete the School AMPS varies depending upon the task and student skills. A 5-day training course and calibration as a reliable rater is required.

Psychometric properties

The School AMPS provides normative data based on >200 children, including those with developmental disabilities, as well as a cross-cultural study of children residing in the USA and in Brazil. Scores are based on a multifaceted Rasch model used during test development. Rater reliability was established with five of six raters demonstrating goodness of fit to the Rasch model (mean squared error ≤ 1.4 and $z < 2$). Internal scale validity was based on all 36 motor and process skills demonstrating goodness of fit. Using School AMPS results of 208 students, person response validity was supported, with 93.7% demonstrating goodness of fit on the School AMPS Motor Scale and 88.9% with goodness of fit on the School AMPS Process Scale.[123] Discriminative construct validity was established, with significant differences identified between students at risk and control children on the School AMPS.[124] Concurrent validity between the School AMPS and Peabody Fine Motor Developmental Scales 2 (PDMS-2 FM) resulted in a higher correlation with the School AMPS Motor Scale ($r=0.45$) than the School AMPS Process Scale ($r=0.35$).[125]

School Function Assessment

Overview and purpose

The SFA is a criterion-referenced, judgement-based questionnaire completed by the school team.[126] It measures an elementary school student's performance on functional tasks that support participation in academic and social aspects of the school programme. It can be applied to older children, bearing in mind that there may be some content insufficiencies. The SFA facilitates collaborative programme planning for students in the school environment and can be used across a variety of physical and cognitive disabilities. It was also designed to be used as an outcome measure, tracking change over the course of a goal period or school term.

The SFA takes a top-down approach where the child's participation in aspects of the school day is determined (Section I), the task and environmental supports (assistance and adaptations) that are in place are documented

SCHOOL FUNCTION ASSESSMENT (SFA)	
Purpose	To measure a student's performance on functional tasks that supports his or her participation in academic and social aspects of an elementary school programme
	May be used to facilitate collaborative programme planning for students with a variety of disabling conditions
Population	Kindergarten to sixth grade, any diagnosis
Description of domains (subscales)	Three domains (sections):
	Participation: rates participation in six areas: (1) regular/special education classroom, (2) playground/recess, (3) transportation to and from school, (4) bathroom activities, (5) transitions to and from class and (6) mealtime or snacktime (six items)
	Task supports: rates two types of support students may require for success in school: (1) assistance (adult help) and (2) adaptations (special equipment or materials) when completing 12 physical tasks and nine cognitive/behavioural tasks which are school-related (21 items)
	Activity performance: rates the ability to perform 12 physical tasks and nine cognitive/behavioural tasks which are school related (171 items)
Administration and test format	Time to complete: may vary from 1.5 to 2h, with individual scales each 5–10min for administration. Since several respondents are involved with completing the SFA, the assessment may take days but should not exceed 2–3 weeks to control for maturation in children
	Testing format: school personnel familiar with the student's performance complete the SFA rating forms
	Scoring: rating of participation section is on a six-point scale ('limited' to 'full participation'). Rating of task supports section is on a four-point scale ('extensive' to 'no' assistance or adaptation). Rating of activity performance section is on a four-point scale ('does not perform' to 'consistent performance'). Individual items are added for a total raw score in each scale. Raw scores are converted to criterion scores. Criterion cut-off scores are outlined for each grade level. These scores can be mapped on Rasch-scaled map (by item difficulty order)
	Training: no specialized training is required
Psychometric properties	Normative sample: 363 students with disabilities and 315 regular education included from 112 different sites in 40 US states and Puerto Rico. Urban (23%), suburban (52%) and rural (26%) areas were represented as well as good representation of sex, ethnicity/race, socioeconomic status and disabling conditions
	Reliability
	Internal consistency excellent: Cronbach's alpha coefficients from 0.92 to 0.98. Test–retest reliability excellent: Pearson r and intraclass correlation coefficient range of 0.80–0.99 for each of the three sections and the individual subscales
	Validity
	30 content experts and 40 professionals participated in a content validity study. Authors provide support for the SFA based on four theoretical concepts outlined in the manual (construct validity). Discriminant validity demonstrated with various groups (integrated vs special classes; Gross Motor Function Classification System levels)
	Responsiveness
	Authors recommend that future research be conducted
How to order	Harcourt Assessment (www.PsychCorp.com)
	Cost: US$210 for the complete test kit including a package of score sheets

Key references	Coster W, Mancini M, Ludlow L (1999) Factor structure of the School Function Assessment. *Ed Psychol Measure* 59: 665–677.
	Davies PL, Soon PL, Young M, Clausen-Yamaki A (2004) Validity and reliability of the School Function Assessment in elementary school children with disabilities. *Phys Occup Ther Pediatr* 24: 23–43.
	Hwang JL, Davies PL (2009) Rasch analysis of the School Function Assessment provides additional evidence for the internal validity of the activity performance scales. *Am J Occup Ther* 63: 369–373.
	Schenker R, Coster WJ, Parush S (2005) Neuroimpairments, activity performance, and participation in children with cerebral palsy mainstreamed in elementary schools. *Dev Med Child Neurol* 47: 808–814.

(Section II) and a rating of the child's activity/performance of a series of 171 physical and cognitive activities is assessed (Section III). The child is given credit if alternative methods are used to perform a task. The SFA encourages consideration of the 'confluence' of the child, environmental and task factors rather than looking at the child's limitations in isolation. Details relating to the components of three sections of the SFA are provided in the summary chart in this chapter.

Administration and scoring

Time to complete the entire SFA varies from 1.5 to 2 hours, with individual subscales each requiring 5 to 10 minutes. Completion can be done by assigning sections to a designated staff member or done collaboratively at a team meeting. No SFA training is required. The SFA does not need to be completed in its entirety: single sections (I, II or III) can be completed because validation work was done separately for each.[127]

The participation section is rated on a six-point scale ('limited' to 'full participation'), task supports on a four-point scale ('extensive' to 'no' assistance or adaptation) and activity performance on a four-point scale ('does not perform' to 'consistent performance'). Individual items are added for a total raw score in each scale. Raw scores are converted to criterion scores. While the measure is not norm-referenced, criterion cut-off scores allow determination of whether the child is at, above or below their grade level. Results can be graphed onto an item map in the scoring booklet to give an idea of the child's strengths and challenges. These maps are derived from Rasch scaling work by the SFA's developers.

Psychometric properties

Item refinement was based on experts' content validity review and on the results of item response analysis with the SFA Try-out edition.[126] The developers concluded that internal consistency was high across sections (0.92–0.98). They also confirmed the two-factor structure of the

activity performance scale (physical function and cognitive/behavioural function) with children who had a physical or cognitive disability.[126] Test–retest reliability was excellent (ICCs 0.82–0.98) for the activity performance section,[126] and pilot work on inter-rater reliability (teacher vs occupational therapist) with a small sample of children with mental retardation,[a] autism or acquired brain injury revealed fair to good reliability across all three sections (from 0.68 to 0.73).[128]

From a validity perspective, discriminant validity evaluation has received the most attention. Each of the SFA's three sections differentiated between children with autism and mental retardation (i.e. 92.3% overall correct classification among the two groups),[128] children with cognitive and physical impairments,[129] typically developing children and those who had a learning disability or CP,[130] children with CP in fully integrated versus self-contained classrooms,[131] and among those with CP in GMFCS levels II, III and IV.[132] Translation to Chinese and Hebrew with related cultural adaptations have been done using rigorous methods.[132,133] For construct validity, there is a high degree of correlation with the Vineland Adaptive Behavior Scale[130] and fair to moderate association between the PODCI mobility scales and the various activity subscales of the SFA (r=0.35–0.65) in children with CP.[134] Rasch analysis supported internal construct validity of the activity performance subscales.[127]

Responsiveness has yet to be studied in depth. One study that evaluated school-based outcomes in the context of a conductive education intervention noted gains in the task supports (Section 2) but not in overall participation (Section 1) in a sample of six children with CP.[135] Section 3 (activity performance) was not evaluated owing to incomplete data. The other study looking at the effectiveness of school-based occupational therapy services on children with handwriting issues found that the written work subscale showed gains (p<0.001) alongside

---

[a] UK usage: learning disability.

EVALUATION TOOL OF CHILDREN'S HANDWRITING (ETCH)

Purpose	Evaluates a child's legibility and speed in a number of different writing tasks which are similar to those required of children in the classroom
Population	Children in grades 1–6 ETCH-Manuscript (ETCH-M) for children in grades 1 and 2 ETCH- Cursive (ETCH-C) for children in grades 3–6
Description of domains (subscales)	Alphabet and/or writing of upper and lower case letters and numerals from memory, near-point copying, far-point copying, manuscript to cursive transition, dictation and sentence composition. Manuscript or cursive writing is evaluated
Administration and test format	Time to complete: 15–25min for administration; 15–20min for scoring Testing format: the child is observed and timed while completing each task Scoring: word and letter legibility percentages determined by the readability of each writing area Writing speed per task is measured in letters per minute. Qualitative judgements related to the legibility components of letter formation, size, horizontal alignment and spacing. Qualitative observations addressing biomechanical aspects of writing: pencil grasp, positional consistency of pencil, pencil pressure, manipulation of pencil, and upper body stability and mobility Training: not required, but tutorials are available in the manual to gain 90% agreement prior to using the test
Psychometric properties	Normative sample: criterion-referenced test Preliminary normative data collected support the speed and legibility ranges for first graders. In one sample ($n=30$), 83% of children scored >80% on ETCH total word legibility and 90% scored >80% on the ETCH total letter legibility *Reliability* Inter-rater reliability (intraclass correlation coefficient) total scores, $r=0.47$–0.96; ETCH-M for inexperienced examiners ($r=0.47$) and between experienced examiners ($r=0.84$) Test–retest reliability high (r 0.84–0.95); ETCH-M ($r=0.63$–0.77) *Validity* ETCH results for children with less than average handwriting scored significantly lower than children with better than average handwriting for discriminative validity. Mean ETCH-C legibility percentage scores improved as handwriting grades improved with a significant moderate correlation reported
How to order	O.T. KIDS (www.alaska.net/~otkids) Cost: US$150
Key references	Feder KP, Majnemer A (2003) Children's handwriting evaluation tools and their psychometric properties. *Phys Occup Ther Pediatr* 23: 65–83. Koziatek SM, Powell NJ (2002) A validity study of the Evaluation Tool of Children's Handwriting-Cursive. *Am J OccupTher* 56: 446–453. Sudsawad P, Trombly CA, Henderson A, Tickle-Degnen L (2000) The relationship between the Evaluation Tool of Children's Handwriting and teachers' perceptions of handwriting legibility. *Am J Occup Ther* 55: 518–523.

a significant gain on the Evaluation Tool of Children's Handwriting (ETCH-M).[136] While both of these studies show that the SFA has potential to detect change, formal responsiveness evaluation is required to elucidate the meaning of the observed change scores.

The SFA has not been adopted by clinical investigators as much as might have been anticipated. While it remains the only measure that broadly covers activity and participation entirely in the school environment context, its length can prove daunting for school teams. As the three sections of the SFA were validated separately, these can be used on their own if this fits with the team's goal focus. Caution is needed if using selected subsections of Section 3 (activity performance), as the reliability of these smaller sections is not known.

Evaluation Tool of Children's Handwriting – Manuscript

Overview and purpose
The ETCH-M is a criterion-referenced, standardized tool designed to evaluate a child's legibility and speed in a number of different writing tasks that are required in the classroom. Children in grades 1 and 2 are the target group for the ETCH-M, while the cursive version, ETCH-C, is for grades 3 to 6.[137] Children tested with the ETCH-M need to have experience with manuscript writing for at least 10 to 12 weeks before evaluation. Although the ETCH has a manuscript and cursive version, the ETCH-M is more frequently cited in the literature. No formal training is required; however, the manual provides tutorials and quizzes to assist the examiner in achieving the recommended 90% scoring competency before using the test in their practice. This review will focus on ETCH-M, anticipating that children with developmental delays will more frequently be administered this version.

Six writing tasks make up the ETCH-M: Task I – writing the alphabet in sequence from memory in lower case and then in upper case; Task II – writing numerals 1 to 12 in sequence from memory; Task III – near-point copying of a short sentence from a preprinted model placed 3 inches from the top of response booklet; Task IV – far-point copying of a short sentence from a preprinted model on a wall chart 1.8 to 2.4 metres from the child's desk; Task V – a dictation task in which the child prints two nonsense words of five letters and one postal code of two numbers which are recited by the examiner; and Task VI – a sentence composition task in which the child is asked to write a sentence containing at least five words.

Administration and scoring
The test is administered individually in the order of the outlined tasks. Legibility is the focus of scoring, with illustrations of legible and illegible letters and numbers and words provided in the manual. Legibility components include letter formation, size, horizontal alignment and spacing. Within each task domain, legibility scores are determined by subtracting the number of illegible letters, numbers and words from the total possible points and converting them to task percentage scores and total legibility percentage scores. Writing speed is calculated for near- and far-point copying and sentence composition and converted to a number of letters per minute calculation. Observations are made of the quality of biomechanical aspects of writing: pencil grasp, positional consistency of pencil, pencil pressure, manipulation of pencil, and upper body stability and mobility. The ETCH-M takes 15 to 25 minutes for test administration and an additional 15 to 20 minutes for scoring.

Psychometric properties
Early development of the ETCH consisted of three pilot editions with revision and review by a panel of experts. Preliminary normative data collected support the speed and legibility ranges for first graders. Eighty-three per cent of children in the sample ($n=30$) scored >80% on ETCH-M total word legibility and 90% scored >80% on the ETCH-M total letter legibility. Further collection of normative data is needed. Inter-rater reliability for the (ICC) total scores of the ETCH is $r=0.47$–0.96. Inter-rater reliability for the ETCH-M is lower for inexperienced raters ($r=0.79$) as compared with experienced raters ($r=0.84$) by Pearson coefficients, and lower by ICCs (0.66). The test's author outlines specific recommendations around total score use based on the lower reliability on task scores.[138] Test–retest reliability was established with a group of 31 first and second graders, with the two tests administered within a 7-day interval. Reliability coefficients varied from $r=0.63$ to 0.77, with upper case legibility more consistent than other ETCH-M tasks. Based on these results, the authors did not recommend the use of individual task scores.[139] Discriminative (construct) validity has been supported by ETCH results of preterm children having significantly lower legibility and slower speed scores than control children born at term.[140] Concurrent validity of the ETCH-C with cursive practice and review worksheets was moderately supported with coefficients of 0.61 to 0.65.[141] A relationship between the ETCH and teachers' perceptions of handwriting legibility has also been established.[142]

Minnesota Handwriting Assessment

Overview and purpose

The Minnesota Handwriting Assessment (MHA, previously the Minnesota Handwriting Test) is a norm-referenced test designed to measure small changes in manuscript handwriting performance of younger children. The MHA may be used as a discriminative/descriptive measure to identify children with handwriting difficulties in grades 1 and 2 and may also be used as an evaluative measure over time to document the outcomes of children receiving services. The MHA evaluates near-point copying and speed of handwriting. Using the test sheet with the sentence 'the quick brown fox jumped over lazy dogs' on top, the child is asked to copy the sentence in the space below. The sentence represents the alphabet in jumbled form. Two forms of the test sheets are available, one in D'Nealian printing and one in standard manuscript to match the printing style used in the classroom. Small triangles are printed on the left side of the page to help the child find the starting point.

Administration and scoring

The child is seated at an appropriate table height for writing and are asked to write the sentence. The stopwatch is started and the child is instructed to stop writing at 2.5 minutes, to put his or her pencil down and circle the last letter completed. He or she is then allowed to finish the sample so that the entire handwriting sample is available for scoring. The child's handwriting sample is rated for quality in five categories: legibility, form, alignment, size and spacing. Legibility is first scored, requiring the letter to be recognizable out of context, be completed with all strokes present and contain no reversals. If legibility criteria are not met, scoring for that letter is discontinued. Specific criteria are also outlined for the other four categories with one point possible for each letter in each category (five total points possible per letter). The rate score is calculated by the number of letters completed in 2.5 minutes. The time limit and paper used in the test were determined through pilot studies.[143] The MHA can be ordered through Pearson Education, Inc. (www.pearson-assessments.com/HAIWEB/Cultures/en-us/Productdetail.htm?Pid=076–1637–001&Mode=summary) at a cost of US$180 at the time of writing.

Psychometric properties

Inter-rater reliability between experienced scorers was established, resulting in a high correlation ($r=0.99$) for total scores and category scores ($r=0.90$–0.99). Correlations of inexperienced scorers were also good for total ($r=0.98$) and category ($r=0.87$–0.98) scores. Test–retest reliability was established with 99 second-grade males tested with a 5- to 7-day window of time between tests. Correlation coefficients for total accuracy scores was $r=0.50$ with a between-school range of $r=0.47$ to 0.67. Differences in testing environments, attention and motivation may have contributed to the between-school differences.[143]

REFERENCES

1. Young NL, Williams JI, Yoshida KK, Bombardier C, Wright JG (1996) The context of measuring disability: does it matter whether capability or performance is measured? *J Clin Epidemiol* 49: 1097–1101.
2. Krumlinde-Sundholm L (2008) Choosing and using assessments of hand function. In: Eliasson AC, Burtner PA, editors. *Improving Hand Function in Children with Cerebral Palsy: Theory, Evidence and Practice*. London: Mac Keith Press, pp. 176–197.
3. Russell D, Palisano R, Walter S, et al (1998) Evaluating motor function in children with Down syndrome: validity of the GMFM. *Dev Med Child Neurol* 40: 693–701.
4. Russell DJ, Avery LM, Rosenbaum PL, Raina PS, Walter SD, Palisano RJ (2000) Improved scaling of the Gross Motor Function Measure for children with cerebral palsy: evidence of reliability and validity. *Phys Ther* 80: 873–885.
5. Russell DJ, Rosenbaum PL, Avery LM, Lane M (2002) *Gross Motor Function Measure (GMFM-66 & GMFM-88) User's Manual*. London: Mac Keith Press.
6. LaForme Fiss A, Effgen SK, Page J, Shasby S (2009) Effect of sensorimotor groups on gross motor acquisition for young children with Down syndrome. *Pediatr Phys Ther* 21: 158–166.
7. Looper J, Ulrich DA (2010) Effect of treadmill training and supramalleolar orthosis use on motor skill development in infants with Down syndrome: a randomized clinical trial. *Phys Ther* 90: 382–390.
8. Palisano RJ, Walter SD, Russell DJ, et al (2001) Gross motor function of children with Down syndrome: creation of motor growth curves. *Arch Phys Med Rehabil* 82: 494–500.
9. van den Heuvel ME, de Jong I, Lauteslager PE, Volman MJ (2009) Responsiveness of the Test of Basic Motor Skills of children with Down syndrome. *Phys Occup Ther Pediatr* 29: 71–85.
10. Gemus M, Palisano R, Russell D, et al (2001) Using the Gross Motor Function Measure to evaluate motor development in children with Down syndrome. *Phys Occup Ther Pediatr* 21: 69–79.
11. Harvey A, Robin J, Morris ME, Graham HK, Baker R (2008) A systematic review of measures of activity limitation for children with cerebral palsy. *Dev Med Child Neurol* 50: 190–198.
12. Damiano DL, Gilgannon MD, Abel MF (2005) Responsiveness and uniqueness of the Pediatric Outcomes Data Collection Instrument compared to the Gross Motor Function Measure for measuring orthopaedic and neurosurgical outcomes in cerebral palsy. *J Pediatr Orthop* 25: 641–645.
13. Josenby AL, Jarnlo GB, Gummesson C, Nordmark E (2009) Longitudinal construct validity of the GMFM-88 total score and goal total score and the GMFM-66 score in a 5 year follow-up study. *Phys Ther* 89: 342–350.
14. Wang HY, Yang YH (2006) Evaluating the responsiveness of 2 versions of the gross motor function measure for children with cerebral palsy. *Arch Phys Med Rehabil* 87: 51–56.

15. Vos-Vromans DC, Ketelaar M, Gorter JW (2005) Responsiveness of evaluative measures for children with cerebral palsy: the Gross Motor Function Measure and the Pediatric Evaluation of Disability Inventory. *Disabil Rehabil* 27: 1245–1252.

16. Wilson A, Kavanaugh A, Moher R, et al (2011) Development and pilot testing of the Challenge Module: a proposed adjunct to the Gross Motor Function Measure for high functioning children with cerebral palsy. *Phys Occup Ther Pediatr* 31: 135–149.

17. Christiansen AS, Lange C (2008) Intermittent versus continuous physiotherapy in children with cerebral palsy. *Dev Med Child Neurol* 50: 290–293.

18. Fowler EG, Knutson LM, Demuth SK, et al (2010) Pediatric endurance and limb strengthening (PEDALS) for children with cerebral palsy using stationary cycling: a randomized controlled trial. *Phys Ther* 90: 367–381.

19. Lowing K, Bexelius A, Carlberg EB (2010) Goal-directed functional therapy: a longitudinal study on gross motor function in children with cerebral palsy. *Disabil Rehabil* 32: 908–916.

20. Meyer-Heim A, Ammann-Reiffer C, Schmartz A, et al (2009) Improvement of walking abilities after robotic-assisted locomotion training in children with cerebral palsy. *Arch Dis Child* 94: 615–620.

21. Grunt S, Becher JG, van SP, van Ouwerkerk WJ, Ahmadi M, Vermeulen RJ (2010) Preoperative MRI findings and functional outcome after selective dorsal rhizotomy in children with bilateral spasticity. *Childs Nerv Syst* 26: 191–198.

22. Brunton L, Bartlett D, Russell D (2009) Validity and reliability of two abbreviated versions of the Gross Motor Function Measure. *Dev Med Child Neurol* 51: 25(F7).

23. Russell DJ, Avery LM, Walter SD, et al (2010) Development and validation of item sets to improve efficiency of administration of the 66-item Gross Motor Function Measure in children with cerebral palsy. *Dev Med Child Neurol* 52: e48–e54.

24. Hanna SE, Bartlett DJ, Rivard LM, Russell DJ (2008) Reference curves for the Gross Motor Function Measure: percentiles for clinical description and tracking over time among children with cerebral palsy. *Phys Ther* 88: 596–607.

25. Rosenbaum PL, Walter SD, Hanna SE, et al (2002) Prognosis for gross motor function in cerebral palsy: creation of motor development curves. *JAMA* 288: 1357–1363.

26. Gorter JW, Ketelaar M, Rosenbaum P, Helders PJ, Palisano R (2009) Use of the GMFCS in infants with CP: the need for reclassification at age 2 years or older. *Dev Med Child Neurol* 51: 46–52.

27. Bourke-Taylor H (2003) Melbourne Assessment of Unilateral Upper Limb Function: construct validity and correlation with the Pediatric Evaluation of Disability Inventory. *Dev Med Child Neurol* 45: 92–96.

28. Klingels K, Jaspers E, Van de Winckel A, De Cock P, Molenaers G, Feys H (2010) A systematic review of arm activity measures for children with hemiplegic cerebral palsy. *Clin Rehabil* 10: 887–900.

29. Klingels K, De CP, Desloovere K, et al (2008) Comparison of the Melbourne Assessment of Unilateral Upper Limb Function and the Quality of Upper Extremity Skills Test in hemiplegic CP. *Dev Med Child Neurol* 50: 1–6.

30. Randall M, Carlin JB, Chondros P, Reddihough D (2001) Reliability of the Melbourne assessment of unilateral upper limb function. *Dev Med Child Neurol* 43: 761–767.

31. Davids JR, Peace LC, Wagner LV, Gidewall MA, Blackhurst DW, Roberson WM (2006) Validation of the Shriners Hospital for Children Upper Extremity Evaluation (SHUEE) for children with hemiplegic cerebral palsy. *J Bone Jt Surg – Am* 88: 326–333.

32. Jebsen RH, Taylor N, Trieschmann RB, Trotter MJ, Howard LA (1969) An objective and standardized test of hand function. *Arch Phys Med Rehabil* 50: 311–319.

33. Bonnier B, Eliasson AC, Krumlinde-Sundholm L (2006) Effects of constraint-induced movement therapy in adolescents with hemiplegic cerebral palsy: a day camp model. *Scand J Occup Ther* 13: 13–22.

34. Charles JR, Wolf SL, Schneider JA, Gordon AM (2006) Efficacy of a child-friendly form of constraint-induced movement therapy in hemiplegic cerebral palsy: a randomized control trial. *Dev Med Child Neurol* 48: 635–642.

35. Charles JR, Gordon AM (2007) A repeated course of constraint-induced movement therapy results in further improvement. *Dev Med Child Neurol* 49: 770–773.

36. Gordon AM, Charles J, Wolf SL (2006) Efficacy of constraint-induced movement therapy on involved upper-extremity use in children with hemiplegic cerebral palsy is not age-dependent. *Pediatrics* 117: e363–e373.

37. Taylor N, Sand PL, Jebsen RH (1973) Evaluation of hand function in children. *Arch Phys Med Rehabil* 45: 129–135.

38. Folio MR, Fewell RR (2000) *Peabody Developmental Motor Scales*, 2nd edition. San Antonio, TX: Pearson.

39. Jones NL, Apling RN, Smole DP (2004) *Individuals with Disabilities Education Act (IDEA)*. Hauppauge: Nova Science Publishers.

40. Connolly BH (2006) Concurrent validity of the Bayley Scales of Infant Developemt II (BSID-II) Motor Scale and the Peabody Developmental Motor Scale II (PDMS-2) in 12-month old infants. *Pediatr Phys Ther* 18: 190–196.

41. Goyen T-A, Lui K (2002) Longitudinal motor development of 'apparently normal' high-risk infants at 18 months, 3 and 5 years. *Early Hum Dev* 70: 103–115.

42. Tieman BL, Palisano RJ, Sutlive AC (2005) Assessment of motor development and function in preschool children. *Ment Retard Dev Disabil Res Rev* 11: 189–196.

43. van Hartingsveldt MJ, Cup EH, Oostendorp RA (2005) Reliability and validity of the fine motor scale of the Peabody Developmental Motor Scales-2. *Occup Ther Int* 12: 1–13.

44. Wang HH, Liao HF, Hsieh CL (2006) Reliability, sensitivity to change, and responsiveness of the Peabody Developmental Motor Scales – second edition for children with cerebral palsy. *Phys Ther* 86: 1351–1359.

45. Wiepert SL, Stemmons V (2002) Effects of an increased number of practice trials on Peabody Developmental Gross Motor Scale Scores in children of preschool age with typical development. *Pediatr Phys Ther* 14: 22–28.

46. Chien CW, Bond TG (2009) Measurement properties of fine motor scale of Peabody Developmental Motor Scales – Second Edition. *Am J Phys Med Rehabil* 88: 376–386.

47. Provost B, Heimerl S, McClain C, Kim NH, Lopez BR, Kodituwakku P (2004) Concurrent validity of the Bayley Scales of Infant Development II Motor Scale and the Peabody Developmental Motor Scales-2 in children with developmental delays. *Pediatr Phys Ther* 16: 149–156.

48. Palisano R (1986) Concurrent and predictive validities of the Bayley Motor Scale and the Peabody Developmental Motor Scales. *Phys Ther* 66: 1714–1719.

49. Maring JR, Elbaum L (2007) Concurrent validity of the Early Intervention Developmental Profile and the Peabody Developmental Motor Scale-2. *Pediatr Phys Ther* 19: 116–120.

50. Snyder P, Eason JM, Philibert D, Ridgway A, McCaughey T (2008) Concurrent validity and reliability of the Alberta Infant Motor Scale in infants at dual risk for motor delays. *Phys Occup Ther Pediatr* 28: 267–282.

51. Kolobe TH, Palisano RJ, Stratford PW (1998) Comparison of two outcome measures for infants with cerebral palsy and infants with motor delays. *Phys Ther* 78: 1062–1072.

52. Palisano RJ, Kolobe TH, Haley SM, Lowes LP, Jones SL (1995) Validity of the Peabody Developmental Gross Motor Scale as an evaluative measure of infants receiving physical therapy. *Phys Ther* 75: 939–951.

53. Coker P, Lebkicher C, Harris L, Snape J (2009) The effects of constraint induced movement therapy for a child less than one year of age. *Neurorehabilitation* 24: 199–208.

54. Olesch CA, Greaves S, Imms C, Reid SM, Graham HK (2010) Repeat botulinum toxin-A injections in the upper limb for children with hemiplegia: a randomized controlled trail. *Dev Med Child Neurol* 52: 79–86.

55. Chen YP, Kang LJ, Chuang TY, et al (2007) Use of virtual reality to improve upper extremity control in children with cerebral palsy: a single subject design. *Phys Ther* 87: 1441–1457.

56. Bruininks RH (1978) *Bruininks–Oseretsky Test of Motor Proficiency. Examiner's Manual Edition*. Circle Pines, MN: American Guidance Service.

57. Bruininks RH, Bruininks B (2005) *Bruininks–Oseretsky Test of Motor Proficiency*. Minneapolis, MN: NCS Pearson.

58. Hattie J, Edwards H (1987) A review of the Bruininks–Oseretsky Test of Motor Proficiency. *Br J Edu Psychol* 57: 104–113.

59. Kambas A, Aggeloussis N (2006) Construct validity of the Bruininks–Oseretsky Test of Motor Proficiency – short form for a sample of Greek preschool and primary school children. *Percept Mot Skill* 102: 65–72.

60. Wilson BN, Polatajko HJ, Kaplan BJ, Faris P (2001) Use of the Buininks–Oseretsky Test of Motor Proficiency in occupational therapy. *Percept Mot Skill* 92: 157–166.

61. Wuang YP, Lin YH, Su CY (2009) Rasch analysis of the Bruininks–Oseretsky Test of Motor Proficiency – second edition in intellectual disabilities. *Res Dev Disabil* 30: 1132–1144.

62. Dietz JC, Kartin D, Kopp K (2007) Review of the Bruininks–Oseretsky Test of Motor Proficiency, Second Edition (BOT-2). *Phys Occup Ther Pediatr* 27: 87–102.

63. Ketelaar M, Vermeer A, Helders PJ (1998) Functional motor abilities of children with cerebral palsy: a systematic literature review of assessment measures. *Clin Rehabil* 12: 369–380.

64. Hassan MM (2001) Validity and reliability for the Bruininks–Oseretsky Test of Motor Proficiency – Short Form as applied in the United Arab Emirates culture. *Percept Mot Skill* 92: 157–166.

65. Wiart L, Darrah J (2001) Review of four tests of gross motor development. *Dev Med Child Neurol* 43: 279–285.

66. Liao HF, Mao PJ, Hwang AW (2001) Test–retest reliability of balance tests in children with cerebral palsy. *Dev Med Child Neurol* 43: 180–186.

67. Wang TN, Tseng MH, Wilson BN, Hu FC (2009) Functional performance of children with developmental coordination disorder at home and at school. *Dev Med Child Neurol* 51: 817–825.

68. Beitel PA (1980) Bruininks–Oseretsky Test of Motor Proficiency: a viable measure for 3 to 5 year old children. *Percept Mot Skill* 51: 919–923.

69. Duger T, Bumin G, Uyanik M, Aki E, Kayihan H (1999) The assessment of Bruininks–Oseretsky test of motor proficiency in children. *Pediatr Rehabil* 3: 125–131.

70. Venetsanou F, Kambas A, Aggeloussis N, Fatouros I, Taxildaris K (2009) Motor assessment of preschool aged children: a preliminary investigation of the validity of the Bruininks–Oseretsky test of motor proficiency – short form. *Hum Mov Sci* 28: 543–550.

71. Wilson BN, Polatajko HJ, Kaplan BJ, Faris P (1995) Use of the Bruininks–Oseretsky test of motor proficiency in occupational therapy. *Am J Occup Ther* 49: 8–17.

72. Ziviani J, Poulsen A, O'Brien A (1982) Correlation of the Bruininks–Oseretsky Test of Motor Proficiency with the Southern California Sensory Integration Tests. *Am J Occup Ther* 36: 519–523.

73. Yoon DY, Scott K, Hill MN, Levitt NS, Lambert EV (2006) Review of three tests of motor proficiency in children. *Percept Motor Skill* 102: 543–551.

74. Crawford SG, Wilson BN, Dewey D (2001) Identifying developmental coordination disorder: consistency between tests. *Phys Occup Ther Pediatr* 20: 29–50.

75. Flanagan A, Krzak J, Peer M, Johnson P, Urban M (2009) Evaluation of short-term intensive orthotic garment use in children who have cerebral palsy. *Pediatr Phys Ther* 21: 201–204.

76. Bumin G, Kavak ST (2008) An investigation of the factors affecting handwriting performance in children with hemiplegic cerebral palsy. *Disabil Rehabil* 30: 1374–1385.

77. Gordon AM, Schneider JA, Chinnan A, Charles JR (2007) Efficacy of a hand-arm bimanual intensive therapy (HABIT) in children with hemiplegic cerebral palsy: a randomized control trial. *Dev Med Child Neurol* 49: 830–838.

78. Hurvitz EA, Conti GE, Brown SH (2003) Changes in movement characteristics of the spastic upper extremity after botulinum toxin injection. *Arch Phys Med Rehabil* 84: 444–454.

79. Yang TF, Fu CP, Kao NT, Chan RC, Chen SJ (2003) Effect of botulinum toxin type A on cerebral palsy with upper limb spasticity. *Am J Phys Med Rehabil* 82: 284–289.

80. Cairney J, Hay J, Veldhuizen S, Missiuna C, Faught BE (2009) Comparing probable case identification of developmental coordination disorder using the short form of the Bruininks–Oseretsky Test of Motor Proficiency and the Movement ABC. *Child Care Health Dev* 35: 402–408.

81. Miller LT, Polatajko HJ, Missiuna C, Mandich AD, Macnab JJ (2001) A pilot trial of a cognitive treatment for children with developmental coordination disorder. *Hum Mov Sci* 20: 183–210.

82. Martin K (2004) Effects of supramalleolar orthoses on postural stability in children with Down syndrome. *Dev Med Child Neurol* 46: 406–411.

83. Lewis CL, Fragala-Pinkham MA (2005) Effects of aerobic conditioning and strength training on a child with Down syndrome: a case study. *Pediatr Phys Ther* 17: 30–36.

84. Connolly BH, Morgan SB, Russell FF, Fulliton WL (1993) A longitudinal study of children with Down syndrome who experienced early intervention programming. *Phys Ther* 73: 170–179.

85. Harvey A, Graham HK, Morris ME, Baker R, Wolfe R (2007) The Functional Mobility Scale: ability to detect change following single event multilevel surgery. *Dev Med Child Neurol* 49: 603–607.

86. Graham HK, Harvey A, Rodda J, Nattrass GR, Pirpiris M (2004) The Functional Mobility Scale (FMS). *J Pediatr Orthop* 24: 514–520.

87. Harvey AR, Morris ME, Graham HK, Wolfe R, Baker R (2010) Reliability of the functional mobility scale for children with cerebral palsy. *Phys Occup Ther Pediatr* 30: 139–149.

88. Harvey A, Baker R, Morris ME, Hough J, Hughes M, Graham HK (2010) Does parent report measure performance? A study of the construct validity of the Functional Mobility Scale. *Dev Med Child Neurol* 52: 181–185.

89. Cobeljic G, Bajin Z, Lesic A, Tomic S, Bumbasirevic M, Atkinson HD (2009) A radiographic and clinical comparison of two soft-tissue procedures for paralytic subluxation of the hip in cerebral palsy. *Int Orthop* 33: 503–508.

90. Svehlik M, Slaby K, Soumar L, Smetana P, Kobesova A, Trc T (2008) Evolution of walking ability after soft tissue surgery in cerebral palsy patients: what can we expect? *J Pediatr Orthop B* 7: 107–113.

91. McNee AE, Gough M, Morrissey MC, Shortland AP (2009) Increases in muscle volume after plantarflexor strength training

in children with spastic cerebral palsy. *Dev Med Child Neurol* 51: 429–435.

92. Novacheck TF, Stout JL, Tervo R (2000) Reliability and validity of the Gillette Functional Assessment Questionnaire as an outcome measure in children with walking disabilities. *J Pediatr Orthop* 20: 75–81.

93. Amichai T, Harries N, Dvir Z, Patish H, Copeliovitch L (2009) The effects of femoral derotation osteotomy in children with cerebral palsy: an evaluation using energy cost and functional mobility. *J Pediatr Orthop* 29: 68–72.

94. Gunel MK, Tarsuslu T, Mutlu A, Livanelioðlu A (2010) Investigation of interobserver reliability of the Gillette Functional Assessment Questionnaire in children with spastic diparetic cerebral palsy. *Acta Orthop Traumatol Turc* 44: 63–69.

95. Hillman SJ, Hazlewood ME, Schwartz MH, van der Linden ML, Robb JE (2007) Correlation of the Edinburgh Gait Score with the Gillette Gait Index, the Gillette Functional Assessment Questionnaire, and dimensionless speed. *J Pediatr Orthop* 27: 7–11.

96. Viehweger E, Haumont T, de Lattre C, et al (2008) Multidimensional outcome assessment in cerebral palsy: is it feasible and relevant? *J Pediatr Orthop* 28: 576–583.

97. Yap R, Majnemer A, Benaroch T, Cantin MA (2010) Determinants of responsiveness to botulinum toxin, casting, and bracing in the treatment of spastic equinus in children with cerebral palsy. *Dev Med Child Neurol* 52: 186–193.

98. Rodda JM, Graham HK, Nattrass GR, Galea MP, Baker R, Wolfe R (2006) Correction of severe crouch gait in patients with spastic diplegia with use of multilevel orthopaedic surgery. *J Bone Jt Surg – Am* 88: 2653–2664.

99. Trost JP, Schwartz MH, Krach LE, Dunn ME, Novacheck TF (2008) Comprehensive short-term outcome assessment of selective dorsal rhizotomy. *Dev Med Child Neurol* 50: 765–771.

100. Gorton GE III, Stout JL, Bagley AM, Bevans K, Novacheck TF, Tucker CA (2011) Gillette Functional Assessment Questionnaire 22-item skill set: factor and Rasch analyses. *Dev Med Child Neurol* 53: 250–255.

101. Daltroy LH, Liang MH, Fossel AH, Goldberg MJ (1998) The POSNA pediatric musculoskeletal functional health questionnaire: report on reliability, validity, and sensitivity to change. Pediatric Outcomes Instrument Development Group. Pediatric Orthopaedic Society of North America. *J Pediatr Orthop* 18: 561–571.

102. McCarthy ML, Silberstein CE, Atkins EA, Harryman SE, Sponseller PD, Hadley-Miller NA (2002) Comparing reliability and validity of pediatric instruments for measuring health and well-being of children with spastic cerebral palsy. *Dev Med Child Neurol* 44: 468–476.

103. McMulkin ML, Baird GO, Gordon AB, Caskey PM, Ferguson RL (2007) The Pediatric Outcomes Data Collection Instrument detects improvements for children with ambulatory cerebral palsy after orthopaedic intervention. *J Pediatr Orthop* 27: 1–6.

104. Oeffinger DJ, Tylkowski CM, Rayens MK, et al (2004) Gross Motor Function Classification System and outcome tools for assessing ambulatory cerebral palsy: a multicenter study. *Dev Med Child Neurol* 46: 311–319.

105. Haynes RJ, Sullivan E (2001) The Pediatric Orthopaedic Society of North America pediatric orthopaedic functional health questionnaire: an analysis of normals. *J Pediatr Orthop* 21: 619–621.

106. Barnes D, Linton JL, Sullivan E, et al (2008) Pediatric Outcomes Data Collection Instrument scores in ambulatory children with cerebral palsy: an analysis by age groups and severity level. *J Pediatr Orthop* 28: 97–102.

107. Pencharz J, Young NL, Owen JL, Wright JG (2001) Comparison of three outcomes instruments in children. *J Pediatr Orthop* 21: 425–432.

108. Sullivan E, Barnes D, Linton JL, et al (2007) Relationships among functional outcome measures used for assessing children with ambulatory CP. *Dev Med Child Neurol* 49: 338–344.

109. Cuomo AV, Gamradt SC, Kim CO, et al (2007) Health-related quality of life outcomes improve after multilevel surgery in ambulatory children with cerebral palsy. *J Pediatr Orthop* 27: 653–657.

110. Wright FV, Rosenbaum PL, Goldsmith CH, Law M, Fehlings DL (2008) How do changes in body functions and structures, activity, and participation relate in children with cerebral palsy? *Dev Med Child Neurol* 50: 283–289.

111. Allen DD, Gorton GE, Oeffinger DJ, Tylkowski C, Tucker CA, Haley SM (2008) Analysis of the Pediatric Outcomes Data Collection Instrument in ambulatory children with cerebral palsy using confirmatory factor analysis and item response theory methods. *J Pediatr Orthop* 28: 192–198.

112. Kimmerle M, Mainwaring L, Borenstein M (2003) The functional repertoire of the hand and its application to assessment. *Am J Occup Ther* 57: 489–498.

113. Krumlinde-Sundholm L, Holmefur M, Kottorp A, Eliasson AC (2007) The Assisting Hand Assessment: current evidence of validity, reliability, and responsiveness to change. *Dev Med Child Neurol* 49: 259–264.

114. Gilmore R, Sakzewski L, Boyd R (2010) Upper limb activity measures for 5- to 16-year-old children with congenital hemiplegia: a systematic review. *Dev Med Child Neurol* 52: 811–816.

115. Buffart LM, Roebroeck ME, van H, V, Pesch-Batenburg JM, Stam HJ (2007) Evaluation of arm and prosthetic functioning in children with a congenital transverse reduction deficiency of the upper limb. *J Rehabil Med* 39: 379–386.

116. Holmefur M, Krumlinde-Sundholm L, Eliasson AC (2007) Interrater and intrarater reliability of the Assisting Hand Assessment. *Am J Occup Ther* 61: 79–84.

117. Holmefur M, Aarts P, Hoare B, Krumlinde-Sundholm L (2009) Test–retest and alternate forms reliability of the Assisting Hand Assessment. *J Rehabil Med* 41 886–891.

118. Krumlinde-Sundholm L, Eliasson AC (2003) Development of the Assisting Hand Assessment: a Rasch-built measure intended for children with unilateral upper limb impairments. *Scand J Occup Ther* 10: 16–26.

119. Holmefur M, Krumlinde-Sundholm L, Bergstrom J, Eliasson AC (2010) Longitudinal development of hand function in children with unilateral cerebral palsy. *Dev Med Child Neurol* 52: 352–357.

120. Vandervelde L, Van den Bergh PYK, Penta M, Thonnard JL (2010) Validation of the ABILHAND questionnaire to measure manual ability in children and adults with neuromuscular disorders. *J Neurol Neurosurg Psychiatr* 81: 506–512.

121. Arnould C, Penta M, Render A, Thonnard J-L (2004) ABILHAND-Kids: a measure of manual ability in children with cerebral palsy. *Neurology* 63: 1045–1052.

122. Fisher AG, Bryze K, Hume V, Griswold LA (2005) *School AMPS: School Version of the Assessment of Motor and Process Skills.* Fort Collins, CO: Three Star Press.

123. Fisher AG, Bryze K, Atchison BT (2000) Naturalistic assessment of functional performance in school settings: reliability and validity of the School AMPS scales. *J Outcome Meas* 4: 504–522.

124. Fisher A, Duran G (2004) School task performance for students at risk of delays. *Scand J Occup Ther* 11: 191–198.

125. Fingerhut P, Madill H, Darrah J, Hodge M, Warren S (2002) Classroom-based assessment: validation for the school AMPS. *Am J Occup Ther* 56: 210–213.

126. Coster W, Deeney T, Haltiwanger J, Haley S (1998) School Function Assessment. San Antonio, TX: The Psychological Corporation.

127. Coster WJ, Mancini MC, Ludlwo LH (1999) Factor structure of the School Function Assessment. *Ed Psychol Meas* 59: 665–677.

128. Davies PL, Soon PL, Young M, Clausen-Yamaki A (2004) Validity and reliability of the school function assessment in elementary school students with disabilities. *Phys Occup Ther Pediatr* 24: 23–43.

129. Eligson S, Coster WJ (2004) School Function Assessment: performance of Icelandic students with special needs. *Scand J Occup Ther* 11: 163–170.

130. Hwang J, Davies PL, Taylor MP, Gavin WJ (2002) Validation of School Function Assessment with elementary school children. *Occup Ther J Res* 22: 1–11.

131. Schenker R, Coster WJ, Parush S (2006) Personal assistance, adaptations and participation in students with cerebral palsy mainstreamed in elementary schools. *Disabil Rehabil* 28: 1061–1069.

132. Schenker R, Coster WJ, Parush S (2005) Neuroimpairments, activity performance, and participation in children with cerebral palsy mainstreamed in elementary schools. *Dev Med Child Neurol* 47: 808–814.

133. Hwang JL, Nochajski SM, Linn RT, Wu YW (2004) The development of the School Function Assessment Chinese version for cross-cultural use in Taiwan. *Occup Ther Int* 11: 26–39.

134. Gates PE, Otsuka NY, Sanders JO, Gee-Brown J (2008) Relationship between parental PODCI questionnaire and School Function Assessment in measuring performance in children with CP. *Dev Med Child Neurol* 50: 690–695.

135. Wright FV, Boschen K, Jutai J (2005) Exploring the comparative responsiveness of a core set of outcome measures in a school-based conductive education programme. *Child Care Health Dev* 31: 291–302.

136. Case-Smith J (2002) Effectiveness of school-based occupational therapy intervention on handwriting. *Am J Occup Ther* 56: 17–25.

137. Amundson SJ (1995) *Evaluation Tool of Children's Handwriting*. Homer, AK: OT KIDS.

138. Feder KP, Majnemer A (2003) Children's handwriting evaluation tools and their psychometric properties. *Phys Occup Ther Pediatr* 23: 65–84.

139. Diekema SM, Deitz J, Amundson SJ (1998) Test–retest reliability of the Evaluation Tool of Children's Handwriting – manuscript. *Am J Occup Ther* 52: 248–255.

140. Feder KP, Majnemer A, Bourbonnais D, Platt R, Blayney M, Synnes A (2005) Handwriting performance in preterm children compared with term peers at age 6 to 7 years. *Dev Med Child Neurol* 47: 163–170.

141. Koziatek SM, Powell NJ (2002) A validity study of the Evaluation Tool of Children's Handwriting – Cursive. *Am J Occup Ther* 56: 446–453.

142. Sudsawad P, Trombly CA, Henderson A, Tickle-Degnen L (2000) The relationships between the Evaluation Tool of Children's Handwriting and teachers' perceptions of handwriting legibility. *Am J Occup Ther* 55: 518–523.

143. Reisman JE (1993) Development and reliability of the research version of the Minnesota Handwriting Test. *Phys Occup Ther Pediatr* 13: 41–55.

24
SELF-CARE (D510–D572)

Laurie M. Snider and Vasiliki Darsaklis

What is the construct?

The World Health Organization (WHO), by describing the spectrum of the effects of disease and disability on health, has emphasized that health can be affected by the inability to carry out activities and to participate in life situations.[1] Daily life activities, such as self-care, link individuals to meaningful patterns of engagement in occupations that allow participation in desired roles and life situations in the home, school, workplace and community. Activity limitations in the area of self-care are therefore an essential consideration in the measurement of the child's functional repertoire.

WHAT ARE SELF-CARE ACTIVITIES?

The construct of self-care addresses a range of activities such as grooming, bathing and hygiene, toileting, dressing, and eating and drinking. Activities attributed to self-care by the WHO International Classification of Functioning, Disability and Health for Children and Youth (ICF-CY) classification include washing oneself, caring for body parts (skin, teeth, hair, nails), toileting (including menstrual care), dressing (clothing and footwear), eating, drinking and looking after one's health (ensuring one's physical comfort, managing diet and fitness, maintaining one's health). Aspects particular to infants and children suggest issues of maturation and dependency, for example indicating the need for eating or drinking or drinking from the bottle/breast.[1] Self-care activities are identified as a component of activities of daily living (ADL). The younger the child, the more likely it is that ADL will be facilitated by parents, caregivers or service providers.

The ability or inability to carry out self-care can be interpreted as a measurement of the child's functional status. Performance of self-care is contingent on multiple factors, which include the interactions between the unique attributes of the individual, the context of the physical and sociocultural environment, and the specific demands of the task.[2] For example, difficulties with postural control and fine motor skills in school-aged children with developmental coordination disorder were reported to contribute to poorer performance of ADL.[3] Functional ability was found to be a significant predictor of participation intensity in both formal and informal activities in children with physical disabilities, such that children with greater functional limitations participated less.[4] Including factors such as level of assistance and technical aids provides a means to estimate the contribution of the environment in the performance of self-care.

General factors to consider when measuring this domain

ISSUES RELATED TO MEASUREMENT OF SELF-CARE IN CHILDREN

Measurement of self-care is carried out through either child self-report (e.g. Activities Scale for Kids[5] [ASK]/ Canadian Occupational Performance Measure[6] [COPM]) and/or through the proxy report of an informed observer such as a parent, teacher or clinician (e.g. Pediatric Evaluation of Disability Inventory[7] [PEDI], Functional Independence Measure for Children[8] [WeeFIM], Battelle Developmental Inventory[9] [BDI], Vineland Adaptive Behavior Scale[10] [VABS], COPM). While self-report by children as early as 6 years of age[11] is potentially feasible and informative for the measurement of satisfaction and other subjective experiences (e.g. performance of self-care), the use of proxy report may be more accurate in very young children whose performance in self-care is typically facilitated by family members/caregivers or in children with severe cognitive or communication challenges.

Measures currently in use vary widely in content. While a few measures have been developed more specifically for the purpose of measuring self-care (ASK), this construct is most commonly measured as a subdomain within a global functional assessment (e.g. VABS, BDI, WeeFIM, COPM). Furthermore, items which relate directly to self-care activities may be categorized into other subdomains. For example, the WeeFIM has six domains which include self-care, sphincter control, transfers, locomotion, communication and social cognition. In this case, the child's abilities in self-care are not only measured in one domain of this test. While some measurement tools clearly name self-care as a domain (WeeFIM, PEDI, COPM), others use different names for this domain, such as personal care, dressing (ASK), adaptive behaviour (BDI) or daily living skills (VABS). Some measures have been developed with a specific population in mind (e.g. Juvenile Arthritis Functional Status Index [JASI]).[12] Some measures are more global (e.g. VABS), while other take into consideration the degree of physical limitations by reporting the level of assistance required through assistive devices or increased caregiver time (e.g. PEDI, Assessment of Life Habits [LIFE-H]). Thus, it is important for the examiner to interpret the profile of the test accordingly. Measures with domains specifically in self-care that can be interpreted separately from the total test scores are useful in the planning and execution of appropriate intervention to improve self-care abilities. Some tests have been developed for younger children (e.g. PEDI) while others span a wider age range (e.g. VABS, LIFE-H).

Tests of feeding abilities examining the different components of feeding (nutritive, non-nutritive sucking, orofacial structure, orofacial motor function) have been developed for neonates (Neonatal Oral-Motor Assessment Scale[13]) and children with feeding disorders (Multidisciplinary Feeding Profile[14]).

Finally, in so far as the construct of self-care includes 'looking after one's health', only the LIFE-H addresses 'fitness' and 'nutrition'. Other aspects of 'maintaining one's health' through self-regulation are not addressed by the traditional self-care assessments, which are generally focused on the physical aspects of function. This area is of interest for the future development of methods and measurement tools which adequately address these components of the construct of self-care.

Overview of recommended measures

For the purposes of this chapter, an exhaustive survey of assessments for children and young people that address self-care was carried out. The results of this search are summarized in Figure 24.1. A brief overview of the primary global assessments (i.e. self-care as one domain among several domains of functioning) felt to be most commonly in use is briefly characterized below. These global measures are described in detail in Chapter 19. A more detailed depiction of measures that focus on self-care is presented in tabular format. In addition, descriptions of the properties of the self-care domain in several of the global measures are also included in the tables.

GLOBAL MEASURES THAT INCLUDE A SELF-CARE DOMAIN

The VABS[10] was one of the earliest measures to be developed that covers the spectrum of adaptive functioning in children and young people. Psychometric properties were established first on typically developing children and then in children and young people with cognitive impairment.[15] In 2005, a revised version with updated normative data based on the current US census demographics was developed.[16] The VABS-II addresses three domains (daily living, communication, socialization) and is administered by proxy report. As part of daily living skills, personal items related to eating, drinking, toileting, dressing, bathing, grooming and health care are included. Domestic items relate to safety at home, kitchen chores and housekeeping; community items include telephone skills, rules, rights and safety, time and dates, television and radio, and going to places independently; and skills relate to a job, computer use, money and going to restaurants. The psychometric properties of the VABS are presented in detail in Chapter 19. In terms of the reliability of the daily living subscale, the internal consistency split-half reliability coefficient ranges from 0.80 to 0.89, depending on age. Test–retest reliability intraclass correlation coefficient (ICC) is >0.90 for all age groups, except 14 to 21 years, where ICC=0.79. Inter-rater reliability ranges from 0.75 to 0.87. The daily living skills subscale correlates strongly (>0.88) with relevant subscales on the VABS, BDI and PEDI, demonstrating concurrent validity.

Designed as a self-report measure of childhood physical disability for children aged 5 to 15 years with musculoskeletal disorders, the ASK[17] can be completed by the child or the parent, either by mail or by computer. It is one of the measures of self-care that has been demonstrated to be very responsive to change over time.[5] The ASK has also been used in populations without musculoskeletal disability,[18] but its primary focus on physical function may be a limitation in its use on populations who are not physically disabled. The seven domains addressed are personal care, dressing, eating and drinking, mobility, play, stairs and standing skills. Two versions assess performance (ASKp: what the child 'does do' in a standardized environment) and capability (ASKc: what the child 'could do') across the various activities. Thus, the

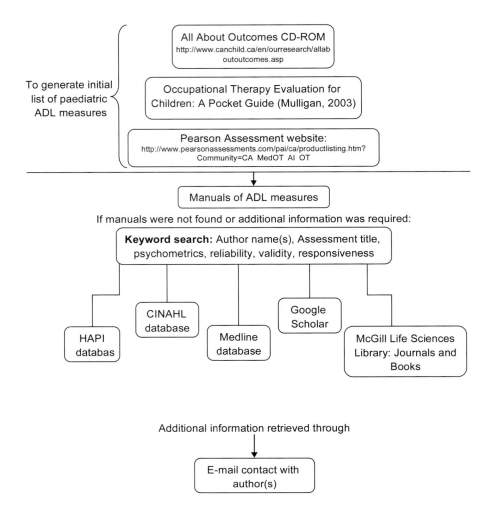

Figure 24.1 Flowchart of search strategy. ADL, Activities of daily living.

ASK combines both the objective and subjective aspects of the measurement of self-care (personal care, dressing and other skills).

Using parental/caregiver report, often through semi-structured interview, the PEDI[7] measures self-care, mobility and social function as part of the Functional Skills Scale in children under 8 years of age. The self-care domains include eating, toothbrushing, hairbrushing, nose care, washing, dressing upper body and lower body, and toileting. In addition there is a Caregiver Assistance Scale (level required) and a Modification Scale, the latter focusing on the equipment and environmental modifications needed. The LIFE-H uses both self-report and parent-proxy report to address 'accomplishment of life habits' using six domains of daily activities (communication,

personal care, housing, mobility, nutrition, fitness) and five domains of social roles for children with disabilities from 5 to 13 years of age.[19] Based on the disability creation process model,[20-22] the LIFE-H reflects the domains of the ICF.

The purpose of the WeeFIM[7,23] is to evaluate and monitor performance in functional (daily living) skills in infants and young children with congenital or acquired disabilities between 6 months and 7 years of age. It may also be used in older children (7–18y) who are functioning below 7 years of age. The measure provides a measure of severity of disability in terms of how much assistance is required beyond what would be considered age appropriate. Intended as a minimal data set, the WeeFIM does not evaluate why children are experiencing activity limitations, and therefore it is not a diagnostic tool. Rather, it is an evaluative tool that measures change over time. Typically, the WeeFIM is administered by interview and/or direct observation,

ASSESSMENT OF MOTOR AND PROCESS SKILLS (AMPS)	
Purpose	To evaluate independence in activities of daily living
	Can help identify the reasons why an individual is experiencing difficulties in particular activities
	To establish the level of task challenge that can be managed by an individual
	Helps to determine needs and set realistic rehabilitation goals
	May be used to track improvement
Population	Individuals aged >3y with any functional limitation
Description of domains (subscales)	Divided into two domains:
	Motor skills (16 items) – posture, mobility, coordination, strength and effort, energy
	Process skills (20 items) – energy, using knowledge, temporal organization, space and objects, adaptation
	A school version is also available (21 items) – writing tasks, drawing and colouring tasks, cutting and pasting tasks, computer writing tasks and maths manipulative tasks
Administration and test format	Time to complete: 30–60min to administer
	Testing format: begin with client/caregiver interview, client chooses two or three purposeful tasks to perform
	Scoring: criterion-referenced. Each item on the two scales is scored on a four-point rating scale (considers difficulty, efficiency, safety and independence). Results are computer analysed to adjust for severity of rater. Normalized standard scores, z-scores and centile ranks available in school version
	Training: certification required. Course registration is available through the website: www.ampsintl.com/
Psychometric properties	Normative sample: >50000 children from a variety of cultures, ages and diagnostic groups
	Reliability
	Reliability is enhanced by a computerized scoring system
	Validity
	Face: supported by comparing motor and process ability scores with normative data in a sample of 33 children with a variety of disabilities
	Discriminant: detected significant deficits in motor and process abilities in a sample of 54 children with cerebral palsy
How to order	To be able to purchase the computer software, the user must have undergone a 5-day training session and completed the requirements for certification. Materials may be ordered from: www.ampsintl.com/Merchant/merchant.mvc?Screen=PLST&Store_Code=API
	Cost: ranges between $315 and $365 plus tax, shipping and handling
Key references	AMPS Project International. Available at: www.ampsintl.com/index.htm (accessed 15 July 2009).
	Law M, Baum C, Dunn W (2001) *Measuring Occupational Performance: Supporting Best Practice in Occupational Therapy*. Thorofare, NJ: SLACK Incorporated.
	Van Zelst BR, Miller MD, Russo RN, Murchland S, Crotty M (2006) Activities of daily living in children with hemiplegic cerebral palsy: a cross-sectional evaluation using the Assessment of Motor and Process Skills. *Dev Med Child Neurol* 48: 723–727.

together with a primary caregiver who is very familiar with the child's functional abilities.

The COPM[24,25] is used to generate child-centred priorities to set performance and satisfaction goals for the domains of self-care, productivity and leisure. While the goals are established by the child and the family, and the scores are responsive to change over time, there is a lack of ability to compare performance across individuals at a particular point in time.

Tabulated format

Detailed tables of the VABS, WeeFIM, PEDI, LIFE-H and ASK appear in Chapter 19. Other measures that evaluate self-care are tabulated below.

BARTHEL INDEX	
Purpose	To evaluate the level of independence in activities of daily living
Population	Originally developed for adults, more specifically inpatients. It has also been used with adolescents with chronic disabilities
Description of domains (subscales)	Two subscales: self-care (nine items) and mobility (six items)
Administration and test format	Time to complete: 1h by observation
	Testing format: can be completed by observation or by interview with the caregiver or client
	Scoring: three-point ordinal scale (self, some aid, cannot do). Each item is individually weighted; maximum score 100
	'Norms' provided by Granger are as follows:
	100 Independent in self-care and mobility
	91–99 Slightly dependent in self-care and mobility
	61–90 Slightly to moderately dependent in self-care and mobility
	21–60 Moderately to markedly dependent in self care and mobility
	0–20 Totally dependent in self care and mobility
	Training: no training is specified
Psychometric properties	*Reliability*
	None reported for paediatric populations
	Validity
	Construct: established in a small sample of children with cerebral palsy between the ages of 5 and 16y
	Responsiveness
	None reported for paediatric populations
How to order	May be used free of charge for non-commercial purposes, with the inclusion of the following acknowledgement:
	Mahoney FI, Barthel D (1965) Functional evaluation: the Barthel Index. *Maryland State Med J* 14: 56–61. Used with permission.
	Permission is required from the Maryland State Medical Society to modify the Barthel Index or to use it for commercial purposes
Key references	Law M, Baum C, Dunn W (2001) *Measuring Occupational Performance: Supporting Best Practice in Occupational Therapy.* Thorofare, NJ: SLACK Incorporated.
	Mulligan S (2003) *Occupational Therapy Evaluation for Children: A Pocket Guide.* Baltimore, MD: Lippincott Williams & Wilkins.
	Young NL, Wright JG (1995) Measuring paediatric physical function. *J Paediatr Orthop* 15: 244–253.

Canadian Occupational Performance Measure (COPM)

Purpose	The COPM is a measure of self-perception of occupational performance. It may also be used for programme evaluation purposes
Population	Across all ages – no diagnostic group is specified. However, it is difficult to administer to children aged <8y, or to those who have cognitive or language impairments
Description of domains (subscales)	Three domains in performance: self-care, productivity, leisure There is also a satisfaction section
Administration and test format	Time to complete: time may vary; on average 30–40min Testing format: interview with client or with caregiver/parent (proxy). In performance section, elicit areas of occupational performance not being performed satisfactorily. Client then identifies up to five of the most important activities, and is asked to rate their perception of their performance, their satisfaction with their performance and the importance of the task on a scale from 1 to 10 Scoring: visual analogue scale of 1–10 Training: available with credentialing of institutions
Psychometric properties	*Reliability* Test–retest: intraclass correlation coefficient of 0.63 for performance and 0.84 for satisfaction *Validity* Content: established during assessment development Criterion: Behavioural Observation Scale and COPM demonstrated similar changes in children with developmental coordination disorder. Children with cerebral palsy undergoing interventions. Changes in COPM were correlated with rating of changes in hand function and quality of movement of the upper extremity. Changes in hand function as reported by parents on a seven-point Likert scale correlated with 0.32 with COPM performance and 0.28 with COPM satisfaction. Quality of movement (as reported by parents) correlated 0.29 with COPM performance and 0.28 with COPM satisfaction Convergent: the Goal Attainment Scale and COPM were found to evaluate different constructs *Responsiveness* COPM was effective in detecting change when clinically meaningful change existed in children with spastic hemiplegia
How to order	Available to order online from the Canadian Association of Occupational Therapists at: https://www.caot.ca/ebusiness/source/orders/index.cfm?section=unknown&ETask=1&Task=1&SEARCH_TYPE=FIND&FindIn=0&FindSpec=COPM&x=0&y=0 Cost: approximately US$52.45 plus tax, shipping and handling
Key references	Cusick A, McIntyre S, Novak I, Lannin N, Lowe K (2006) A comparison of goal attainment scaling and the Canadian Occupational Performance Measure for paediatric rehabilitation research. *Paediatr Rehabil* 9:149–157. Law M, Baptiste S, Carswell A, McColl MA, Polatajko H, Pollock N (1994) *Canadian Occupational Performance Measure,* 2nd edition. Toronto: CAOT Publications ACE. Law M, Baum C, Dunn W (2001) *Measuring Occupational Performance: Supporting Best Practice in Occupational Therapy.* Thorofare, NJ: SLACK Incorporated.

CHILD OCCUPATIONAL SELF-ASSESSMENT (COSA)

Purpose	Allows clients to indicate personal values and set priorities May be used for follow-up purposes in order to document changes over time
Population	Ages 3mo to >80y, no diagnostic group specified
Description of domains (subscales)	Lists various activities that children complete on a daily basis Two scales: 1, performance; 2, importance
Administration and test format	Time to complete: children take 20–30min to complete the form; therapists should plan 15min to discuss responses and 5min to score. In all, 40–50min is required Testing format: the child can fill out the checklist and then discuss responses with the therapist. The child can also complete the assessment with sorting cards Scoring: four-point ordinal scale Performance: 'I have a big problem doing this', 'I have a little problem doing this', 'I do this ok', 'I am really good at doing this' Importance: 'Not really important to me', 'Important to me', 'Really important to me', 'Most important of all to me' Training: none required
Psychometric properties	*Reliability* Not specified in studies reviewed *Validity* Content: good content validity (acceptable fit to the Rasch model on the Occupational Competence Scale) External validity: children who used translators reported higher values
How to order	COSA manual is available to order online. Assessment forms are in the manual. A password is provided to print coloured assessment forms from the website: www.moho.uic.edu/assessments.html Cost: approximately $40, plus tax, shipping and handling
Key references	Kielhofner G (2008) *Model of Human Occupation*, 4th edition. Baltimore, MD: Lippincott, Williams & Wilkins. Kramer J (2008) *Rating Scale Use by Children with Disabilities on a Self Report of Competence and Value for Everyday Activity: A Profile of Four Users*. Chicago, IL: University of Illinois. Kramer J (2008) *Validity Evidence for the Child Occupational Self Assessment*. Chicago, IL: University of Illinois.

JUVENILE ARTHRITIS FUNCTIONAL STATUS INDEX (JASI)

Purpose	To evaluate the functional status of children with juvenile rheumatoid arthritis
Population	Ages 8–18y with juvenile rheumatoid arthritis
Description of domains (subscales)	Five domains: self-care (38 items), domestic (15 items), mobility, school, extracurricular

Administration and test format	Time to complete: 30–45min
	Testing format: self-report; child interview
	Scoring: seven-point ordinal scale, criterion-referenced. Two components – child rates his or her own performance on tasks and child identifies five tasks that are most difficult to accomplish with interviewer
	Training: no need for training is specified
Psychometric properties	*Reliability*
	Test–retest reliability was established (intraclass correlation coefficient ≥0.95). In Part 1, inter-rater reliability, examined according to American College of Rheumatology (ACR) functional rating categories, was lower for individuals with mild disease. In Part 2, kappa=0.57 (fair)
	Validity
	Content: test content reviewed by 17 different clinicians
	Construct: JASI correlated strongly with rheumatology measures (n=36): joint count (r=−0.51), grip strength (r=0.60), hip synovitis (r=−0.62), timed walk (r=−0.66) and run (r=−0.79), (ACR) functional rating (r=−0.75), etc. Relationship to pain only r=−0.15. Comparison between children's scores and clinician's scores (n=30) using mean weighted kappa=0.66; children as young as 8y can provide a realistic report of their functional status
	Responsiveness/sensitivity
	Comparing the Childhood Health Assessment Questionnaire, Juvenile Arthritis Functional Assessment Report and JASI – no statistically significant differences between tests regarding responsiveness between two groups of treated children (intra-articular steroid injection group and methotrexate/hip surgery group). All tests sufficiently responsive. 57% agreement at 2–3 weeks and 53% agreement at 3mo when children were asked to rate the amount of change in their ability since baseline
How to order	E-mail vwright@hollandbloorview.ca. Paper version of the questionnaire and Excel scoring template can be obtained for US$30
Key references	Brown GT, Wright V, Lang BA, et al (2005) Clinical responsiveness of self-report functional assessment measures for children with juvenile idiopathic arthritis undergoing intraarticular corticosteroid injections. *Arth Rheum* 53: 897–904.
	Law M, Baum C, Dunn W (2001) *Measuring Occupational Performance: Supporting Best Practice in Occupational Therapy*. Thorofare, NJ: SLACK Incorporated.
	Wright FV, Law M, Crombie V, Goldsmith CH, Dent P (1994) Development of a self-report functional status index for juvenile rheumatoid arthritis. *J Rheumatol* 21: 536–544.
	Wright FV, Kimber JL, Law M, Goldsmith CH, Crombie V, Dent P (1996) The Juvenile Arthritis Functional Status Index (JASI): a validation study. *J Rheumatol* 23: 1066–1079.

School Function Assessment (SFA)

Purpose	To evaluate children's functioning in school. May be useful in guiding programme planning
Population	Kindergarten to grade 6
Description of domains (subscales)	Three domains: participation (bathroom and toileting activities, mealtime or snack time), task supports (assistance and adaptations), activity performance

Administration and test format	Time to complete: not specified
	Testing format: questionnaire. Completed by one or more school professionals
	Scoring: criterion-referenced. Cut-off score provided to establish whether or not student is functioning at or below grade-level expectations
	Training: no training is mentioned
Psychometric properties	Normative sample: 678 students in two groups (one group consisted of children with activity limitations)
	Reliability
	Not mentioned in studies reviewed
Psychometric properties	*Validity*
	Convergent: correlation with VABS r=0.56–0.72 (n=64: 29 healthy, 18 with specific learning disabilities, 17 with cerebral palsy)
	Construct: significant differences across all parts of SFA among the three groups
	Discriminant: 55.8–93.1% of children were correctly classified in their respective groups
How to order	Complete kit (including user's manual, 25 record forms, and three eight-page rating scale guides) can be purchased from:
	http://psychcorp.pearsonassessments.com/haiweb/cultures/en-us/productdetail.htm?pid=076-1615-709&Community=CA_MedOT_AI_OT
	Cost: approximately US$215, plus tax, shipping and handling
Key references	Coster W, Deeney TA, Haltiwanger T, Haley SM (1998) *School Function Assessment, User's Manual.* San Antonio, TX: Therapy Skill Builders.
	Coster WJ, Deeney T, Haltiwanger J, Haley S (2008) *Technical Report School Function Assessment (SFA).* San Antonio, TX: Pearson
	Hwang J, Davies PL, Taylor MP, Gavin WJ (2002) Validation of School Function Assessment with elementary school children. *OTJR Occup Participation Health* 22: 48–58.

SKILLS OF INDEPENDENT BEHAVIOUR – REVISED (SIB-R)	
Purpose	This assessment is a descriptive measure of adaptive skills and maladaptive behaviours
Population	Individuals aged 3mo to >80y. No diagnostic group is specified
Description of domains (subscales)	Full form: five domains – motor skills (38 items), social and communication skills (56 items), personal living skills (88 items), community living skills (seven skills), maladaptive behaviour (24 items)
	Short Form and Early Development Scale also available (40 items each)
Administration and test format	Time to complete: 45–60min to administer full scale; 15–20min for Short Form or Early Development Form
	Testing format: questionnaire or structured interview
	Scoring: four-point ordinal scale, criterion-referenced, as follows:
	Rarely or never performs (0), performs about 25% of the time (1), does fairly well or about 75% of the time (2), does very well without being asked almost all the time (3)
	Training: none specified

Psychometric properties	Normative sample: 2182 individuals between age 0 and 90y. A supplemental standardization group consisting of children and adults with disabilities was also included (n=1681). For problem behaviour scale, normative group consisted of 778 individuals aged 0–50y. The same supplemental standardization group consisting of children and adults with disabilities was also included
	Reliability
	Internal consistency: for 14 subscales (Cronbach's alpha=0.87–0.96)
	Test–retest: established (intraclass correlation coefficient [ICC]=0.98 for full scale; 0.86 for problem behaviours scale)
	Inter-rater: established for full scale and maladaptive behaviours scale (ICC=0.95; ICC=0.86)
	Validity
	Construct: correlation with ages 0–18y (0.91)
	Criterion: correlation with IQ (0.20–0.78). Correlated with other adaptive behaviour scales (0.66–0.81)
	Responsiveness
	Not reported in studies reviewed
How to order	Available to order online at:
	www.riverpub.com/products/sibr/index.html
	www.assess.nelson.com/test-ind/sib-r.html
	Cost: approximately CAN$396 for assessment; CAN$498 for software, plus tax, shipping and handling
Key references	Azaula M, Msall ME, Buck G, Tremont MR, Wilczenski F, Rogers BT (2000) Measuring functional status and family support in older school-aged children with cerebral palsy: comparison of three instruments. *Arch Phys Med Rehabil* 81: 307–311.
	Hill B. n.d. *Adaptive and Maladaptive Behaviour Scales*. Available at: www.come-over.to/FAS/VinelandCompare.htm (accessed 15 July 2009).
	Lecavalier L, Leone S, Wiltz J (2006) The impact of behaviour problems on caregiver stress in young people with autism spectrum disorders. *J Intel Disabil Res* 50: 172–183.
	Msall ME (2005) Measuring functional skills in preschool children at risk for neurodevelopmental disabilities. *Mental Retard Dev Disabil Res Rev* 11: 263–273.
	Nelson Education; n.d. *Scales of Independent Behaviour – Revised*. Available at: www.assess.nelson.com/test-ind/sib-r.html (accessed 15 July 2009).

MULTIDISCIPLINARY FEEDING PROFILE

Purpose	This tool provides a quantitative assessment of feeding disorders in children with severe disabilities
Population	Children with feeding disorders
Description of domains (subscales)	Six domains: physical/neurological, orofacial structure, orofacial sensory inputs, orofacial motor function, ventilation/phonation, functional feeding assessment

Administration and test format	Time to complete: 30–45min to administer
	Testing format: 136 items with an additional 56 items that are included for clinical value but not computed in final score. Assessment is done through observation, which may be videotaped and played back
	Scoring: five-point ordinal scale, criterion-referenced. Criteria for each item vary
	Training: training to facilitate scoring is recommended
Psychometric properties	*Reliability*
	Inter-rater and intrarater reliability established (intraclass correlation coefficient=0.86 and 0.90, respectively)
	Validity
	Experts are involved in establishing content validity
How to order	Available at www.sickkids.ca/dentistry under 'Resources'
Key references	Judd PL, Kenny DJ, Koheil RM, Miller LJ, Moran R (1989) The Multidisciplinary Feeding Profile: a statistically-based protocol for the assessment of dependent feeders. *Dysphagia* 4: 29–34.
	Kenny DJ, Koheil RM, Greenberg J, et al (1989) Development of a Multidisciplinary Feeding Profile for children who are dependent feeders. *Dysphagia* 4: 16–28.

NEONATAL ORAL-MOTOR ASSESSMENT SCALE (NOMAS)

Purpose	To assess the nutritive sucking (NS) and non-nutritive sucking (NNS) skills of infants
	May be used as an outcome measure of treatment effectiveness
	Utilized as a record of developmental progression
	Used to confirm oromotor dysfunction
Population	Infants from birth to 8wk post term
Description of domains (subscales)	28 items divided into rate, rhythm, consistency of degree of jaw excursion, direction of tongue movement, range of motion of tongue movement, timing of tongue movement, tongue configuration
Administration and test format	Time to complete: varies according to the time required to observe
	Testing format: observation during NNS and during first 2min of regular feeding. May be videotaped and played back
	Scoring: checklist– normal sucking pattern, disorganized sucking pattern, dysfunctional sucking pattern. Severity ratings for disorganized sucking pattern and dysfunctional sucking pattern: mild (1), moderate (2–3), severe (4)
	Training: training and certification required

Psychometric properties	*Reliability*
	Test–retest: fair to high (kappa=0.33–0.94; r=0.67–0.82)
	Inter-rater: moderate to high (kappa=0.40–0.65; intraclass correlation coefficient= 0.93–0.97)
	Internal consistency: Cronbach's alpha >0.70
	Validity
	Convergent: moderate correlations between feeding performance and NOMAS score for all age groups except at age >6wk
	Predictive: predictive of neurological outcomes at 6 and 12mo
	Responsiveness
	Standard response mean >0.5 in every 2-wk period
How to order	Details regarding training and certification may be obtained through www.marjoriemeyerpalmer.com/index.html
Key references	da Costa SP, van der Scahns CP (2007) The reliability of the Neonatal Oral-motor Assessment Scale. *Acta Paediatr* 97: 21–26.
	Howe T, Sheu C, Hsieh Y, Hsieh C (2007) Psychometric characteristics of the Neonatal Oral-motor Assessment Scale in healthy preterm infants. *Dev Med Child Neurol* 49: 915–919.
	Howe T-H, Lin K-C, Fu C-P, Su C-T, Hsieh C-L (2008) A review of psychometric properties of feeding assessment tools used in neonates. *J Obstet Gynecol Neonatal Nurs* 37: 338–349.
	Tsai S-W, Chen C-H, Lin M-C (2009) Prediction for developmental delay by Neonatal Oral Motor Assessment Scale in preterm infants without brain lesion. *Pediatrics International* 52: 65–68.

REFERENCES

1. World Health Organization (2007) *International Classification of Functioning, Disability, and Health – Children and Youth.* Geneva: WHO.
2. Law M, Cooper B, Strong S, Stewart D, Rigby P, Letts L (1996) The Person–Environment–Occupation Model: a transactive approach to occupational performance. *Can J Occup Ther* 63: 9–23.
3. Rodger S, Ziviani J, Watter P, Ozanne A, Woodyatt G, Springfield E (2003) Motor and functional skills of children with developmental coordination disorder: a pilot investigation of measurement issues. *Human Mov Sci* 22: 461–478.
4. Law M, King G, King S, et al (2006) Patterns of participation in recreational and leisure activities among children with complex physical disabilities. *Dev Med Child Neurol* 48: 337–342.
5. Young NL, Williams JI, Yoshida KK, Wright JG (2000) Measurement properties of the Activities Scale for Kids. *J Clin Epidemiol* 53: 125–137.
6. Law M, Baptiste S, Carswell A, McColl MA, Polatajko H, Pollock N (1994) *Canadian Occupational Performance Measure,* 2nd edition. Toronto: CAOT Publications ACE.
7. Haley SM, Coster WJ, Ludlow LH, Haltiwanger J, Adrellos PJ (1992) *Pediatric Evaluation of Disability Inventory (PEDI): Development, Standardization and Administration Manual.* Boston, MA: New England Medical Center Hospitals, Inc & PEDI Research Group.
8. State University of New York (1993) Guide for the Uniform Data Set for Medical Rehabilitation for Children (WeeFIM), Version 4.0 – Community/Outpatient. Buffalo, NY: State University of New York at Buffalo.
9. Newborg J, Stock JR, Wnek L, Guidubaldi J, Svinicki J (1988) *Battelle Developmental Inventory, Examiner's Manual.* Chicago, IL: Riverside.
10. Sparrow S, Balla D, Cichetti D (1984) *Vineland Adaptive Behavior Scales* (survey edition). Circle Pines, MN: American Guidance Service.
11. Riley A (2004) Evidence that school-age children can report on their health. *Ambulatory Pediatr* 4: 371–376.
12. Wright FV, Law M, Crombie V, Goldsmith CH, Dent P (1994) Development of a self-report functional status index for juvenile rheumatoid arthritis. *J Rheumatol* 21: 536–544.
13. Palmer M, Crawley K, Blanco I (1993) Neonatal Oral-Motor Assessment Scale: a reliability study. *J Perinatol* 13: 28–35.
14. Kenny DJ, Koheil RM, Greenberg J, et al (1989) Development of a multidisciplinary feeding profile for children who are dependent feeders. *Dysphagia* 4: 16–28.
15. de Bildt A, Kraijer D, Sytema S, Minderaa R (2005) Psychometric properties of the Vineland Adaptive Behavior Scales in children and adolescents with mental retardation. *J Autism Dev Disord* 35: 53–62.
16. Sparrow SS, Cicchetti DB, Balla DA (2005) *Vineland Adaptive Behavior Scales,* 2nd edition. Circle Pines, MN: AGS Publishing.
17. Young N, Yoshida K, Williams J, Bombardier C, Wright J (1995) The role of children in reporting their physical disability. *Arch Phys Med Rehabil* 76: 913–918.

18. Plint A, Gaboury I, Owen J, Young N (2003) Activities Scale for Kids: an analysis of normals. *J Paediatr Orthopaed* 23: 788–790.

19. Noreau L, Lepage C, Boissière L, et al (2007) Measuring participation in children with disabilities using the Assessment of Life Habits. *Dev Med Child Neurol* 49: 666–671.

20. Morris C, Kurinczuk JJ, Fitzpatrick R (2005) Child or family assessed measures of activity performance and participation for children with cerebral palsy: a structured review. *Child Care Health Dev* 31: 397–407.

21. McConachie H, Colver AF, Forsyth RJ, Jarvis SN, Parkinson KN (2006) Participation of disabled children: how should it be characterised and measured? *Disabil Rehabil* 28: 1157–1164.

22. Sakzewski L, Boyd R, Ziviani J (2007) Clinimetric properties of participation measures for 5- to 13-year-old children with cerebral palsy: a systematic review. *Dev Med Child Neurol* 49: 232–240.

23. Feldman AB, Haley SM, Coryell J (1990) Concurrent and construct validity of the Pediatric Evaluation of Disability Inventory. *Phys Ther* 70: 602–610.

24. Law M, Baptiste S, McColl M, Opzoomer A, Polatajko H, Pollock N (1990) The Canadian Occupational Performance Measure: an outcome measure for occupational therapy. *Can J Occup Ther* 57: 82–87.

25. Missiuna C, Pollock N (2000) Perceived efficacy and goal setting in young children. *Can J Occup Ther* 67: 101–109.

25
DOMESTIC LIFE (D610–D699)

Mónica Silveira-Maia, Kylee Miller and Rune J. Simeonsson

What is the construct?

Active participation in everyday tasks is a significant part of every child's development.[1–3] These domains of involvement – involving having a place to live, food to eat, clothing and other necessities, as well as the experience of domestic assistance and care – are essential and valued by children with disabilities and their families alike.[4] With this priority, the focus of intervention and habilitation for children with disabilities is moving beyond improvement of their body functions and acquisition of skills to include their social participation in home, school and community.[5]

Participation in domestic life has been increasingly recognized not only as a domain of importance in the child's development but also as having a significant influence on the child's functioning in other areas of life.[1–3,6,7] The domestic life domain, defined in the International Classification of Functioning, Disability and Health for Children and Youth (ICF-CY) as 'carrying out domestic and everyday actions and tasks' (p.172), includes activities such as acquisition of necessities, household tasks, caring for household objects and assisting others.[8]

Documentation of domestic life is also acknowledged in the literature under the concept of 'instrumental activities of daily living' (IADL).[8–10] The IADL concept incorporates the domestic life activities listed in the ICF-CY such as meal preparation, caring for others and shopping, but also includes others such as using public transportation, managing finances and using the phone.[9–11] These activities are represented in the ICF-CY framework under other domains of mobility, major life areas and communication.[8]

In this context, it is important to distinguish IADL from general activities of daily living (ADL). The word *instrumental* in IADL corresponds to tasks that are essential for independent community living, while the more basic ADL tasks refer to life-sustaining and basic self-care practices such as feeding, bathing and dressing.[11] The IADL concept includes complex multistep activities that require a high level of social, physical and mental skills – such as

judgement, imitation, sequencing and problem solving.[11,12] As frameworks for assessing disability, Spector et al[13] refer to a hierarchical relationship between IADL and ADL items, with assessment of limitations of ADL representing more severe disability than limitations of IADL.

Another point of clarification needs to be made with reference to the terms 'household tasks' and 'housework'; both have been used to describe activities such as food shopping, preparing meals and children taking care of their own toys.[2,6,14,15] These terms are often used synonymously in the literature in discussions related to the activities included in the domestic life domain of the ICF-CY.[6,14,15] The engagement of children in household work[3,16] is supported by studies demonstrating that the majority of American school-aged children perform some type of housework as a part of their daily routine, spending an average of 6 to 7 hours per week on household tasks.[6] Similarly, the results from a study by Cogle and Tasker[17] demonstrated that 88% of children between the ages of 6 and 17 years old perform at least one household chore on a regular basis, specifically house cleaning, food preparation or dishwashing. In light of the significant role of work performed by children in the home setting, further investigation of a child's participation in domestic life is warranted. Nevertheless, the importance and level of participation in household tasks is, historically and socioculturally, enormously associated with factors such as the child's sex,[3,18–21] birth order (i.e. being first or second child in the family),[6,14,22] adults' occupation (e.g. whether or not mother works),[23,24] family size,[3,6,18,19] rural/urban status of the family[6] and the child's age.[19]

Although the research specifically investigating domestic life participation at different ages is limited, evidence points towards a greater level of participation between the ages of 5 and 18 years,[2,6,14,15,18] with perhaps a significant increase once the child has reached adolescence between the ages of 13 and 18 years.[19]

There have been a number of perspectives on the relationship between participation in housework and a child's developmental outcome. Perspectives focused on children's perceptions about the importance of their own participation in domestic life, with the conclusion that household work is viewed as integral to a child's independence.[16] Some researchers have maintained that housework increases the child's responsibility and unity within the family[17,25,26] and Leonard[16] found that housework influences children's social development. A survey of adults found that a child's participation in household work was perceived as essential to anticipated independent living.[16,27] Additionally, parents report that the opportunity of scaffolding the successful completion of chores provides vital teaching moments throughout development.[7,28,29]

Within the context of cultural differences, White and Brinkerhoff[30] proposed a distinction between self-care and family-care household tasks and their implications on the development of responsibility in the child. According to Dunn,[2] self-care household tasks involve 'managing one's own needs, belongings and space (e.g. making own meal, putting away own toys)' (p. 180). Family-care household tasks, on the other hand, involve 'caring for other's needs, belongings and common space (e.g. caring for younger siblings, setting the table, doing the dishes)'[2] (p. 180). Bowes and colleagues[29] have suggested that different levels of involvement in these two types of household tasks have implications for the development of a more individualistic responsibility (self-reliance and care of one's own things) and/or of a socially orientated responsibility (concern for the welfare of others) in the child. The authors[29] also hypothesized that such differentiation may also reflect cultural divergence between individualist/capitalist societies and those with a collectivist orientation.

As Tomanovic[31] has emphasized, the family constitutes the basic social context for children's participation – through participation in family life, children become conscious of a substantial part of their participatory rights while training for participation in the larger society. Accordingly, studies demonstrated a strong relationship between the development of a child's sense of control and autonomy and the nature and quality of a child's participation within his or her family.[32,33] This is supported by findings that the degree to which parents recognize the child's competences will influence the creation or constriction of participation opportunities at home and consequently will play an important role in the development of the child's autonomy.[31]

Related findings have shown that the participation of younger children depends on the opportunities that are provided by parents, caregivers or service providers which are not isolated, but rather immersed in the context of the family system.[34]

The link between participation in household tasks and further independence has been highlighted by Dunn,[2] who stresses that 'learning opportunities available through participation in household tasks appear to contribute to development of a variety of behaviors and skills needed for successful independent living' (p.179). Participation in these learning experiences as a family member offers the child opportunities to set goals, plan, self-monitor, make decisions and problem solve.[2] These learning opportunities have been empirically related to positive child outcomes of greater self-control, development of prosocial behaviours and even to a decreased likelihood of problem behaviours in childhood and adolescence.[1,2] In the field of disability research, participation in household tasks has been strongly associated with the development of self-determination (e.g. autonomy, self-regulation) and participation as a family member.[35,36]

Given the significant role of children's participation in household tasks, focus should be placed on the development of interventions that address strategies and support to promote the participation of children in household life and family routines.[1] It is important to recognize that participation in domestic life by children with disabilities may require adaptations in terms of providing services to assist families in their children's preparation for independent living.[2] The importance of this view is reinforced in articles of the United Nations Convention on the Rights of the Child[37] and Standard Rules on Equalization of Opportunity for Persons with Disabilities.[38] These articles endorse the importance of providing support to children and young people in their natural environment and empowering families and significant others.[39] The implications for interventions planning are thus for an assessment approach that emphasizes the child's everyday functioning.[5] However, despite recognition of the relevance of participation in household tasks, it is a domain that is often disregarded in a comprehensive functional assessment for children and young people with disabilities.[6] As a developmental indicator, it is therefore important that assessment is made to provide a better understanding of the nature and extent of the participation of the child with disabilities in home routines and to identify the extent and types of support required by the child and family.[1]

To this end, an assessment approach is needed that captures the interaction between the child and the environment and identifies what supports children need to be able to participate.[1,5,40] The ICF-CY can serve as a useful framework and tool to document the interaction between the environment and the child, defining the focus of assessment and guiding the selection of assessment tools.[41,42] As such, the ICF-CY can define the approach to assessment and provide the basis for systematic selection of tools to measure aspects of the child's functioning within the domain of domestic life.[41,42] In Table 25.1, we have identified a set of categories from the ICF-CY domestic life domain that are described in studies measuring domestic life activities of children and young people (Table 25.1).

DOMESTIC LIFE ON TRANSITION PLANNING

A central feature of the development of children and adolescents is the experiences that prepare them for the transition to adulthood.[43] These experiences involve health and social services as well as other services that facilitate independent living, social support and informed decision-making.[44] The importance of transition planning is acknowledged for children and young people with disabilities[45] to 'facilitate the child's movement from school to postschool activities'[43] (p. 60) in order to promote independent living and community inclusion. To this end, significant efforts have been invested in the development of transition plans for children and young people, with common agreement being that best practices in this field focus on assessment initiated in elementary and middle school years and no later than the age of 14 years.[46–48]

Expected outcomes of successful transition planning for adolescents with disabilities include employment, participating in postsecondary education, becoming appropriately involved in the community, experiencing satisfactory personal and social relationships and other roles, and home maintenance, as described in various studies.[49–51]

A review by Alwell and Cobb[52] examined interventions based on functional life skill curricula for secondary-aged young people with developmental disabilities. A finding was that *domestic skills* training was integrated in general characteristics of life skills interventions, particularly in studies aimed at measuring strategies to improve and teach cleaning skills, cooking and meal preparation skills, laundry skills and sewing-machine use. These intervention strategies, using pictorial cues, colour-coding and task simplification,[53] can be conceptualized within the ICF-CY framework as environmental facilitators or barriers found mainly in chapter 1 of the environmental factors component.[8]

Halpern[54] focused on a number of aspects that influence transition success. These include the importance of the family context, the quality and impact of the student's school programme, and the nature and quality of transition services available for the student and his or her family.[54] In addition, opportunities actually available in the community for the young person, and the promptness and motivation revealed by the young person to move forward with his or her life, are other important factors.[54]

Currently, a key characteristic of quality transition programmes contributing to improved independent life outcomes for young people with disabilities is the acquisition of housekeeping work skills.[55] The relevance of immersing skills training in the context of real-life activities that are functional for the individual is recognized.[56] Given the context-immersed nature of domestic skills, standardized tests may not adequately cover every need and expected transition outcomes of children and young people.[2] Luft et al[57] have emphasized that professionals should be acquainted with ecological and situational approaches to assess students' needs and to implement intervention plans.

In this regard, guidelines for programme success have been identified, including effective interagency

TABLE 25.1

International Classification of Functioning, Disability and Health for Children and Youth categories of domestic life domain described in representative studies of children and young people

Domestic life domain	Category from domestic life domain	Description	Examples of literature sources
Acquisition of necessities (d610–d629)	Acquisition of goods and services (d620)	To do the shopping and gather daily necessities – selecting and obtaining food, drinks, water, etc. – with or without exchange of money	Antill et al;[14] Blair[6]
Household tasks (d630–d649)	Preparing meals (d630)	Helping others to cook, getting together ingredients for preparing meals, cooking such as making a snack or planning a meal with several dishes	Antill et al;[14] Blair;[6] Cheal;[18] Peña et al;[15] Dunn et al[1]
	Doing housework (d640)	Managing a household such as cleaning his or her own room, washing clothes, storing food, disposing of garbage	Antill et al;[14] Blair;[6] Cheal;[18] Peña et al;[15] Dunn et al[1]
Caring for household objects and assisting others (d650–d669)	Caring for household objects (d650)	Maintaining and repairing household and other personal objects, such as play material, clothes and assistive devices, and caring for plants and animals	Antill et al;[14] Blair;[6] Peña et al;[15] Dunn et al[1]
	Assisting others (d660)	Assisting household members and others such as looking after younger sisters and brothers	Antill et al;[14] Blair;[6] Peña et al[15]

collaboration, natural support within the community and person-centred planning strategies.[44,54,57] With recognition of the significant role of environmental factors on domestic life participation of transition-aged young people, assessment tools need to address the quality of transition programmes and services.[44]

Assessment of family and home context plays an essential role in a comprehensive approach to domestic life participation of children and young people.[34] Such assessment draws mainly on the third and fourth chapters of the ICF-CY environmental factors component[8] (see some recommended measures in Chapters 30 and 31). The broader contexts of neighbourhood, school and community also play important roles in quality assessment tools for transition planning (e.g. National Secondary Transition Technical Assistance Center Indicator 13 Checklist;[58] National Standards and Quality Indicators: Transition Toolkit for Systems Improvement;[59] Transition Quality Indicators[60]). Such assessments allow schools, teams and other agencies to identify transition plans based on the young person's strengths and difficulties that may be in need of improvement.[58] In the description of the child's domestic life participation, this approach to transition services quality can be documented with codes from chapter 5 of the ICF-CY environmental factors component.[8]

General factors to consider when measuring this domain

Regarding the factors to consider when measuring the domestic life of children, the following measurement factors were identified upon reflection on the principles of the ICF-CY framework and on the current understanding of domestic life participation. The environmental and task characteristics defining the child's engagement in domestic life activities may either promote or hinder participation.[2] These interactions are reflected in the description of the child's functioning, classified with codes in the domains of body functions, activities and participation in life roles and situations.[8,42,61] As the ICF-CY classifies environmental factors influencing child functioning,[8] it is a framework that supports an assessment process within a holistic model of human development.[61–63] In measuring the child's participation in the domestic life domain, environmental factors need to be recognized as undeniable influences and moderators.[63]

Thus, assessment results should provide information about the contextual changes required to meet a child's needs instead of being centred only on the identification of skills needed to be developed by the child in order to meet household system demands.[64] By identifying the additions or modifications that need to be made in the

environment to maximize participation, this assessment approach reflects an implementation of the *environmental habilitation* philosophy.[40] Within this perspective, children's participation in domestic life can be maximized if the necessary support services and supplementary aids are provided, to assure their success and to increase their opportunities to participate as a full contributing member of the family.[65]

By considering the interaction between the person and the environment, the ICF-CY enables descriptions that go beyond the documentation of impairments, limitations and restrictions, and supports documentation of what a child is able to do when embedded within certain environmental facilitators.[40] Comprehensive assessment measures of children's domestic life participation must therefore cover variations across environmental factors on the nature and extent of children's participation in household tasks.[34]

A limitation of many existing measures is that they only provide an account of the frequency of the child's engagement in domestic chores, not capturing the influence of the environment on the child's performance.[2] There is a need to measure children's participation patterns. For example, although they may participate in the same tasks over many years, their performance in doing these tasks by their own initiative and without help may change over time.[2] Thus, while legislation and classification schemes promote the concept of participation in context as a central component to address disability, the development of measures for capturing the essence of participation is still in its early stages.[66] With this recognition, the selection of measures for review in this chapter were based on consideration of Schneider's[67] statements that 'the effective operationalization of the ICF-CY framework in current measures is mainly dependent of (1) explicit questions on environmental factors and a better understanding of its role in functioning and disability and (2) using the format of the information matrix to develop a comprehensive and minimal set of questions on functioning and disability' (pp. 9–10).

Overview of recommended measures

Having the ICF-CY as a 'model to help guide and organize the practitioner's thoughts about what information is needed and why'[41] and to identify appropriate assessment tools, we selected five tools which seem to meet and support 'workable' functioning and disability descriptions of children's domestic life participation congruent with the ICF-CY model (see Table 25.2 for selected measures). The selection of instruments was based on correspondence of the instrument items to the closest ICF-CY domestic life domain. It also took into consideration the extent to which

TABLE 25.2
Overview of selected measures

Children Helping Out: Responsibilities, Expectations and Supports (CHORES)

Life Habits Assessment (LIFE-H for Children)

Supports Intensity Scale (SIS) for Children

Pediatric Care and Needs Scale (PCANS)

The Short Child Occupational Profile (SCOPE)

they reflected the formulation of functioning and disability framed by the ICF-CY framework, specifically child–environment interactions that define domestic life participation.

CHILDREN HELPING OUT: RESPONSIBILITIES, EXPECTATIONS AND SUPPORTS

The Children Helping Out: Responsibilities, Expectations and Supports (CHORES) is framed within child–environment interaction and assesses the process of the child's engagement in home activities and routines.[2] A unique feature of the CHORES is that it emerged from the development of a scale for examining the degree of assistance with household tasks, which allows the acknowledgement of the operationalization of 'transfer of responsibility'.[2] Specifically, as the child takes greater responsibility for a task and demonstrates increased competence, the caregiver progressively removes his or her assistance.[68] By measuring the assistance score, the changes on the child participation patterns and the work of families in facilitating their child's participation in household tasks can both be assessed.[2] The CHORES thus offers a useful resource for practitioners and families in designing and planning interventions for future independent living.[2]

ASSESSMENT OF LIFE HABITS FOR CHILDREN

The Assessment of Life Habits for Children (LIFE-H) was developed to assess the quality of participation in 12 domains of the Disability Creation Process.[66] Social participation is viewed through the concept of life habits and understood as daily activities and social roles associated with adaptive survival and development of a person in society.[66] The LIFE-H provides a measure for assessment based on two concepts: the level of difficulty when performing a life habit and the type of assistance required.[66] The scale includes ADL such as maintaining the home (e.g. cleaning, laundry), the level of accomplishment (e.g. no difficulty, with difficulty, performed by substitution) and the types of assistance needed (e.g. technical aids, adaptation, human assistance).[66] In this way, the LIFE-H offers a conceptually relevant assessment approach that captures the interaction of the individual and his or her environment, which is consistent with the ICF-CY framework.[66] The LIFE-H captures

multiple domains of activities and participation within the ICF-CY, and a detailed description of the LIFE-H may be found in Chapter 19.

SUPPORTS INTENSITY SCALE FOR CHILDREN

A traditional approach to measure a person's level of developmental disability has been to focus on the individual's limitations or skills that he or she lacks.[64,69] This focus on *lacks* is reframed to *needs* in the Supports Intensity Scale (SIS), developed by the American Association on Intellectual and Developmental Disabilities.[69] The SIS for children offers a standardized procedure and a reliable and valid means to measure the relative intensity of support needs of children with intellectual disabilities and related developmental disabilities.[64] It involves reflection on the frequency, duration and type of supports needed for a child to participate successfully in an extensive set of life activities.[64,69] Therefore, the use of the SIS-Children demands focusing not on the specific skills or tasks the child is capable of doing, but on the types of support required by the child to accomplish full participation in diverse activities.[64] Defined by these features, the SIS-Children may be a useful tool for planning teams and organizations to arrange resources and strategies for promoting a child's personal independence and productivity.[64]

PEDIATRIC CARE AND NEEDS SCALE

The Pediatric Care and Needs Scale (PCANS) is a recently developed measure adapted from the CANS to assess support needs with children with acquired brain impairment.[70] Important features of the PCANS are that it covers a wide scope with respect to disability severity and provides a needs checklist, offering a comprehensive sampling of the activities and participation domains of the ICF.[70] Both the type of needs as well as the checklist items map to the activity and participation component of the ICF-CY.[70,71] Contextual factors are also recognized in the PCANS with items mapping to domains of the environmental factors component of the ICF-CY.[70,71]

THE SHORT CHILD OCCUPATIONAL PROFILE

The Short Child Occupational Profile (SCOPE) is a measure developed to assess dimensions of occupational

CHILDREN HELPING OUT: RESPONSIBILITIES, EXPECTATIONS AND SUPPORTS (CHORES)	
Purpose	Data collection on the performance of individual children on tasks at home and assessment of assistance needed for child's participation
Population	School-aged children
Description of domains	Items comprise household tasks and reflect the distinction between self-care tasks (e.g. making own meal, putting away own toys) and family-care tasks (e.g. caring for younger siblings, doing the dishes) established by White and Brinkerhoff[30]
Administration and test format	Time to complete: 15–20min
	Testing format: parents are asked to score a 33-item survey with 12 items forming a self-care subscale and 21 items forming a family-care subscale. Each item is composed of two types of questions: one that aims to verify whether the child carries out the household task (or not), and the other to acknowledge the assistance level required on its performance. Moreover, two other general questions are included: (1) importance to parents of their child's participation in household tasks, and (2) the satisfaction level with their child's participation in household tasks
	Scoring: two types of response are elicited for each item: (1) a dichotomous yes/no response for performance of each household task; (2) a seven-point Likert scale for the level of assistance needed on each task (7=on own initiative; 6=with a verbal prompt; 5=with supervision; 4=with some help; 3=with lots of help; 2=cannot do the task; and 1= not expected to do the task). Each time parents indicate that some task is not performed by their child, an additional question is included in order to specify its motives: whether it is due to child's inability to perform it (child-specific reasons, e.g. the child's intellectual or physical development) or they do not expect that task to be performed by their child (socio-environmental reasons, e.g. time available, other family members perform the task). Additionally, two general items in a six-point Likert scale quantify the importance level perceived by parents on their child's participation in household tasks and parents' satisfaction level with their child's participation in household tasks
	Training: no specific training needed
Psychometric properties	Internal consistency: self-care subscale α=0.92; family-care subscale α=0.95
	Validity
	Face: all parents reported that the items and rating scales were easy to understand and relevant on their family routines
	Discriminant: moderate low and positive correlation was obtained between summed total of Child Routine Inventory and summed performance total of CHORES (r=0.38; p<0.05)
	Reliability
	Temporal stability. Intraclass correlation coefficients for performance scores: r=0.92. Intraclass correlation coefficients for assistance scores: r=0.88
How to order	The CHORES can be ordered from Louise Dunn (louise.dunn@hsc.utah.edu)
Key reference	Dunn L (2004) Validation of the CHORES: a measure of school aged children's participation in household tasks. *Scand J Occup Ther* 11: 179–190.

participation and the influence of personal and environmental factors on such participation.[72] The measure is based on the Model of Human Occupation theory, defining participation in terms of the influence of multiple factors, including the person's volition, habituation, skills and the role of environmental factors.[72] The SCOPE involves the use of a four-point rating scale to specify the influence of the variables represented in the child's participation. In this way, the measure generates a profile of strengths and challenges affecting the child's occupational participation, which in the present chapter can be defined as domestic life participation.[72] The profile derived from use of the SCOPE may contribute to the identification of specific person or person–environment factors to be addressed in intervention.[72]

ASSESSMENT OF LIFE HABITS (LIFE-H) FOR CHILDREN (DOMESTIC LIFE DOMAIN)

Purpose	Measures life habits at home and school and in the neighbourhood
Population	Children with disabilities aged 5–13y
Description of domains	Organized under daily activity domain and social roles domain, the LIFE-H includes 11 dimensions corresponding to the first domain (nutrition, fitness, personal care, communication, housing, mobility) and to the second (responsibilities, interpersonal relationships, community life, education and recreation). Considering the aim of this chapter, the dimensions related to the International Classification of Functioning, Disability and Health for Children and Youth domestic life domain are (1) nutrition, namely 'selecting appropriate food for snacks and meals' and 'taking part in meal preparation'; (2) housing, specifically 'taking part in housekeeping tasks' and 'taking part in maintaining the grounds'; and (3) responsibilities, namely 'shopping' and 'helping out at home'
Administration and test format	Time to complete: approximately 45min Testing format: LIFE-H is a questionnaire completed by the parent/caregiver about the child. Two versions of the instrument were developed: a short version (64 items) and a long version (197 items). The measure also encompasses a second scale, the objective of which is to evaluate the individual's level of satisfaction with the accomplishment of life habits Scoring: these versions use an item score ranging from 0 to 9 that conjugates two concepts on the scale degree of difficulty and types of required assistance, where 0 indicates total impairment (meaning that the activity or role is not accomplished or achieved) and 9 indicates optimal social participation (meaning that the activity or role is performed without difficulty and without assistance). A transformation of scores (on a 0–10 scale) can be applied to give similar weighting to each category of life habits in order to allow for the variable number of items in each category, and the number of non-applicable items for the respondent. On the second scale that evaluates the individual's level of satisfaction with the accomplishment of life habits, the score varies from 1 (very unsatisfied) to 5 (very satisfied) Training: the International Network on the Disability Creation Process provides training sessions on LIFE-H
Psychometric properties	Internal consistency: $\alpha=0.73–0.90$ for categories, 0.97 for daily activities and 0.90 for social roles *Validity* Face: most of the experts judged items as adequate to cover the different dimensions of social participation. Parents reported that the items were easy to understand Convergent and divergent: correlations of LIFE-H with Pediatric Evaluation of Disability Inventory (PEDI) and Functional Independence Measure for Children (WeeFIM) dimensions were high in categories with similar constructs such as LIFE-H personal care and housing dimensions with PEDI self-care and mobility dimensions ($0.79<r<0.88$) and with WeeFIM self-care ($r=0.90–0.94$). A weaker association was found of all PEDI dimensions with some LIFE-H dimensions, supporting distinctiveness between the constructs of activities of daily living and social roles. WeeFIM cognitive dimensions showed a lower association with LIFE-H motor dimensions ($r=0.43–0.49$) *Reliability* Intrarater $r=0.83–0.95$ for daily activities. Inter-rater $r=0.80–0.91$ for daily activities and $r=0.63–0.90$ for social roles
How to order	The long and short versions can be ordered from the website of the International Network on the Disability Creation Process: www.ripph.qc.ca/
Key reference	Noreau L, Lepage C, Boissiere L, et al (2007) Measuring participation in children with disabilities using the Assessment of Life Habits. *Dev Med Child Neurol* 49: 666–671.

SUPPORTS INTENSITY SCALE (SIS) FOR CHILDREN	
Purpose	Measures the relative intensity of support needs of children with disabilities
Population	Children with intellectual disabilities and related developmental disabilities
Description of domains	The SIS-Children comprises two sections: (1) Exceptional and Medical Support Needs, evaluating the relative intensity of support needed associated with a variety of medical conditions (e.g. respiratory care, feeding assistance, skin care) and behavioural problems (e.g. self-directed destructiveness, external-directed destructiveness, sexual); and (2) Support Needs Across Life Areas Scale, evaluating the relative intensity of support needs in home living, community living, school learning, health and safety, social and advocacy activities. Bearing in mind the purpose of this chapter, the dimensions related to the International Classification of Functioning, Disability and Health for Children and Youth domestic life domain are placed on the Support Needs Scale, namely on: 'Part A: Home Living Activities' (taking care of clothes, preparing food, housekeeping and cleaning); and 'Part B: Community Living Activities' (shopping and purchasing goods and services)
Administration and test format	Time to complete: the interview takes approximately 2h to complete
	Testing format: the SIS-Children is scored by an interviewer who collects information from at least two respondents who can be interviewed (a) separately or (b) at the same time, in a group interview. These respondents are individuals who know the child very well and thus may include parents and other family members, teachers or direct support staff, and even the child with a disability his or herself. In Part 2 (Support Needs Scale) the interviewer must rate the child in relationship the following: (1) How frequently is support needed for this activity?; (2) On a typical day when support in this area is needed, how much time should be devoted?; and (3) What kind of support should be provided?
	Scoring: the Support Needs Scale is rated across three dimensions of support intensity – frequency, time and type. For rating the type of support the options are 0=none; 1=monitoring; 2=verbal/gestural prompting; 3=partial physical assistance; 4=full physical assistance. For rating the frequency of support the options are 0=negligible; 1=infrequently; 2=frequently; 3=very frequently; 4=always. For rating the daily support time the options are 0=none; 1=<30 min; 2=30 min–<2h; 3=2h–<4h; 4=4h or more
	Training: interviewers should have completed at least a bachelor-level degree and generally be individuals who have experience in conducting assessments and possess an extensive knowledge of behaviour rating or psychological testing principles. Moreover, interviewers should also have several years of direct work experience with people with intellectual and closely related developmental disabilities. Lastly, interviewers should know how to request and verify information from respondents
Psychometric properties	Psychometric properties of the SIS-Children are under study, but preliminary results show inter-rater correlations of 0.91
	The original measure (SIS) shows:
	Internal consistency of $\alpha > 0.90$ in all SIS subscales
	Validity
	Criterion related: correlation coefficients between a rater estimation on a five-point Likert scale about the overall support needed in each of the SIS domains and SIS subscales scores exceeded 0.35 in all SIS scores except protection and advocacy scale
	Construct: correlation coefficients between each SIS subscale and the other SIS subscales range from 0.45 to 0.87. As expected, SIS subscales scores correlate less with Inventory for Client and Agency Planning – adaptive behaviour scale – than another measure of support needs (i.e. rated estimated of support needs)
	Reliability
	Interinterviewer: from $r=0.51$ to $r=0.92$
	Inter-respondent: from $r=0.60$ to $r=0.87$

How to order	Available soon to order from SIS website: www.siswebsite.org/
Key references	Thompson J, Hughes C, Schalock R, et al (2002) Integrating supports in assessment and planning. *Mental Retard* 40: 390–405.
	Thompson J, Tassé M, McLaughlin C (2008) Interrater reliability of the Supports Intensity Scale (SIS). *Am J Mental Retard* 113: 231–237.
	Thompson J, Wehmeyer M, Copeland S, et al (2009) *Supports Intensity Scale for Children – Field Test Version 1.1*. Washington, DC: American Association on Intellectual Disabilities.

PEDIATRIC CARE AND NEEDS SCALE (PCANS)

Purpose	Assesses support needs following childhood acquired brain injury
Population	Children with acquired brain injury
Description of domains	Type of support is determined into four broad domains: special needs, activities of daily living (ADL), instrumental ADL (IADL) and psychosocial. For the purposes of the present chapter, the dimensions related to the International Classification of Functioning, Disability and Health for Children and Youth domestic life domain are placed namely on the IADL domain
Administration and test format	Time to complete: interview format takes approximately 30min to complete
	Testing format: the PCANS checklist of activities can be either self-completed by a clinician or other respondent based on their knowledge or completed through an 'interview style' with a person who has current knowledge of the child's functioning level. For each activity, it is asked whether the child is independent in his or her performance or requires support. In the case of support being needed, it is classified as needing physical assistance and/or supervision. PCANS comprises 130 activities nested within the 25-item checklist, classified into four domains: special needs, ADL, IADL and psychosocial. The list of activities was clustered according to four age ranges, resulting in four separate forms: (1) Form A: 5–7y; (2) Form B: 8–11y; (3) Form C: 12–14y; and (4) Form D: 15–18y. In addition to a supports needs scale, within each age band, three levels of skill are identified for each activity: independence expected for age, emerging independence and independence not expected for age.
	Scoring: based on the activities which the child is expected to be independent for his or her particular age group, three summary scores are calculated: (1) the overall level of support is represented by the single highest rating obtained across all activities (range 0–2), regardless of the number of activities which require such support; (2) the extent of support is calculated by summing the number of items (range 0–25) in which support is required; (3) the intensity of support is calculated by multiplying the number of items endorsed (maximum 25) by the support rating (maximum 2; thus, the score range for intensity is 0–50). Owing to the structure of the rating system, scores can be generated separately for physical assistance and supervision, as well as the four main domain groups (special needs, ADL, IADL and psychosocial)
	Training: no specific training is needed
Psychometric properties	*Validity*
	Criterion related: correlation coefficients of moderate to strong magnitude were found between the PCANS support intensity score and most of the Vineland Adaptive Behaviour Scale (VABS), Wee-FIM and King's Outcome Scale of Childhood Head Injury (KOSCHI) variables ($r=-0.46$ to $r=-0.77$; $p<0.01$)
	Convergent and divergent: correlation coefficients between similar domains of the PCANS and other scales were moderately high (e.g. VABS socialization vs PCANS psychosocial items, $r=-0.64$; $p<0.01$). Correlation coefficients between dissimilar domains were low (e.g. Wee-FIM self-care vs PCANS psychosocial items, $r=-0.29$)

Psychometric properties	Discriminant: PCANS support extent and intensity scores were able to distinguish between subgroups dichotomized by VABS and KOSCHI scores *Reliability* The original measure (CANS) shows inter-rater reliability from r=0.93 to r=0.96, and intrarater reliability of r=0.98
How to order	Available soon to order from Cheryl Soo (cheryl.soo@mcri.edu.au)
Key reference	Soo C, Tate R, Williams L, Waddingham S, Waugh M (2008) Development and validation of the Paediatric Care and Needs Scale (PCANS) for assessing support needs of children and youth with acquired brain injury. *Dev Neurorehabil* 11: 204–214.

THE SHORT CHILD OCCUPATIONAL PROFILE (SCOPE)

Purpose	Assesses the extent to which each personal and environmental factors influence occupational participation
Population	Children between 2 and 21y of age with a range of abilities and diagnosis
Description of domains	Organized within four items, the influence of personal and environmental factors assessed in any child's occupational participation – which in this chapter and accordingly to its purpose – will be conceived within the domestic life areas of volition (referred to as 'motivation for occupation' in the SCOPE), habituation (referred to as 'pattern of occupation' in the SCOPE), communication and interaction skills, process skills, motor skills and environment
Administration and test format	Time to complete: gathering information could take from 5 to 30min. Additionally, rating the SCOPE items typically takes 5–10min for a therapist familiar with Model of Human Occupation (MOHO) concepts. The time for completion is also dependent on the amount of information a therapist wants to include on the SCOPE rating forms Testing format: using a four-point rating scale, the SCOPE indicates the influence of 25 factors – related to a person's volition, habituation, performance and environment – on the child's occupational participation. In order to gather useful information to complete the SCOPE rating, therapists can make use of any combination of the following methods: observation, conversation, proxy report, team feedback or medical records. Although its rating process generates a profile of strengths and challenges affecting the client's occupational participation, it is fundamentally an observational therapist-rated tool. The SCOPE may be used in clinical, community and school settings Scoring: the therapist rates each item as to whether the factor represented by the item facilitates (F), allows (A), inhibits (I) or restricts (R) the child's occupational participation Training: formal training in the administration and scoring of the SCOPE is not required. Therapists can learn how to use this assessment tool by reviewing the administration manual and becoming familiar with MOHO concepts
Psychometric properties	*Validity* Results from Rash analysis showed that the SCOPE items represent the construct of occupational participation in a valid way. The SCOPE discriminated between clients who had varying levels of occupational participation *Reliability* Therapists used the SCOPE in a similar way and analysis demonstrated that there was limited variability among therapists
How to order	Order from the website: www.moho.uic.edu/assess/scope.html

Key references   Bowyer P, Kramer J, Kielhofner G, Maziera-Barbosa V, Girolami G (2007) Measurement properties of the Short Child Occupational Profile (SCOPE). *Phys Occup Ther Paediatr* 27: 67–85.

Kramer J, Bowyer P, Kielhofner G, O'Brien J, Maziero-Barbosa V (2009) Examining rater behaviour on a revised version of the Short Child Occupational Profile (SCOPE). *OTJR Occup Participation Health* 29: 88–96.

REFERENCES

1. Dunn L, Coster W, Orsmond G, Cohn E (2009) Household task participation of children with and without attentional problems. *Phys Occup Ther Pediatr* 29: 258–273.
2. Dunn L (2004) Validation of the CHORES: a measure of school-aged children's participation in household tasks. *Scand J Occup Ther* 11: 179–190.
3. Riggio H, Valenzuela A, Weiser D (2010) Household responsibilities in the family of origin: relations with self-efficacy in young adulthood. *Personality Individual Diff* 48: 568–573.
4. Law M, Finkeman S, Hurley P, et al (2004) Participation of children with physical disabilities: relationships with diagnosis, physical function, and demographic variables. *Scand J Occup Ther* 11: 156–162.
5. Simeonsson R, Carlson D, Huntington G, McMillen J, Brent J (2001) Students with disabilities: a national survey of participation in school activities. *Disabil Rehabil* 23: 49–63.
6. Blair L (1992) Children's participation in household labor: child socialization versus the need for household labor. *J Youth Adolesc* 21: 241–258.
7. Goodnow J (1988) Children's household work: its nature and functions. *Psychol Bull* 103: 5–28.
8. Wiener J, Hanley R, Clark R, Nostrand J (1990) Measuring the activities of daily living. *J Gerontol Soc Sci* 45: 229–237.
9. Medeiros M, Guerra R (2009) Tradução, adaptação cultural e análise das propriedades psicométricas do Activities of Daily Living Questionnaire (ADLQ) para avaliação funcional de pacientes com a doença de Alzheimer. *Revista Brasileira Fisioterapia* 13: 257–266.
10. Graf C (2007) The Lawton Instrumental Activities of Daily Living (IADL) Scale. *Ann Long-Term Care* 15: 21–22.
11. World Health Organization (2007) *International Classification of Functioning, Disability and Health for Children and Youth (ICF-CY)*. Geneva: World Health Organization.
12. Seidel D, Jagger C, Brayne C, Matthews F (2009) Recovery in instrumental activities of daily living (IADLs): findings from the Medical Research Council Cognitive Function and Ageing Study. *Age Ageing* 38: 663–668.
13. Spector W, Katz S, Fulton J (1987) Hierarchical relationship between activities of daily living and instrumental activities of daily living. *J Chronic Dis* 40: 481–490.
14. Antill J, Goodnow J, Russel G, Cotton S (1996) The influence of parents and family context on children's involvement in household tasks. *Sex Roles* 34: 215–236.
15. Peña J, Menéndez C, Torío S (2010) Family and socialization processes: parental perception and evaluation of their children's household labor. *J Comparative Family Studies* 41: 131 –148.
16. Leonard M (2009) Helping with housework: exploring teenagers' perceptions of family obligations. *J Sociol* 17: 1–18.
17. Cogle F, Tasker G (1982) Children and housework. *Family Relations* 31: 395–399.
18. Cheal D (2003) Children's home responsibilities: factors predicting children's household work. *Social Behav Personality* 31: 789–794.
19. Gager C, Sanchez L, Demaris A (2009) The effect of employment and work/family stress on children's housework. *J Family Issues* 30: 1459–1485.
20. Crouter C, Head R, Bumpus F, McHale M (2001) Household chores: under what conditions do mothers lean on daughters? *New Directions Child Adolesc Dev* 94: 23–41.
21. Raley S, Bianchi S (2006) Sons, daughters, and family processes: does gender of children matter? *Annu Rev Sociol* 32: 401–421.
22. Punch S (2001) Household division of labour: generation, gender, age, birth order and sibling composition. *Work Employment Soc* 15: 803–823.
23. Coltrane S (2000) Research on household labor: modeling and measuring the social embeddedness of routine family work. *J Marriage Fam* 62: 1208–1233.
24. Meil G (2006) *Padres e Hijos en la España Actual*. Barcelona: Fundación 'La Caixa'.
25. Elder W, Conger D (2000) *Children of the Land: Adversity and Success in Rural America*. Chicago: University of Chicago Press.
26. Weisner S (2001) Children investing in their families: the importance of child obligation in successful development. *New Directions Child Adolesc Dev* 94: 177–183.
27. Klein W, Graesch A, Izquierdo C (2009) Children and chores: a mixed-methods study of children's household work in Los Angeles families. *Am Anthropol Assoc* 30: 98–109.
28. Grusec E, Goodnow J, Cohen L (1996) Household work and the development of concern for others. *Dev Psychol* 32: 999–1007.
29. Bowes J, Flanagan C, Taylor A (2001) Adolescents' ideas about individual and social responsibility in relation to children's household work: some international comparisons. *Int J Behav Dev* 25: 60–68.
30. White LK, Brinkerhoff DB (1981) Children's work in the family: its significance and meaning. *J Marriage Family* 43: 789–798.
31. Tomanovic-Mihajlovic S (2000) Young people's participation within the family: parents' account. *Int J Child Rights* 8: 151–167.
32. Alanen L, Mayal B (2001) *Conceptualizing Child–Adult Relations*. London: Routledge and Kegan Paul.
33. Brannen J (1996) Discourses of adolescence: young people's independence and autonomy within families. In: Brannen J, O'Brien M, editors. *Children in Families: Research and Policy*. London: Falmer Press, pp. 114–130.
34. Rama S, Richter M (2007) Children's household work as a contribution to the well-being of the family and household. In: Amoateng A, Heaton T, editors. *Families and Households in Post-Apartheid South Africa: Socio-Demographic Perspectives*. Cape Town: HSRC Press, pp. 135–170.
35. Zhang D (2005) Parent practices in facilitating self-determination skills: the influences of culture, socioeconomic status, and children's special education status. *Res Pract Persons Severe Disabil* 30: 154–162.

36. Wehmeyer M (1999) A functional model of self-determination: describing development and implementing instruction. *Focus Autism Dev Disabil* 14: 53–62.

37. United Nations Convention on the Rights of the Child, Res 44/25 (20 November 1989). Available at: www.unicef.org/crc (accessed 17 July 2012).

38. United Nations Standard Rules on Equalization of Opportunities for Persons with Disabilities, Res 48/96 (20 December 1993). Available at: www.un.org (accessed 17 July 2012).

39. Ibragimova N, Granlund M, Björck-Åkesson E (2009) Field trial of ICF version for children and youth (ICF-CY) in Sweden: logical coherence, developmental issues and clinical use. *Dev Neurorehabil* 12: 3–11.

40. Silveira-Maia M, Lopes-dos-Santos (2010) Práticas em educação especial à luz do modelo biopsicossocial: o uso da CIF-CJ como referencial na elaboração dos programas educativos individuais. Proceedings of the 7th Simpósio Nacional de Investigação em Psicologia; 4–7 February 2010. Porto: Universidade do Minho.

41. Simeonsson R, Sauer-Lee A, Granlund M, Björck-Åkesson E (2010) Developmental and health assessment in habilitation with the ICF-CY. In: Mpofu E, Oakland T, editors. *Rehabilitation and Health Assessment: Applying to ICF Guidelines*. New York: Springer, pp. 27–46.

42. Simeonsson R, Leonardi M, Björck-Åkesson E, Hollenweger J, Lollar D (2003) Applying the International Classification of Functioning Disability and Health to measure childhood disability. *Disabil Rehabil* 25: 602–610.

43. Johnson D (2005) Supported employment trends: implications for transition-age youth. *Res Pract Persons Severe Disabil* 29: 243–247.

44. Manteuffel B, Stephens R, Sondheimer D, Fisher S (2008) Characteristics, service experiences and outcomes of transition-aged youth in systems of care: programmatic and policy implications. *J Behav Health Serv Res* 35: 469–487.

45. United Nations Convention on the Rights or Persons with Disabilities (13 December 2006). Available at: www.un.org (accessed 17 July 2012).

46. Ministry of Children and Family Development (2005) *Transition Planning for Youth with Special Needs.* Victoria, BC: Ministry of Children and Family Development.

47. Individuals with Disabilities Education Act of 1997, Pub. L. No. 105–17, 111 Stat. 37 (4 June 1997).

48. Ministério da Educação (2008) *Educação Especial: manual de apoio à prática*. Lisbon: Direcção Geral de Inovação e Desenvolvimento Curricular.

49. Scruggs T, Michaud K (2009) The 'surplus' effect in developmental disability: a function of setting or training (or both)? *Life Span Disabil* 12: 141–149.

50. Haber M, Karpur A, Deschênes N, Clark H (2008) Predicting improvement of transitioning young people in the partnerships for youth transition iniciative: findings from a multisite demonstration. *J Behav Health Serv Res* 35: 488–513.

51. Kirk S (2008) Transitions in the lives of young people with complex healthcare needs. *Child Care Health Dev* 34: 567–575.

52. Alwell M, Cobb B (2009) Functional life skills curricular interventions for youth with disabilities: a systematic review. *Career Dev Exceptional Ind* 20: 1–12.

53. Arnold-Reid G, Schloss P, Alper S (1997) Teaching meal planning to youth with mental retardation in natural settings. *Remedial Special Edu* 18: 166–173.

54. Halpern A (1993) Quality of life as a conceptual framework for evaluating transition outcomes. *Exceptional Child* 59: 486–498.

55. Domaracki W, Lyon R (1992) A comparative analysis of general case simulations instruction and naturalistic instruction. *Res Dev Disabil* 13: 363–379.

56. Singh N, Oswald D, Ellis C, Singh S (1995) Community-based instruction for independent meal preparation by adults with profound mental retardation. *J Behav Edu* 5: 77–91.

57. Luft P, Rumrill P, Snyder J, Hennessey M (2001) Transition strategies for youth with sensory impairments: educational, vocational and independent living considerations. *Sensory Impair* 17: 125–134.

58. National Secondary Transition Technical Assistance Center (NSTTAC) (2006) NSTTAC Indicator 13 Checklist. Available at: www.edresourcesohio.org/transition/indicator_13.php

59. National Alliance for Secondary Education and Transition (2005) *National Standards and Quality Indicators: Transition Toolkit for Systems Improvement*. Minneapolis, MN: University of Minnesota, National Center on Secondary Education and Transition.

60. Employment and Disability Institute – Cornell University (2006) Transition Quality Indicators. Available at: www.ilr. cornell.edu/edi/transqual/docs/TQIndicators0906.pdf

61. Florian L, Hollenweger J, Simeonsson R, et al (2006) Cross-cultural perspectives on the classification of children with disabilities. *J Special Edu* 40: 36–45.

62. Bickenback JE, Chatterji S, Badley EM, Ustun TB (1999) Models of disablement, universalism, and the international classification of impairments, disabilities and handicaps. *Social Sci Med* 48: 1173–1187.

63. Whiteneck G (2006) Conceptual models of disability: past, present and future. In: Field MJ, Jette AM, Martin L, editors. *Disability in America – A New Look.* Washington, DC: The National Academies Press, pp. 50–66.

64. Thompson J, Hughes C, Schalock R, et al (2002) Integrating supports in assessment and planning. *Mental Retard* 40: 390–405.

65. Lopes-dos-Santos P, Silveira-Maia M, Tavares A, Santos M, Sanches-Ferreira M (2008) Virtual reality and associated technologies in disability research and intervention. Proceedings of the 7th ICDVRAT, 8–11 September 2008, Reading, UK.

66. Noreau L, Lepage C, Boissiere L, et al (2007) Measuring participation in children with disabilities using the Assessment of Life Habits. *Dev Med Child Neurol* 49: 666–671.

67. Schneider M (2001) Participation and environment in the ICF. WHO presentation to UN meeting on measurement of disability. New York, 4–6 June.

68. Rogoff B (1996) Developmental transitions in children's participation in sociocultural activities. In: Sameroff AJ, Haith MM, editors. *The Five to Seven Year Shift.* Chicago: University of Chicago Press, pp. 273–294.

69. Thompson J, Wehmeyer M, Copeland S, et al (2009) *Supports Intensity Scale for Children – field test version 1.1.* Washington DC: American Association on Intellectual Disabilities.

70. Soo C, Tate R, Williams L, Waddingham S, Waugh M (2008) Development and validation of the Pediatric Care and Needs Scale (PCANS) for assessing support needs of children and youth with acquired brain injury. *Dev Neurorehabil* 11: 204–214.

71. Tate R, Soo C (2007) *Developing an Assessment Tool for Traumatic Brain Injury: The Care and Needs Scale (CANS).* Sydney: MAA Final Report: The Care and Needs Scale.

72. Bowyer P, Kramer J, Kielhofner G, Maziera-Barbosa V, Girolami G (2007) Measurement properties of the Short Child Occupational Profile (SCOPE). *Phys Occup Ther Pediatr* 27: 67–85.

INTERPERSONAL INTERACTIONS AND RELATIONSHIPS (D710–D799)

Sacha N. Bailey, Lucyna M. Lach and Katie Byford-Richardson

What is the construct?

One of the ways in which the 'social' dimension of the International Classification of Functioning, Disability and Health – Children and Youth Version (ICF-CY)[1] is addressed is through the consideration of the child's interpersonal interactions and relationships with individuals in their more proximal social environment. *General interpersonal interactions* (d710–d729) refer to *skills* that the child/adolescent demonstrates in basic and more complex interactions such as showing and demonstrating warmth in relationships or initiating social interactions whereas *particular interpersonal interactions* (d730–d799) is a more relational construct that refers to the *quality of the child's relationships* or his or her *level of impairment in relationships* with specific individuals such as strangers (d730), family members (d760) and intimate others (d770), as well in relationships that are both formal (d740) and informal (d750).

This same differentiation between skills and quality of relationships is evident in the way that activities and participation are dealt with in this chapter of the ICF-CY. Given that this chapter is located in the activities/participation component of the ICF-CY framework, the *activity* component of interpersonal interactions and relationships refers to the extent to which the child carries out or is limited in 'the actions and tasks required for basic and complex interactions with people (strangers, friends, relatives, family members and lovers)' (p. 173).[1] Among these actions and tasks are the social skills that the child brings into interactions with others. The *participation* component refers to the extent to which the child is engaged or involved in interpersonal interactions and relationships and could be reflected in the level of impairment in, or quality of, those interactions and relationships. This suggests that measures that evaluate the child's social abilities or skills are different from those that evaluate the quality of relationships with peers and

parents. These will therefore be dealt with separately in this chapter (Fig. 26.1).

SOCIAL SKILLS

Among all children, effective social skills and peer relationships are increasingly important predictors of success in school.[2] Children with developmental disorders present with a range of impairments in social skills.[3] In their Social Information Processing (SIP) model, Crick and Dodge[4] delineate the steps involved in generating a behavioural response in social situations. All children enter into social situations with biologically informed capabilities as well as a database of memories of past experiences upon which to interpret social cues. As they receive social cues, they selectively attend to those cues and interpret their meaning. Almost simultaneously, they attend to a goal or desired outcome, access and select a potential response from their bank of possibilities and enact a response. This process is highly automatic but breaking it down in this manner allows us to examine how the social skills of children with developmental delays or disabilities may be affected.

The core deficit among children diagnosed with autism spectrum disorder (ASD) is their impairment in social behaviour and interactions.[5] Using the SIP model to understand this impairment, we can hypothesize that there are a number of ways in which the generation of a behavioural response in social situations is impaired. Malformation or malfunctioning of physical structures associated with the neurobehavioural system, the child's capacity to access and use past experiences, the extent to which he or she selectively attends to social cues, interprets the meaning of social cues and/or selects a behavioural response may be differentially involved. This is further supported by 'Theory of Mind', which posits that communication impairment among children with autism, as well as their inability to represent the mental state of

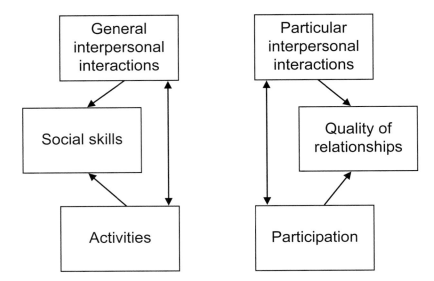

Figure 26.1 Connection between ICF-CY framework, social skills and relationships.

others due to a deficit in abstraction, probably contributes to the way in which their social skills are expressed.[6]

A recent study tested the SIP model and found that children with mild to borderline intellectual disabilities had a small response repertoire, and had more problems with perspective taking, problem recognition, interpretation, inhibiting their responses and emotion recognition than their typically developing peers.[7,8] Other studies have tested different aspects of this model and found that children with various developmental disorders differ from their typically developing peers in the extent to which they interpret others' intentions as benign/hostile,[9] in the encoding of information, and in the extent to which they focus on negative and emotional information in social situations.[10] These impairments are associated with how various parts of the brain are configured and therefore operate, and are further informed by the social context within which the child functions.[3]

QUALITY OF INTERACTIONS

The level of impairment in a child's interactions and relationships, hereinafter referred to as the quality of relationships, refers to the nature and quality of the child's interactions with his or her friends as well as his or her status among peers. The formation of friendships and integration into peer groups provide all children with an opportunity to develop social skills and to experience a sense of social belonging to their communities.[11] In typically developing children, having a friend, friendship quality and group acceptance make separate contributions to a child's experience of loneliness.[12] Children between the ages of 8 and 14 with autism report being

lonelier and the quality of their friendships (i.e. experience of companionship, security and help) is poorer than in typically developing children.[13] Friendship quality is also poorer among children with cerebral palsy,[14] ASD[15] and Asperger syndrome.[16]

The question of whether children with developmental disorders such as autism are capable of appraising their loneliness was recently addressed in a study by Lasgaard et al,[17] who contributed to the growing evidence that youth with ASD can appraise their loneliness and experience higher levels of loneliness. In a study of adolescents with Asperger syndrome, individuals with Asperger syndrome similarly displayed higher levels of loneliness than age-matched controls. In that study, having a higher level of best-friendship quality was associated with a lower level of loneliness.[18] Loneliness is a major mental health issue given its relationship to concurrent as well as longer-term psychosocial implications.[19]

The peer status of children with developmental disorders is generally more compromised than that of their typically developing peers. Their peer social networks are more limited:[20–22] those with ASD are more likely to be isolated or to have peripheral peer group status; they are nominated fewer times as a friend by peers, and they have fewer overall classroom connections and fewer reciprocated best friends than their typically developing peers[15]; those with neurofibromatosis are viewed by their peers and teachers as displaying less leadership ability and being more sensitive and isolated relative to their peers.[23] Although the skills that children with mild developmental delays demonstrate in dyadic friendships evolve and improve over a 2-year period, these changes are not evident in more complex social interactions in larger peer-group settings.[24] These challenges appear to continue, and even worsen in the young adult years when individuals with developmental disorders are likely to show more interest in social exchanges. In a study of 235 adolescents and young adults with autism, almost half (46.4%) of the sample was reported to have no same-aged friends with whom they had a reciprocal relationship, either within or outside of prearranged settings.[25]

QUALITY OF PARENT–CHILD INTERACTION

The study of the parent–child interaction is subsumed under the larger umbrella of the study of parenting. Studies that address parenting are challenging to summarize as the concept of parenting is complex and there is no universally accepted definition of what it means. As a result, there is a multiplicity of conceptualizations underlying how parenting is studied[26] and evaluated.[27] It may refer to *parenting behaviours* such as sensitivity;[28] *cognitions* such as beliefs, expectations and attributions;[29] *affect* such as worry;[30] or *style* such as permissive/authoritarian/authoritative.[31] The conceptual basis of measures used to evaluate parenting is one way of understanding implicit assumptions about what is meant by parenting. However, even then there is no consensus on what any single measure is evaluating as it may be referred to in a number of ways. For example, the Parenting Sense of Competence Scale is referred to as a measure of parental cognition,[32] self-esteem[33] or skills and knowledge.[34]

In an effort to classify measures of parenting and the parent–child relationship, a typology has been developed to facilitate the meaningful grouping of studies for a systematic review currently in progress. The typology has two layers: one that classifies generic parenting measures and another that classifies disability-related parenting measures. Generic parenting measures are further broken down into the following: parenting-as-enacted, parenting-as-experienced and parent–child interactions. The disability-related layer similarly breaks down into the following: parenting-as-enacted – disability-related; parenting-as-experienced – disability-related; and impact of disability. The following paragraphs clarify each of these concepts.

Parenting-as-enacted refers to measures that evaluate what parents do when they parent, observable acts that are directed at their child towards the achievement of a particular goal or measures that evaluate a parent's pattern of parenting (e.g. parenting style). For example, the Parental Tasks subscale of the Daily Parenting Hassles Scale (DPH)[35,36] asks parents to identify how often they have engaged in specific parenting behaviours (e.g. continually cleaning up messes of toys and food, refereeing

sibling arguments or fights, changing their plans because of unprecedented child needs). The Parent Protection Scale (PPS)[37] has three subscales that evaluate parenting behaviour: supervision, dependence and control. The supervision subscale includes items such as 'I comfort my child immediately when he or she cries' and 'I encourage my child to depend on me'; the dependence subscale includes items such as 'I let my child make his or her own decisions' and 'I urge my child to try new things'; the control subscale includes items such as 'I decide when my child eats' and 'I dress my child even if he or she can do it alone'. All of these items refer to what parents do when they parent; thus the term parenting-as-enacted. The measures that we have included as 'parenting-as-enacted' are the Children's Report of Parental Behaviour Inventory (CRPBI-56),[38] the Parental Acceptance/Rejection Questionnaire (PARQ)[39] and the Parenting Scale.[40] They have similar items that capture different aspects of parenting behaviour.

Parenting-as-experienced is a term used for measures that capture parents' cognitions, thoughts, beliefs, expectations and feelings about their experience of themselves as parents to their child. Similarly, it includes cognitions that capture their experience of their child. Measures that evaluate a parent's self-efficacy, locus of control and satisfaction with parenting would be included in the former whereas measures that evaluate attributions related to their child's behaviour refer to the latter. An example of a parenting-as-experienced measure is the Caregiver Self-Efficacy Scale.[41] Although the subscales are behaviour management, school issues, advocacy, emotional support and provider issues, the scale asks parents to rate their level of comfort with their ability to perform specific parenting tasks. In other words, it asks about their parenting experience. Another example of parenting-as-experienced is the Family Impact Questionnaire.[42] Although authors state that it assesses parents' perceptions of their child's impact on their family, four of the six subscales are in fact evaluating the parent's feelings and attitudes about his or her child. The measure asks parents to evaluate situations or feelings indicative of their experience of their child. For example, 'Compared with children and parents with children the same age as my child…my child is more stressful', 'I enjoy the time I spend with my child more', 'My child brings out feelings of frustration and anger more', etc. The Parenting Sense of Competence (PSOC) Scale[43] is similar to these in so far as it evaluates parenting-as-experienced.

Parent–child interaction refers to measures that capture the quality of the interaction/relationship, the nature of the transaction between the parent and child, and aspects of attachment. An example of a parent–child interaction measure is the conflict subscale of the Parental Environment Questionnaire.[44] The child is asked to reflect on the extent to which a number of statements are true. Statements reflect the nature of the transaction between parent and child: 'I often seem to anger or annoy my parent', 'Often there are misunderstandings between my parent and myself'. The Parent Development Interview (PDI)[45] is reviewed as an example of a parent–child interaction measure.

The *disability-related* layer refers to measures that evaluate parenting a child with a disability. These measures specifically ask parents to reflect on their child's disability when answering the questions, or may specifically enquire about what parents do, believe or feel as a result of being a parent to a child with a disability.

Parenting-as-enacted – disability-related therefore refers to what parents do and the patterns that best describe their parenting behaviour and style that occur as a result of their child's disability. For example, the Maternal Agency Questionnaire[46] was developed to evaluate the maternal behaviour associated with promoting the development of her child with autism. The questionnaire asks mothers to indicate how often they engage in the following actions: 'learn new ways to encourage your child's language and cognitive development' or 'teach your child social skills'. The Parent Response to Child Illness (PRCI) Scale[47] similarly includes subscales that invite the parent to reflect on how his or her parenting promotes child autonomy and supports his or her child.

As expected, *parenting-as-experienced – disability-related* refers to parents' cognitions, beliefs, expectations and feelings about their experience of themselves as a parent to a child with a disability or their experience of their child who has a disability. Emphasis of the instructions or items is on the child's diagnosis, and therefore factors such as their experience of stigma, worry or the extent to which their child's limitations are disability-related fall into this category. There are numerous measures that fall into this category, as researchers are often interested in how the developmental disability impacts on parental experience. For example, the Family Empowerment Scale[48] is deceiving by its title, as it suggests that what is being measured is the level of empowerment in the *family*. However, the scale in fact measures the *parents'* perception of adequacy of services received (e.g. 'I know the steps I need to take when I am concerned my child is receiving poor services') and their perception of their involvement in the community (e.g. 'I feel that my knowledge and experience as a parent can be used to improve services for children and families'), revealing little about how the *family* interacts in a way that is empowering. Each item

refers to an aspect of parenting-as-experienced but in relation to their child who has a disability. The PRCI[47] subscales, condition management and child discipline, are further examples of measures of parenting-as-experienced – disability-related.

Finally, measures of impact of disability are unique in so far as they capture the immense challenges faced by parents who have a child with a disability. These measures document what parents do because they are a parent of a child with a disability, but they measure parenting that does not directly involve the child. Impacts may refer to work hours, finances, housing and parental health or actions that parents engage in such as advocacy and community involvement. The Parent Advocacy Scale[49] describes parent advocacy actions undertaken in the last 9 months, such as making telephone calls, office visits or meetings related to their child's disability. Another example is the Impact-on-Family Scale,[50] which measures the parent's perception of the social and familial impact of a child's developmental disorder. It includes items such as 'additional income is needed in order to cover medical expenses' and 'I am cutting down on the hours I work to care for my child'. Among the measures reviewed below, one of the subscales of the PRCI,[47] the family life/leisure subscale, evaluates the impact of the child's condition on the activities of the family.

Factors to consider when measuring this domain

The selection of a measure for clinical purposes or for a research study requires critical reflection on what aspect of the parent–child interaction the practitioner or researcher wishes to measure. In the case of peer interactions, there are a number of possibilities to choose from. First, a decision must be made as to whether social skills or some aspect of peer relationships are to be evaluated. In the case of parent–child interactions, a decision must similarly be made about whether parenting in general or disability-related parenting is of interest, and then whether parenting as enacted or experienced, the parenting interaction or the impact of the disability are to be assessed.

The second decision requires practitioners and researchers to determine whether they are interested in a parent report, a child report, a teacher report or an interview- or observation-based measure. These last types of measure tend to require multiple raters and specialized training, which can be costly. Administering measures that enquire about the child's subjective experience of different aspects of his or her life to younger children has been questioned by some.[51] Younger children may give more extreme responses on Likert-type items than older children[52] and little is known about how children with developmental disorders respond to Likert-type items.

A number of measures that look promising are actually specific to younger children and so attention must be paid to the age group for which they were validated. Furthermore, most measures have been developed for children without developmental disorders but are being used in this population. This is reflective of the underdeveloped nature of the field. Much more work is needed to ensure that generic measures adequately reflect the underlying concepts in this population. Often measures have been adapted by hand-picking items, shortening scales or adapting questions, without considering the impact this has on the reliability or validity of the measure. Virtually none of the measures reviewed addresses responsiveness to change or indicates a clinical cut-off. This means that their sensitivity to evaluate changes made as a result of intervention or a practitioner's/researcher's capacity to identify 'at-risk' parenting is limited or unknown.

Finally, some of these measures are publicly available whereas others can be obtained only through a distributor who holds the licence. The latter involves a cost that must be absorbed by practitioners, agencies or research grants. Some professions (e.g. psychologists and occupational and physical therapists) may be set up to purchase measures as they are trained to use them, whereas other professions (e.g. social work, psychotherapists) are less inclined to do so. The selection of a measure is therefore contingent on the availability of financial resources.

The evaluation of activities and participation is an integral component of the ICF-CY framework. Measures that address interpersonal interactions and relationships exist but clearly require further development, particularly for children with developmental disorders.

Overview of recommended measures: social skills and relationships

Given the complexity associated with conceptualizing peer-related aspects of interpersonal relationships, it is not surprising that there is no agreed-upon definition of key concepts and measures associated with this social domain.[53] The typology developed in this chapter differentiates social behaviour from social skills, peer acceptance, loneliness and friendship quality, each of which represents a different aspect of a child's general and interpersonal interactions. A number of measures have been selected to illustrate the various ways in which these can be evaluated (see Table 26.1) and the following sections provide a brief description of each.

CHILDREN'S SELF-EFFICACY FOR PEER INTERACTION[54]

Crick and Dodge's[4] reformulated social information processing model postulates that when children receive

social cues, they engage in a process of interpreting those cues. In this part of the model, children evaluate the goal they wish to attain as well as their past performance (e.g. how they have previously managed similar kinds of cues/goals). Furthermore, prior to generating a behavioural response to the social cue, children draw on outcome expectations and evaluate their self-efficacy to enact their decision. The self-efficacy that the Children's Self-efficacy for Peer Interaction (CSPI) model evaluates is defined as the 'belief that one can successfully perform behavior required to produce desired outcomes' (p. 795).[54] The evaluation of self-efficacy is therefore entirely consistent with these components of the SIP model.

A review of the literature indicates that this measure has not been widely used among children with developmental disorders. One study was found that used the CSPI to evaluate self-efficacy among children with sickle cell disease.[55] This is surprising given the importance of self-efficacy for the well-being of any child.[56] Nevertheless, in their review of measures used to evaluate social skills, Matson and Wilkins[57] identify the CSPI as a valid and reliable measure that should be considered for use among children and adolescents. It is an easy to administer 22-item self-report that asks children to evaluate their ability to enact pro-social verbal persuasive skills/tactics used in peer situations. Developed and tested among children in grades three to five, it requires an ability to be able to understand and respond to questions such as 'Your class is going on a trip and everyone needs a partner. Asking someone to be your partner is _____ (insert HARD! hard, easy, EASY!) for you'. This is a potential limitation for children with developmental disorders whose level of cognitive function is below that typical of the third grade.

SOCIAL SKILLS RATING SYSTEM

There are many measures that seek to assess the behavioural enactment component of Crick and Dodge's[4] SIP model. Among these are measures that evaluate social skills.[58] The SSRS is one of the most widely used measures for this purpose.[57] Although the age range covered by the SSRS is broad, it has most frequently been used with preschool- and school-aged children.[57] This measure has been used in studies with children who have Asperger syndrome,[59] epilepsy,[60] developmental delay[61] or intellectual disability.[62]

There are many advantages to using this measure: it covers a broad age spectrum; there are child/adolescent-, parent- and teacher-rated forms available to evaluate the child's social skills, problematic behaviours and academic competence; raw scores can be converted into standard scores and centile rankings; and a computer program for scoring and reporting is available. It appears to be

TABLE 26.1
Selected measures of social skills and peer relationships

Name of measure	Aspect of interpersonal interaction evaluated
Children's Self-Efficacy for Peer Interaction Scale	Social behaviour
Social Skills Rating System	Social skills
Revised Class Play	Peer acceptance
UCLA Loneliness Scale	Loneliness
Friendship Quality Questionnaire	Friendship quality

CHILDREN'S SELF-EFFICACY FOR PEER INTERACTION SCALE (CSPI)

Purpose	The 22-item CSPI scale assesses children's perceptions of their ability to enact pro-social verbal persuasive skills/tactics used in peer situations. There is also a teacher-rated version that consists of 11 items
Population	The scale was originally tested with six classrooms of children in grades three to five. The scale has been used with adolescents up to age 17y
Description of domains (subscales)	There are two subscales in this measure: conflict (12 items that reflect conflict peer situations) and non-conflict (10 items that reflect non-conflict peer situations) A total score of self-efficacy is calculated whereby higher ratings reflect higher levels of self-efficacy
Administration and test format	Time to administer: 10–15min Testing format: paper and pencil. Each item describes a social situation, followed by an incomplete statement requiring the child to evaluate his or her ability to perform the persuasive skill involved in the social situation on a four-point scale (e.g. HARD! hard, easy, EASY!) Scoring: response ratings are summed to generate an overall self-efficacy score ranging from 22 to 88 Training: none required
Psychometric properties	Normative sample: 243 school-aged children in New York and Indiana. The CSPI has not been validated for use with children with disabilities *Reliability* Cronbach's alpha of 0.85 for the conflict component and 0.73 for the non-conflict component Test–retest reliability established over a 2-wk period (0.90 for males, 0.80 for females), indicating stability over this time period *Validity* Correlates with Peer Rating Scale of Social Influence, Play Nominations Sociometric Measure and Piers–Harris Children's Self-concept Scale
How to order	The scale is published in Wheeler and Ladd (1982)
Key reference	Wheeler VA, Ladd GW (1982) Assessment of children's self-efficacy for social interaction with peers. *Dev Psychol* 18: 795–805.

sensitive enough to the social challenges that children with developmental disorders face as group differences were established for children with and without disabilities[63] and children with 22q11 deletion syndrome and their siblings.[64]

Other related measures include the following:

SOCIAL SKILLS RATING SYSTEM (SSRS)

Purpose	The SSRS evaluates a broad range of socially validated behaviours that affect teacher–student relationships, peer acceptance and academic performance
Population	The SSRS has been developed for use in 3 to 18 year olds. There are self, parent and teacher versions for the social skills subscales; teacher and parent versions for the problem behaviour subscales; and a teacher version for only the academic competence subscales
Description of domains (subscales)	Social skills scale: co-operation, empathy, assertion, self-control, responsibility Problem behaviours scale: externalizing and internalizing problems, hyperactivity Academic competence scale: performance, general cognitive functioning, motivation, parental support
Administration and test format	Time to complete: 15–25min per form Testing format: the test consists of parent, teacher and self-report forms for children at different academic levels (preschool, elementary or secondary). Each form has 34–55 items, depending on the subscale, and each item is rated on a three-point scale except for the teacher-rated academic competence score, which ranges from 1 to 5 Scoring: subscale scores are the sum of the item raw scores for a subscale. The sum of all subscale raw scores is the total raw score for a scale. Raw scores can be transformed into standard scores and centile rankings using tables provided in the manual Training: Master's-level education and completion of the training package
Psychometric properties	Normative sample: the test was normed with an American sample of 4000+ children and adolescents in grades 3–10 (including 'learning-disabled', 'behaviourally disordered' and 'mentally handicapped' children), 1000+ parents and 250+ teachers *Reliability* Internal consistency was 0.90 for the social skills scale, 0.84 for the problem behaviours scale and 0.95 for the academic competence scale Test–retest reliability was 0.84–0.93 for all scales on the teacher form, 0.65 for the problem behaviour scale and 0.80 for the social skills scale on the parent form, and 0.68 for the social skills scale on the self-report form *Validity* Extensive validity information is published in the manual. Correlations with other standardized measures (including the Child Behavior Checklist, Piers–Harris Children's Self-concept Scale and the Walker–McConnell Scale of Social Competence and School Adjustment) range between 0.50 and 0.75
How to order	PsychoCorp, Pearson Assessments (www.pearsonassessments.com/pai/)
Key reference	Gresham FM, Elliott SN (1990) *The Social Skills Rating System*. Circle Pines, MN: American Guidance Service.

- Preschool and Kindergarten Behavior Scales. See Merrell KW (2003) *Preschool and Kindergarten Behavior Scales*, 2nd edition. Austin, TX: Pro-Ed.
- Early Social Communication Scales. See Seibert JM, Hogan AE, Mundy PC (1982) Assessing interactional competences: the early social-communication scales. *Infant Ment Health J* 3: 244–258.
- Matson Evaluation of Social Skills with Youngsters (MESSY). See Matson JL, Rotatori AF, Helsel WJ (1983) Development of a rating scale to measure social skills in children: the Matson Evaluation of

Social Skills with Youngsters (MESSY). *Behav Res Ther* 21: 335–340; and Matson JL, Stabinsky-Compton LS and Sevin JA (1991) Comparison and item analysis of the MESSY for autistic and normal children with autism spectrum disorders. *Res Autism Spectr Disord* 1: 28–37.

REVISED CLASS PLAY[65]
Sociometric evaluations are used to assess the extent to which children are accepted or rejected by their peers.[65] The Revised Class Play (RCP) was developed

and validated as comprising three subscales: sociability/ leadership, aggressive/disruptive and sensitive/isolated.[65] However, a more recent analysis indicates that there are four subscales: popular-leader, prosocial, aggressive-disruptive and sensitive-isolated.[66] Children are asked to cast their classmates into each specific role and the rating that each child receives is based on the number of times they are nominated for that particular role. There are 15 positive roles such as 'polite', 'plays fair' or 'makes new friends easily' and 15 negative roles such as 'teases other children too much' or 'shows off a lot', and each role is assigned to one of the subscales. Each child would therefore receive a rating on the frequency with which he or she was cast into a sociability/leadership, aggressive/disruptive and sensitive/isolated role by their peers. Other typologies that use similar techniques include popular, average, rejected and neglected, based on peer ratings of who is liked the most/ least[67] or who is the most popular or liked.[68]

REVISED CLASS PLAY (RCP)	
Purpose	Requires children to assess peers' reputation
Population	Original RCP was based on a study with third- to sixth-grade students
Description of domains (subscales)	Sociability-leadership (15 items): e.g. 'good leader', 'has many friends' Aggressive-disruptive (eight items): e.g. 'bossy', 'gets into a lot of fights' Sensitive-isolated (seven items): e.g. 'feelings get hurt easily', 'very shy'
Administration and test format	Time to complete: 20min Testing format: 30-item scale where each item represents a different role, with 15 positive 'roles' and 15 negative 'roles' (e.g. '____ has good ideas for things to do'; '____ picks on other kids'). Children are provided with an alphabetical class register and asked to nominate one student for each role. The instructions given to students are the following: Now what we want each of you to do is to pretend that you are a director of a play starring the students in this classroom. The director of a play has to do many things but the most important job is to select the right people to act in the play. So, your job is to choose the students who could play each part or role best. Try to pick the students who seem to fit each part in real life. Children are instructed to select only one classmate per role, although the same classmate could be selected for more than one role. In some studies, children are instructed to select three classmates per role Scoring: the number of votes received by each child for each role is tallied and then standardized within classroom and sex to adjust for variations in class size and sex distribution. Scores are generated for positive reputation and disruptive and isolated behaviours Training: none required
Psychometric properties	Normative sample: 600+, in American elementary schools *Reliability* Test–retest=0.63–0.87; internal consistency=0.81–0.93 *Validity* Results of the RCP correlated with other measures, including teacher ratings, academic achievement scores and IQ
How to order	Contact the author, Ann Masten (amasten@umn.ed; www.cehd.umn.edu/icd/faculty/ Masten.html)
Key references	Masten AS, Morison P, Pellegrini DS (1985) A Revised Class Play method of peer assessment. *Dev Psychol* 21: 523–533. Zeller M, Vannatta K, Schafer J, Noll RB (2003) Behavioural reputation: a cross age perspective. *Dev Psychol* 39: 129–139.

Studies of children with developmental disabilities have used modified versions of the original RCP. For example, one of the subscales of the RCP was used in a study of children between the ages of 9 and 12, to compare the social isolation of four groups: preterm with cerebral palsy, preterm without cerebral palsy, term with cerebral palsy and term without cerebral palsy. Females born pre-term with or without cerebral palsy and females born at term with cerebral palsy were rated by their peers as more socially isolated than females born at term without cere-bral palsy.[69] In another study, 11 roles from the RCP were selected to explore the relationship between peer status and whether teachers would select/nominate a classmate to be a peer buddy of a child with autism.[70] Others have found a three-factor solution for the sensitive-isolated scale (six items in total) and a two-factor solution for the sociability/leadership subscale (nine items in total),[71] or have used 11 individual items from the RCP,[72] or have taken items from the RCP and combined them with items from other sociometric measures, for example refs 67 and 73.

Other sociometric measures include the following:

- Crick NR, Grotpeter JK (1995) Relational aggres-sion, gender, and social–psychological adjustment. *Child Dev* 66: 710–722.
- Coie JD, Dodge KA, Coppotelli H (1982) Dimensions and types of social status: a cross-age perspective. *Dev Psychol* 18: 557–570.
- Lease AM, Kennedy CA, Axelrod JL (2002) Children's social constructions of popularity. *Social Dev* 11: 87–109.
- Pekarik EG, Prinz RJ, Liebert DE, Weintraub S, Neale JM (1976) The pupil evaluation inventory: a sociometric technique for assessing children's social behaviour. *J Abnorm Child Psychol* 4: 83–97.

University of California Los Angeles Loneliness Scale[74]

The University of California Los Angeles (UCLA) ver-sion of the Loneliness Scale was tested using a diverse population: college students, hospital-based nurses, public school teachers and elderly individuals.[74] The chart that follows provides detailed information about this measure.

This measure has not been highly subscribed to in the childhood disability literature. However, Lasgaard[75] translated this version into Danish and established it as a reliable and valid measure of loneliness in a national sample of 13- to 17-year-old youth. Recently, Lasgaard et al[17] used this measure with adolescent males with ASD and established its reliability with this sample. Previous debates regarding the factor structure of this measure were not evident, indicating that this is indeed a one-factor measure evaluating extent of loneliness along a continuum. Among adolescent males with ASD, higher levels of loneliness were associated with lower levels of perceived social support from classmates, parents and a close friend, but were not associated with the amount of contact with peers outside of school.[17]

Friendship Quality Questionnaire[12]

Counting the number of friends that a child has may address the density of a child's social network, but it does not address the quality of those relationships. In fact, having a friend, friendship quality and group acceptance made separate contributions to the prediction of loneli-ness.[12] The Friendship Quality Questionnaire (FQQ) is a measure designed to address the second factor, namely the quality of friendships that a child has. The initial set of items was informed by a measure initially developed by Bukowski, Hoza and Boivin in 1987 and published in 1994.[76] Parker and Asher made changes to the wording of some items and to the response scale. The extent to which relationships are validating and caring, conflicts are resolved, help and guidance is obtained, companion-ship and recreation are evident and intimate exchange is experienced are measured using this scale. Children are asked to think of a specific best friend when responding to the items in the measure. The five-point scale ranges from 'not at all true' to 'really true'.

Generally, the study of quality of peer relationships among children with developmental disorders is not as advanced as it is among typically developing children.[77] The constructs identified in this section of the chapter rep-resent distinct concepts that warrant future investigation in this highly undersubscribed field of study.

Other related measures include the following:

- Friendship Quality Scale. See Bukowski WM, Hoza B, Boivin M (1994) Measuring friendship quality during pre- and early adolescence. The develop-ment and psychometric properties of the Friendship Qualities Scale. *J Soc Pers Relat* 11: 471–484.

Overview of recommended measures: parent–child interactions

Children's Report of Parental Behaviour Inventory[38]

Parental behaviour can be rated by the parent, a third party or the child. The CRPBI is a well-established measure that captures the child's perception of his or her parent's behaviour. Some have argued that this is more predic-tive of child adjustment than actual parental behaviour.[78]

UNIVERSITY OF CALIFORNIA LOS ANGELES (UCLA) LONELINESS SCALE

Purpose	The UCLA Loneliness Scale is a 20-item self-report of loneliness
Population	The scale was originally developed and validated with college students, nurses, teachers and the elderly. Lasgaard translated it into Danish and validated it for use with adolescents and more recently for use with adolescent males with autism spectrum disorder
Description of domains (subscales)	There are no subscales in this measure. There are 11 positively worded items and nine negatively worded items. A total score of loneliness is generated by reverse-scoring the 11 positively worded items so that higher scores reflect higher levels of loneliness
Administration and test format	Time to complete: 5min Testing format: this is a self-administered questionnaire that can be completed by children/adolescents Scoring: each item is scored from 1 (never) to 4 (always); scores range from 20 to 80 Training: none required
Psychometric properties	*Reliability* In a study of adolescent males with autism spectrum disorder, Cronbach's alpha was 0.85 for males with autism spectrum disorder and 0.91 for typically developing males (Lasgaard et al, 2010) *Validity* Convergent validity with New York University Loneliness Scale and Differential Loneliness Scale was 0.65 and 0.72, respectively. Correlations with social support measures were negative. Discriminant validity has been established with a measure of social support and construct validity has been established with measures of neuroticism and introversion–extroversion, self-esteem and depression
How to order	The scale is published in Russell (1996)
Key references	Lasgaard M (2007) Reliability and validity of the Danish version of the UCLA Loneliness Scale. *Pers Individ Dif* 42: 1359–1366. Lasgaard M, Nielsen A, Eriksen ME, Goossens L (2010) Loneliness and social support in adolescent males with autism spectrum disorder. *J Autism Dev Disord* 40: 218–226. Russell DW (1996) UCLA Loneliness Scale (version 3): reliability, validity, and factor structure. *J Pers Assess* 66: 20–40.

In order to measure children's perceptions of specific, observable parenting behaviours (parenting as enacted), the CRPBI asks children to report on whether their mother and father are similar or different from the descriptors provided in the scale (e.g. 'Feels hurt when I don't follow his or her advice'; 'Almost always speaks to me in a warm and friendly voice') on a three-point Likert scale ('like', 'somewhat like' and 'not like').

The CRPBI was originally developed by Schaefer[78–80] and consisted of 260 items. Based on the developmental and empirical literature, Schaefer conceptualized parenting behaviour using a circumplex model, in which maternal behaviour was thought to fall into two dimensions of parenting behaviour: love versus hostility and autonomy versus control. Further study using this model revealed three dimensions: acceptance versus rejection, psychological autonomy versus psychological control, and firm control versus lax control.[38] Margolies and Weintraub's 56-item version[38] includes separate and identical forms for the child to complete about his or her mother and father and includes six subscales of parenting behaviour: acceptance, child-centredness, non-enforcement, instilling persistent anxiety, controlling through guilt, and lax discipline. The 56-item version has shown good reliability and accuracy in relation to the original 260-item version. The CRPBI has been used in a study of children with spina bifida.[81] This study used the intrusiveness subscale from the CRPBI-108 to compare parental overprotection among parents of 8- and 9-year-old children with spina bifida to a matched sample of parents of typically

FRIENDSHIP QUALITY QUESTIONNAIRE (FQQ)	
Purpose	The FQQ evaluates children's perceptions of various aspects of their best friendship
Population	Originally developed by Parker and Asher (1993) with typically developing children in grades three to six, this 40-item, six-subscale measure is used with adolescents with developmental disorders up to age 18y (Whitehouse et al, 2009)
Description of domains (subscales)	There are six subscales in this self-report measure: Validation and caring (10 items): e.g. '(friend) would like me even if others do not' Conflict resolution (three items): e.g. '(friend) and I get over arguments really quickly' Conflict and betrayal (seven items): e.g. '(friend) and I get mad a lot' Help and guidance (nine items): e.g. '(friend) and I help each other with school work a lot' Companionship and recreation (five items): e.g. '(friend) and I always sit together at lunch' Intimate exchange (six items): e.g. '(friend) and I tell each other secrets' Higher scores indicate greater perceived friendship quality except for conflict/betrayal subscale where lower scores indicate greater perceived friendship quality
Administration and test format	Time to complete: 15–25min Testing format: this is a self-administered questionnaire that can be completed by the child alone or with the support of an interviewer The child identifies the name of his or her best friend and then responds to 40 statements about how true that statement is, on a five-point Likert scale, about their friendship with this person Scoring: each item is scored from 0 (not at all true) to 4 (really true) Training: none required
Psychometric properties	Normative sample: 800+ elementary school children from a range of socioeconomic and ethnic backgrounds. Norms for children with disabilities not provided *Reliability* Cronbach's alpha for subscales is as follows: validation and caring, 0.90; conflict resolution, 0.73; conflict and betrayal, 0.84, help and guidance, 0.90; companionship and recreation, 0.75; intimate exchange, 0.86 *Validity* All subscales correlate with low-accepted children on a sociometric measure of acceptance by peers
How to order	Contact the primary author, Jeffrey G. Parker (jgparker@psu.edu; http://parker.psych.psu.edu/default.htm)
Key references	Parker JG, Asher SR (1993) Friendship and friendship quality in middle childhood: links with peer group acceptance and feelings of loneliness and social dissatisfaction. *Dev Psychol* 29: 611–621. Whitehouse AJO, Durkin K, Jaquet E, Ziatas K (2009) Friendship, loneliness and depression in adolescents with Asperger's syndrome. *J Adolesc* 32: 309–322.

developing children. In a study examining the impact of parenting style and disease severity on quality of life (QOL) in children aged 6 to 18 years with cerebral palsy, parenting, as measured by a Hebrew version of the CRPBI, was significantly related to child QOL and child psychological health.[82]

CHILDREN'S REPORT OF PARENTAL BEHAVIOUR INVENTORY (CRPBI) AND CRPBI-56

Purpose	The CRPBI is a 56-item designed to assess how a child perceives his or her mother's or father's parenting behaviour
Population	The original 260-item scale was developed by Shaefer (1965) and tested on children aged 12–18y. The 56-item version was validated by Margolies and Weintraub (1977) with children in grades four to six. Children must be able to read to complete the measure. Previous versions were used with college students
Description of domains (subscales)	The CRPBI comprises six subscales that yield three factors: acceptance/rejection – the degree to which the child perceives positive involvement versus hostile detachment in the parent (acceptance subscale and child-centredness subscale); psychological control/ psychological autonomy – the degree to which the child perceives the parent's covert use of control through guilt, intrusiveness and parental direction (control through guilt subscale and instilling persistent anxiety subscale); and firm control/lax control – the degree to which parents make the rules and enforce them (lax discipline subscale and non-enforcement of rules subscale)
Administration and test format	Time to complete: 20min Testing format: the CRPBI is a child self-report (paper and pencil) measure containing 56 items. The child indicates whether his or her parent is 'like', 'somewhat like' or 'not like' each of the items identified. The child completes separate, but identical, forms for his or her mother and father Scoring: the CRPBI generates a score for each of the three factors. Acceptance/rejection: 16 items from acceptance subscale, eight items from child-centredness subscale; scores range from 0 to 48, where a higher score indicates less acceptance and more rejection Psychological control/psychological autonomy: eight items from control through guilt subscale, eight items from instilling persistent anxiety subscale; scores range from 0 to 32, a higher score indicatimg less psychological control and more psychological autonomy Firm control/lax control: eight items from lax discipline subscale, eight items from nonenforcement of rules subscale; scores range from 0 to 32, where a higher score indicates more firm control and less lax control Training: none required
Psychometric properties	Normative sample: available for the 108-item version with a high school and college age sample *Reliability* Test–retest reliability: 0.66–0.93 at 1-wk and 5-wk intervals in children from 9y to 11y of age Internal consistency of original Shaefer scale (26 scales): 0.60–0.90 (median=0.76). Factor analysis found factors I and II (acceptance/rejection and psychological autonomy/control) held up very well, but factor III (lax/firm control) was less stable than the others *Validity* Discriminant validity has been demonstrated
How to order	The CRPBI-56 can be made available through researchers who have used it. Dr Weintraub and Dr Margolies do not recommend contacting them
Key references	Margolies PJ, Weintraub S (1977) The revised 56-item CRPBI as a research instrument: reliability and factor structure. *J Clin Psychol* 33: 472–476. Schaefer ES (1959) A circumplex model for maternal behaviour. *J Abnorm Soc Psychol* 59: 226–235. Schaefer ES (1961) Multivariate measurement and factorial structure of children's perceptions of maternal and paternal behaviour. *Am Psychol* 16: 345–346.

Schludermann E, Schludermann S (1970) Replicability of factors in Children's Report of Parent Behaviour (CRPBI). *J Psychol* 76: 239–249.

The original CRPBI-260 is published in Schaefer ES (1965) Children's Reports of Parental Behaviour: an inventory. *Child Dev* 36: 413–424.

PARENTAL ACCEPTANCE–REJECTION QUESTIONNAIRE (PARQ)

Purpose	Designed to assess the degree of warmth in the parent–child relationship as evaluated by the child, the parent about his or her behaviour, and the parent about the parenting that he or she received as a child/adolescent. There is a 60-item standard form version and a 24-item short-form version
Population	This self-administered measure can be given to children from age 7y to 18y. There is a kindergarten version for children aged 4–6y that can be administered by an evaluator. There is also a version for parents to evaluate the parenting they received as children/ adolescents
Description of domains (subscales)	This measure comprises four subscales:
	Warmth/affection (20 items on standard form; eight items on short form): describes parent–child relationships in which parents give love and affection without qualification, but not necessarily with great demonstration. Demonstrated when parents show approval of their child, play with their child, enjoy their child and praise him or her
	Hostility/rejection (15 items on standard form; six items on short form): describes parent–child relationships that lack warmth and affection, in which the parent seems to reject the child, disapproves of them and views them as a burden. Demonstrated by parents who are impatient, irritable and antagonistic towards the child; parents may nag, scold and ridicule their child. This also includes parents who handle their child abruptly and roughly and who hit and curse the child
	Indifference/neglect (15 items on standard form; six items on short form): describes parent–child relationships in which the parent is seen as being unconcerned or uninterested in the child and may be viewed as cold or distant. Demonstrated by parents who pay little attention to the child, do not spend much time with their child and may ignore the child's requests for help, attention or comfort
	Undifferentiated rejection (10 items on standard form; four items on short form): refers to forms of rejection in which children perceive their parents to be rejecting or unloving without necessarily seeing them as being hostile, aggressive, indifferent or neglectful
Administration and test format	Time to complete: 15–20min for child PARQ; 10–15min for adult and parent version; short forms take about 7–10min
	Testing format: self-report. Three formats: adult PARQ – adults' perceptions of their mother's or father's treatment of them when they were 7–12y; parent PARQ – parents' assessment of how they treat their child currently; and child PARQ – child's perception about how their mother or father treats him or her now. Two forms: long (standard) form containing 60 items; short form containing 24 items (long form is recommended; it is recommended that reliability and validity are assessed when using the short form)
	Scoring: respondents are asked if an item is 'almost always true', 'sometimes true', 'rarely true' or 'almost never true'. The measure produces subscale and total scores. The total score ranges from 60 (maximum perceived acceptance) to 240 (maximum perceived rejection) on the standard form and from 24 to 96 on the short form. Higher scores indicate greater perceived parental rejection. Scoring can be done online at no cost using the PARSCORE VI, a programme used for scoring all standard full-length versions of the PARQ (available from Rohner Research Publications)
	Training: none required

Psychometric properties	Normative sample: adult and child PARQ (US sample): scores usually range from 90 to 110; mean=105 (SD=25). Approximately 7–10% of children's and adults' scores fall at or above 150 (midpoint)
	Reliability
	Extensively reported in the manual (internal consistency, test–retest reliability; meta-analysis of reports about reliability). Internal consistency reliability for the mother version of the adult and child PARQ: Warmth/Affection=0.95 (Adult), 0.90 (Child); Hostility/Aggression=0.93 (Adult), 0.87 (Child); Indifference/Neglect=0.88 (Adult), 0.77 (Child); Undifferentiated Rejection=0.86 (Adult), 0.72 (Neglect). Mean weighted effect sizes (diversity of samples from the USA, as well as other regions such as Africa, Caribbean, Europe, Middle East and South Asia): 0.89 (total PARQ), 0.91 (warmth/affection), 0.89 (hostility/aggression), 0.80 (indifference/neglect), 0.81 (undifferentiated rejection). Mean weighted alpha coefficients: 0.89 (child PARQ), 0.95 (adult PARQ), 0.84 (parent PARQ)
	Validity
	Extensively reported in the manual (convergent and discriminant validity, factor analyses). The PARQ has been validated in many languages and diverse cultures
	Convergent validity: PARQ hostility/aggression with a measure of physical punishment=0.43 (adult PARQ), 0.55 (child PARQ). PARQ warmth/affection with CRPBI acceptance subscale=0.90 (adult PARQ), 0.83 (child PARQ)
	Discriminant validity: every subscale in the adult and child PARQ is correlated more highly with its validation scale than with any other scale in a given PARQ scale
How to order	The PARQ can be ordered using the order form on the website: http://home.earthlink.net/~rohner_research/
	Cost: handbook for the study of parental acceptance and rejection, which includes copies of all versions of the measures and all forms, costs $35 USA; $45 international; $55 global priority or international air; $20 ebook payment (cheque/money order or credit by Paypal) and order form can be sent by mail or email (rohner_research@earthlink.net)
Key references	Rohner RP, Khaleque A (2005) *Handbook for the Study of Parental Acceptance and Rejection*, 4th edn. Storrs, CT: Rohner Research Publications.
	There is a website that contains a comprehensive list of studies employing the PARQ: www.csiar.uconn.edu/bibliographies.html

PARENTAL ACCEPTANCE–REJECTION QUESTIONNAIRE[39]

Based on a great deal of cross-cultural research on parenting behaviour, Rohner and Khaleque[39] conceptualized parental acceptance–rejection as a bipolar dimension. They developed a measure that taps into four elements of parental warmth: warmth/affection, hostility/rejection, indifference/neglect and undifferentiated rejection; each of these being bipolar. The PARQ assesses perceptions of parental behaviour (parenting as enacted) in the family of origin. This measure has three formats: the Adult PARQ asks parents about their perceptions of their own parents' behaviour; the Parent PARQ asks parents about their current behaviour towards their child; and the Child PARQ asks children about their perceptions of their parents' behaviour. The 'Child PARQ: Father' version asks children how true the statement about how their father treats them is (e.g. 'Praises me to others'; 'Pays no attention to

me') on a four-point scale. The Parent PARQ asks parents to note how well the statement describes how they parent their own child (e.g. 'I am harsh with my child'; 'I make my child feel what [s]he does is important') on a similar four-point scale. Kourkoutas and Erkman[83] have used the PARQ extensively in their work in Greece. It has also been used in studies of parents of children with neurodevelopmental delay in Turkey and Pakistan (personal communication with Dr Rohner, March 2011). The PARQ is available in several languages, as noted on the website (http://home.earthlink.net/~rohner_research/r_instruments.htm).

PARENTING SCALE[40]

The basis for the development of the Parenting Scale was parenting discipline 'mistakes' that relate theoretically to externalizing problems and/or studies that substantiated this relationship. This measure asks parents to specify the

PARENTING SCALE (PS)

Purpose	The 30-item PS assesses the discipline practices of parents. This measure asks about actual parenting practices rather than parental beliefs and attitudes regarding discipline. Parents rate their probabilities of using specific discipline strategies in response to child misbehaviours
Population	Originally developed for use with parents of preschool children (Arnold et al, 1993), but has since been validated for use with middle-school children (Collett et al, 2001; Irvine et al, 1999) and children aged 2–9y with neurodevelopmental disorders (autism spectrum disorder) (Whittingham et al, 2009)
Description of domains (subscales)	There are three subscales and a total scale score: Laxness (11 items): permissive and inconsistent discipline Over-reactivity (10 items): authoritarian parenting style which includes threats and physical punishment and emotional and harsh discipline, equivalent to coercive discipline practices Verbosity (seven items): giving lengthy verbal responses to misbehaviour rather than taking direct action
Administration and test format	Time to complete: 10min Testing format: the PS is a parent self-report measure with 30 items Scoring: each item is rated on a seven-point scale that is anchored by one effective and one ineffective discipline strategy. Some items are reverse scored. Higher scores indicate more ineffective discipline. The scale generates three subscale scores as well as a total score Training: none required
Psychometric properties	Normative sample: none reported *Reliability* Internal consistency (alpha)=0.83 (Laxness), 0.82 (Over-reactivity), 0.63 (Verbosity), 0.84 (Total score); test–retest reliability over a 2-wk period=0.83 (Laxness), 0.82 (Over-reactivity), 0.79 (Verbosity), 0.84 (Total score) (from a sample of 168 mothers of children aged 2–4y) Internal consistency (alpha)=0.78 (Laxness), 0.78 (Over-reactivity), 0.65 (Verbosity), 0.81 (Total score) (from a sample of children aged 2–9y with autism spectrum disorder) *Validity* Correlated with Battelle Developmental Inventory, Marital Adjustment Test and the Child Behavior Checklist. The PS distinguished between mothers who were attending a behaviour clinic to improve their child-management skills and mothers who were not attending such a clinic. High scores on the PS also distinguished parents of children with attention-deficit–hyperactivity disorder (ADHD) and comorbid conduct problems from parents of children with ADHD alone. The measure has also been correlated with observational measures of inadequate parental discipline and child misbehaviour
How to order	A copy of the PS can be obtained free of charge by sending a self-addressed, stamped envelope to: Susan G. O'Leary, Department of Psychology, Stony Brook University, Stony Brook, NY 11794–2500, USA. Email: susan.oleary@stonybrook.edu
Key references	Arnold DS, O'Leary SG, Wolff LS, Acker MM (1993) The Parenting Scale: a measure of dysfunctional parenting in discipline situations. *Psychol Assess* 5: 137–144. Collett BR, Gimpel GA, Greenson JN, Gunderson TL (2001) Assessment of discipline styles among parents of pre-school through school-age children. *J Psychopathol Behav Assess* 23: 163–170.

Irvine AB, Biglan A, Smolkowski K, Ary DV (1999) The value of the Parenting Scale for measuring the discipline practices of parents of middle school children. *Behav Res Ther* 37: 127–142.

Rhoades KA, O'Leary S (2007) Factor structure and validity of the Parenting Scale. *J Clin Child Adolesc Psychol* 36: 137–146.

Whittingham K, Sofronoff K, Sheffield J (2009) Stepping Stones Triple P: an RCT of a oarenting programme with parents of a child diagnosed with an autism spectrum disorder. *J Abnorm Child Psychol* 37: 469–480.

extent to which specific disciplinary behaviours are used. For each item, two anchors are used, one effective and the other ineffective. Parents must situate their perception of their parenting practice along a seven-point continuum. The original measure was developed for use with parents of preschool children[40] and had three factors: laxness, over-reactivity and verbosity. A sample item from the laxness subscale is 'When I want my child to stop doing something…I firmly tell my child to stop/I coax or beg my child to stop'. These two parenting behaviours represent the anchors and parents indicate at what point along the seven-point continuum their parenting behaviour is reflected.

The psychometric properties of the Parenting Scale were originally assessed on a sample of mothers of children aged 18 to 48 months. The factor structure has since been examined with other populations, including parents (mostly mothers) of older children, children with attention-deficit–hyperactivity disorder (ADHD), African American children, low-income African American children, and mothers and fathers of children aged 3 to 7 years (see ref. 84 for a review). Each of these studies supported a two-factor solution: laxness and over-reactivity. The verbosity factor, which had initially been identified in the development study of the scale, was never replicated. A hostile factor was identified and supported in a study of mothers and fathers of children aged 3 to 7 years.[84] This factor included physical punishment, cursing and name-calling. A sample item from the hostility subscale includes 'When my child does something I don't like, I insult my child, say mean things, or call my child names'. The anchors related to that item are 'never or rarely' and 'most of the time'. It is important to note that this factor was not frequently endorsed in a community sample of parents, but represents parenting behaviours that are related to parent characteristics and contributed to unique variance in the prediction of child behaviour problems. Rhoades and O'Leary,[84] therefore, recommend a two-factor structure, with the option of including the hostile subscale. Some authors have noted that a potential shortcoming of using the Parenting Scale with adolescents is that only one item on the measure relates to parental monitoring.[85] The

Parenting Scale has been used in an intervention study to evaluate the efficacy of the Stepping Stones Triple P for parents of children aged 2 to 9 years with ASD,[86] and in a randomized clinical trial of the Stepping Stones Triple P programme for parents of preschoolers with developmental and behavioural problems.[87] Caution should therefore be exercised in considering the use of this scale for adolescents.

PARENTING SENSE OF COMPETENCE SCALE[43]

The Parenting Sense of Competence Scale (PSOC) was originally developed by Gibaud-Wallston and Wandersman[88] to measure parenting self-esteem, defined as a parent's perceived self-efficacy as a parent (efficacy subscale) and the satisfaction derived from parenting his or her child (satisfaction subscale). The measure asks parents to rate their level of agreement with statements such as 'A difficult problem in being a parent is not knowing whether you're doing a good job or a bad one' (satisfaction) and 'I meet my own personal expectations for expertise in caring for my child' (efficacy). Although the original scale had two factors/subscales (efficacy and satisfaction), a subsequent study revealed three factors: satisfaction, efficacy and interest.[89] The interest subscale reflects a parent's engagement in the parenting role. The authors of this factor analysis study conducted analyses separately for mothers and fathers in a normative community sample of parents of children under the age of 18 years. The three factors accounted for more of the variance than that accounted for by the two-factor structure originally put forward by Johnston and Mash.[43]

The PSOC has been used in studies of parents of older children as well as in clinical samples. The scale is used frequently in studies of children with ADHD, conduct disorder and oppositional defiant disorder and has shown validity in studies of parents of children with neurodevelopmental disorders. For example, it was used with younger and older children with hyperactivity.[90] Hudson, Cameron and Matthews[91] used the PSOC in an evaluation of Signposts for Building Better Behavior, a support programme for parents of children with intellectual disabilities aged 3 to 16 years.

PARENTING SENSE OF COMPETENCE SCALE (PSOC)

Purpose	The PSOC was developed to measure parenting self-esteem or parenting efficacy and satisfaction
Population	The measure is completed by parents of children (aged 0–9y)
Description of domains (subscales)	There are two subscales and a total score: Skill-knowledge (referred to by Johnston and Mash [1989] as efficacy): efficacy is an instrumental dimension and refers to the degree to which the parent feels competent, capable of problem solving and familiar with parenting Value-comforting (referred to by Johnston and Mash [1989] as satisfaction): satisfaction is an affective dimension and refers to the degree to which the parent feels frustrated, anxious and poorly motivated in the parenting role Total score: evaluates overall competence
Administration and test format	Time to complete: 5–10min Testing format: the PSOC is a 17-item, parent self-report scale. Mother and father versions exist, differing only in their use of the words 'mother' and 'father'. Each item is answered on a six-point Likert scale Scoring: some items are reverse scored. Higher scores correspond to greater efficacy, satisfaction and overall competence Training: none required
Psychometric properties	Normative sample: normative data are available for a community-based sample of mothers and fathers of children aged 4–9y *Reliability* Alpha=0.82 (satisfaction), 0.70 (efficacy). Satisfactory 6-wk test–retest correlations ranged from 0.46 to 0.82. Internal reliability=0.72 (efficacy scale in a sample of mothers of infants) *Validity* Evidence exists for the efficacy and satisfaction dimensions of the PSOC by the differential relationships to parent and child characteristics and by interparent differences on the two scales. Internal consistency (alpha)=0.79 (total score), 0.75 (satisfaction), 0.76 (efficacy) 0.82 (total score), 0.71 (satisfaction), 0.77 (efficacy) in a sample of parents of children aged 2–9 years with ASD. Parent perceptions of child behaviour significantly correlated with PSOC scores. Interparental differences were found, where fathers reported higher levels of parenting self-esteem than mothers, particularly on the satisfaction dimension
How to order	The PSOC is in the public domain and is free to use. Contact Dr Johnston (cjohnston@psych.ubc.ca)
Key references	Gibaud-Wallston J, Wandersman LP (1978) Development and utility of the Parenting Sense of Competence Scale. Paper presented at the annual meeting of the American Psychological Association, Toronto. Hudson A, Cameron C, Matthews J (2008) The wide-scale implementation of a support programme for parents of children with an intellectual disability and difficult behaviour. *J Intellect Dev Disabil* 33: 117–126. Ohan JL, Leung DW, Johnston C (2000) The Parenting Sense of Competence Scale: evidence of a stable factor structure and validity. *Can J Behav Sci* 32: 251–261. For the development of the measure, see Johnston C, Mash EJ (1989) A measure of parenting satisfaction and efficacy. *J Clin Child Psychol* 18: 167–175.

PARENT DEVELOPMENT INTERVIEW (PDI)	
Purpose	The PDI is a structured interview-based measure that uses a coding template to evaluate six dimensions of parent–child interaction. The interview focuses on three central themes: a parent's view of her experiences in the parent–child relationship; a parent's view of the child's experiences in the relationship; and a parent's overall awareness of the relationship. Interview questions enquire about a parent's description of their relationship in general and about specific topics such as discipline, achievement, separation and affect. Parents are probed to provide examples for characteristics of their child and for thoughts and feelings associated with these examples. Parents are asked to provide adjectives describing their child and memories supporting those adjectives, to describe positive and negative interactions with their child and other typical parenting situations, and to discuss a variety of emotions typically experienced by parents
Population	The interview is to be used with parents of children with disabilities and typically developing children between the ages of 1y and 10y
Description of domains (subscales)	Six dimensions of the parent–child relationship are evaluated and generate a score: Compliance: the extent to which interactions involve the child's response to maternal requests or demands Achievement: the child's developmental process Comfort/safety: the extent to which the mother acts as a source of comfort and security for the child Enmeshment: boundary confusion between mother and child Worry about child's future: for example, whether the child will live independently Emotional pain: for example, sadness, grief
Administration and test format	Time to complete: 45min Testing format: semi-structured interview; 13 items. There are several versions of the PDI: the original (toddler version), an infancy version, a revised version (PDI-R) and a brief version (PDI-R brief). The authors recommend using the PDI-R Scoring: interviews are coded based on a manual. Three aspects of parent narratives are coded: content or themes represented (what parents say about caregiving); process or how the parents represent themselves and the content (how they say it); and affective tone of representations (what emotions they express or exhibit as they discuss caregiving themes). Content codes include the following: mentions compliance, ineffectiveness with control/compliance, mentions business of caregiving, mentions child's achievement, mentions comfort/safe haven. Process codes include the following: perspective taking, enmeshment, neutralizing/defensive, confusion of response. Affect codes include the following: anger, pleasure, guilt, worry/anxiety about the future, sadness/pain. Confusion (Global scale). Responses to each of the 13 questions are coded on a set of six four-point rating scales developed to reflect the six dimensions of the parent–child relationship listed above. Training: training in administration, transcription and scoring is suggested. The PDI itself comes with extensive instructions. However, training in using the interview is also offered by Dr Slade and colleagues
Psychometric properties	Normative sample: none *Reliability* Inter-rater reliability using intraclass correlations ranged from 0.73 to 0.83 with standard error ranging from 0.10 to 0.17; inter-rater reliability based on cells from 0.68 to 0.90 depending on whether non-zero codes were considered. Reliability varies the version of the PDI used. In a three-factor version, Cronbach's alpha was 0.84 for joy-pleasure/coherence; 0.82 for anger; and 0.68 for guilt-separation distress *Validity* No information available

How to order	A copy of the PDI can be requested from Arietta Slade (arietta.slade@gmail.com)
Key references	Aber L, Slade A, Berger B, Bresgi I, Kaplan M (1985) The Parent Development Interview. Unpubished manuscript, Barnard College, Columbia University, New York.
	Pianta R, O'Conner T, Marvin RS (1993) *Adapted Parent Development Interview*. Charlottesville, VA: University of Virginia.
	Pianta R, O'Conner T, Morog M, Button S, Dimmock J, Marvin RS (1995) *Parent Development Interview: Coding Manual*. Charlottesville, VA: University of Virginia.

PARENT DEVELOPMENT INTERVIEW

The PDI was originally developed by Aber, Slade and colleagues (unpubished material, 1985 and 2003) to assess parents' representation of their relationship with their toddler. The original PDI was a 45-item semi-structured clinical interview taking between 1 and 2 hours to administer. The authors subsequently developed a toddler version, an infancy version, a revised version (PDI-R) and a brief version (PDI-R brief). The authors recommend using the PDI-R as it has demonstrated validity and they feel that parents need the longer time required of the full-length version to warm up. The PDI-R asks parents to describe their child (e.g. 'In an average day, what would you describe as his or her [child's] favourite moments?'). Parents provide five adjectives describing their relationship to their child and are asked to offer evidence in support of these descriptors. They are also asked what they like and dislike about their child and to describe similarities and differences between the child and both parents. Parents are then asked about their relationship to the child, specifically pleasures and difficulties, moments of harmony and dissention (e.g. 'Describe a time in the last week when you and [your child] really weren't clicking'). Parents are then asked about their representations of themselves as parents, including their own strengths and weaknesses. Lastly, parents are asked to describe their child's reactions to normal separations from them and about routine upsets (e.g. 'What is it like for you when your child refuses to do what you ask him/her to, or deliberately provokes you?'). Following their responses, parents are often probed to offer more information about their behavioural and emotional responses to the situation presented.

Pianta and colleagues[45] adapted the original PDI to assess parents' representation of themselves as parents and of their relationship with their child. The interview was shortened to 13 items, and takes about 45 minutes to administer. Pianta's version of the PDI taps into dimensions of parenting that have been found to be particularly salient to parents of children with disabilities[28]: compliance, achievement, comfort/safety, enmeshment, worry about the child's future, and emotional pain such as sadness and grief associated with parenting the child. Parent responses to the questions are scored on a set of six four-point rating scales reflecting content, process and affect of their responses. This version of the PDI has been used in studies of children with cerebral palsy[92] and epilepsy.[28] Slade has been using the PDI to measure reflective functioning, which is the 'parent's capacity to reflect upon her and her child's internal mental experience' (p. 269).[93] She and her colleagues have developed a coding scale to evaluate parental reflective functioning using the original PDI.[93]

PARENT RESPONSE TO CHILD ILLNESS[47,94]

The 35-item PRCI was developed to measure parenting behaviours and perceptions related to parenting a child with a chronic illness. The subscales that evaluate 'parenting-as-experienced – disability-related' include child support and child autonomy; the subscales that evaluate 'parenting-as-enacted – disability-related' include condition management and child discipline. The sample used to develop this measure consisted of caregivers (mostly mothers) of children aged 4 to 14 years of age with new-onset seizures or new-onset asthma. Ronen et al[60] used the autonomy subscale of the PCRI in a study of children with epilepsy and found that it correlated with the child-reported present worries subscale of the health-related quality of life measure as well as the secrecy subscale. This measure is reliable and valid, and although it was developed for use with children aged 4 to 14 years of age with epilepsy, it shows some promise for use with children who have other types of neurodevelopmental disorders.

PARENT RESPONSE TO CHILD ILLNESS SCALE (PRCI)	
Purpose	The PRCI is a 35-item disability-related measure that evaluates parents' perceptions and behaviours related to parenting a child with a chronic illness
Population	This self-administered measure is intended for parents of children between the ages of 4y and 14y but has been used for adolescents up to the age of 18y
Description of domains (subscales)	There are five subscales: Child support (eight items): parental provision of emotional support to the child relative to the health condition Family life/leisure (10 items): family participation in leisure activities Condition management (five items): parental confidence in their ability to manage child's health condition Child autonomy (six items): parental encouragement of their child's independence Child discipline (six items): parental confidence in their ability to manage their child's behaviour
Administration and test format	Time to complete: 10min Testing format: the PRCI is a parent self-report measure that uses a five-point Likert scale response Scoring: the PRCI generates five individual subscale scores, where higher scores on each subscale connote more adaptive aspects of parenting Training: none required
Psychometric properties	Normative sample: no norms *Reliability* Internal consistency reliability: good (ranging from 0.67 to 0.85) for the five subscales in a sample of children with seizures; good (ranging from 0.72 to 0.89) for child support, family life/leisure and condition management; and low for child autonomy (0.57) and discipline (0.59) in a sample of children with asthma Test–retest reliability: three factors (child support, child autonomy and child discipline) had good test–retest reliability (ranging from 0.60 to 0.74) and two factors (condition management and family life/leisure) had fair test–retest reliability (ranging from 0.40 to 0.59) for the seizure sample; moderate test–retest for the asthma sample (child autonomy was good, the other four subscales were fair) *Validity* The measure was developed and validated with children with new-onset seizures or asthma, and was later tested with children with chronic epilepsy. Construct validity has been explored between PRCI and related constructs, such as parent mood, family environment, child behaviour problems, parent perceptions of stigma, parent worry and parents' need for information
How to order	Free to use. Contact Paul Buelow (pbuelow@iupui.edu); cc. Joan Austin (joausti@iupui.edu). For the published scale see Austin et al (2008)
Key references	Austin JK, Dunn DW, Johnson CS, Perkins SM (2004) Behavioural issues involving children and adolescents with epilepsy and the impact of their families: recent research data. *Epilepsy Behav* 5: 33–41. Austin J, Shore CP, Dunn DW, Johnson CS, Buelow JM, Perkins SM (2008) Development of the Parent Response to Child Illness (PRCI) scale. *Epilepsy Behav* 13: 662–669.

REFERENCES

1. World Health Organization (2007) *International Classification of Functioning, Disability, and Health – Children and Youth Version*. Geneva: WHO.

2. NICHD Early Child Care Research Network (2006) The relations of classroom contexts in the early elementary years to children's classroom and social behavior. In: Huston AC, Ripke MN, editors. *Developmental Contexts in Middle Childhood: Bridges to Adolescence and Adulthood*. New York: Cambridge University Press, pp. 217–236.

3. Yeates KO, Bigler ED, Dennis M, et al (2007) Social outcomes in childhood brain disorder: a heuristic integration of social neuroscience and developmental psychology. *Psychol Bull* 133: 535–556.

4. Crick NR, Dodge KA (1994) A review and reformulation of social information-processing mechanisms in children's social adjustment. *Psychol Bull* 115: 74–101.

5. Travis LL, Sigman M (1998) Social deficits and interpersonal relationships in autism. *Ment Retard Dev Disabil* 4: 65–72.

6. Baron-Cohen S, Leslie AM, Frith U (1985) Does the autistic child have a 'theory of mind'? *Cognition* 21: 37–46.

7. van Nieuwenhuijzen M, Orobio de Castro B, van Aken MAG, Matthys W (2008) Impulse control and aggressive response generation as predictors of aggressive behaviour in children with mild intellectual disabilities and borderline intelligence. *J Intellect Disabil Res* 53: 233–242.

8. van Nieuwenhuijzen M, Vriens A, Scheepmaker M, Smit M, Porton E (2011) The development of a diagnostic instrument to measure social information processing in children with mild to borderline intellectual disabilities. *Res Dev Disabil* 32: 358–370.

9. Leffert JS, Siperstein GN, Widaman KF (2010) Social perception in children with intellectual disabilities: the interpretation of benign and hostile intentions. *J Intellect Disabil Res* 54: 168–180.

10. Embregts P, van Nieuwenhuijzen M (2009) Social information processing in boys with autistic spectrum disorder and mild to borderline intellectual disabilities. *J Intellect Disabil Res* II: 922–931.

11. Newcomb AF, Bagwell CL (1995) Children's friendship relations: a meta-analytic review. *Psychol Bull* 117: 306–347.

12. Parker JG, Asher SR (1993) Friendship and friendship quality in middle childhood: links with peer group acceptance and feelings of loneliness and social dissatisfaction. *Dev Psychol* 29: 611–621.

13. Bauminger N, Kasari C (2000) Loneliness and friendship in high-functioning children with autism. *Child Dev* 71: 447–456.

14. Cunningham SD, Warschausky S, Thomas PD (2009) Parenting and social functioning of children with and without cerebral palsy. *Rehabil Psychol* 54: 109–115.

15. Kasari C, Locke J, Gulsrud A, Rotheram-Fuller E (2011) Social networks and friendships at school: comparing children with and without ASD. *J Autism Dev Disord* 41: 533–544.

16. Chamberlain B, Kasari C, Rotheram-Fuller E (2007) Involvement or isolation? The social networks of children with autism in regular classrooms. *J Autism Dev Disord* 37: 230–242.

17. Lasgaard M, Nielsen A, Eriksen ME, Goossens L (2010) Loneliness and social support in adolescent boys with autism spectrum disorder. *J Autism Dev Disord* 40: 218–226.

18. Whitehouse AJO, Durkin K, Jaquet E, Ziatas K (2009) Friendship, loneliness and depression in adolescents with Asperger's syndrome. *J Adolesc* 32: 309–322.

19. Heinrich LM, Gullone E (2006) The clinical significance of loneliness: a literature review. *Clin Psychol Rev* 26: 695–718.

20. Guralnick MJ (1997) Peer social networks of young boys with developmental delays. *Am J Ment Retard* 101: 595–612.

21. Guralnick MJ, Connor RT, Johnson LC (2009) Home-based peer social networks of young children with Down syndrome: a developmental perspective. *Am J Intellect Dev Disabil* 114: 340–355.

22. Stoneman Z, Brody GH, Davis CH, Crapps JM (1988) Childcare responsibilities, peer relations, and sibling conflict: older siblings of mentally retarded children. *Am J Ment Retard* 93: 174–183.

23. Noll RB, Reiter-Purtill J, Moore BD, et al (2007) Social, emotional, and behavioral functioning of children with NF1. *Am J Med Genet* Part A143A: 2261–2273.

24. Guralnick MJ, Neville B, Hammond MA, Connor RT (2007) The friendships of young children with developmental delays: a longitudinal analysis. *J Appl Dev Psychol* 28: 64–79.

25. Orsmond G, Krauss MW, Seltzer MM (2004) Peer relationships and social and recreational activities among adolescents and adults with autism. *J Autism Dev Disord* 34: 245–256.

26. Patterson GR, Fisher PA (2002) Recent developments in our understanding of parenting: bidirectional effects, causal models, and the search for parsimony. In: Bornstein MH, editor. *Handbook of Parenting: Practical Issues in Parenting*, 2nd edition. Mahwah, NJ: Lawrence Erlbaum Associates, Inc., pp. 59–88.

27. Hoghughi M (2004) Parenting: an introduction. In: Hoghughi M, Long N, editors. *Handbook of Parenting: Theory and Research for Practice*. London: Sage.

28. Button S, Pianta RC, Marvin RS (2001) Mothers' representations of relationships with their children: relations with parenting behavior, mother characteristics, and child disability status. *Soc Dev* 10: 455–472.

29. Bugental DB, Johnston C (2000) Parental and child cognitions in the context of the family. *Ann Rev Psychol* 51: 315–344.

30. Pianta R, O'Conner T, Morog M, Button S, Dimmock J, Marvin RS (1995) *Parent Development Interview: Coding Manual*. Charlottesville, VA: University of Virginia.

31. Baumrind D (1968) Authoritarian v. authoritative parental control. *Adolescence* 3: 255–271.

32. Hassall R, Rose J, McDonald J (2005) Parenting stress in mothers of children with an intellectual disability: the effects of parental cognitions in relation to child characteristics and family support. *J Intellect Disabil Res* 49: 405–418.

33. Walker LS, VanSlyke DA, Newbrough JR (1992) Family resources and stress: a comparison of families of children with cystic fibrosis, diabetes, and mental retardation. *J Pediatr Psychol* 17: 327–343.

34. Rodrigue JR, Morgan SB, Geffken GR (1992) Psychosocial adaptation of fathers of children with autism, Down syndrome, and normal development. *J Autism Dev Disord* 22: 249–263.

35. Crnic KA, Greenberg MT (1980) Minor parenting stresses with young children. *Child Dev* 61: 1628–1637.

36. Crnic KA, Greenberg MT, Robinson NM, Ragozin AS (1984) Maternal stress and social support: effects of the mother–infant relationship from birth to eighteen months. *Am J Orthopsychiatry* 54: 224–235.

37. Thomasgard M, Metz WP, Edelbrock C, Shonkoff JP (1995) Parent–child relationship disorders: parental overprotection and the development of the Parent Protection Scale. *J Dev Behav Pediatr* 16: 244–250.

38. Margolies PJ, Weintraub S (1977) The revised 56-item CRPBI as a research instrument: reliability and factor structure. *J Clin Psychol* 33: 472–476.

39. Rohner RP, Khaleque A (2005) *Handbook for the Study of Parental Acceptance and Rejection*, 4th edition. Storrs, CT: Rohner Research Publications.

40. Arnold DS, O'Leary SG, Wolff LS, Acker MM (1993) The Parenting Scale: a measure of dysfunctional parenting in discipline situations. *Psychol Assess* 5: 137–144.

41. Boothroyd RA (1997) *Preliminary Manual for the Caregiver Self-efficacy Scale*. Tampa, FL: Department of Mental Health Law & Policy, University of South Florida.

42. Donenberg G, Baker BL (1993) The impact of young children with externalizing behaviours on their families. *J Abnorm Child Psychol* 21: 179–198.

43. Johnston C, Mash EJ (1989) A measure of parenting satisfaction and efficacy. *J Clin Child Psychol* 18: 167–175.

44. Elkins IJ, McGue M, Iacono WG (1997) Genetic and environmental influences on parent–son relationships: evidence for increasing genetic influence during adolescence. *Dev Psychol* 33: 351–363.

45. Pianta R, O'Conner T, Marvin RS (1993) *Adapted Parent Development Interview*. Charlottesville, VA: University of Virginia.

46. Kuhn JC, Carter AS (2006) Maternal self-efficacy and associated parenting cognitions among mothers of children with autism. *Am J Orthopsychiatry* 76: 564–575.

47. Austin JK, Dunn DW, Johnson CS, Perkins SM (2004) Behavioral issues involving children and adolescents with epilepsy and the impact of their families: recent research data. *Epilepsy Behav* 5: 33–41.

48. Koren PE, DeChillo N, Friesen BJ (1992) Measuring empowerment in families whose children have emotional disabilities: a brief questionnaire. *Rehabil Psychol* 37: 305–321.

49. Nachshen J, Anderson L, Jamieson J (2001) The Parent Advocacy Scale: measuring advocacy in parents of children with special needs. *J Dev Disabil* 8: 93–105.

50. Stein REK, Jessop DJ (2003) The Impact on Family Scale revisited: further psychometric data. *Dev Behav Pediatr* 24: 9–16.

51. Fredricks JA, Blumenfeld P, Friedel J (2005) School engagement. In: Moore KA, Lippman L, editors. *What do Children Need to Flourish?* New York: Springer Science, pp. 305–321.

52. Chambers CT, Johnston C (2002) Developmental differences in children's use of rating scales. *J Pediatr Psychol* 27: 27–36.

53. Cook F, Oliver C (2011) A review of defining and measuring sociability in children with intellectual disabilities. *Res Dev Disabil* 32: 11–24.

54. Wheeler VA, Ladd GW (1982) Assessment of children's self-efficacy for social interaction with peers. *Dev Psychol* 18: 795–805.

55. Gold JI, Mahrer NE, Treadwell M, Weissman L, Vichinsky E (2008) Psychosocial and behavioral outcomes in children with sickle cell disease and their healthy siblings. *J Behav Med* 31: 506–516.

56. Bandura A (1993) Perceived self-efficacy in cognitive development and functioning. *Educ Psychol* 28: 117–148.

57. Matson JL, Wilkins J (2009) Psychometric testing methods for children's social skills. *Res Dev Disabil* 30: 249–274.

58. Wilkins J, Matson JL (2007) Handbook of assessment in persons with intellectual disabilities. *Int Rev Res Ment Retard* 34: 321–363.

59. Castorina LL, Negri LJ (2011) The inclusion of siblings in social skills training groups for boys with Asperger's syndrome. *J Autism Dev Disord* 41: 73–81.

60. Ronen GM, Streiner DL, Verhey LH, et al (2010) Disease characteristics and psychosocial factors: explaining the expression of quality of life in childhood epilepsy. *Epilepsy Behav* 18: 88–93.

61. Fenning RM, Baker BL, Juvonen J (2011) Emotion discourse, social cognition, and social skills in children with and without developmental delays. *Child Dev* 82: 717–731.

62. Green S, Baker B (2011) Parents' emotion expression as a predictor of child's social competence: children with and without intellectual disability. *J Intellect Disabil Res* 55: 324–338.

63. Lyon MA, Albertus C, Birkinbine J, Naibi J (1996) A validity study of the Social Skills Rating System – Teacher Version with disabled and nondisabled preschool children. *Percept Mot Skills* 83: 307–316.

64. Kiley-Brabeck K, Sobin C (2006) Social skills and executive function deficits in children with the 22q11 deletion syndrome. *Appl Neuropsychol* 13: 258–268.

65. Masten AS, Morison P, Pellegrini DS (1985) A revised class play method of peer assessment. *Dev Psychol* 21: 523–533.

66. Zeller M, Vannatta K, Schafer J, Noll RB (2003) Behavioral reputation: a cross-age perspective. *Dev Psychol* 39: 129–139.

67. Coie JD, Dodge KA, Coppotelli H (1982) Dimensions and types of social status: a cross-age perspective. *Dev Psychol* 18: 557–570.

68. Lease AM, Kennedy CA, Axelrod JL (2002) Children's social constructions of popularity. *Soc Dev* 11: 87–109.

69. Nadeau L, Tessier R (2009) Social adjustment at school: are children with cerebral palsy perceived more negatively by their peers than other at-risk children? *Disabil Rehabil* 31: 302–308.

70. Jackson JN, Campbell JM (2009) Teachers' peer buddy selections for children with autism: social characteristics and relationship with peer nominations. *J Autism Dev Disord* 39: 269–277.

71. Gest SD, Sesma A, Masten AS, Tellegen A (2006) Childhood peer reputation as a predictor of competence and symptoms 10 years later. *J Abnorm Child Psychol* 34: 509–526.

72. Lindstrom WA, Lease AM, Kamphaus RW (2007) Peer- and self-rated correlates of a teacher-rated typology of child adjustment. *Psychol Schools* 44: 579–599.

73. Estell DB, Farmer TW, Irvin MJ, Crowther A, Akos P, Boudah DJ (2009) Students with exceptionalities and the peer group context of bullying and victimization in late elementary school. *J Child Fam Stud* 18: 136–150.

74. Russell DW (1996) UCLA Loneliness Scale (version 3): reliability, validity, and factor structure. *J Pers Assess* 66: 20–40.

75. Lasgaard M (2007) Reliability and validity of the Danish version of the UCLA Loneliness Scale. *Pers Individ Diff* 42: 1359–1366.

76. Bukowski WM, Hoza B, Boivin M (1994) Measuring friendship quality during pre- and early adolescence. The development and psychometric properties of the friendship qualities scale. *J Soc Pers Relat* 11: 471–484.

77. Webster AA, Carter M (2007) Social relationships and friendships of children with developmental disabilities: implications for inclusive settings. A systematic review. *J Intellect Dev Disabil* 32: 200–213.

78. Schaefer ES (1965) Children's report of parental behavior: an inventory. *Child Dev* 36: 413–424.

79. Schaefer ES (1959) A circumplex model for maternal behavior. *J Abnorm Soc Psychol* 59: 226–235.

80. Schaefer ES (1961) Multivariate measurement and factorial structure of children's perceptions of maternal and paternal behavior. *Am Psychol* 16: 345–346.

81. Holmbeck GN, Johnson SZ, Wils KE, et al (2002) Observed and perceived parental overprotection in relation to psychosocial adjustment in preadolescents with a physical disability. *J Consult Clin Psychol* 70: 96–110.

82. Aran A, Shalev RS, Biran G, Gross-Tsur V (2007) Parenting style impacts on quality of life in children with cerebral palsy. *J Pediatr* 151: 56–60.

83. Kourkoutas EE, Erkman F (2011) *Interpersonal Acceptance–Rejection: Social, Emotional, and Educational Contexts*. Boca Raton, FL: BrownWalker Press.

84. Rhoades KA, O'Leary S (2007) Factor structure and validity of the Parenting Scale. *J Clin Child Adolesc Psychol* 36: 137–146.

85. Irvine AB, Biglan A, Smolkowski K, Ary DV (1999) The value of the Parenting Scale for measuring the discipline practices of parents of middle school children. *Behav Res Ther* 37: 127–142.

86. Wittingham K, Sofronoff K, Sheffield J (2009) Stepping Stone Triple P: an RCT of a parenting program with parents of a child diagnosed with an autism spectrum disorder. *J Abnorm Child Psychol* 37: 469–480.

87. Roberts C, Mazzucchelli T, Studman L, Sanders MR (2006) Behavioral family intervention for children with developmental disabilities and behavioral problems. *J Clin Child Adolesc Psychol* 35: 180–193.

88. Gibaud-Wallston J, Wandersman LP (1978) Development and utility of the Parenting Sense of Competence Scale. Paper presented at the annual meeting of the American Psychological Association; Toronto.

89. Gilmore L, Cuskelly M (2008) Factor structure of the Parenting Sense of Competence Scale using a normative sample. *Child Care Health Dev* 35: 48–55.

90. Mash EJ, Johnston C (1983) Parental perceptions of child behavior problems, parenting, self-esteem and mothers' reported stress in younger and older hyperactive and normal children. *J Consult Clin Psychol* 51: 86–99.

91. Hudson A, Cameron C, Matthews J (2008) The wide-scale implementation of a support program for parents of children with an intellectual disability and difficult behavior. *J Intellect Dev Disabil* 33: 117–126.

92. Sayre JM, Pianta RC, Marvin RS, Saft EW (2001) Mothers' representations of relationships with their children: relations with mother characteristics and feeding sensitivity. *J Pediatr Psychol* 26: 373–384.

93. Slade A (2005) Parental reflective functioning: an introduction. *Attach Hum Dev* 7: 269–281.

94. Austin J, Shore CP, Dunn DW, Johnson CS, Buelow JM, Perkins SM (2008) Development of the Parent Response to Child Illness (PRCI) scale. *Epilepsy Behav* 13: 662–669.

27

MAJOR LIFE AREAS: PLAY AND EDUCATION (D810– D880)

Margareta Adolfsson, Rune J. Simeonsson, Andrea Lee and Kirsten M. Ellingsen

What is the construct?

Participation is a central concept in the International Classification of Functioning, Disability and Health for Children and Youth (ICF-CY),[1] defined and viewed as the universal human experience of involvement in societal roles and situations. In order to assess participation in children using the ICF-CY, it is important to distinguish it from the related concept of activity in the classification. In this regard, activity is defined as that which 'represents the individual perspective of functioning' whereas participation as that which 'represents the societal perspective of functioning' (p. 228).[1] A second clarification that reinforces the distinction between individual and societal functioning is the differentiation of ICF-CY components into health domains, which include such activities as walking, learning and remembering and health-related domains that include education and social interactions (p. 7).[1] For the purpose of this chapter, participation in major life areas will build on these clarifications, and will be defined by children's engagement in societal roles and situations of play, family life and education.

The concept of participation for children in the ICF-CY is similar to its use in the two universal declarations for human rights. Framed within the United Nations Convention on the Rights of the Child,[2] the importance of participation is endorsed as a right for all children, including *children with disabilities* to engage in play (Article 31), family life (Article 18) and free, compulsory education (Article 28). Paragraph 1 of Article 23 states that '…a mentally or physically disabled child should enjoy a full and decent life in conditions which ensure dignity, promotes self reliance and facilitates the child's active participation in the community'. Specifically, paragraph 3 specifies that such participation should involve '… effective access to and receives education, training, health care services, rehabilitation services, preparation for employment and recreation opportunities…conducive to…achieving the fullest possible social integration and individual development, including… cultural and spiritual development'.

The underlying principle of 'full and effective participation and inclusion in society' is similarly endorsed in the third Article of the United Nations Convention on the Rights of Persons with Disabilities.[3] With reference to participation in *major life areas*, the best interests of children (Article 7) are specified for involvement in family life (Article 23, paragraph 3), participation in education (Article 24, paragraph 2) and participation in play (Article 30, paragraph 5).

Taken together, the ICF-CY and the UN Convention on the Rights of Children and Persons with Disabilities can be seen as complementary documents. The two conventions define universal human rights of societal involvement, and the ICF-CY provides a standard language for defining and classifying the essential rights of children and adults to participate in the society of which they are a part. Although the major life areas of children that have been identified above are by no means exhaustive of roles and situations that may be found across societies, they are ones that are essential and common to children's lives in most, if not all, societies. This is evident by the fact that countries all over the world believe and are committed to the rights to participation in major areas of family life, community and education. These rights are defined by national laws and policies that either protect the child from neglect or exploitation or provide essential experiences such as free, compulsory education.[4]

The importance of these major life areas to children is documented in literature across various disciplines. It is commonly believed that children demonstrate cognitive, social, linguistic and emotional growth through play.[5] Play has long been considered a primary activity for children and a primary means of expression.[6,7] As such, play is even utilized within therapy to teach skills and provide children with an outlet for acting out feelings and behaviours they may otherwise withhold.[8,9] Family life is no less integral to understanding children and their participation in the world. Indeed, the family represents a large part of the care and consistency in the child's world[10] and provides many of the early learning opportunities for the infant, toddler and young child. Stressors in family life or in familial relationships are associated with challenges in development and psychological functioning, with some arguing that the child's functioning can never be fully understood in isolation from his or her family.[11] Educational systems typically represent another primary influence in a child's life, and a domain of particular importance throughout the world.[4] The influence of families and schools on children's participation is evidenced in their shared provision of support for children, emphasized in many settings as the need for home–school collaboration to fully promote child development and participation.[12–15] The fundamental nature of these three major life areas is evidenced by the fact that some programmes combine therapeutic support for families and children with prevention programmes in schools.[16]

Experiences embedded within home or early childhood education environments provide a foundation for children's development. Measuring children's engagement in important life situations in infancy and early childhood involves relationships with caregivers, peers and objects or materials. Determining the level of engagement in informal and early educational settings necessitates evaluating the opportunities available as well as environmental facilitators and barriers.

In the context of the ICF-CY, participation can be seen as the engagement of children in common activities with others. In this chapter, the major life areas of children as defined in the ICF-CY are involvement in play with others, involvement in informal learning opportunities at home with family members, and participation in formal and informal roles and situations of preschool and school life. For the purpose of this chapter, the ICF-CY is proposed to contribute to the assessment of children's participation by (a) providing a framework for defining dimensions and categories of participation; (b) identifying tools suitable to measure these dimensions; and (c) summarizing assessment results in a standard language in the form of profiles of ICF-CY categories (Table 27.1).

ENGAGEMENT IN PLAY

For children, play is the most important occupation. Play is integrated with many aspects of a child's daily life such as at home with or without siblings, in the school playground with classmates, during domestic activities with the family such as cooking, or during free time with neighbourhood peers. In parallel, involvement in play provides incidental opportunity for honing skills such as physical coordination, language, sociability, thinking and problem solving.[17] Depending on age, play is characterized in different ways. It can be to explore or pretend, or it can be to engage in games or sports, and pursuing hobbies. Play is the earliest occupation, persisting throughout life. In proportion to the whole lifespan, an activity undertaken for its own sake belongs to play.[18] Within the ICF-CY, the concept of play is found in two different domains: d8 (Major life areas) and d9 (Community, social and civic life).[1] Play in childhood is seen as the major life area (d880) described as 'purposeful, sustained engagement in activities with objects, toys, materials or games, occupying oneself or with others' (p. 184).[1] It is about shared co-operative, developmental play without special rules. Play in adolescence or adulthood is seen as recreational activities. It is about engagement in games with a set of rules or competitive play, such as playing cards or chess, performed during leisure time (d9200; see Chapter 28). Other recreational activities can be sports, arts and culture, crafts, hobbies and socializing.[19,20] Play has a central role in life involvement, enjoyment, pleasure and learning. As such, it is important to provide methods for children, parents, and teachers to be able to think about and evaluate play engagement and skills over a range of contexts.

Assessment of play is very important in that children with disabilities have been found to be the least preferred playmates of typically developing children.[21] 'In particular, children with disabilities have special difficulty mastering the social tasks of gaining entry into peer groups, maintaining play and resolving conflicts' (p. 174).[21] Compared with typically developing children, even children with minor delays spend less time in sustained play and interactions with other children during playtime.[22]

INFORMAL AND PRESCHOOL EDUCATION

Home and early caregiving environments provide the foundational experiences that young children need to develop. The resources and important relationships available within these environments meaningfully influence child outcomes across all developmental domains. For young children, informal education occurs through interactions with caregivers and other children as well as through exploration and use of material objects. Yet, participation in the home and early childcare and educational settings is highly dependent on the opportunities that adults make available to young children. Consequently, differential child outcomes have been found to occur based on the quality and types of experiences provided. Thus, the quality of early caregiving environments is

TABLE 27.1

Categories and content appropriate for children from the ICF-CY domain of 'Major life areas' with reference to articles in the United Nations Conventions on the Rights of the Child (UNCRC) and Persons with Disabilities (UNCRPWD)

Category	Description	Rights basis (Convention: references)
1. Engagement in play (d880)	Purposeful, sustained engagement in activities with objects, toys, materials or games, alone or with others	UNCRC: 31 UNCRPWD: 30.5
2. Informal education (d810)	Learning at home or in the immediate environment in the acquisition of physical, social, pre-academic and academic skills from parents and members of the family or community	UNCRC: 18 UNCRPWD: 23.3
3. Preschool education (d815 and d816)	Learning at an initial level of organized instruction in the home or in the community, designed primarily to introduce a child to the school-type environment and prepare the child for compulsory education, such as by acquiring skills in daycare or similar setting as preparation for advancement to school (e.g. educational services provided in the home or community settings, designed to promote health and cognitive, motor, language and social development and readiness skills for formal education)	UNCRC: 23.3 UNCRPWD: 24.2
4. School education (d820)	Gaining admission to school, education, engaging in all school-related responsibilities and privileges, and learning the course material, subjects and other curriculum requirements in a primary or secondary education programme, including attending school regularly, working co-operatively with other students, taking direction from teachers, organizing, studying and completing assigned tasks and projects, and advancing to other stages of education	UNCRC: 23.3 UNCRC: 28 UNCRPWD: 24.2

important to consider when investigating the nature and level of child participation.

Research has established that 'young children's competences are embedded within relationships and contexts' (p. 5).[23] Findings have clearly demonstrated the central role of parent–child interactions in facilitating development, with recent attention also given to the role of the father's involvement in child outcomes. In addition, young children's exposure to language and early literacy experiences in the home environment has been found to be linked to preparedness for formal school and language development. As such, a measure of contextual resources and experiences would provide valuable information to better understand a young child's informal learning in the home setting (see Chapter 30 for information on the Home Observation for Measurement of the Environment [HOME]).

Child care

In addition, over the past few decades there has been an increase in the number of children who routinely participate in non-parental child care before entering preschool. The increased rates of involvement in child care and types of care arrangements have led to considerable research about effects on child outcomes. While evidence is mixed regarding the impact of age of entry and amount of care on development, there is consensus about the necessary dimensions of experience that reflect quality of care. Repeatedly, studies find that high-quality child care has been linked to more positive developmental outcomes for children. While both structural and process variables

have been used to define high-quality care, the responsiveness and sensitivity to needs of individual children has been found to be particularly important.[23] Although this chapter focuses on child participation in major life areas, assessment of the environments in which they participate can be done with measures such as the Infant Toddler Environmental Rating Scale (ITERS), Family Day Care Rating Scale (FDCRS) and Early Childhood Environment Rating Scale (ECERS). (For information on these measures, see www.fpg.unc.edu/~ECERS/). Involvement of children with special needs in non-parental child care is an area that needs further study[23] as participation in early educational settings for children may be hindered by a lack of available settings and a lack of training of childcare providers to address special healthcare or developmental needs of these children. In addition, limited information is available about factors that promote or hinder the engagement of young children with disabilities within a childcare setting, as well as how differences in level of impairment or severity of disability and family resources may influence access to care.[21]

PRESCHOOL

With development in the early years, children are increasingly able to initiate engagement with peers and materials and exhibit different levels of child-directed participation in early educational settings. While still influenced by the amount of available and accessible resources, typically developing young children enter preschool or prekindergarten settings with increased language and mobility, which allows them more choice in the nature of involvement. Children's experiences in preschool settings prepares them for the transition to formal schooling and positive peer and learning experiences have been connected to later social competence and readiness to be successful in formal education classrooms.

Traditionally, parent and teacher rating scales have been used to measure dimensions of child involvement and participation in early childhood settings. However, given that studies often find a low level of agreement between raters, direct measurement based on observation would be a complement to rating measures. A measure that uses a standardized process to document an individual child's experience in the preschool setting is the Individualized Classroom Assessment Survey (InCLASS).[23] This tool has been used to link observable indicators of involvement and provides information relevant for instructional planning and intervention. 'Growing consensus in the field indicates that children engage in classroom interactions that reflect patterns of adaptation to three core developmental tasks, competent exchanges with teachers, peers, and tasks – that in turn relate to building effective social relationships and acquiring skills and knowledge through instructional opportunities'(p. 2).[23]

General factors to consider when measuring this domain

Valid assessment of the strengths and difficulties of a child's engagement and participation in home and community life is the starting point for any programme of prevention and intervention for children with disabilities. Assessment of the nature and extent of children's participation represents a significant challenge in that many existing measures have focused on specific cognitive functions or psychological traits intrinsic to the child rather than the child's engagement in social roles and situations with others. In particular, there has been a lack of tools and measures based on a comprehensive conceptual framework of functioning for assessment of participation in family, school and community life.

With reference to assessment of participation, Forsyth and Jarvis[24] maintain that participation must focus on what the child actually experiences, not what the child might experience. Such experiences are defined not only by environmental factors but also by the child's age, access to objects and events, and the ability to exercise choice. The developmental nature of life areas for participation varies across the stages of infancy, early childhood, middle childhood and adolescence. Access and choice may vary with the age of the child and relate to participation in the home, school and community. Participation in home, school and community situations for children with disabilities may also be influenced by limitations they may experience in

performing activities. Of relevance are ICF-CY activities covered in chapters in this volume related to the child's learning (Chapter 20) and communication (Chapter 22), mobility (Chapter 23) and self-care (Chapter 24) skills. Of particular significance are variations in interpersonal relationships (Chapter 26), a domain in which many developmental disabilities manifest significant difficulties.

To address the problems of assessing children's participation, tools are needed that measure how children function and behave in environments involving shared activities with others. Specifically, such measurement should take developmental considerations into account, recognizing that the major life areas of children change rapidly over the period of a few years, with social play characterizing the toddler and young child, shifting to engagement in the roles and situations defined within preschool and school settings. Results of assessment should yield a profile of assets and limitations of functioning of direct relevance for intervention and support of children in home, school and communal settings. Current research indicates that activities and participation of children are facilitated or limited by environmental factors[25], such as fewer neighbourhood facilities contributing to fewer instances of play or physical acitivty.[26] A critical role is played by the social and physical environment in expanding opportunities for independence and social participation of the child. A priority for assessment is thus to identify aspects of the child's participation in the context of environments that may be significant for promoting their independence and social engagement.

Overview of recommended measures

The measures selected for this section reflect individual children's involvement in play, and informal and formal education (see Table 27.2 for selected measures). For three of the measures, child self-report versions are available (i.e. the Play Skills Self Report Questionnaire [PSSRQ], Availability of Activities and Participation and Pediatric Interest Profiles [PIP]). They provide opportunities for children to express their own experience of play skills,

TABLE 27.2
Selected measures described in this overview

Transdisciplinary Play-based Assessment (TPBA2)

The Play Skills Self Report Questionnaire (PSSRQ)

Pediatric Interest Profiles (PIP)

Code for Active Student Participation and Engagement Revised (CASPER III)

Availability of Activities and Participation

Classroom Assessment Scoring System (CLASS)

interests or experienced degree of participation in school life.

It should be noted that a number of these measures have been developed with limited documentation of psychometric properties available. Additional psychometric testing is likely in the future, in terms of validity and reliability of the measures.

TRANSDISCIPLINARY PLAY-BASED ASSESSMENT – A FUNCTIONAL APPROACH TO WORKING WITH YOUNG CHILDREN, SECOND EDITION

The Transdisciplinary Play-based Assessment – A Functional Approach to Working with Young Children, second edition (TPBA2) is a natural, functional approach to assessment and intervention, with parents actively involved throughout the process.[27] It is the first step in a comprehensive transdisciplinary play-based system. The TPBA2 is divided into six phases providing information about self-initiated play, play that is not spontaneously initiated, child–child interaction, parent–child interaction, motor play and snack time. Initially, the child engages in natural play with a parent until the child is comfortable with a play facilitator. A parent-facilitator observes and discusses sessions with the parents. The TPBA2 ends with a programme planning meeting. The system also offers the Transdisciplinary Play-based Intervention (TPBI2) for professionals and parents, to choose playful interventions that help children progress across domains and generalize their new skills in different situations and settings. Team Ideas for Play (TIP) sheets link programme objectives to home intervention and the classroom curriculum. The last step in the system is Read, Play, and Learn! Storybook Activities for Young Children, helping teachers plan further for a transdisciplinary play-based classroom.

THE PLAY SKILLS SELF-REPORT QUESTIONNAIRE

The PSSRQ is a self-report measure on play skills for 5- to 10-year-old children and their parent.[17,20,28] The entire questionnaire is about play and is based on the theoretical principle that only the child decides if what they are doing is playing.[29] Therefore, parents or teachers cannot say it is play. To gather a comprehensive picture of the perceptions of a child's play in most aspects of his or her daily life, the PSSRQ has been designed to tap play skills in a range of contexts – home, school and community. The PSSRQ gathers children's perceptions of their current ability and provides the ability to compare each child to him- or herself over time. It can be used in either an intervention or a research context, and hence does not aim to produce a meaningful summative score. The PSSRQ also provides a parent/caregiver version aiming to gather the current parent or caregiver's perception of the child's ability on the same set of play skills. Thus, the parent/caregiver's and child's views can be compared for meaningful difference in either an intervention or research situation, and over time.

PAEDIATRIC INTEREST PROFILES

The PIP is a self-report general measure of participation in play and leisure activities.[19,28] It can be used for children with or without disabilities and covers a broad range of activities: sports, outdoors, winter, summer, indoor, creative, lessons/classes and socialization. There are three versions: Kid Profile for young school-aged children, Preteen Play Profile for older school-aged children and Adolescent Leisure Interest Profile for adolescents. The two versions for lower ages are created as booklets supported by pictures. Instructions can be read for children who cannot read and they may also receive physical assistance if needed. The questions are grouped in eight categories. After finishing each category, an interview is conducted. The version for adolescents is a traditional questionnaire. All three profiles can be administered to the individual child or to small groups of three to five children or adolescents. The PIP was designed with an emphasis on participation due to influences of the predecessor to the ICF-CY (ICIDH-2).[19] Five perspectives of participation are considered: interest, frequency, competence, enjoyment and with whom activities are done. PIP helps providers gain an understanding of an individual child's or adolescent's participation in play and leisure, to identify individuals at risk for play-related problems. A child's profile might be a 'red flag' if, for example, the child has very few interests, has play interests deviant from other children's of the same age, lacks joy in play or tends to play only by himself. By using the PIP, providers identify the play activities of special interest for the individual child, so as to use them during intervention. This self-report measure might facilitate a conversation with the child. The age ranges on the three profiles overlap. The decision about which profile to use for a particular child must be based on the child's life experiences, maturity and disability (if applicable).

CODE FOR ACTIVE STUDENT PARTICIPATION AND ENGAGEMENT REVISED

The Code for Active Student Participation and Engagement Revised (CASPER III) aims to examine the social participation of young children in preschool programmes.[30–32] As an eco-behavioural tool, it assesses both ecological and behavioural variables in preschool settings. CASPER III is a direct observational system focusing on a single child at a time and considering two perspectives: (1) the environmental context and (2) the behaviour of the focal child

TRANSDISCIPLINARY PLAY-BASED ASSESSMENT – A FUNCTIONAL APPROACH TO WORKING WITH YOUNG CHILDREN, SECOND EDITION (TPBA2)	
Purpose	To examine developmental skills, underlying developmental processes, learning style and interaction patterns To identify service needs, develop intervention plans and evaluate progress
Population	Birth to 6y
Description of domains	Four developmental domains: cognitive, social-emotional, communication and language, and sensorimotor development
Administration and test format	Time to complete: 60–90min Testing format: checklist/worksheets for each domain. Observational data about performance from a developmental perspective are collected throughout a structured play session implemented based on prereported information from parents. Questions are used to address qualitative aspects of 'how' the child performs a task, not just 'if'. Three professionals are engaged: speech–language pathologist, occupational or physical therapist and a teacher or psychologist. The TPBA can be conducted in any creative play environment. A preschool or infant intervention room is usually used as there are materials present to encourage play Scoring: observational guidelines and age ranges are used to examine the child's performance in the categories of each domain Training: no specific training is needed. The assessment process can be conducted by anyone with knowledge of child development
Psychometric properties	Content validity: all of the developmental domains were judged favourably by both users and non-users Concurrent validity: accurate in identifying and determining whether a child was eligible for special services *Reliability* Well supported in test–retest and inter-rater conditions
How to order	North America: www.amazon.com Cost: approximately US$50 The assessment materials can be ordered together with the Transdisciplinary Play-based Intervention (US$42) and Administration Guide for TPBA and TPBI (US$39) Also available at web-book stores in Europe
Key references	Friedli C (1994) Transdisciplinary Play-based Assessment: a study of reliability and validity. Unpublished doctoral dissertation, University of Colorado at Boulder. Linder TW (2008) *Transdisciplinary Play-based Assessment: A Functional Approach to Working with Young Children.* Baltimore, MD: Paul H. Brookes Publishing Co.

THE PLAY SKILLS SELF REPORT QUESTIONNAIRE (PSSRQ) (CHILD SELF REPORT, PARENT/CAREGIVER REPORT)	
Purpose	The purpose of the children's questionnaire is to gather a child's perception of his or her current ability in a set of 29 play skills that have been found to be valid. It is designed to be able to compare a child to him- or herself over time on each item in either an intervention or a research context, and hence does not aim to produce a meaningful summative score

Population	Children with or without disabilities aged 5–10y who have problems with play or social skills
Administration and test format	Time to complete: approximately 15min
	Testing format: booklet. The 29 items are presented on one page each and with animated pictures. The child is asked about whether he or she is good at a particular play skill, for example 'How good are you at trying to fix up arguments or fights when you are playing with other kids?' The child answers by choosing a star symbol which represents Not good, OK, Good or Very good.
	The parent/caregiver report contains similar questions organized with three items per page
	Scoring: the aim is not to produce a meaningful summative score
	Training: users should have read the manual thoroughly and had practice administering the PSSRQ with a number of children of varying ages prior to use in professional situations. Users should also have assisted several adults in completing the questions, and have talked over the information, prior to formal use
Psychometric properties	Statistical analysis of the data gathered centred on the description of the sample and the pattern of responses by age and sex, similarities and differences between parent and child responses, and the influence of relevant independent variables on parent–child agreement. In brief, there were more items on which parent and child disagreed (n=17) than items on which they agreed (n=13). This was interpreted as supporting the hypothesis that the child self-report would produce unique information about play skills
	Test–retest reliability: stability over time for the small sample (n=16) was shown for both parents and children
How to order	Email Dr Jennifer Sturgess (jenny.sturgess@gmail.com) for an order form
	Cost: AU$145 (plus postage for international sales) for manual (64 pages), questionnaire booklet, child score sheet – photocopy master, and parent/caregiver version – photocopy master (see http://playskillsselfreport.com/)
Key references	Sturgess J (2003) A model describing play as a child-chosen activity – is this still valid in contemporary Australia? *Aus Occupat Ther J* 50: 104–108.
	Sturgess J (2007) The development of a Play-skills Report Questionnaire (PSSRQ) for 5–10 year old children and their parents/caregivers. PhD thesis, University of Queensland, School of Health and Rehabilitation Sciences.

PAEDIATRIC INTEREST PROFILES (PIP) SURVEYS OF PLAY FOR CHILDREN AND ADOLESCENTS: KID PROFILE PRETEEN PLAY PROFILE AND ADOLESCENT LEISURE INTEREST PROFILE	
Purpose	To identify play activities of special interest for the individual child to be used during intervention
Population	Children and youth aged 6–9y, 9–12y and 12–21y, with and without disabilities
Description of domains	Activities grouped into eight categories in each profile:
	Kid Profile and Preteen Play Profile – sports, outside, summer, winter, indoor and creative activities; lessons/classes; and socializing
	Adolescent Leisure Interest Profile – sports, outside, exercise, relaxation, intellectual, creative, socializing, and club/community organizations
Administration and test format	Time to complete: around 15, 20 and 30min, respectively, for the different profiles.

Administration and test format	Testing format: *Kid profile* Booklet. Fifty items are presented with animated pictures. The child is asked up to three questions: Do you do this activity? (Yes/No). If the answer is Yes, the child is asked: Do you like this activity? (A lot/A little/Not at all) Who do you do this activity with? (By myself/With friends/With a grown-up) The response alternatives are symbolized by stick figure drawings. The child replies by marking with a circle, colouring or in some other manner. Each group of questions is followed up with an interview. *Preteen play profile* Booklet. Fifty-nine items are presented with an animated picture. The child is asked up to five questions: Do you do this activity? (Yes/No). If the answer is Yes, the child is asked: How often do you do this activity? (Once a week or more/Once a month or more/Once a year or more) How much do you like this activity? (A lot/A little/Not at all) How good are you at this activity? (Very good/So-so/Not so good) Who do you do this activity with? (By myself/With friends/With a grown-up) The response alternatives are in written text for each item. The child answers by circling a response. Each group of questions is followed up with an interview. *Adolescent leisure interest profile* Questionnaire. Eighty-three items are listed. The adolescent is asked up to five questions: How interested are you in this activity? How often do you do this activity? (3–7 times a week/Less than 3 times a week/Once or twice a month/Never) How well do you do this activity? (Very well/Well/Not very well) How much do you enjoy this activity? (Very much/Somewhat/Not at all) Who do you do this activity with? (By myself/With friends/With family) The adolescent ticks one response for each question. They are also asked why they do an activity. Scoring: a total profile and scores for sections can be examined Training: no required training is reported
Psychometric properties	Information available from pilot testing only: test–retest reliability calculated with Pearson correlation and internal consistency with Cronbach's alpha *Kid profile* Test–retest reliability acceptable for the first two questions (total score 0.91 and 0.70), modest for the third (0.45) Internal consistency reliable for the first question (total score 0.80) *Preteen play profile* Test–retest reliability acceptable for three of the five questions (No. 1 [0.92], No. 2 [0.75], No. 4 [0.72]), moderate for two questions (No. 3 [0.51], No. 5 [0.57]) Internal consistency for the first question showed a value of 0.72 *Adolescent leisure interest profile* Test–retest reliability acceptable for all questions together (0.62–0.78) for children with and without disabilities Internal consistency reliable for the first question (total score 0.93)

How to order	The manual with questionnaires and score sheets is available at www.moho.uic.edu/images/assessments/PIPs%20Manual.pdf
Key reference	Henry AD (2000) *Paediatric Interest Profiles. Surveys of Play for Children and Adolescents, Kid Play Profile, Preteen Play Profile, and Adolescent Leisure Interest Profile*. San Antonio, TX: Therapy Skill Builders.

CODE FOR ACTIVE STUDENT PARTICIPATION AND ENGAGEMENT REVISED (CASPER III)

Purpose	Collects information about preschool environments and behaviour of participants in those environments (e.g. children, adults)
Population	Preschool children
Description of domains	Two coding categories: The focal child's environmental context: this category includes four variables – group arrangement, group composition, activity area and activity and initiator of the activity The behaviour of the focal child or peers' and adults' behaviour in reference to the focal child: this category includes three variables – child behaviour, child social behaviour and adult behaviour Each variable consists of a set of behavioural categories
Administration and test format	Time to complete: 30min to 1h for each session Testing format: prior to the observation, two environmental variables are noted – group arrangement and group composition For the additional five variables, observers record a single category during a 2s point in time every 30s. The observations are repeated across a specific period of time Each activity and behaviour variable has 5–15 coding symbols, consisting of the acronym for the category. Data are collected on laptop computers and later downloaded to a database Training: comprehensive observer training for observers is required to recall environmental and behavioural categories and become reliable users of the coding system. A suggested training format is presented at the end of the CASPER *Training Manual for Observers*
Psychometric properties	*Reliability* Observers have to obtain 80–85% interobserver agreement on each of the recorded variables during training and before they can begin collecting data. However, psychometric data on the measure were not found, defining a limitation of its use
How to order	The manual may be ordered from Samuel L Odom (slodom@unc.edu)
Key references	Odom SL, Zercher C, Li S, Marquart J, Sandall S, Brown WH (2000) Approaches to understanding the ecology of inclusive early childhood settings for children with disabilities. In: T. Thompson, D. Felce and F. Symons, editors. *Behavioural Observation: Innovations in Technology and Application in Developmental Disabilities*. Baltimore, MD: Paul H Brookes Publishing Co., pp. 193–214. Tsao L, Odom SL, Brown WB (2001) *Code for Active Student Participation and Engagement – Revised (CASPER III): A Training Manual for Observers*. Bloomington, IN: Indiana University.

or the behaviour of peers and adults in the current setting. Observations are momentary. Repeatedly, observers watch a child for a brief period of time and immediately record one category for each of the seven variables. A positive social behaviour includes verbal or motor actions made towards another child. A negative social behaviour is any kind of aggressive behaviour towards others. In addition to collecting information about children's preschool environments and their behaviour in those environments, the temporal relationships among environmental and behavioural events can be analysed.

AVAILABILITY OF ACTIVITIES AND PARTICIPATION

This is a self- or teacher-report questionnaire to rate students' degree of availability and participation in school activities.[33,34] The questionnaire contains a variety of common school activities, such as breaks/gym classes, science laboratories, school dances, library use, art classes and playground games. Each activity is rated on a four-point scale. The questionnaire has been adapted to Swedish school contexts and the activities were adapted for different age groups.[34] This questionnaire is not a standardized test but the availability index has been determined to be reliable.

CLASSROOM ASSESSMENT SCORING SYSTEM

The Classroom Assessment Scoring System (CLASS) is an observational instrument developed to assess the quality of teacher–student interactions in preschool to third-grade classrooms. Recently it has been adapted and trialled for younger children in toddler child care.[35] The teacher–child relationship is described as a regulatory system that contributes to children's social, behavioural and academic competences in school.[36] The overall aim of the assessment is to help teachers improve their competences and become more effective teachers. In that way, the instrument might belong to Chapter 30, which covers environmental factors. However, the teachers influence children's participation. Effective teachers tend to establish routines for themselves and their students so that children know the expectations for behaviour and work. This improves the child's opportunities to participate in school activities. La Paro et al[36] refer to studies showing that when children's disruptive and off-task behaviour is prevented, they are able to spend more time engaged in productive learning activities. Highly skilled teachers monitor students' performance and engagement in activities and provide additional explanations and ideas, leading to continued engagement. The CLASS includes three major areas of classroom characteristics. The emotional support area considers peer interactions in addition to interaction with the teacher. The classroom organization area includes, for example, classroom routines, how well children understand routines, and how teachers foster autonomous behaviour in children. The instructional support area focuses on interaction with children

AVAILABILITY OF ACTIVITIES AND PARTICIPATION	
Purpose	To measure the degree of availability and participation in school activities
Population	School-aged children (5–17y)
Description of domains	Questions cover a variety of activities occurring during school days, both inside and outside of the classroom
Administration and test format	Time to complete: 10–15min Testing format: questionnaire with a list of approximately 25 school activities, each activity connected to two questions: How available are activities? How much do you/does this student participate? Scoring: the two scales for availability and participation are each rated on a four-point Likert scale (0=not available/no participation; 1=minimally available/minimal participation; 2=somewhat available/some participation; 3=fully available/full participation) Training: none required
Psychometric properties	Cronbach's alpha for participation: 7–12y, α=0.71; 13–17y, α=0.71 Cronbach's alpha or availability index: 7–12y, α=0.75; 13–17y, α=0.79. No validity data are available
How to order	The protocol may be ordered from Rune J Simeonsson (rjsimeon@email.unc.edu)
Key reference	Simeonsson RJ, Carlsson D, Huntington G (1999) *Participation of Students with Disabilities: A National Survey of Participation in School Activities*. Chapel Hill, NC: Frank Porter Graham Child Development Center.

CLASSROOM ASSESSMENT SCORING SYSTEM (CLASS)	
Purpose	Observe and assess the quality of interactions between teachers and students in classrooms
Population	Children in prekindergarten and kindergarten to third grade (3–9y) Adapted version is likely to be available soon for toddler child care (15–36mo)

Description of domains	Classroom quality is defined by three crucial domains of effective interactions with a total of 10 subscales:
	
	     Emotional Support – Positive Climate, Negative Climate, Teacher Sensitivity and Regard for Student Perspectives
	
	     Classroom Organization – Behaviour Management, Productivity and Instructional Learning Formats
	
	     Instructional Support – Concept Development, Quality of Feedback and Language Modelling

Administration and test format	Time to complete: the performance requires 30-min cycles for observation and scoring, repeated up to six times over 3h Testing format: classroom observation. Two manuals (prekindergarten, kindergarten to third grade) provide system overview, procedures and scoring. The observation is completed by administrators, supervisors, principals, programme directors or researchers Scoring: each subscale is scored on a seven-point scale considered to be low range (1–2), mid-range (2–5) and high range (6–7). Training: at least a 2-day training session is required to gain familiarity with the CLASS system and to become skilled at observing in classrooms. An overview of training programmes, types and costs can be found at www.classobservation.com/training
Psychometric properties	*Reliability* Average inter-rater reliability (agreement) for the 10 subscales was 87% Updated information on psychometric properties is available in a technical manual. See www.teachstone.org/research-and-evidence
How to order	Materials are ordered from Paul H. Brookes Publishing Co. (www.brookespublishing.com/store/books/pianta-class/index.htm) or at www.classobservation.com/contact/CLASS_order_form2009.pdf Manuals cost approximately US$50 (2008); CLASS forms cost US$28 for packs of 10
Key reference	La Paro KM, Pianta RC (2003) *CLASS: Classroom Assessment Scoring System.* Charlottesville, VA: University of Virginia.

such as engagement in activities, problem solving and discussions.

Conclusions

Engagement in play and participation in formal and informal education are essential to children and youth's lives. Their salience is evidenced by their recognition in international documents, including the ICF-CY, as well as international commitment to protect youth's rights to participate in these major life areas. Documenting participation by youth in play, informal education, pre-school education, and school education is an important task for the development of prevention and individualized intervention programmes that support the engagement

of children with disabilities in these important every-day contexts. Although play and schooling are central to youth's lives, truly capturing youth's participation within the ICF-CY codes identified in this chapter is challenged by the few measures that conceptually and practically focus on a child's actual engagement in these areas. It is important to reiterate that the process of documenting a child's participation in these contexts would be most useful if conducted with consideration of environmental factors, which may provide salient information as to how a child's participation was facilitated or which components of the environment provided a barrier to full participation. The measures described in this chapter provide a useful and important foundation for describing participation by youth in play and informal and formal education. Given the importance of the identified major life areas, further research on the utility and psychometric properties of

the listed measures would be a helpful activity, as would consideration of how to apply the collected information to prevention or intervention programme development.

REFERENCES

1. World Health Organization (2007) *International Classification of Functioning, Disability and Health for Children and Youth (ICF-CY)*. Geneva: WHO.
2. United Nations (1989) *UN Convention on the Rights of the Child*. New York: United Nations.
3. United Nations (2009) *UN Convention on the Rights of Persons with Disabilities*. New York: United Nations.
4. UNESCO (2000) *The Dakar Framework for Action*. Paris: UNESCO.
5. Ginsberg KR (2007) Committee on Communications, Committee on Psychosocial Aspects of Child and Family Health. *Pediatrics* 119: 182–191.
6. Axline V (1947) *Play Therapy: The Inner Dynamics of Childhood*. Boston, MA: Houghton Mifflin.
7. Lowenfield M (1991) *Play in Childhood*. London: Mac Keith Press. (Original work published 1935.)
8. Landreth GL (1993) Child-centered play therapy. *Elementary School Guidance & Counseling* 28: 17–29.
9. Buser JK (2007) Play therapy. In: Thompson CL, Henderson DA, editors. *Counseling Children*, 7th edition. Belmont, CA: Thomson Brooks/Cole, pp. 414–456.
10. Roberts RN, Wasik BH, Casto G, Ramey CT (1991) Family support in the home. *Am Psychol* 46: 131–137.
11. Wagner BM, Reiss D (1995) Family systems and developmental psychopathology: courtship, marriage, or divorce? In: Cicchetti D, Cohen DJ, editors. *Developmental Psychopathology: Vol 1., Theory and Methods*. New York: Wiley, pp. 696–730.
12. Adams J, Biss C, Burrell-Mohammad V, Meyers J, Slaton E (1998) *Family–Professional Relationships: Moving Forward Together*. Alexandria, VA: Federation of Families for Children's Mental Health.
13. Epstein JL (1995) School/family/community partnerships: caring for the children we serve. *Phi Delta Kappan* May: 701–711.
14. Fine MJ, Nissenbaum MS (2000) The child with disabilities and the family: implications for professionals. In: Fine MJ, Simpson, RL, editors. *Collaboration with Parents and Families of Children and Youth with Exceptionalities*, 2nd edition. Austin, TX: Pro-Ed, pp. 3–26.
15. Simpson RL, Zurkowski JK (2000) Parent and professional collaborative relationships in an era of change. In: Fine MJ, Simpson RL, editors. *Collaboration with Parents and Families of Children and Youth with Exceptionalities*, 2nd edition. Austin, TX: Pro-Ed, pp. 89–102.
16. McDonald L, Morgan A (1997) Families and schools together (FAST): integrating community development with clinical strategies. *Families in Society* 78: 140–156.
17. Sturgess J (2003) A model describing play as a child-chosen activity – is this still valid in contemporary Australia? *Aust Occup Ther J* 50: 104–108.
18. Kielhofner G, Forsyth K, Federico J, et al (2002) Self-report assessments. In: Kielhofner G, editor. *Model of Human Occupation: Theory and Application*, 3rd edition. Netherlands: Wotters Kluwer Health, pp. 212–236.
19. Henry AD (2000) *Pediatric Interest Profiles. Surveys of Play for Children and Adolescents, Kid Play Profile, Preteen Play Profile, Adolescent Leisure Interest Profile*. San Antonio, TX: Therapy Skill Builders.
20. Sturgess J (2007) *The Development of a Play-skills Report Questionnaire (PSSRQ) for 5–10 Year Old Children and their*

Parents/carers. University of Queensland, School of Health and Rehabilitation Sciences.
21. Shonkoff JP, Phillips DA (eds) (2000) *From Neurons to Neighborhoods: The Science of Early Childhood Development*. Washington, DC: The National Academy Press.
22. Almqvist L (2006) Children's health and developmental delay: Positive functioning in every-day life. PhD thesis, Örebro University.
23. Downer JT, Booren LM, Lima OK, Luckner AE, Pianta RC (2010) The Individualized Classroom Assessment Scoring System (inCLASS): preliminary reliability and validity of a system for observing preschoolers' competence in classroom interactions. *Early Child Res Q* 25: 1–16.
24. Forsyth R, Jarvis S (2002) Participation in childhood. *Child Care Health Dev* 28: 277–279.
25. Malone K, Tranter PJ (2003) School grounds as site for learning: making the most of environmental opportunities. *Environ Educ Res* 9: 283–303.
26. Giles-Corti B, Donovan RJ (2003) Socioeconomic status differences in recreational physical activity levels and real and perceived access to a supportive physical environment. *Prev Med* 25: 601–611.
27. Linder TW (2008) *Transdisciplinary Play-based Assessment: A Functional Approach to Working with Young Children*. Baltimore, MD: Paul H. Brooks.
28. Sturgess J, Rodger S, Ozanne A (2002) A review of the use of self-report assessment with young children. *Br J Occup Ther* 65: 108–116.
29. Sturgess J (2009) Play as child-chosen activity. In: Stagnitti K, Cooper R, editors. *Play as Therapy*. London: Jessica Kingsleys Publishers, pp. 20–30.
30. Tsao L, Odom SL, Brown WB (2001) *Code for Active Student Participation and Engagement – Revised (CASPER III): A Training Manual for Observers*. Bloomington, IN: Indiana University.
31. Tsao L-L, Odom SL, Buysse V, Skinner M, West T, Vitztum-Komanecki J (2008) Social participation of children with disabilities in inclusive preschool programs: program typology and ecological features. *Exceptionality* 16: 125–140.
32. Odom SL, Zercher C, Li S, Marquart J, Sandall S, Brown WH (2000) Approaches to understanding the ecology of inclusive early childhood settings for children with disabilities. In: Thompson T, Felce D, Symons F, editors. *Behavioral Observation: Innovations in Technology and Application in Developmental Disabilities*. Baltimore, MD: Paul Brookes, pp. 193–214.
33. Eriksson L (2005) The relationship between environment and participation for students with disabilities. *Pediatr Rehabil* 8: 130–139.
34. Simeonsson RJ, Carlsson D, Huntington G (1999) *Participation of Students with Disabilities; A National Survey of Participation in School Activities*. Chapel Hill, NC: Frank Porter Graham Child Development Center.
35. Thomason AC, La Paro LM (2009) Measuring the quality of teacher–child interactions in toddler care. *Early Educ Dev* 20: 285–304.
36. La Paro LM, Pianta RC, Stuhlman M (2004) The Classroom Assessment Scoring System: findings from the prekindergarten year. *Elementary School Journal* 104: 409–426.

28
COMMUNITY, SOCIAL AND CIVIC LIFE (D910–D950)

Gary Bedell, Mary A. Khetani, Wendy J. Coster, Mary Law and Martha Cousins

What is the construct?

Participation has been broadly defined in the International Classification of Functioning (ICF)[1] and International Classification of Functioning for Children and Youth (ICF-CY)[2–4] as a person's involvement in a life situation. The concept of *involvement* is further described in the ICF as 'taking part in, being included or engaged in an area of life, being accepted or having access to needed resources' (p. 213).[1] There are no specific guidelines in the ICF or ICF-CY about how to define or characterize the relevant life situations of children and youth. Researchers and measurement developers may use varying criteria to define life situations and identify the situations that are important to measure for children and youth. For example, McConachie and colleagues[5] proposed that measurement of participation should address life situations related to key themes that are important to children's well-being: (1) essential for survival, (2) supportive of child development, (3) discretionary and (4) educational activities. Coster and Khetani[6] defined life situations as organized sequences of activities directed towards a personally or socially meaningfully goal. They proposed that goals are setting specific and focus on the following: (1) sustenance and physical health, (2) development of skills and capacities and (3) enjoyment and emotional well-being.

Participation is differentiated from the ICF-CY construct of *activity*, which focuses on the execution and performance of tasks and actions. The ICF-CY uses the same nine domains to classify activity and participation, making it difficult to distinguish between these two constructs and the measures that assess them.[6,7] In this chapter, we focus solely on available measures that include content that address children's participation and specifically children's participation in one of the nine ICF-CY domains: *Community, Social and Civic Life*. Some of the measures described also assess the ICF-CY activity construct; however, a description of the activity content is not provided in this chapter.

Participation in Community, Social and Civic Life encompasses a child's engagement in social situations outside of the family and home life. This domain is further categorized in the ICF-CY[2] (Chapter d9, pp. 186–188) according to five main categories: (1) community life (d910); (2) recreation and leisure (d920); (3) religion and spirituality (d930); (4) human rights (d940); and (5) political life and citizenship (d950) (see Table 28.1). The measures described in this chapter to varied extents address the range of life situations depicted in all but one of the categories: category four, human rights. Category two (recreation and leisure) has the greatest representation in content whereas categories three (religion and spirituality) and five (political life and citizenship) have the least representation in content in the measures described.

General factors to consider when measuring this domain

The nature and extent of participation is influenced by a number of child, family and environment factors such as the child's age, abilities and preferences; the family's sociocultural background, resources and preferences; and the physical, social and attitudinal environmental features of settings where children and youth live their lives.[8–12] Thus, these factors need to be considered in order to interpret the meaning of scores from assessments of children's participation. The reader is referred to other chapters in this book that describe measures of these factors.

When selecting a specific participation measure, *stakeholders* (individuals with a vested interest in the child's participation such as children, families, teachers, clinicians, researchers, programme directors and policy makers) have to consider a number of factors. First, stakeholders consider what type of information is needed about the child's participation. For example, stakeholders might be interested in documenting the type of life situations the child is and is not participating in, the amount of time the child spends participating in life situations, or the

TABLE 28.1
Categories and content from the ICF-CY domain of community, social and civic life

Category	Description
1. Community life	Engaging in community social life including informal and formal clubs, organizations and events
2. Recreation and leisure	Engaging in any form of play, recreational or leisure activity (organized, competitive or informal sports done in groups or individually); physical fitness activities; arts and cultural activities and events such as going to the cinema or museums, painting, dancing, singing, playing a musical instrument; crafts; hobbies; socializing (informal or casual gathering; visiting friends or relatives); and games
3. Religion and spirituality	Engaging in religious or spiritual activities, organizations and practices (e.g. attending church, temple, mosque, synagogue; praying; chanting; meditating)
4. Human rights	Enjoying all nationally and internationally recognized rights that are accorded to people by virtue of their humanity, including the right to self-determination or autonomy and control over one's destiny
5. Political life and citizenship	Engaging in social, political and governmental life of a citizen, having legal status as a citizen and enjoying the rights, protections, privileges and duties associated with that role

degree to which the child is able or not able to participate. Also, they may want or need to know about multiple domains of participation, or specific domains of participation, such as recreation and leisure or school life. The relevant information may vary according to child-related factors (age; diagnosis; level of physical, cognitive and psychological functioning and development), sociocultural factors, country of residence and geographic location. Stakeholders can examine the specific content of the measures described in the next section to ensure that the domains and ways they are assessed are relevant to their information goals.

Second, stakeholders consider what the overall purpose is for using the measure. Measurement can be viewed as having three broad purposes that are linked to stakeholders' specific information goals. Each purpose has a somewhat different level of focus: (1) individual child and family, (2) programme or intervention group and (3) population or society. Stakeholders often have more than one purpose and the measures often support more than one focus. *Individualized or person-centered assessment* is used to describe a child's profile or extent of participation. The purpose is to inform decisions about appropriate services or specific interventions, or to evaluate change over time or change due to provision of services or specific interventions. *Programme evaluation or outcomes-based assessment* is used to assess the effects of programmes on groups of clients, and to identify where programme improvements and resources might be needed. *Population-based assessment* is often used to identify and compare trends and patterns of larger groups of individuals to guide policy decisions directed at prevention, intervention and effective use of resources.

Once stakeholders have determined what type of information they need and for what measurement purposes, additional practical questions are considered to inform measurement selection. For example, will the measure be acceptable to stakeholders (i.e. does it meet their specific information goals and do so in a way that maximizes relevance and usefulness and minimizes burden and discomfort)? Can the measure feasibly be used given the resources and constraints of the programme or research study? Is there available and supportive research evidence about each assessment (reliability, validity)? If the measure is designed as an evaluative measure, is there evidence to suggest that it can detect change over time or change related to specific services and interventions? If the measure is designed as a discriminative measure, is there evidence to suggest that it is able to distinguish among groups of children who are likely to differ in scores in some way (e.g. due to the child's age, type of diagnosis or impairment, level of functioning)?

As illustrated in the next section, measures of participation have specific characteristics that may be more or less relevant to stakeholders' information goals. Some measures are comprehensive and detailed; others may be global and general. Additionally, some measures have been designed for children in specific age groups (e.g. preschoolers) or for a broader age range of children. All of the measures described could be used generically for children with a variety of disabilities and, in many instances, for children without disabilities.

Methods to obtain information about participation vary and include both quantitative and qualitative approaches.[7] The measures described assess quantitative aspects of participation using interviews, rating scales, activity card sorts or surveys administered to or completed by self-report by the child, family caregiver or professional based on observation of or familiarity with the child's participation. Therefore, stakeholders need to consider whose perspectives are desired and represented by the measure (e.g. the child, family, professional).

Another important issue when assessing participation, quantitatively, is that a greater extent of participation (in terms of amount or frequency) is not necessarily better unless the life situation is one that matters to the child or family. Some of the measures address this issue by asking about child and family preferences or satisfaction regarding particular life situations, or asking the child and family to select life situations that are of most importance to them. Additionally, some of the measures use item ratings that compare the child's participation with that of same-age peers, whereas others do not. Measures that are age referenced might be less responsive to quantitative change in a child's participation (e.g. because of intervention, development, injury/illness recovery) because the child may increase his or her level of participation but never reach the levels of his or her same-age peers. Along similar lines, measures that are not age referenced might be more responsive to change because the child serves as his or her own control or source of comparison.

Finally, stakeholders also need to assess whether the measures described are socioculturally and linguistically sensitive to the children and families with whom they serve or conduct research. Similarly, because children with disabilities are not a homogeneous group, measures of children's participation, especially those administered to or completed by children, must consider the child's age, development, receptive and expressive language, and overall physical, cognitive and psychological functioning. Certain measures can be modified or tailored to accommodate the child's specific learning and performance needs and in some instances a proxy for the child, such as the family caregiver or teacher, could complete or be administered the assessment.[7]

Overview of recommended measures
The measures selected for discussion in this chapter and described in this section include content (items, sections or scales) that represent the broad ICF-CY domain of participation in community, social and civic life (see Table 28.2 for a list of selected measures). Many of the measures include content from other ICF-CY domains, and therefore are also described in other chapters. Only the content relevant to this chapter will be described in this section. All but two measures (Vineland Adaptive Behavior Scales, 2nd Revision [VABS II][13] and the Child Behavior Checklist [CBCL])[14] were designed based on the ICF-CY or its predecessors, and thus explicitly assess either multiple or specific participation domains. The VABS II and CBCL are described because they include relevant items or sections that implicitly assess participation.

The measures described are standardized instruments that range in their degree of structure and flexibility in procedures and testing materials required. They vary in the type of information they obtain, their purposes, and the extent to which they have been developed and tested and have reported evidence about their usefulness, reliability, validity and responsiveness to change. Also, they may provide different levels of scoring. For example, scores could be item-level, subsection or subscale scores that examine specific domains, or total scores that summarize the child's overall participation.

Detailed description of selected measures
This section provides more detailed descriptions (including available psychometric evidence) of all of the measures described in the prior section except for the two comprehensive measures that assess multiple content domains: VABS II[13] and the CBCL.[14] These measures, as well as the LIFE-H, are presented in detail in Chapters 9 and 19.

CHILDREN'S ASSESSMENT OF PARTICIPATION AND ENJOYMENT/PREFERENCES FOR ACTIVITIES OF CHILDREN
The Children's Assessment of Participation and Enjoyment (CAPE)/Preferences for Activities of Children (PAC)[15] measures participation in recreation and leisure activities outside of mandated school activities. These measures were designed for children and youth, with and without disabilities, aged 6 to 21. The PAC is an extension of the CAPE and measures activity preference. The PAC and CAPE can be used concurrently or independently. For the CAPE, the child either completes a self-administered questionnaire booklet containing 55 items with activity drawings or is interviewed using activity drawings on cards and visual response forms. Assistance from a parent or guardian can be provided if needed for either version. There are three levels of scoring: one overall participation score, two domain scores that reflect participation in informal and formal activities, and five scores related to types of activities (recreational, active physical, social, skill-based and self-improvement). Responses to specific items can be examined as well. The CAPE assesses five dimensions of participation: (1) diversity of activities (participates? yes/no); (2) intensity or how often the child participates across all activities (seven-point scale); (3) with whom the child participates; (4) where the child participates; and (5) extent of enjoyment in activities (five-point scale). For the PAC, the child is asked to rate the extent to which he or she would like to be doing the 55 CAPE activities, using a three-point scale.

The purpose of the CAPE/PAC is to obtain a comprehensive picture of the child's participation in leisure and recreation outside of school from the child's perspective.

TABLE 28.2
Selected measures described in this overview

Children's Assessment of Participation and Enjoyment/Preferences for Activities of Children (CAPE/PAC)

Assessment of Life Habits for Children (LIFE-H)

Child and Adolescent Scale of Participation (CASP)

Pediatric Activity Card Sort (Pediatric ACS)

Preschooler Activity Card Sort (Preschooler ACS)

Perceived Efficacy and Goal Setting System (PEGS)

Canadian Occupational Performance Measure (COPM)

Vineland Adaptive Behavior Scales II (VABS II)

Child Behavior Checklist (CBCL)

Participation and Environment Measure for Children and Youth (PEM-CY)

CHILDREN'S ASSESSMENT OF PARTICIPATION AND ENJOYMENT/PREFERENCES FOR ACTIVITIES OF CHILDREN (CAPE/PAC)	
Purpose	CAPE: designed to document how children with or without disabilities participate in everyday activities outside of mandated school activities
	PAC: designed to determine activity preferences for the same set of activities as the CAPE
	The PAC is an extension of the CAPE but was designed for concurrent use. Both measures can be used independently. The CAPE should be used first, followed by the PAC, when used together. The authors are also developing a preschool version of the CAPE
Population	Children and youth between 6y and 21y who are cognitively able to comprehend the associated tasks of recognizing and sorting cards (can be completed by parents if the child is unable to respond)
Description of domains (subscales)	CAPE/PAC: two domains outside of mandated school activities – formal and informal. Five types of activities (recreational, active physical, social, skill-based and self-improvement/educational)
	CAPE: five dimensions and ratings for each item: (1) diversity (performed in last 4 months – yes/no); (2) intensity/how often (seven-point scale); (3) with whom; (4) where; and (5) extent of enjoyment (five-point scale)
	PAC: addresses the child's preferences for an activity (three-point scale)
Administration and test format	Time to complete: CAPE: approximately 30–45min; PAC: approximately 15–20min
	Testing format: CAPE: 55 items; child report (ages 6–21y), assistance can be provided by caregiver
	Two domains: informal (40 items) or formal (15 items) activities
	Five activities: recreational (12 items), active physical (13 items), social (10 items), skill-based (10 items) and self-improvement/educational (10 items)
	Format includes a self-assessment or interview version
	Self-assessment version
	Children look at drawings of other children performing 55 different activities
	If performed in the last 4mo the child identifies on a Likert-type scale with whom and how often the activity was performed
	Interviewer-assisted version
	The child's responses are recorded directly onto the CAPE Summary Score Sheet

	PAC
	Self-administered version:
	Children look at drawings of other children performing 55 different activities
	Children record their preference for each activity by circling one of three facial expressions (I would not like to do at all, I would sort of like to do and I would really like to do)
	Interviewer-assisted version:
	Child sorts drawings into one of three piles using the same three facial expressions as in the self-administered version
	A card containing enlarged facial expressions with corresponding written descriptions assists them in their sorting
	CAPE/PAC
	Scoring: the CAPE and PAC include scores for the six dimensions of participation: diversity, intensity, with whom, where, enjoyment and preference. Overall, domain or activity type scores are provided in these six dimensions
	Training: review of the CAPE/PAC manual and practice administering and scoring the assessment should be sufficient for use. No additional training is required
	Note: the CAPE/PAC has been translated into Dutch, Hebrew and Swedish
Psychometric properties	CAPE:
	Reliability
	Test–retest: intraclass correlation coefficients (ICCs) for overall participation and two domain scores ranged from 0.64 to 0.77 (diversity, intensity and enjoyment)
	ICCs for enjoyment ranged from 0.12 (active physical activities) to 0.73 (recreational activities), which indicates poor to good reliability
	ICCs ranged from 0.64 to 0.81 (diversity and intensity)
	Internal consistency: Cronbach's alpha ranged from 0.30 to 0.62 for the five activity-type scores and 0.42 for the formal and 0.77 for the informal activity domain scores
	Validity
	Content: extensive literature and expert review
	Construct: small to moderate significant correlations were found between participation intensity and enjoyment scores from the CAPE and relevant outcome variables. Small to moderate significant correlations were found between intensity scores and scores from measures of environmental, familial and child factors
	Criterion: relationships between the CAPE and measures of family and child functioning were significant
	Responsiveness: further testing is needed to measure responsiveness over time
	PAC:
	Reliability
	Internal consistency: Cronbach's alpha was calculated for the domains and activity types. The calculation shows reliable values of 0.84 for the formal domain and 0.76 for the informal domain of the PAC. Values from the five activity types/scales ranged from 0.67 to 0.77
	Test–retest: N/A
	Validity
	Content: extensive review of the literature on participation, expert review and pilot work demonstrate validity evidence
	Construct: factor analyses were performed with two sets of data. Time 1 shows 34.2% variance and revealed the presence of five factors and Time 2 accounts for 36.1% variance. CAPE and PAC scores vary by age, sex and disability status (and severity of disability)

	Concurrent validity: Correlations among PAC scores and CAPE intensity and enjoyment scores ranged from 0.22 to 0.61. PAC scores demonstrate small to moderate significant correlations between intensity scores and measures of environmental, familial and child factors
	Responsiveness: further testing is needed to measure responsiveness over time
	Note: psychometric findings based on children from Ontario, Canada; Quebec, Canada; and Victoria State, Australia
How to order	Internet order only. Manual and toolkit available at Harcourt Assessment (http://harcourtassessment.com) (English version only)
	Cost: US$109
	The CAPE/PAC assessment tool is purchased as a package
Key references	Imms C (2008) Review of the Children's Assessment of Participation and Enjoyment and the Preferences for Activity of Children. *Phys Occupat Ther Paediatr* 28: 389–404.
	King G, Law M, King S, Rosenbaum P, Kertoy M, Young NL (2003) A conceptual model of the factors affecting the recreation and leisure participation of children with disabilities. *Phys Occupat Ther Paediatr* 23: 63–90.
	King G, Law M, King S, et al (2004) *Children's Assessment of Participation & Enjoyment (CAPE) and Preferences for Activities of Children (PAC)*. San Antonio, TX: PsychCorp.

However, family caregivers could be administered the CAPE/PAC to obtain their participation profiles if their child is unable to self-report owing to cognitive and communication impairments. The primary purpose of the CAPE/PAC is individualized assessment; however, it could be used for program-level and population-based assessment. Most CAPE/PAC items address participation in community and social life (hobbies, crafts, games, social activities, active and quiet recreation, organized sports, clubs, groups and organizations, arts and entertainment) with the exception of jobs and chores.

ASSESSMENT OF LIFE HABITS FOR CHILDREN

The Assessment of Life Habits (LIFE-H)[16,17] was initially developed for adults with disabilities and has been adapted for use with children aged 5 years and older. Its purpose is to identify disruptions in the accomplishment of life habits (daily activities and social roles) in persons with disabilities. The LIFE-H for Children was designed to be completed by parent or guardian report but could be completed by children and youth who have the requisite comprehension and communication skills. The LIFE-H is a comprehensive tool that examines multiple domains of participation. The most recent revision has a long form (197 items) and short form (64 items) that include two broad domains (daily activities and social roles) and 12 life habit categories. The *daily activities* domain includes six categories (communication, personal care, housing, mobility, nutrition, fitness) and the

social roles domain includes five categories (recreation, responsibility, education, community life, interpersonal relationships). The LIFE-H assesses both activity and participation and taps all of the ICF domains except for learning and applying knowledge. Two categories in the *social roles* domain are most relevant for this chapter's domain of focus: *community life* (items that address community participation; and spiritual life and religious practice) and *recreation* (items that address sports and games; arts and culture; socio-recreational activities). Also of relevance to this chapter is an item about civic life in the *responsibility* category (*social roles* domain) and items in the *fitness* category (*daily activities* domain).

The LIFE-H assesses level of accomplishment using a 'difficulty' scale (no difficulty, some difficulty, performed by substitution, not performed, not applicable) and 'type of assistance' scale (no help, technical aid, adaptation, human assistance). A 'not applicable' response is selected if the life habit is not part of the person's lifestyle by choice. The difficulty and assistance scales are combined to create a nine-point modified life accomplishment scale. The LIFE-H also assesses level of satisfaction for each life habit category using a five-point scale ('very satisfied' to 'very dissatisfied'). Level of accomplishment and satisfaction scores can be computed for items, life habit categories and global scores. The LIFE-H can be used for all three purposes: individualized, programme- and population-based assessment.

CHILD AND ADOLESCENT SCALE OF PARTICIPATION

The Child and Adolescent Scale of Participation (CASP)[12,18] was initially developed as part of a follow-up survey to monitor outcomes and needs of children with traumatic brain injury (TBI) and other acquired brain injuries after inpatient rehabilitation, as reported by family caregivers. More recently, the CASP has been used alone or for follow-up of children and youth with varied diagnoses.[19] The CASP measures the extent to which children, compared with those of the same age, participate in home, school and community activities. It consists of four subsections: (1) home participation, (2) school participation, (3) community participation and (4) home and community living activities. Twenty items are rated on a four-point scale: 'age expected', 'somewhat restricted', 'very restricted' and 'unable'. A 'not applicable' response is selected when the item reflects an activity (e.g. work) in which the child would not be expected to participate because of his or her age. Most items are applicable to children who are aged 5 years and older. Each item examines a broad participation domain and examples are provided for each domain. Open-ended questions are included that ask about supports and barriers to participation. The CASP broadly taps all participation domains except for 'learning and applying knowledge' and can be used for all three purposes: individualized, programme- and population-based assessment. Item, subsection and total summary scores can be examined. Three CASP items address community and social life, and thus are relevant to this chapter's domain of focus: (1) social, play and leisure activities, (2) structured events and activities and (3) communicating with others in the community.

PEDIATRIC ACTIVITY CARD SORT

The Pediatric Activity Card Sort (Pediatric ACS)[20] is an adaptation of the Activity Card Sort,[21] a measure developed for adults. The Pediatric ACS is used to determine levels of occupational performance and engagement in children and youth to assist occupational therapists in determining appropriate goals and intervention strategies. It has many items (83 activity cards) reflecting discrete activities that are organized into four main categories: personal care, school/productivity, hobbies/social activities and sports. The last two categories are of relevance to this chapter as they address community and social life. The majority of items are in the hobbies and social activities areas – areas that are also addressed in two other ICF chapters, major life areas and interpersonal interactions and relationships. The Pediatric ACS is administered by occupational therapists to children or parents using Q-sort methodology. Cards are presented one at a time and the examiner asks if and how often the child engages in the activity depicted. The child/proxy is instructed to place the card in a 'yes' or 'no' pile based on whether he or she has participated in the activity within the last 4 months. Children are asked if they participate and, if so, how often (daily, weekly, monthly or annually). Scoring involves recording the five activities that are most important to or for the child and the activities the child would like to do the most. Total scores highlight the child's activity level prior to therapy and assist the therapist in developing a client-centred intervention plan. The measure was designed primarily as an individualized assessment, but appears useful for programme-level assessment.

PRESCHOOLER ACTIVITY CARD SORT

The Preschooler Activity Card Sort (Preschooler ACS)[22,23] was developed for preschool-aged children (2–6y) whereas the previously described Pediatric ACS[21] was designed for children aged 5 to 14 by a different research team. Both measures are adaptations of the ACS that was developed for adult clients.[21] The purpose and content of the Preschooler ACS is different from that of the Pediatric ACS. The primary purpose of the Preschooler ACS is to develop an occupational profile of a child based on the parent's perspective and to determine if limited participation is due to child, family or environmental barriers. The Preschooler ACS assesses seven areas: self-care, domestic chores, social interaction, high-demand leisure, low-demand leisure, community mobility and education. Many items (73 picture cards) address discrete activities in these areas. Four of these areas – social interaction, high-demand leisure, low-demand leisure and community mobility – include items that are relevant to this chapter's domain of focus. The community mobility area is included here because it has items related to engaging in community life such as going to the library or grocery store.

The Preschooler ACS also uses Q-sort methodology. A parent interview is conducted by showing the different pictures of children participating in everyday activities at home, school or in the community. Parent responses include: 'yes, my child participates'; 'yes, with adult assistance'; 'yes, with environmental accommodation'; or 'no, my child does not participate'. If the parent gives a 'no' response, follow-up discussion questions are asked to examine if the barrier for participation is related to the child, parent or environment.

The measure was designed as an individualized assessment. An occupational profile is developed by the therapist and parents based upon the card sort and the six domains. The parent is then asked to identify five goals for treatment based upon this profile.

CHILD AND ADOLESCENT SCALE OF PARTICIPATION (CASP)

Purpose	To assess the extent to which children participate in home, school and community activities in comparison with children of the same age, as reported by family caregivers. Initially designed as part of the Child and Family Follow-up Survey (CFFS), used to assess outcomes and needs of children and youth with acquired brain injuries (ABIs) as reported by parents or other primary guardians
Population	Initially designed for children with ABI between the ages of 3y and 22y. Now used for children and youth with other disabling conditions. The majority of items are applicable to children who are 5y and older
Description of domains (subscales)	Four sections: (1) home, (2) school, (3) community participation and (4) home and community living. Four-point scale (4=age-expected, 3=somewhat limited, 2=very limited, 1=cannot participate) includes not-applicable response. The CASP broadly examines all participation domains from the ICF-CY except for learning and applying knowledge. Examples are provided for each participation domain. Open-ended questions that ask about supports and barriers to participation are included
Administration and test format	Time to complete: the CASP (20 items) can be administered in 10–15min
	Testing format: can be done as part of the larger CFFS or separately. Can be done as a self-report, or administered as part of an in-person or phone interview (by family caregiver). A youth-report version and Spanish translation are currently being tested
	Scoring: total scores, subsection scores and item level scores can be examined
	Training: no training is required other than familiarity with the content and format
	Note: a youth report version and Spanish, Hebrew, Arabic and Dutch translated versions are currently being tested
Psychometric properties	*Reliability*
	Internal consistency: Cronbach's alphas=0.98 and 0.96 (two studies)
	Test–retest: intraclass correlation coefficient=0.94
	Validity
	Construct: moderate correlations found between CASP scores and variables hypothesized to be associated with participation (activity performance, and extent of child impairment and problems in physical and social environment). Typically developing children, on average, had significantly higher CASP scores than children with disabilities
	Factor analyses: three factors contributed 63% of the variance explained: (1) participation in social, leisure and communication items (50%); (2) participation in advanced daily living items (7%); and (3) participation in basic daily living and mobility items (6%)
	Rasch analyses: findings suggest that the CASP is probably measuring essentially one unidimensional construct. The item difficulty order closely matched the expected pattern of life situations that children would find more or less challenging to participate in. Children were more restricted in school and community activities that required more developmentally complex skills and social interactions and children were less restricted in simpler and more routine mobility, communication and personal care activities done at home and school
	Responsiveness: has not been examined
How to order	The administration and scoring guidelines are available for free by contacting Dr Gary Bedell (gary.bedell@tufts.edu)
Key references	Bedell G (2004) Developing a follow-up survey focused on participation of children and youth with acquired brain injuries after inpatient rehabilitation. *NeuroRehabilitation* 19: 191–205.
	Bedell G (2009) Further validation of the Child and Adolescent Scale of Participation (CASP). *Dev Neurorehabil* 12: 342–351.
	Bedell G, Dumas H (2004) Social participation of children and youth with acquired brain injuries discharged from inpatient rehabilitation: a follow-up study. *Brain Injury* 18: 65–82.

PEDIATRIC ACTIVITY CARD SORT (PEDIATRIC ACS)	
Purpose	To determine levels of occupational performance and engagement in children/youth to assist therapists in goal planning and designing intervention strategies
Population	Children/youths aged 5–14y with various diagnoses and physical disabilities
Description of domains (subscales)	Four subdomains assessed: personal care, school/productivity, hobbies/social activities and sports
Administration and test format	Time to complete: 20–25min
	Testing format: 83 cards depicting 75 activities. Organized into four categories: personal care, school/productivity, hobbies/social activities and sports. Administered to children or parents using Q-sort methodology. Cards are presented one at a time; the examiner asks if/how often children engage in the activity depicted. The child is instructed to place the card in a 'yes' or 'no' pile if he or she has participated in the activity within the last 4mo. If he or she participates, then the child is asked how often he or she participates (daily, weekly, monthly, yearly)
	Scoring: the five most important activities to the child and the activities the child would like to do most are recorded. The total scores highlight the child's activity level prior to therapy and assist the therapist in developing a client-centred intervention plan
	Training: no specific training other than having a client-centred focus and being familiar with the content (activity cards) and format. The manual specifies that the Pediatric ACS is meant for use by occupational therapists and certified occupational therapy assistants
Psychometric properties	*Reliability*
	Internal consistency: no reported evidence found
	Test–retest: no reported evidence found
	Validity
	Evidence reported in test manual and based on a number of studies conducted as Master's theses
	Content validity: activities identified based on clinical experiences of authors and literature review. Item validation was undertaken in one study with 13 children aged 6–12y. In another study, parents corroborated their children's responses (n=11) (percentage agreements among parent–child pairs ranged from 86% to 96% and averaged 91.6%)
	Construct/discriminant validity: in one study differences were found in activity patterns related to age. In another study differences were found in occupational profiles between children with developmental coordination disorder (DCD) and typically developing children (n=10; aged 6–10y)
	Responsiveness: no reported evidence was found
How to order	Mail order from Canadian Association of Occupational Therapists, CTTC Building, Suite 3400, Ottawa, Ontario K1S 5R1, Canada
	www.caot.ca; publications@caot.ca
	Cost: CA$169.95
	Mandich AD, Polatajko HJ, Miller LT, Baum C (2004) *Paediatric Activity Card Sort*. Ottawa, ON: CAOT Publications ACE.

PRESCHOOLER ACTIVITY CARD SORT (PRESCHOOLER ACS)

Purpose	To develop an occupational profile of a child using the parent's perspective and to determine if a lack of child/youth participation in everyday preschool activities is due to child, family or environmental barriers
Population	Children/youth with disabilities between 3y and 6y of age
Description of domains (subscale)	Seven domains assessed: self-care, domestic chores, social interaction, high-demand leisure, low-demand leisure, community mobility and education
Administration and test format	Time to complete: 30min Testing format: parent interview is conducted by showing 73 different pictures of children participating in everyday activities at home, school or in the community. Parent responses: 'yes, my child participates'; 'yes, with adult assistance'; 'yes, with environmental accommodation'; or 'no, my child does not participate'. If the parent gives a 'no' response, follow-up questions are asked to determine if the barrier for participation is related to the child, parent or environment. An occupational profile is developed by the therapist and parents based upon the card sort and the six domains. The parent is then asked to identify five goals for treatment based upon this profile Scoring: occupational profile developed during card sort and follow-up interview. No normative comparisons made. The profile is specific to the child based on parental perspective Training: no training needed other than familiarity with the content and format Note: the Preschooler ACS has been translated into Spanish
Psychometric properties	*Reliability* Inter-rater: intraclass correlation=0.91; test–retest: r=0.93 *Validity* Content: thorough literature, expert and parental review of photographs to determine accurate representation of preschool-aged activities Construct/discriminant: differences were found between preschoolers with autism spectrum disorder (ASD) and typically developing preschoolers; preschoolers with ASD participated in significantly fewer activities in all domains except for low-demand leisure Responsiveness: no current evidence of responsiveness
How to order	Mail order only from Christine Berg, Campus Box 8505, 4444 Forest Park Ave., St. Louis, MO 63108, USA Cost: US$50 for cards and scoring forms made payable to Washington University (no manual is available at this time)
Key references	Berg C, LaVesser P (2006) The Preschool Activity Card Sort. *Occupat Ther J Res* 26: 143–151. Stoffel A, Berg C (2008) Spanish translation and validation of the Preschool Activity Card Sort. *Phys Occupat Ther Paediatr* 28: 171–189.

PERCEIVED EFFICACY AND GOAL-SETTING SYSTEM

The Perceived Efficacy and Goal Setting System (PEGS)[24] is an assessment tool adapted from the All About Me (AAM) assessment.[25] Three areas are assessed: self-care, school and leisure. The PEGS includes items in two ICF-CY categories that are relevant to this chapter: (1) community life and (2) recreation and leisure. It was designed for children aged 6 to 9 years to be used with their occupational therapist, but can be used by other health professionals. During the assessment, 24 pairs of cards with pictures depicting children performing everyday activities 'more competently' and 'less competently' are presented sequentially to the child. Children are asked to report which picture best illustrates their ability to perform the activity and then if they are 'a lot' or 'a little' like the child in the picture. Activities illustrated in the PEGS drawings are those that take place at school and outside of school: self-care, school and leisure. The child is able to report on additional activities that he or she feels less competent in performing. The occupational therapist has a discussion with the child and reviews activities he or she reported as being less competent at performing. The child chooses activities in which he or she desires improvement, allowing the process of goal setting to take place collaboratively. Family caregiver and teacher versions of the PEGS are available. Adults are asked to report on their perception of their child's competence in the same activities and identify goals they believe to be most important, using sentences rather than pictures. The measure is used for individualized assessment.

CANADIAN OCCUPATIONAL PERFORMANCE MEASURE

The Canadian Occupational Performance Measure (COPM)[26] was developed as a client-centred outcome measure to assess clients' perception of their occupational performance (activity and participation) and satisfaction with their performance over time. The COPM assesses three subdomains: self-care, productivity and leisure. Two subdomains, leisure and productivity, are particularly relevant for this chapter. Productivity is relevant because it encompasses play activities. Although originally designed for adult clients, the COPM is used with children via family/proxy report.[27] Children and youth with requisite understanding and communication skills can complete the COPM as well. The family caregiver/proxy identifies his or her child's occupational performance problems that reflect activities that he or she (or the child) wants or needs the child to do in daily life. Using a semi-structured interview format, family caregivers rate the importance of these occupational performance problems using a 10-point scale, where 1 is not important at all and 10 is extremely important. The five most important problems are rated using 10-point scales to assess the family caregiver's perception of the child's performance, where 1 is not able to do at all and 10 is able to do extremely well, and their satisfaction with the child's performance, where 1 is not satisfied at all and 10 is extremely satisfied. The COPM can be used for all three purposes: individualized and programme- and population-based assessment. Item level scores can be generated for each activity rated in terms of the family caregiver's perception of the child's performance and his or her satisfaction with performance. Summary performance scores and satisfaction with performance scores can also be generated by averaging performance and satisfaction ratings for all activities rated.

VINELAND ADAPTIVE BEHAVIOR SCALES, SECOND EDITION

The Vineland Adaptive Behavior Scales, Second Edition (VABS II)[13] was released in 2005 and examines the same four domains of functioning as the original version (communication, daily living, socialization and motor) using parent/caregiver and teacher report versions. The parent versions can be used to follow children from infancy into older adulthood. There are items in the daily living domain that implicitly assess participation, such as extent of involvement in personal activities (e.g. self or personal care items), domestic activities (e.g. household items such as preparing meals, washing clothes) and community living activities (e.g. managing money, employment, transportation items). However, most participation items relevant for this chapter's domain are located in the *socialization domain* and particularly in two socialization subdomains: 'interpersonal relationships' (friendships, dating, social communication and responding to others) and 'playing and using leisure time' (playing and going places with friends). The reader is also referred to Chapter 26, on interpersonal interactions and relationships, for further description given that these items are also of particular relevance to content covered in that chapter. The items ask whether the child does the activity using a three-point scale, where 2=yes, usually; 1=sometimes or partially; 0=no, never; or N=no opportunity. A number of scores are available including a total score as well as scores for each domain. The VABS II can be used for all three purposes: individualized and programme- and population-based assessment. Item, subsection and total summary scores also can be examined.

CHILD BEHAVIOR CHECKLIST

The Child Behavior Checklist (CBCL)[14] assesses multiple content domains and includes parent/caregiver report (for children aged 2–3 and 4–18y), youth report (11–18y) and teacher report versions (ages 2–18y). Domains assessed include the child's social competence, academic performance, internalizing/externalizing behaviours and specific strengths and needs. The social competence subscale includes subsections that measure aspects of participation that are relevant to this chapter's domain of focus: participation in activities, number of friendships and frequency of contact with friends. The reader is also referred to Chapter 26, on interpersonal interactions and relationships, for further description given that the friendship items are also of particular relevance to content covered in that chapter. Participation in activities is assessed by asking the parent or youth to list three activities the child most likes to take part in under the following four categories: (1) sports; (2) hobbies, activities or games other

PERCEIVED EFFICACY AND GOAL SETTING SYSTEM (PEGS)	
Purpose	To obtain children's perspective on their ability to perform everyday activities and identify areas needing improvement to assist with goal setting
Population	Children with disabilities aged 6–9y. Parent and caregiver versions that elicit the adult perspective on the child's ability and what goals should be set are also available
Description of domains (subscale)	Children are shown pictures of a child of their age performing activities related to self-care, school and leisure
Administration and test format	Time to complete: 20min Testing format: *Child* Twenty-four pairs of cards depicting pictures of children performing everyday activities. The child is shown two pictures of a child doing the same activity: one shows a child doing the activity 'more competently' and the other 'less competently'. The child is asked to identify which picture best depicts his or her ability to do a task and if it is 'a lot' or 'a little' like them. The tester reviews and discusses with the child the activities that he or she reported as being less competent at, to help identify goals for therapy *Parent and caregiver* The content is the same as the child version but a questionnaire format is used instead of pictures. Adults report from their own perspective what the child's competences are, what areas need improvement and what goals should be attained Training: no training is required other than familiarity with the content and format Note: the PEGS has been translated into Hebrew, Swedish and Norwegian
Psychometric properties	*Reliability* Internal consistency: Cronbach's alphas of 0.85 for fine motor and 0.91 for gross motor scales Test–retest: 92% of children chose two to four of the same activities when asked to complete the PEGS a second time in a standardization study of the PEGS (Missiuna et al 2006a) *Validity* Content: many items were derived from the previously validated All About Me (AAM) measure. Additional items were added through pilot testing and expert review Criterion: scores on the AAM measure correlated significantly with the Pictorial Scale of Perceived Competence and Social Acceptance for Young Children (PCSA) (r=0.80), the Developmental Test of Visual Motor Integration (r=0.64), and the Bruininks–Oseretsky Test of Motor Proficiency (r=0.73). The AAM discriminated significantly between children with and without disabilities Responsiveness: no current evidence of responsiveness
How to order	The PEGS can be ordered from Pearson Assessments Online In North America: http://pearsonassess.com/HAIWEB/Cultures/en-us/Productdetail.htm?Pid=076–1606–211&Mode=summary Cost: US$121 In the UK: www.psychcorp.co.uk/product.aspx?skey=2964 Cost: £104
Key references	Missiuna C (1998) Development of the All About Me, a scale that measures children's perceived motor competence. *Occupat Ther J Res* 18: 85–108.

Missiuna C, Pollock N (2000) Perceived efficacy and goal setting in young children. *Can J Occupat Ther* 67: 101–109.

Missiuna C, Pollock N, Law M (2004) *The Perceived Efficacy and Goal Setting System.* San Antonio, TX: Psychcorp.

Missiuna C, Pollock N, Law M, Walter S, Cavey N (2006a) Examination of the Perceived Efficacy and Goal Setting System (PEGS) with children with disabilities, their parents, and teachers. *Am J Occupat Ther* 60: 204–214.

Missiuna C, Pollock N, Law M (2006b) *Perceived Efficacy and Goal Setting in Young Children (PEGS) Hebrew Manual.* Translation and research by Annya Miller-Hillel. Jerusalem: PsychTec.

CANADIAN OCCUPATIONAL PERFORMANCE MEASURE (COPM)

Purpose	Designed to be used by occupational therapists (but can be used by multidisciplinary team) as an outcome measure based on a client-centred service model. Assesses a person's self-perception of occupational performance over time
Population	All children receiving paediatric services
Description of domains (subscale)	Three subdomains: self-care, productivity and leisure. (Assesses importance, performance and satisfaction with performance in self-identified activities within these three domains.)
Administration and test format	Time to complete: 30–40min
	Testing format: semi-structured interview by an experienced therapist. Can be completed by children with sufficient cognitive ability to understand the measure or by family caregivers
	The family caregiver identifies occupational problems that reflect activities that he or she (or the child) wants or needs the child to do in daily life
	Occupational problems are rated in terms of importance using a 10-point scale (1=not important at all; 10=extremely important)
	The five most important problems are rated using 10-point scales to assess the family caregiver's perception of the child's performance (1=not able to do at all; 10=able to do extremely well) and his or her satisfaction with child's performance (1=not satisfied at all; 10=extremely satisfied)
	Re-assessment (time period decided by family caregiver and therapist) using the performance and satisfaction rating scales
	Scoring: item level scores can be generated for each activity rated in terms of the family caregiver's perception of child's performance and their satisfaction with performance. Summary performance scores and satisfaction with performance scores can also be generated by averaging performance and satisfaction ratings for all activities rated
	Training: good interviewing skills are necessary; designed for use by experienced occupational therapists. Can be used by multidisciplinary teams but training is required. Guidelines for use can be found in the manual (Law et al, 2005)
	Note: the COPM has been translated into 29 languages
Psychometric properties	*Reliability*
	Internal consistency:
	Adult population: Cronbach's alphas=0.56 (performance); 0.71 (satisfaction) (Law et al, 2005)
	Paediatric population: Cronbach's alphas=0.86 (performance); 0.82 (satisfaction) (Cusick et al, 2007)

	Test–retest:
	Adult population: $r=0.80$ for both subscales (Carswell et al, 2004). Paediatric population: $r=0.79$ for performance scores and 0.75 for satisfaction scores in a sample of young children with disabilities (the COPM was completed with their parents) (Law and Stewart, 1996)
	Validity
	Content:
	Adult population: extensive content validation procedures have been conducted throughout the process of development. The COPM is now in its fourth version (Law et al, 2005)
	Paediatric population: preliminary evidence based on review by and feedback from families of children of cerebral palsy (Cusick et al, 2007)
	Criterion and construct validity:
	Adult population: associations found between COPM scores and similar scores from other measures (Carswell et al, 2004; Law et al, 2005)
	Paediatric population: moderate correlations with Goal Attainment Scale (GAS) scores from related domains (Cusick et al, 2007)
	Responsiveness
	Adult population: many studies conducted and have shown change over time (Carswell et al, 2004; Law, et al, 2005)
	Paediatric population: Cusick et al (2007) found the COPM to be responsive to intervention-related change in a randomized clinical trial of intervention for children with cerebral palsy. The COPM was able to detect change above the reported minimally important difference of two points. Also, moderate correlations were found between COPM change scores and GAS change scores
How to order	Mail order from:
	The Canadian Association of Occupational Therapists, CTTC Building, Suite 3400, 1125 Colonel By Drive, Ottawa, Ontario K1S 5R1, Canada
	www.caot.ca
Key references	Carswell A, McColl MA, Baptiste S, Law M, Polatajko H, Pollock N (2004) The COPM: a research and clinical review. *Can J Occupat Ther* 71: 210–222.
	Cusick A, McIntyre S, Novak I, Lannin N, Lowe K (2006) A comparison of goal attainment scaling and the Canadian Occupational Performance Measure for paediatric rehabilitation research. *Paediatr Rehabil* 9: 49–157.
	Cusick A, Lannin NA, Lowe K (2007) Adapting the Canadian Occupational Performance Measure for use in a paediatric clinical trial. *Disabil Rehabil* 29: 761–766.
	Law M, Stewart D (1996) Test retest reliability of the COPM with children. Unpublished manuscript.
	Law M, Baptiste S, Carswell A, McColl MA, Polatajko H, Pollock N (2005) *Canadian Occupational Performance Measure*, 4th edition. Ottawa, ON: CAOT Publications.

than sports; (3) organizations, clubs, teams or groups; and (4) jobs or chores. (The first three categories are relevant for this chapter.) The respondent can select up to three activities for each category or tick 'none'. The respondent is asked how much time the child spends in each selected activity ('less than average', 'average', 'more than average', 'don't know') compared with others of the same age. The CBCL friendship items ask about how many friends the child has ('none', '1', '2 or 3', '4 or more') and how many times a week the child does things with friends outside of regular school hours ('less than 1', '1 or 2', '3 or more'). The CBCL can be used for all three purposes: individualized and programme- and population-based assessment. Item, subsection and total summary scores also can be examined.

PARTICIPATION AND ENVIRONMENT MEASURE FOR CHILDREN AND YOUTH

The Participation and Environment Measure for Children and Youth (PEM-CY)[28,29] is the most recently developed of all the measures included in this chapter. It is a parent/guardian report measure that examines both participation and environmental factors that support or hinder participation. The decision to have a combined participation and environment measure was informed by interviews with parents of children with and without disabilities from the USA and Canada.[30]

The PEM-CY participation items reflect broad types of activities that are typically done in three settings: home (e.g. indoor play and games, household chores); school (e.g. classroom activities, school-sponsored teams, clubs and organizations, and getting together with peers outside of class); and community activities (e.g. neighbourhood outings, unstructured physical activities, organizations, groups, clubs and volunteer or leadership activities).

Each participation item is rated in three ways: (1) frequency/how often (seven-point scale: 0=never to 7=daily; (2) involvement (five-point scale: 1=minimally to 5=very involved); (3) desire for change (parents are asked if they want any aspect of their child's participation to change [Yes or No?]). If yes, the parent is asked to indicate the type of change desired: more or less frequency, more or less involvement and/or more variety).

A separate set of environment items are asked after each set of participation items for each setting. Parents are asked questions about whether physical and social features of the environment (e.g. physical layout, activity demands, attitudes of others) help or hinder their child's participation and whether there are available or adequate resources (e.g. services, equipment, time and money) to support their child's participation.[28] Refer to Chapter 30, on physical, social and attitudinal environment, for further discussion on environmental measures.

There are many PEM-CY items that address participation in community and social life (e.g. hobbies, crafts, games, social activities, active and quiet recreation, organized sports, clubs, groups and organizations, arts and entertainment). There are three items that address aspects of participation in civic life (e.g. volunteer and leadership roles, activities and organizations at school and in the community). The PEM-CY was originally designed for population-based assessment, but can also be used for individualized and programme-level assessment.

In summary, it is clear that there are a number of measures that assess participation in community and social life. However, only a few of the measures described address participation in civic life and do so in a limited way. There are strengths, limitations and trade-offs associated with the use of any one measure. Moreover, there is scant research evidence that supports the selection of a specific participation measure over another at this point in time. However, certain measures are probably better than others depending on the specific situation or purpose.

Measures such as the CAPE/PAC,[15] PEGS[24] and Pediatric and Preschool Activity Card Sorts[20,22] might be better at individualized assessment than some of the other measures because they focus on participation in a comprehensive set of discrete activities. The LIFE-H,[16,17] CASP[19] and PEM-CY[28,29] could be used for individualized assessment as well, but might be better at population-based assessment than some of the other measures because they address fewer and broader categories of participation (however, the CAPE/PAC has also been used to assess participation at the population level). Measures such as the COPM[26,27] or other approaches that focus on the goals and needs of the child and family (e.g. assessing achievement of intervention objectives, goal attainment scaling[31]) or using specific items or subsections from larger measures (e.g. VABS II[13] and CBCL[14]) might be better at assessing change over time or as a result of intervention because measurement can be tailored to reflect intervention or programme-specific outcomes.[7]

Ultimately, stakeholders will have to find the measure or measures that can best address their own information goals and clinical, research or policy questions. This process will involve consideration of the available research evidence and some of the practical, conceptual and methodological issues described in this chapter.

PARTICIPATION AND ENVIRONMENT MEASURE FOR CHILDREN AND YOUTH (PEM-CY)

Purpose	To examine the participation of children and youth in three settings (home, school and community) and environmental factors that support or hinder participation specific to these three settings
Population	Children and youth with and without disabilities aged 5–17y
Description of domains (subscale)	There are PEM-CY summary scores for each setting: (1) home (participation=10 items, environment=12 items); (2) school (participation=5 items, environment=17 items); and (3) community (participation=10 items, environment=16 items). Participation summary scores can be created for each setting to indicate: (1) percentage of activities the child participates in (or never participates in); (2) frequency of participation; (3) extent of involvement; and (4) desire for change
Administration and test format	Time to complete: about 30min
	Testing format: completed by parents or primary guardians. Only the online survey has been tested. A paper and pencil version will be available in the near future.
	Scoring: summary scores and item-level scores can be created for each domain of participation and for each setting as described above. Other composite scores can be created depending on the specific research or clinical question. (There are separate environment scores for each setting as well – see Chapter 30.)
	Training: no formal training is required other than knowledge of the PEM-CY content and format, conceptual foundation and administration and scoring guidelines
Psychometric properties	*Reliability*
	Internal consistency: Cronbach's alphas ranged from 0.59 to 0.91 for the different PEM-CY summary rating scales across settings
	Test–retest: intraclass correlation coefficients ranged from 0.58 to 0.95 for the different PEM-CY summary scores across settings
	Validity
	Significant differences and moderate to large effect sizes were found comparing summary scores in each setting for children with and children without disabilities. Children with disabilities had significantly lower frequencies of participation in activities, lower general level of involvement when participating in these activities, and less overall environmental supportiveness as perceived by caregivers
	Responsiveness: not yet examined
How to order	The paper and pencil version and scoring guidelines will be available free of charge in the near future. Please check the following websites that describe the Participation and Environment Project for further information:
	Boston University (Dr Wendy Coster; Sargent College – Kids in Context Research Lab): www.bu.edu/kidsincontext/pep/
	McMaster University (Dr Mary Law; *CanChild* Center for Childhood Disability Research): www.canchild.ca/en/ourresearch/pep.asp
Key references	Bedell G, Khetani MA, Cousins MA, Coster WJ, Law MC (2011) Parent perspectives to inform development of measures of children's participation and environment. *Arch Phys Med Rehabil* 92: 765–773.
	Coster W, Bedell G, Law M, Khetani MA, Teplicky R, Liljenquist K, Gleason K, Kao YC (2012) Psychometric evaluation of the Participation and Environment Measure for Children and Youth (PEM-CY). *Dev Med Child Neurol* 53: 1030–1037.
	Coster W, Law M, Bedell G, Khetani MA, Cousins M, Teplicky R (2012). Development of the Participation and Environment Measure for Children and Youth (PEM-CY): conceptual basis. *Disabil Rehabil* 34: 238–246.

REFERENCES

1. World Health Organization (2001) *International Classification of Functioning, Disability and Health (ICF)*. Geneva: WHO.
2. World Health Organization (2007) *International Classification of Functioning, Disability and Health: Children and Youth Version (ICF-CY)*. Geneva: WHO.
3. Lollar DJ, Simeonsson RJ (2005) Diagnosis to function: classification for children and youths. *Dev Behav Paediatr* 26: 323–330.
4. Simeonsson RJ, Leonardi M, Lollar D, Bjorck-Akesson E, Hollenweger J, Martinuzzi A (2003) Applying the International Classification of Functioning, Disability, and Health to measure childhood disability. *Disabil Rehabil* 25: 605–610.
5. McConachie H, Colver AF, Forsyth RJ, Jarvis SN, Parkinson KN (2006) Participation of disabled children: how should it be characterised and measured? *Disabil Rehabil* 28: 1157–1164.
6. Coster W, Khetani MA (2008) Measuring participation of children with disabilities: issues and challenges. *Disabil Rehabil* 30: 639–648.
7. Bedell G, Coster W (2008) Measuring participation of school-aged children with traumatic brain injuries: considerations and approaches. *J Head Trauma Rehabil* 23: 220–229.
8. King G, Law M, King S, Rosenbaum P, Kertoy MK, Young N (2003) Conceptual model of the factors affecting recreation and leisure participation of children with disabilities. *Phys Occup Ther Pediatr* 23: 63–90.
9. Forsyth R, Colver A, Alvanides S, Woolley M, Lowe M (2004) Participation of young severely disabled children is influenced by their intrinsic impairments and environment. *Dev Med Child Neurol* 49: 345–349.
10. Law M, Petrenchik T, King G, Hurley P (2007) Perceived environmental barriers to recreational, community, and school participation for children and youth with physical disabilities. *Arch Phys Med Rehabil* 88: 1636–1642.
11. Mihaylov SI, Jarvis SN, Colver AF, Beresford B (2004) Identification and description of environmental factors that influence participation of children with cerebral palsy. *Dev Med Child Neurol* 46: 299–304.
12. Bedell G, Dumas H (2004) Social participation of children and youth with acquired brain injuries discharged from inpatient rehabilitation: a follow-up study. *Brain Injury* 18: 65–82.
13. Sparrow SS, Cicchetti DV, Balla D (2005) *Vineland Adaptive Behavior Scales, Second Edition*. Circle Pines, MN: American Guidance Service Publishing.
14. Achenbach TM (1991) *Manual for the Child Behavior Checklist/4-18 and 1991 Profile*. Burlington, VT: University of Vermont, Department of Psychiatry.
15. King G, Law M, King S, Hurley P, Rosenbaum P, Hanna S, Kertoy M, Young N (2004) *Children's Assessment of Participation & Enjoyment (CAPE) and Preferences for Activities of Children (PAC)*. San Antonio, TX: PsychCorp.
16. Noreau L, Fougeyrollas P, Tremblay J (2005) *Measure of Life Habits (LIFE-H): User's Manual*. Québec: Réseau International sur le Processus de Production du Handicap (RIPPH).
17. Noreau L, Lepage C, Boissiere L, et al (2007) Measuring participation in children with disabilities using the Assessment of Life Habits. *Dev Med Child Neurol* 49: 666–671.
18. Bedell G (2004) Developing a follow-up survey focused on participation of children and youth with acquired brain injuries after inpatient rehabilitation. *NeuroRehabilitation* 19: 191–205.
19. Bedell G (2009) Further validation of the Child and Adolescent Scale of Participation (CASP). *Dev Neurorehabil* 12: 342–351.
20. Mandich AD, Polatajko HJ, Miller LT, Baum C (2004) *Pediatric Activity Card Sort*. Ottawa, ON: CAOT Publications ACE.
21. Baum CM, Edwards DF (2001) *The Activity Card Sort*. St. Louis, MO: Washington University School of Medicine.
22. Berg C, LaVesser P (2006) The Preschool Activity Card Sort. *Occup Ther J Res* 26: 143–151.
23. Stoffel A, Berg C (2008) Spanish translation and validation of the Preschool Activity Card Sort. *Phys Occup Ther Pediatr* 28: 171–189.
24. Missiuna C, Pollock N, Law M (2004) *The Perceived Efficacy and Goal Setting System*. San Antonio, TX: Psychcorp.
25. Missiuna C (1998) Development of the *All About Me*, a scale that measures children's perceived motor competence. *Occup Ther J Res* 18: 85–108.
26. Law M, Baptiste S, Carswell A, McColl MA, Polatajko H, Pollock N (2005) *Canadian Occupational Performance Measure*, 4th edition. Ottawa, ON: CAOT Publications.
27. Cusick A, Lannin NA, Lowe K (2007) Adapting the Canadian Occupational Performance Measure for use in a pediatric clinical trial. *Disabil Rehabil* 29: 761–766.
28. Coster W, Bedell G, Law M, Khetani MA, Teplicky R, Liljenquist K, Gleason K, Kao YC (2012) Psychometric evaluation of the Participation and Environment Measure for Children and Youth (PEM-CY). *Dev Med Child Neurol* 53: 1030–1037.
29. Coster W, Law M, Bedell G, Khetani MA, Cousins M, Teplicky R (2012) Development of the Participation and Environment Measure for Children and Youth (PEM-CY): conceptual basis. *Disabil Rehabil* 34: 238–246.
30. Bedell G, Khetani MA, Cousins MA, Coster WJ, Law MC (2011) Parent perspectives to inform development of measures of children's participation and environment. *Arch Phys Med Rehabil* 92: 765–773.
31. Cusick A, McIntyre S, Novak I, Lannin N, Lowe K (2006) A comparison of goal attainment scaling and the Canadian Occupational Performance Measure for paediatric rehabilitation research. *Pediatr Rehabil* 9: 49–157.

SECTION V CONTEXTUAL FACTORS

29
PERSONAL FACTORS

Rune J. Simeonsson, Andrea Lee and Kirsten M. Ellingsen

Introduction

Every chapter in this volume, except this one, identifies and describes instruments or procedures that may be used to measure and document specific taxonomic categories in the International Classification of Functioning, Disability and Health (ICF)[1] and the International Classification of Functioning, Disability and Health for Children and Youth (ICF-CY).[2] In the ICF, personal factors are defined as 'contextual factors that relate to the individual, such as age, gender, social status, life experiences and so on, which are not currently classified in ICF but which users may incorporate in their applications of the classification' (p. 229). Given the absence of a taxonomy of personal factors with associated codes, there are no categories to be matched with measures or procedures, as in the remaining chapters of this volume. Further, there is no stated purpose for the documentation of personal factors nor is there a description of how such documentation should be made in classifying an individual's health and functioning in the context of the ICF. Thus, this chapter differs from the rest of the chapters in that the lack of a classification domain and a stated purpose and place for documentation of personal factors precludes the identification of corresponding measurement tools or procedures.

The publication of the ICF and ICF-CY, 11 and 5 years ago respectively, represented an important advance in the documentation of disability within a holistic framework of human functioning. With implementation of the classifications in practice and research, however, a number of conceptual as well as practical problems have been identified in the classifications, which need to be addressed. With reference to broad concerns, Masala and Petretto[3] maintain that the ICF does not fully capture the dynamic of the person–environment interaction process and Conti-Becker[4] has critiqued the ICF for not adequately representing elements of the Biopsychosocial Model. Concerns about other limitations have taken the form of recommendations for a third qualifier for engagement in participation[5] and for standardizing the quantification of the universal qualifier.[6] The nature and role of contextual factors in defining functioning and disability have been seen as issues needing clarification. This has resulted in the suggestion that their role is one of 'scene setters'[7] in which they may act as independent, moderating, mediating or confounding roles[8]. With specific reference to personal factors, proposals have been made for incorporating the domain in a mechanical 'friction model' to measure the dynamics of interaction.[9] Other recommendations have focused on the need to include quality-of-life indices as personal factors.[10,11]

The limited concerns that have been raised in the literature about contextual factors and specifically personal factors in the ICF have not focused on the problems described in the introductory paragraph of this chapter. In fact, there appears to be an unquestioned acceptance of personal factors as an appropriate domain in the ICF. This is a significant problem in that the absence of a conceptual basis, a stated purpose and an associated classification of personal factors are fundamental limitations to the integrity and use of the ICF and ICF-CY as taxonomies. This problem is compounded by the fact that personal factors are identified as a formal domain in the ICF manual, making it likely that users will in fact see documentation of personal factors as appropriate. This likelihood is increased by the statement in the manual that personal factors 'are not currently classified in the ICF, but which users may incorporate in their applications of the classification' (p. 229).[1] This invitation for users to make their own applications is problematic in a number of ways, most notably in that such applications will not be based on the universal and standard language of codes that characterizes the rest of the ICF classifications.

The authors of this chapter are not in a position to change or revise the inclusion of personal factors or the existing descriptions of personal factors in the ICF. Recognizing that users can choose to document personal factors in applying the ICF, however, it is our position that it is important to review the construct as described in the manual, identify limitations and propose qualifications for users to consider if they intend to document personal factors. In the context of this review and chapter development, reference will be made to the ICF and the ICF-CY together as one classification (ICF/ICF-CY), although it should be pointed out that the ICF-CY is fully inclusive of all the information in the ICF.

Personal factors: an incomplete construct

References to personal factors as a component of the ICF/ICF-CY are made in a number of places in the introduction as well as elsewhere in the manual. In the introduction to the volume, personal factors are referenced 11 times and are identified in the graphic model as a component of the contextual factors domain. These references and the remaining content of the manual are framed within the universal scope of the ICF/ICF-CY that encompasses 'all aspects of human health and some health-relevant components of well-being' (p. 7).[1] Further, this framework also seems to be the basis for describing the domains and their relationships in which 'an individual's functioning in a specific domain is an interaction or complex relationship between the health condition and contextual factors (i.e. environmental and personal factors)' (p. 17).[1] However, a formal definition of personal factors is not provided in the table of definitions on page 9 of the manual in which each of the other domains in the classification is fully defined. In the absence of a formal definition of personal factors, this chapter provides a brief review of descriptions available in the manual, in order to identify what, if any, conclusions can be drawn about them and their application.

Contextual factors are described in the manual as 'the complete background of an individual's life and living. They include two components: Environmental Factors and Personal Factors, which may have an impact on the individual with a health condition and that individual's health and health-related states' (p. 15).[1] The manual further refers to personal factors as

the particular background of an individual's life and living, and comprise features of an individual that are not part of a health condition or health states. These factors may include gender, race, age or other health conditions, fitness, lifestyle, habits, upbringing, coping styles, social background, education, profession, past and current experience (past life events and concurrent events), overall behavior pattern and character

style, individual psychological assets and other characteristics, all or any of which may play a role in disability at any level.

(p. 16)[1]

Taken as a whole, these descriptions of personal factors in the ICF/ICF-CY manual do not yield a consistent definition of the construct nor do they specify inclusion and exclusion criteria of the construct. As cited above, personal factors are described with a variety of terms such as 'background', 'features', 'lifestyle', 'habits', 'upbringing', 'experience' and 'characteristics'. These broad terms cover an extremely wide range of characteristics with potential overlap with elements already present in the domains of body functions and activities and participation. Such potential overlap also pertains to the confusing declaration in the manual that personal factors 'comprise features... that are not part of a health condition or health states' but may 'include... other health conditions' (p. 16).[1] These vague and confusing descriptions of personal factors do not define in what way they constitute contextual factors in the ICF/ICF-CY framework, nor their role in accounting for the health and health-related states of a person. Without a definition distinguishing the construct of personal factors and a clearly stated reason for their documentation, it is difficult to specify what, if anything, could or should be documented relative to personal factors with the use of the ICF/ICF-CY.

Despite there being no codes, the fact that personal factors are identified as a domain with descriptive examples gives the impression that the documentation of personal factors is an appropriate use of the ICF/ICF-CY. Such application in the absence of a taxonomy of codes, however, is a significant problem in that the requirement for codes on which to base the classification of personal factors is not met in the ICF/ICF-CY. As stated in the ICF, the criterion for a classification is that it 'should be clear about what it classifies: its universe, its scope, its units of classification, its organization, and how these elements are structured in terms of their relation to each other' (p. 7).[1] The component of personal factors in the ICF/ICF-CY fails to meet these criteria given ambiguities and limitations regarding how the construct is defined, and the overlapping nature of the content with other classification domains.

In addition to the lack of a definition of personal factors noted above, there are other limitations associated with documenting the component of personal factors using the ICF-CY. A limitation in this regard is the absence of an explicit rationale and stated purpose for the inclusion of personal factors in the ICF/ICF-CY. No rationale is provided as to why personal factors are included in the ICF/

ICF-CY nor the purpose they are to serve in the classification. Is the purpose of including personal factors simply to describe characteristics of persons with impairments, limitations and restrictions that are not available in the other domains? As there are no codes it is not clear how or in what way such information would be documented. Some of the examples of personal factors identified in the manual (e.g. age, gender and race) are demographic variables that would typically be recorded in patient records or other data collection forms. The need for documenting these variables within a separate component of the ICF/ICF-CY is not obvious. Some other examples of personal factors, such as profession and health conditions, are also variables that are often collected as background information in clinic or research documents without a need for their identification as a component of contextual factors. In the absence of classification codes for personal factors that parallel those of other domains in the classifications, users are left without information as to what should be recorded and how it should be documented relative to codes of body functions and structures, activities and participation, and environmental factors.

The location of the personal factors within the contextual factors domain is another problematic issue. The nature and role of personal factors in this regard are described as follows:

> The scheme shown in Figure 1 of the manual demonstrates the role that contextual factors (i.e. environmental and personal factors) play in the process. These factors interact with the individual with a health condition and determine the level and extent of the individual's functioning. Environmental Factors are extrinsic to the individual (e.g. the attitudes of the society, architectural characteristics, the legal system) and are classified in the Environmental Factors classification. Personal Factors, on the other hand, are not classified in the current version of ICF. They include gender, race, age, lifestyle, habits, coping styles and other such factors. Their assessment is left to the user, if needed.
>
> (p. 18)[1]

The description and location of personal factors in the graphic 'biopsychosocial' model convey the premise that personal factors serve a purpose similar to that of environmental factors, namely as factors that qualify functional characteristics of the person coded in other domains. If this is the case, a qualifier would be necessary to indicate the valence and intensity of personal factors parallel to the use of the universal qualifier defining the impact of

environmental factors on body functions, body structures, activities and participation. Central to this perspective is the fact that documenting personal factors in a manner parallel to environmental factors would imply that attributes and characteristics of the individual somehow serve as barriers or facilitators for other characteristics of functioning, activities and participation of the individual. In the most benign application, this approach would simply convey the fact that variables such as age or sex play a role in the manifestation of an individual's disability. In less benign applications, there is a danger that assigning a negative qualifier value to an individual's lifestyle, habit or personal style, to account for a significant negative influence (barrier) on the individual's disability, could become a way of 'blaming the victim'. Such application of personal factors would be inconsistent with an underlying ethical principle of the ICF/ICF-CY, namely to objectively describe the health and functioning of an individual without identifying that individual's own characteristics as causal or contributing to the nature and severity of his or her health condition.

The listing of age, sex or race as personal factors is also problematic in that each is, by definition, a characteristic that can be seen as belonging to, or being a part of, the person. Specifically, each of the factors of age, sex and race can be linked to underlying body functions and structures. Other personal factors listed in the ICF/ICF-CY, such as habits, coping styles, behaviour patterns and character style, may similarly be seen to have counterparts in the activities and participation domain. In Table 1 of the manual, personal factors are described in terms of 'internal influences on functioning and disability' and 'impact of attributes of the person' (p. 10).[1] It is problematic logically, that some characteristics or attributes belonging (internal) to the person (e.g. age, sex, race) are identified as external contexts for other intrinsic characteristics classified in the domains of body functions and activities and participation (e.g. mental functions, communication, self-care ability or awareness). This logical problem is illustrated in the 'biopsychosocial' model in which 'internal' personal factors and environmental factors are portrayed together as contextual factors exerting external influences on body functions, body structures and activities and participation domains. From a conceptual standpoint, personal factors in the form of attributes and traits of the individual should be located as appropriate within the domains of body functions, body structures, activities and participation rather than as contextual factors external to the individual. Such an approach would resemble how personal factors are classified and located in another classification, the Disability Creation Process model and classification.[12]

The manual states that a reason for the lack of codes for personal factors is that they 'are not classified in ICF because of the large social and cultural variance associated with them' (p. 16).[1] In the absence of a definition and codes for personal factors, it is not clear what constitutes such cultural and social variance or why they do not apply to other domains. A review of the descriptions and examples of personal factors in the ICF/ICF-CY, however, suggests overlap of personal factors with content in other domains of the classification. In some cases, overlap could be considered on the basis of a broad term such as 'fitness' with linkage to content in several chapters (e.g. mobility, self-care) in the activities and participation domain. In other cases, a more specific example of personal factors, such as 'coping styles', could be seen to link with a number of codes in the second chapter in general tasks and demands in the activities and participation domain (e.g. handling stress and other psychological demands).

Each of the problems noted in this review reflects the lack of clarity of personal factors as a separate domain of the ICF/ICF-CY. The results of this ambiguity are evident in a recent review by Geyh et al[13] of 79 papers that made reference to personal factors and their applications. Within the framework of the review, a wide range of phenomena were described as personal factors, with 52% of the papers identified by the authors as consistent with descriptions in the ICF manual and 30% identified as not consistent. The range of personal factors included not only standard demographic factors such as social class and age, but personality, psychological and lifestyle characteristics. The wide range of personal factors found by Geyh et al can be seen as reflecting the absence of a clear definition and an associated taxonomy.

This variable interpretation of personal factors and overlap of content is problematic at several levels. From a taxonomical perspective, a classification domain should be unique, with distinct and non-overlapping content of information. This requirement is not met with the ICF/ICF-CY in that there is an overlap of characteristics intrinsic to, or 'belonging' to, the individual in the personal factors component with those found in other domains. The content in personal factors is thus not unique with some level of duplication of content with other domains of the classification. Finally, the ambiguity of the domain of personal factors and the lack of actual codes raise the problem that any characteristic perceived as a personal factor by a user will be identified accordingly, as evident in the wide range of elements found in the review by Geyh et al.[13] Such personal factors would be idiosyncratic to a specific user and challenge the fundamental purpose of the ICF/ICF-CY to provide a standard, universal language

for classifying phenomena in terminology with defined inclusion and exclusion criteria.

Implications

The absence of classification codes for personal factors, the lack of a stated purpose for their use and other problems identified above present serious concerns about the documentation of personal factors using the ICF/ICF-CY. Recognizing the challenge these problems impose on the validity of the construct of personal factors, documentation of personal factors as currently described in the ICF/ICF-CY is not recommended. However, for users who may choose to document personal factors using the ICF/ICF-CY, caution should be observed and consideration given to several issues.

As an initial step, it would be useful for the user to approach personal factors from an alternative perspective in which they are not seen as contextual factors qualifying the functioning of the individual. This would avoid the paradox in which one set of characteristics intrinsic to the person in the component of personal factors are identified as external influences on other characteristics of the person in the body functions, body structures and activities and participation domains. Conceptually and graphically, this would mean not viewing personal factors as contexts for other dimensions of the person. For any personal factor currently described in the manual that is not an intrinsic attribute of the person, a concept such as 'situational factors' might be used to denote the fact that they may be contextual in nature. This would include indicators such as social class, cultural factors, school and employment status and other factors[14,15] that are neither intrinsic to the person nor encompassed by the domain of environmental factors. Further, some personal factors may in fact be represented by codes in other domains. Sex, for example, is a characteristic often used as a demographic marker and potential proxy codes can be found in the body functions and body structures domains. Finally, users who intend to use the ICF/ICF-CY to document personal factors are encouraged to consider the following additional issues.

1   The reason for documenting 'personal factors' as currently described in the ICF/ICF-CY should be clearly stated by the user. In this case the user should indicate whether it is to derive demographic or other background characteristics of the individual or to identify personal characteristics that may explain or account for variation of observed functioning in other domains. This provides a context to ensure that consumers will interpret the meaning and significance of documented information appropriately.

2   Having stated the reason for the documentation of personal factors, the user should specify what will be included in the domain, that is define inclusion and exclusion criteria for the construct.

3   In keeping with the ethical guidelines stated for use of the ICF/ICF-CY (Annex 6)[1] no documentation of 'personal factors' should have potential negative or harmful consequences for the individual. As noted earlier, this pertains to documentation of psychological attributes as personal factors that could be seen to 'blame the victim' for an impairment, limitation of functioning or disability. If, in fact, there are psychological characteristics seen as associated with a person's functioning or disability, such characteristics should be assigned appropriate codes under the domains of body functions or activities and participation.

4   The user should specify criteria for what constitutes personal factors and exclude from use any characteristic that is intrinsic to the person. If such characteristics need to be documented, they could be assigned closely related or proxy codes in the domains of body functions, body structures or activities and participation.

5   In setting inclusion criteria, the user is encouraged to identify characteristics and features that are not intrinsic to the person, but rather reflect features that are external to the person. Such factors would include socioeconomic status, education or employment status, family size, family composition, sibling order and other cultural markers.

6   In all instances involving documentation of personal factors using the ICF/ICF-CY, the user should clearly state any limitations that should be taken into account pertaining to the interpretation of the information. This would include stating the purpose for such documentation and how the information will be used. This is an important step to ensure that the information is used appropriately to describe the uniqueness of individuals necessary to understand their needs and thereby fulfil the intended purpose of the ICF/ICF-CY.

REFERENCES

1. World Health Organization (2001) *International Classification of Functioning, Disability and Health (ICF)*. Geneva: WHO.

2. World Health Organization (2007) *International Classification of Functioning, Disability and Health for Children and Youth (ICF-CY)*. Geneva: WHO.

3. Masala C, Petretto DR (2008) From disablement to enablement: conceptual models of disability in the 20th century. *Disabil Rehabil* 30: 1233–1244.

4. Conti-Becker A (2009) Between the ideal and the real: reconsidering the International Classification of Functioning, Disability and Health. *Disabil Rehabil* 31: 2125–2129.

5. Bjorck-Akesson E, Wilder J, Granlund M, et al (2010) The International Classification of Functioning, Disability and Health and the version for children and youth as a tool in child habilitation/early childhood intervention – feasibility and usefulness as a common language and frame of reference for practice. *Disabil Rehabil* 32(Suppl. 1): S125–S138.

6. Simeonsson RJ, Sauer-Lee A, Granlund M, Björck-Åkesson E (2010) Developmental and health assessment in habilitation with the ICF-CY. In: Mpofu E, Oakland T, editors. *Rehabilitation and Health Assessment: Applying ICF Guidelines*. New York: Springer, pp. 27–46.

7. Badley EM (2008) Enhancing the conceptual clarity of the activity and participation components of the International Classification of Functioning, Disability and Health. *Soc Sci Med* 66: 2335–2345.

8. Wang PP, Badley EM, Gignac M (2006) Exploring the role of contextual factors in disability models. *Disabil Rehabil* 28: 135–140.

9. Borg J, Larsson S, Ostergren P, Eide AH (2010) The Friction Model – a dynamic model of functioning, disability and contextual factors and its conceptual and practical applicability. *Disabil Rehabil* 32: 1790–1797.

10. Huber JG, Sillick J, Skarakis-Doyle E (2010) Personal perception and personal factors: incorporating health-related quality of life into the International Classification of Functioning, Disability and Health. *Disabil Rehabil* 32: 1955–1965.

11. McDougall J, Wright V, Schmidt J, Miller L, Lowry K (2011) Applying the ICF framework to study changes in quality-of-life for youth with chronic conditions. *Disabil Rehabil* 14: 41–53.

12. Anaby D, Miller WC, Eng JE, Jarus T, Noreau L, PACC Research Group (2009) Can personal and environmental factors explain participation of older adults? *Disabil Rehabil* 31: 1275–1282.

13. Geyh S, Peter C, Muller R, et al (2011) The personal factors of the International Classification of Functioning, Disability and Health in the literature – a systematic review and content analysis. *Disabil Rehabil* 33: 1089–1102.

14. Punch S (2001) Household division of labour: generation, gender, age, birth order and sibling composition. *Work Employ Soc* 15: 803–823.

15. Zhang D (2005) Parent practices in facilitating self-determination skills: the influences of culture, socioeconomic status, and children's special education status. *Res Pract Persons Severe Disabil* 30: 154–162.

30

ENVIRONMENTAL FACTORS: PHYSICAL, SOCIAL AND ATTITUDINAL ENVIRONMENT (E110–E165, E210–E260, E310–E360, E410–E465, E510–E595)

Mary A. Khetani, Gary Bedell, Wendy J. Coster, Martha Cousins and Mary Law

What is the construct?

A Focus on Environmental Factors for Best Practice in Paediatric Rehabilitation

Best practice in the field of paediatric rehabilitation involves a focus on promoting a child's developmental growth and minimizing disability. The largest group of children with disabilities is those with developmental disorders that were apparent at birth or were identified within the period of early childhood, including intellectual disabilities, communication disorders or movement disorders such as cerebral palsy.[1] Accordingly, rehabilitation services are typically focused on trying to support optimal development and prevent or reduce secondary conditions. Paediatric rehabilitation services are also needed to address disabling consequences of acute-onset conditions in childhood such as traumatic brain injury (TBI), burns or infectious diseases. These services have a dual focus of trying to remediate the immediate effects of the illness or injury and to support the ongoing developmental process. Contemporary theory and scientific evidence suggest that interventions orientated towards these two outcomes are best informed by examining the dynamic interplay of the child within specified environments. In this chapter, we examine how environmental factors have been conceptualized and measured to inform decision-making about environmental modifications that are likely to be effective in promoting positive development and function among children with developmental disabilities.

Environmental Factors Influencing the Development of Children with Disabilities

The environment has become a central feature of contemporary thinking in the field of human development. A major tenet of developmental theories employing a systems approach is that children and youth are embedded in a changing social, cultural and economic environment within which they too are changing as they develop skills and interests in relationships with others.[2–7] In this systems model, specific skills and capacities can be built in a variety of ways as a child interacts with home and community environments in the course of daily life. Accordingly, intervention approaches based on this model emphasize flexibility as they focus on facilitating a child's participation in culturally relevant activities as a means of enhancing developmental outcomes. As children participate in meaningful routines, rituals and activities in specified contexts such as the home, school and community, they are given opportunities to acquire the knowledge, skills and relationships that are purposeful and valued in their culture.[8–14] In this paradigm, children influence and are influenced by their physical and social environment, and both individual and contextual factors contribute to developmental skill acquisition.

Developmentalists recognize that change within an individual is inextricably linked to the immediate and distant forces in the environment, and these forces have been described in several ways. Brofenbrenner[2] described environmental forces as consisting of five distinct levels: microsystem (consisting of the home, family, peer group, classroom, neighbourhood, and sometimes a church, temple or mosque); mesosytem (interactions among elements within the microsystem, such as when a parent co-ordinates efforts with a teacher to educate a child); exosystem (including external networks, such as community organizations and educational, medical and employment services); macrosystem (the cultural values, economic patterns, political philosophies and social conditions); and chronosystem (historical time). Environmental factors are further described as exerting historical, cultural and socioeconomic influence in an individual's development throughout his or her life course.[15] The historical context involves the major historical events, technologies and sociopolitical trends that influence a cohort of individuals as they travel through life together. Cultural contexts account for the diverse ways in which cultural groups encourage values, attitudes and beliefs that will enable individuals to engage effectively in the specific customs and practices of a particular cultural community. Individuals are also influenced by the socioeconomic context in which they live, a climate impacted on by factors such as family income and the educational level of parents in the household. Across the life course, change can occur in both directions as individuals interact with these distinct dimensions of their environment. Just as environmental forces help shape and refine the course of development within a person, changes within the individual can precipitate changes in the environment, as when developmental changes in the child elicit changes in parenting style. This bidirectional relationship implies that individuals and environments are shaped at the same time.

ENVIRONMENTAL FACTORS REPRESENTED WITHIN CONTEMPORARY MODELS OF DISABILITY

Conceptual models of disability have also shifted towards a person-in-context perspective. Influenced in large part by the social model of disability, disability has been recently redefined as a socially constructed experience that can be explained in part by the perceived absence or inadequacy of supports in the individual's external environment, which limits his or her participation.[16-19] Several conceptual models have been proposed for use by practitioners intending to assess and intervene in the lives of children with physical and intellectual disabilities. These models are intended to shift emphasis away from the child's impairment, resulting in a component-focused intervention, and towards top-down approaches to intervention[20] whereby the practitioner considers environmental changes when attempting to facilitate a client's engagement in everyday activities.

Researchers have developed models that draw explicit attention to a range of environmental factors as they contribute to participation in occupations by children and families,[21,22] the presentation of an intellectual disability[23,24] or the overall functioning of children with disabilities.[25] In these models, the environment is conceptualized as external to the individual, consisting of both physical and social elements, which can be classified in up to six areas. Key environmental domains captured across these practice models include the physical (objects, spaces), economic (finances, employment, insurance), social (trained staff, family, siblings, pets), institutional (inclusion policies, information, child care), and cultural (disability awareness, attitudes, group customs) aspects. The social environment has further been described as encompassing activity features that support or challenge a child's participation, such as the ways in which activities are carried out within a school day.[26] These activity features are probably influenced by legal policies and/or cultural customs of a particular community and further broaden the concept of the environment.

TRANSLATING THE CONCEPT OF ENVIRONMENT TO SUPPORT BETTER MEASUREMENT

The environment is considered to play a critical role in developmental and disablement processes for children with and without disabilities. For this reason, researchers and practitioners need to be equipped with measures that address these environmental factors in order to develop, implement and evaluate rehabilitation services directed towards these two outcomes. The International Classification of Functioning, Disability and Health, Children and Youth version (ICF-CY) has emerged as one of the most prominent international models, emphasizing the importance of environmental factors and advancing the research agenda by defining the concept in a way that supports measurement development.[27] Grounded in a biopsychosocial model, the ICF implies a positive and universal perspective of disability. This dynamic view of disability is congruent with the developmental systems model, in that child–environment interactions underlie both the development and disablement processes.[28] The classification of disability is based upon the nature and severity of a child's functional limitations.

The environmental factors represented in the ICF are considered external to the individual but interact with health conditions to support or challenge functional outcomes at the body structure and function, and activity and participation level of analysis. The ICF-CY classifies the environment along five key dimensions. The physical environment is depicted as being composed of both the *products and technology (e110–e165)* in an individual's immediate environment, as well as the *natural and human-made changes to that environment (e210–e260)*. The social dimensions of the environment include the people or animals that provide *support and opportunity for relationships (e310–e360)*, and the cultural aspects of environment include the *attitudes (e410–e465)*, values and beliefs that are consequences of the customs, practices, ideologies and norms within the individual's cultural group. Finally, there is recognition of the broader *services, systems and policies (e510–e595)* that provide structured opportunities designed to meet the needs of an individual in everyday life.

The environmental factors described in the ICF-CY are congruent with the physical, social, cultural and socioeconomic features represented in both contemporary developmental and disablement models. In the remainder of this chapter, we focus on the physical, social and attitudinal dimensions of the environment and use the ICF-CY as a structural guide to inform our search, selection and reporting of the best available measures for capturing these specific domains in research and practice.

General factors to consider when measuring this domain

Researchers and practitioners are seeking environmental measures to gather information about the environmental factors most supportive of children in terms of their development and function in everyday life. Quantitative assessment of the extent to which the environment supports or challenges a child can be accomplished in a variety of ways. In this section, we discuss two issues that are important to consider in the development and use of environmental measures. These issues are (1) the purpose of the assessment and (2) whose voice is represented.

WHAT IS THE PURPOSE?

Environmental measures have been developed for one of three intended purposes, each of which lends itself to a different format according to who is expected to receive the information (i.e. the target audience), and what level of detail and type of information is needed for effective decision-making. According to Bedell and Coster,[29] measures are generally developed to support one or more of the following purposes: (1) individualized assessment, (2) programme evaluation and (3) population-based assessment. Individual assessments of environmental factors would be longer and provide the most depth in terms of content coverage in one or more content areas. The purpose of individual assessment of the environment is to help practitioners, families and researchers identify supports and barriers and provide direction for the purpose of planning interventions directed towards modifying one or more aspects of an environment to promote positive outcomes for children with disabilities. These measures would be developed for the purposes of describing and documenting individual-level change. When using an environment measure developed for the purpose of programme evaluation, a stakeholder (e.g. programme director) can either gather information about the most prevalent supports and barriers among a group of clients or compare groups of clients within a single programme. This information can inform decisions about allocation of resources and programme development. Similarly, measures developed for the purpose of population-based assessment enable one to gather information about environmental factors to assess how and to what extent they predict key functional outcomes in terms of activity engagement, participation and improved quality of life. These measures tend to be short

and general in their coverage of key content areas. The information gleaned from these types of measures can be most directly used to inform policy decisions and the allocation of limited resources.

WHOSE VOICE IS REPRESENTED?

Stakeholders are typically invited into the process of measurement development as content experts. Their perspectives are often used to inform the selection of content areas, item wording and response options to increase the likelihood that information gleaned from these measures is both accurate and meaningful to the needs and priorities of the client population being described as well as the intended user.[29,30] Stakeholders typically include expert researchers, administrators and practitioners who carry scientific and/or service-related expertise. However, constituent perspectives can also include those of the parent and/or child who carry expertise derived through the lived experience. The selection of whose voice is represented is typically determined according to (1) who is expected to be the ultimate respondent for the measure, (2) age and developmental considerations and (3) disability-specific issues and challenges.

PARENT PERSPECTIVE

Parent perspectives about environmental factors have most commonly been captured for descriptive purposes. Parents of children with physical disabilities commonly report on the physical design and accessibility of settings,[17,31] social attitudes,[17,32] institutional policies, services and resources[18,31] and the availability of well-trained staff.[19,32] Qualitative methods have also been used to examine parent-reported strategies for promoting the social participation of adolescents with TBI[33] and the 10 types of accommodations that parents describe employing to enable them to sustain daily life while raising a young child with a developmental delay.[34] In these studies, parents seem to consider a host of child, family and environmental factors in selecting a strategy that will guide their response to a situation.

Additional insights have been gained when parent perspectives have been elicited to inform measurement development in this domain. A recent study of environmental supports and barriers for children with physical disabilities is the first large, quantitative examination of environmental factors.[35] In this research, the Craig Hospital Inventory of Environmental Factors (CHIEF)[36] was used to assess supports and barriers. Results of this research indicated that parents of children with physical disabilities experienced the most pronounced environmental barriers in the areas of school and work that were attributed to the physical/structural environment and institutional policies. The perspectives of parents of children with and without disabilities have provided additional insights about the types of environmental factors associated with the social participation of children and adolescents with physical, intellectual and emotional/behavioural disabilities in the specified settings of home, school and community to inform the development of a new parent-report survey of children's participation and environment.[37] Results of these earlier studies point to the need for greater specificity in the information derived from use of environmental measures, according to setting and/or type of activity. In addition, prior studies involving children with intellectual and emotional/behavioural disabilities have drawn increasing attention to the lack of understanding from peers and adults as a major barrier to inclusion that are seldom addressed adequately through measurement.[38,39]

CHILD PERSPECTIVE

Gathering perspectives about environmental factors from children with and without disabilities is important for informing the design of environment measures but, owing to age and condition-specific factors, has challenged researchers.[29,30] Despite challenges associated with the process of gathering the child's perspective, there is some research evidence to suggest that children provide unique insights and differ in their perspectives about environmental factors when compared with each other and with their parents. Whereas children with physical disabilities commonly report on issues of access, services and resources,[18] adolescents and young adults with intellectual disabilities emphasize choice-making opportunities, social and emotional support (e.g. staff attention and assistance, family involvement in decision-making), assistive technology (i.e. set-up and implementation) and positive staff attitudes (e.g. interactive and motivated staff) as impacting their community participation.[40] Harding et al[41] completed a pilot study of children's perceptions of participation and environment using a measure of participation (Children's Assessment of Participation and Enjoyment), child-taken photographs of activities and semi-structured interviews. Findings indicate that the children's experience of environment and place is closely connected with each specific activity. In a recent study conducted by the authors, a small sample of children with disabilities reported on a broader range of relationships when describing people whose attitudes matter: parents, professionals, extended family, peers, siblings and pets, and they emphasized having the opportunity to make choices as an activity feature influencing participation.[42] Methods for child data collection in these studies varied and included focus group, interview, observation and photography.

Overview of recommended measures

While there is evidence that environmental factors have a major effect on the participation of children with disabilities, the measurement of these environmental factors remains relatively unsophisticated. There is currently a small group of instruments designed to measure the impact of the environments for children with disabilities, including the physical but also the social and attitudinal dimensions that together comprise a primary focus in this chapter. There are various ways to classify and describe the measures that have been developed. As a starting point, we have chosen to search for and sort a set of existing measures according to the extent to which individual items correspond with the key characteristics of the environment as outlined in the ICF-CY. We recognize that some of the measures described in this chapter were developed using different conceptual frameworks that were available before the emergence of the ICF-CY. We examined the match between current measurement tools and the ICF-CY codes, as this type of item review can provide a basis for (1) comparing content across measures, in terms of similarities and differences in item wording and scaling options and (2) identifying areas where new measures may be needed to address gaps or areas of inadequate coverage. This type of review is in line with larger efforts to ensure that new and existing measures of environment are congruent with the scope and terminology of the ICF-CY, to help practitioners and researchers (1) develop functional profiles by documenting the range of environmental factors impacting young children with disabilities in everyday life; (2) facilitate the use of a common language to ease interdisciplinary dialogue around environmental factors, which, in turn, promotes integrated service planning; and (3) design studies to test proposed relationships among the elements of the ICF-CY framework and hypothesized pathways to outcomes (e.g. participation) within and across subgroups receiving rehabilitation services.[30,41,42] In the remainder of this section, we outline the process we used to complete a review of measures for children aged 0 to 18 years. This item review provides an overview of available options for the documentation of environmental factors and answers the question, 'How well do items from existing measures fit with the characterization of environment (i.e. ICF-CY codes) for children with disabilities?'

CONTENT REVIEW OF AVAILABLE MEASURES:
METHOD

The content review consisted of two major phases. First, a comprehensive literature search was conducted using PsycINFO, Hispanic American Periodicals Index (HAPI), PubMed, CINAHL (Cumulative Index to Nursing and

Allied Health Literature) and the Education Resources Information Center (ERIC) databases to identify measures with information about physical, social and attitudinal factors in the environment as they exert influence on the lives of children with disabilities. The following search terms were employed: environment, supports, facilitators, barriers, resources, social factors, social relationships, physical factors, attitudes, child, family, assessment, measurement, instrument development, reliability, validity, outcome measure, consistency, self-report and survey. Search limits included articles published within the past 20 years and English language. In addition, author searches were conducted, and all reference lists from retrieved publications were reviewed to identify additional studies involving the development or use of environment measures, and experts in the field were contacted for feedback in identifying measures that were under development. The search resulted in 21 initial hits, of which 18 measures were retrieved and included for review. Two measures were identified but excluded from this review because of their exclusive focus on the influence of services, systems and policies. Table 30.1 provides a complete list of the measures that were reviewed.

We completed a content review of the retrieved measures using the Outcome Measures Rating Form.[45] This structured form is designed to help a practitioner select an appropriate measure for clinical use and compare instruments that were designed for the same purpose. The form enables the rater to identify the focus of the measure according to ICF dimensions, as well as evaluate the clinical utility, scale construction, standardization, reliability and validity of the measure. For this review, two research assistants independently rated items from each measure according to their fit with the ICF-CY environment codes for each of the five domains and convened to achieve consensus through discussion. No formal assessment of inter-rater reliability was performed. The lead research assistant then transferred the final ratings for each measure to create a summary table (Table 30.1).

OVERVIEW OF SELECTED MEASURES: RESULTS
There are several ways of describing the measures that were identified and retrieved for this content review. To provide a standard for comparison, we will describe measures first according to the extent to which measures achieve broad representation of the five environmental domains depicted by the ICF-CY. This point of comparison yields three major groupings, and within each of these groupings we will briefly highlight other relevant features when considering use of these measures, including their purpose (population, programme, individual) and respondent (self-report, proxy, observation).

As Table 30.1 illustrates, there are six measures that appear to have the most comprehensive coverage of the environmental factors represented by the five content areas outlined in the ICF-CY. Each measure involves report by proxy, focuses explicitly on environmental factors and has been primarily used in large-scale population research. The Child and Adolescent Scale of Environment (CASE) contains three broad items that are intended to capture elements of both aspects of the natural and built environment, including the design and layout of public and private buildings as well as the general layout of spaces in the home, school and community. There are seven measures that capture four of the five content areas depicted by the ICF-CY coding structure. These measures address products and technology as well as types of social supports and relationships but differ with respect to content coverage across the other three domains. The Home Observation for Measurement of the Environment (HOME) explicitly focuses on the documentation of environmental factors and addresses all domains except for characteristics of the natural or built environment. It has been designed for use in large-scale population studies. In contrast, the primary purpose of the Ecocultural Family Interview (EFI), Family Needs Survey, Family Resources Survey and Family Needs Scale is individualized assessment with an explicit focus on environmental factors of families raising young children with developmental disabilities. These measures use the parent as proxy. Based on this item review, there are five measures that capture three or fewer content areas as represented by the ICF-CY coding structure. None of these measures addresses the services, systems and policies domain. Some of these measures focus on environmental factors influencing a child's participation in specified settings (home/housing, school) or situations (play). They vary in terms of their purpose, with some measures being developed for primary use in population assessment, such as the Participation and Environment Inventory, whereas others, such as the Test of Environmental Supportiveness (TOES), have been developed for use in individual assessment and are in the beginning stages of development from a psychometric point of view. This measure is also distinct in terms of being an observational assessment.

DETAILED DESCRIPTION OF KEY MEASURES
In the remainder of this chapter, we highlight a select group of measures to describe in detail. In light of what is currently available in the field for measuring this domain, we propose that these measures best capture the impact of physical, social and attitudinal environments for children with disabilities. The measures selected for inclusion

TABLE 30.1
Items from existing measures and the ICF-CY environmental domains

Name of measure	Products and technology	Natural environment and human-made changes to environment	Support and relationships	Attitudes	Services, systems and policies
Measures addressing environmental factors across *all five* content areas of the ICF-CY (listed alphabetically)					
Child and Adolescent Scale of Environment (CASE)	5	0	5	2	6
European Child Environment Questionnaire (ECEQ)	23	2	17	10	10
Facilitators and Barriers Survey (FABS/M)	50	5	15	9	3
Home Observation for Measurement of the Environment (HOME) – Middle Childhood	16	2	24	12	3
Measure of the Quality of the Environment (MQE)	22	18	5	9	33
Paediatric CHIEF	5	2	4	2	8
Participation and Environment Measure for Children and Youth (PEM-CY)	3	8	3	3	5
Measures addressing environmental factors across *four* content areas of the ICF-CY (listed alphabetically)					
Ecocultural Family Interview	5	0	17	9	10
Family Needs Survey	5	1	7	6	0
Family Resources Survey	14	4	6	0	8
Family Needs Scale	6	0	3	0	8
Home Observation for Measurement of the Environment (HOME) – Infant Toddler	12	0	24	5	4
Home Observation for Measurement of the Environment (HOME) – Early Childhood	18	1	29	1	0
Participation and Environment Inventory	6	1	4	4	0
Measures addressing environmental factors in *up to three* content areas of the ICF-CY (listed alphabetically)					
Designing the Home for Children: A Self-Report Measure	12	2	0	13	0
Housing Enabler	150	0	0	0	0
Multidimensional Scale of Perceived Social Support (MSPSS)	0	0	12	0	0
Test of Environmental Supportiveness (TOES)	12	3	27	0	0

meet the following criteria: (1) the measure includes items that address at least three of the five ICF-CY chapters for environment and address aspects pertaining to the physical (products and technology, natural environment and human-made changes to environment), social (social supports and relationships) and attitudinal (values, beliefs) environment; *and* (2) the measure has reported psychometric evidence to support consideration for use in research and practice with children and youth with disabilities. Family functioning and family needs measures were specifically excluded as they are described in Chapters 31 and 32.

The European Child Environment Questionnaire (ECEQ) is a 60-item measure that covers all five environmental domains as represented in the ICF-CY and is in the earlier stages of development with respect to psychometric evidence. Although the ECEQ is not described

in detail within this last section, there has been, and will probably be, more use of this measure by researchers in the field to gather information about the impact of environmental influences on the participation patterns of large groups of children aged 8 to 12 years with cerebral palsy.[46] The Participation and Environment Inventory[47] is a large-scale survey that has been developed for use in documenting the types of barriers experienced by children nationally as related to their participation in educational activities. Descriptions of this measure as reported in the literature[45] suggest that its validation is in progress and is not yet appropriate for general use. The Facilitators and Barriers Survey for People with Mobility Impairments (FABS/M)[48,49] was developed along with a measure of participation and is intended as a self-report measure to assess the influence of environmental interventions for individual and population-based assessment. This

CHILD AND ADOLESCENT SCALE OF ENVIRONMENT (CASE)	
Purpose	The CASE assesses physical, social and attitudinal environmental barriers of children and youth with disabilities as reported by parents or other primary guardians. It was initially designed as part of the Child and Family Follow-up Survey (CFFS) to monitor outcomes and needs of children and youth with acquired brain injuries discharged from inpatient rehabilitation (*n*=60)
Population	Data have been collected on children and youth with acquired brain injuries and other disabling conditions (*n*=285; personal communication with author)
Description of domains (subscale)	The CASE was adapted from the Craig Hospital Inventory of Environmental Factors (CHIEF; Whiteneck et al, 2004), an existing instrument designed to assess the frequency and impact of environmental barriers experienced by adults with disabilities. The CASE has 18 items addressing the impact of problems experienced with physical, social and attitudinal environment features of the child's home, school and community and problems related to the quality or availability of services or assistance that the child may need in these settings. Items address problems with the physical design and layout of the setting; lack of support and encouragement for the child at the setting; problems with attitudes on the part of others towards the child at the setting; inadequate or lack of resources such as services, equipment, finances; information about the child's condition and/or interventions; family stress; neighbourhood crime/violence; and problems with government agencies/policies
Administration and test format	Time: approximately 10min (if done separately from larger CFFS) Testing format: 18 items. Can be done as part of the larger CFFS or separately. Can be done as self-report or administered as part of an in-person or phone interview Scoring: three-point ordinal scale (1=no problem; 2=little problem; 3=big problem). CASE summary scores are created by summing the item responses, dividing this number by the maximum possible score, and multiplying this number by 100 to conform to a 100-point scale. Higher scores indicate a greater extent of problem Training: no training needed
Psychometric properties	*Reliability* Internal consistency: Cronbach's alpha=0.91 (Bedell and Dumas, 2004) and 0.85 based on recent analyses (*n*=285; personal communication) Test–retest: intraclass correlation coefficient=0.75 and Spearman's rho coefficient=0.78; *n*=33 (Bedell and Dumas, 2004) *Validity* Content: feedback obtained from parents of children with acquired brain injury, measurement and content experts Construct validity: higher CASE scores (greater impact of problems) significantly associated with lower scores on the Child Adolescent Scale of Participation (CASP) (more restricted participation) and Paediatric Evaluation of Disability Index (PEDI) mobility and social function subscales (more limited functional skills). Results from factor analyses and Rasch analyses suggest that the CASE is best viewed as an inventory of environmental factors or multidimensional scale rather than a unidimensional scale (Bedell, 2004). Recent factor analyses identified four main factors explaining 58% of the variance: (1) problems associated with home/community (includes inadequate information, problems with government policies); (2) problems related to school (support, assistance, services, equipment, attitudes); (3) problems with physical design of school, home and community; (5) other family/neighbourhood problems (family stress, problems with finances, inadequate transportation and neighbourhood crime/violence (personal communication with author) Responsiveness: not assessed

How to order	Additional information about the CASE can be obtained by contacting Dr Gary Bedell (gary.bedell@tufts.edu)
Key references	Bedell G (2004) Developing a follow-up survey focused on participation of children and youth with acquired brain injuries after inpatient rehabilitation. *NeuroRehabilitation* 19: 191–205.
	Bedell G, Dumas H (2004) Social participation of children and youth with acquired brain injuries discharged from inpatient rehabilitation: a follow-up study. *Brain Injury* 18: 65–82.
	Whiteneck G, Harrison-Felix CL, Melick D, Brookes CA, Charlifue S, Gerhart KA (2004) Quantifying environmental factors: a measure of physical, attitudinal, service, productivity, and policy barriers. *Arch Phys Med Rehabil* 85: 1324–1335.

HOME OBSERVATION FOR MEASUREMENT OF THE ENVIRONMENT (HOME)

Purpose	The HOME is a tool designed for investigating the stimulation potential of the home (quality and quantity of available social, emotional and cognitive support)
Population	There are three versions of the HOME instrument: Infant/toddler: 0–3y; Early childhood: 3–6y; Middle childhood: 6–10y
Administration and test format	Testing format: Infant/toddler: 45-item checklist divided into six subscales (parental responsivity, acceptance of child, organization of the environment, play materials, involvement with child, variety of stimulation) Early childhood: 55-item checklist with eight subscales Middle childhood: 55-item checklist with eight subscales Time: 60min Scoring: interview and observation, each behaviour assessed based on observation present (+) or absent (−), yielding a sum score Training: workshops and videotapes available for training
Psychometric properties	*Reliability* Internal consistency: infant/toddler, Cronbach's alpha=0.84; early childhood, Cronbach's alpha=0.93; middle childhood, Cronbach's alpha unknown. Test–retest: infant/toddler, intraclass correlation coefficient (ICC)=0.24–0.70; early childhood, ICC=0.05–0.70; middle childhood, ICC unknown. *Validity* Criterion: positively correlates with measures of early cognitive development and IQ Construct: discriminates between supportive and 'at-risk' homes
How to order	See Bradley RH, Caldwell BM (1979) Home observation for measurement of the environment: a revision of the preschool scale. *Am J Ment Deficiency* 84: 235–244.
Key reference	Elardo R, Bradley R, Caldwell BM (1977) A longitudinal study of the relation of infants' home environments to language development at age three. *Child Dev* 48: 595–603.

measure has been primarily validated on adults aged 17 to 92 years across a variety of diagnoses.

The following seven measures will be described in detail within this section (listed alphabetically): Child and Adolescent Scale of Environment (CASE); Home Observation for Measurement of the Environment (HOME) – Infant/Toddler, Early Childhood, and Middle Childhood; Measure of the Quality of the Environment (MQE); Craig Hospital Inventory of Environmental Factors (CHIEF); School Function Assessment (SFA) – Task Supports subscale; Test of Environmental Supportiveness (TOES); and Participation and Environment Measure for Children and Youth (PEM-CY). Each measure is described separately in the tables below.

It should be noted that items from the SFA – Task Supports subscale were difficult to fit directly with the ICF-CY chapter codes. This measure addresses the environment in terms of the use of human assistance and/or adaptations (modifications of equipment, environment, activity, programme) as needed to complete specified school tasks. This measure includes a checklist of nine specific types of adaptations that may be relevant in a set of physical and cognitive/behavioural tasks. The SFA links environmental factors to performance at a more specified level, can be used for population, programme and individual assessment and has psychometric evidence to support its use. For these reasons, this subscale will be included in this section and is described below.

MEASURE OF THE QUALITY OF THE ENVIRONMENT (MQE)	
Purpose	To measure the influence of environmental factors on the realization of life habits in relation to a person's functional capabilities
Population	Developed for use with a heterogeneous group of people with different conditions, to describe participation that takes place in generic settings
Administration and test format	Testing format: 109 items addressing the following six domains: support and attitudes of family; income, job and income security; governmental and public services; physical environment and accessibility; technology; and equal opportunity and political orientations. Response options: seven-point Likert scale ranging from –3 to 3 (–3=major obstacle, –2=medium obstacle, –1=minor obstacle, 0=no influence, 1=minor facilitator, 2=medium facilitator, 3=major facilitator), and each item includes options for 'I do not know' and 'does not apply'
	Timing: approximately 45 min
	Scoring: it is possible for users to aggregate the individual scoring of each item to get the scoring of more general environmental factor categories
	Training: the International Network on the Disability Creation Process (INDCP) is currently in the process of producing a user's guide for those interested in administering the MQE. A training workshop is in development for use of the MQE
Psychometric properties	*Reliability*
	Test–retest: r=0.60–0.85
	Validity
	Validation studies have been completed, and results are available in French. Please contact Francis Charrier for more information
How to order	Can be purchased from www.ripph.qc.ca/ (CA$23)
	For more information about this measure, please contact Francis Charrier, Co-ordinator, International Network on the Disability Creation Process (INDCP) at francis.charrier@ irdpq.qc.ca
Key references	Boschen K, Fougeyrollas P, Noreau L (1997) Measure of the quality of environment – reliability study. *Can J Rehabil* 11: 13–14.
	Fougeyrollas P, Noreau L, Michel G, Boschen K (1999) Measure of the Quality of Environment (MQE) Version 2. Lac Saint Charles, QC: INDCP-C.P. 225.

CRAIG HOSPITAL INVENTORY OF ENVIRONMENTAL FACTORS (CHIEF)

Purpose	Designed to capture five characteristics of the environment that are barriers to participation for people with a disability
Population	This measure was designed for adults aged 16–95y. With permission from the authors, parent proxy versions for children with disabilities have been used (Law et al, 2007)
Description of domains (subscale)	There are five subscales or domains that are measured: Policies subscale: *policies businesses, *policies government, policies employment/education and services community. Physical/structural subscale: *surroundings, *natural environment, design home, design community, design work/school and technology. Work/school subscale: *attitudes work/school, *help work/school and support work/school. Attitudes/support subscale: *attitudes home, *discrimination, support community, attitudes community and support home. Services/assistance subscale: *transportation, *medical care, *help home, *information, education/training, help community and personal equipment. *Items retained in the CHIEF short version
Administration and test format	Testing format: there are two versions of the CHIEF: long version (25 items) and short version (12 items). It can be self-administered or interviewer administered. There is a frequency score that measures how often (daily to never [0–4]) and a magnitude score that measures to what extent (no problem, big problem, little problem [0–2]) each item is a barrier or limitation to participation across the environments of school and work, community, recreational, social and civil activities in the past 12 months. A frequency–magnitude score is the total of frequency and magnitude combined indicating the overall impact of the barrier
Psychometric properties	*Reliability* Total scale score intraclass correlation coefficient (ICC) of 0.926. Parents or family members of adults with a disability were asked to be a proxy that resulted in a total score ICC of 0.618, indicating that proxy versions should not be used for adults. Test–retest reliability is currently being assessed for a paediatric version of the CHIEF *Validity* Most items and subscales showed statistically significant differences among impairment groups when validated with adults (Whiteneck et al, 2004). Parent proxy versions for children have showed significant relationships between age, school and work and natural and built environment characteristics as reported by parents of children with physical disabilities (Law et al, 2007)
How to order	Contact Cindy Harrison-Felix (charrison-felix@craighospital.org)
Key references	Craig Hospital Research Department (2001) *Craig Hospital Inventory of Environmental Factors (CHIEF)*. Englewood, CO: Craig Hospital. Law M, Petrenchik T, King G, Hurley P (2007) Perceived environmental barriers to recreation, community, and school participation for children and youth with physical disabilities. *Arch Phys Med Rehabil* 88: 1636–1642. Whiteneck GG, Harrison-Felix CL, Mellick DC, Brooks CA, Charlifue SB, Gerhart KA (2004) Quantifying environmental factors: a measure of physical, attitudinal, service, productivity, and policy barriers. *Arch Phys Med Rehabil* 85: 1324–1335.

SCHOOL FUNCTION ASSESSMENT (SFA) – TASK SUPPORTS

Purpose	To measure a student's performance of functional tasks that support his or her participation in the academic and social aspects of an elementary school programme (from kindergarten to sixth grade). The SFA was designed to facilitate collaborative programme planning for students with a variety of disabling conditions

Population	Children enrolled in kindergarten to sixth grade
Description of domains (subscales)	The SFA is composed of three parts:
	Part I: Participation examines the student's level of participation in six major school activity settings: regular or special education classroom, playground or break, transportation to and from school, bathroom and toileting activities, transitions to and from class, and mealtime or snack time
	Part II: Task Supports examines supports currently provided to the student when he or she performs school-related functional tasks that are required to participate effectively in an educational programme. Two types of task supports are examined separately: assistance (adult help) and adaptations (modifications to the environment or programme, such as specialized equipment or adapted materials)
	Part III: Activity Performance examines the student's performance of specific school-related functional activities. Each scale includes a comprehensive set of activities that examine in detail one of the tasks addressed globally in Part II, such as moving around the classroom and the school, using school materials, interacting with others, following school rules and communicating needs
Administration and test format	Testing format: a judgement-based (questionnaire) assessment completed by one or more school professionals who know the student well and have observed his or her typical performance on the school-related tasks and activities being assessed. Items are written in measurable behavioural terms that can be used directly in the student's individual educational plan. The Task Supports subscales include 18 tasks that fall into one of two domains: physical or cognitive/behavioural tasks
	Response options: assistance (1=extensive assistance, 2=moderate assistance, 3=minimal assistance, 4=no assistance) and adaptations (1=extensive adaptations, 2=moderate adaptations, 3=minimal adaptations, 4=no adaptations)
	Time: 5–10min
	Scoring: item ratings are summed, then a look-up table is used to transform the raw score total into a score on a 0–100 criterion scale. Each of the four scales is independent; there is no aggregate score
	Training: none required. Detailed instructions are in the manual and in the Rating Scale Guide
Psychometric properties	*Reliability*
	Internal consistency: Cronbach's alpha=0.92–0.98 across all subscales. Consistency also confirmed through examination of results of Rasch analyses (item fit)
	Test–retest: intraclass correlation coefficient =0.92–0.99 across all subscales
	Validity
	Content: structured review conducted on pilot and tryout editions with related service professionals and classroom teachers
	Criterion: SFA positively correlates with related sections of Vineland Adaptive Behaviour Scales – Classroom edition (Hwang et al, 2002)
	Construct: supportive evidence obtained from analyses testing key hypotheses using standardization data: performance varies by context; environmental supports contribute to predicting task performance; participation is predicted by performance of setting-related tasks (Coster et al, 1998); differentiates performance of typical elementary student from children with disabilities; differentiates children with cerebral palsy, learning disabilities and autism (Hwang et al, 2002).
	Responsiveness
	Change in participation and resource requirement scores after intervention, not in mobility (King et al, 1998)
How to order	The SFA can be purchased from Pearson Education at http://pearsonassess.com/

Key references	Coster WJ, Deeney T, Haltiwanger J, Haley S (1998) *School Function Assessment.* San Antonio, TX: The Psychological Corporation/Therapy Skill Builders.
	Hwang J, Davies P, Taylor M, Gavin W (2002) Validation of School Function Assessment with elementary school children. *OTJR: Occupation, Participation and Health* 22: 48–58.
	King G, Tucker M, Alambers P, Gritzan J, MacDougall J, Ogilvie A, et al (1998) The evaluation of functional, school-based therapy services for children with special needs: a feasibility study. *Phys Occupat Ther Paediatr* 18: 1–27.

TEST OF ENVIRONMENTAL SUPPORTIVENESS (TOES)

Purpose	Designed to be administered in conjunction with the Test of Playfulness (ToP) and explicate the ways in which a child's playfulness is affected by the environment to facilitate intervention planning and consultation with caregivers
Population	Children 1.5–15y, both with and without disabilities
Administration and test format	Testing format: 17-item observational assessment addressing caregivers, playmates, play objects, space and quality of the sensory environment. Response options: a descriptive profile is generated by rating each item according to a five-point response scale, ranging from −2 to 2
	Time taken: 15- to 20-min free play session
	Scoring: 5–10min, completed after a 15- to 20-min free play session in the child's natural environment. No summary score available at this time, as the measure is in the early phases of development
	Training: minimal rater training. There is a manual available upon request from the author
Psychometric properties	*Reliability*
	No information
	Validity
	16 of 17 items shown to have acceptable goodness of fit statistics using Rasch analysis and conform to the measurement model. Data from 95% of children, both with and without disabilities, tested (*n*=160) demonstrated goodness of fit to the Rasch model
How to order	Published in Parham LD and Fazio LS, *Play in Occupational Therapy for Children*, 2nd edition. Copies of the text cost US$66.95 and can be ordered from www.us.elsevierhealth.com/index.jsp
	For more information about this measure, please contact Anita Bundy, University of Sydney (anita.bundy@sydney.edu.au)
Key references	Harding P (1997) Validity and reliability of a test of environmental supportiveness. Master's thesis, Colorado State University, Fort Collins, CO.
	Rogers M (1999) A correlational study of a test of playfulness and a test of environmental supportiveness. Master's thesis, Colorado State University, Fort Collins, CO.

PARTICIPATION AND ENVIRONMENT MEASURE FOR CHILDREN AND YOUTH (PEM-CY)

Purpose	To examine children's participation in the home, school and community settings. For each of these three settings, the measure affords an opportunity to examine environmental factors that are perceived by parents/caregivers to support or challenge participation. Factors include activity demands (physical, cognitive, social) as well as physical layout, social supports, attitudes, resources (time, money) and services/policies

Population	Children and youth, with and without disabilities, aged 5–17y
Administration and test format	Testing format: completed by parents or primary guardians. The PEM-CY has been validated using a web-based format. A paper-and-pencil version will be available free of charge in the near future.
	Time: 20–30min
	Scoring: a clinimetric approach has been suggested when using the PEM-CY. The environmental supportiveness summary score can be computed by taking the sum of all the ratings and dividing by the number of items rated
	Training: an administration and scoring manual will be made available in the near future
Psychometric properties	*Reliability*
	Internal consistency: Cronbach's alphas ranged from 0.83 to 0.91 for the environmental supportiveness summary score across settings
	Test–retest: intraclass correlation coefficients ranged from 0.85 to 0.95 for the environmental supportiveness summary score across settings
	Validity
	Negative association between desire for change and environmental supportiveness (–0.42 to –0.59) was found
How to order	For more information about this measure, please contact the authors: Wendy Coster (wjcoster@bu.edu); Mary Law (lawm@mcmaster.ca); or Gary Bedell (gary.bedell@tufts.edu)
Key references	Bedell G, Khetani MA, Cousins MA, Coster WJ, Law MC (2011) Parent perspectives to inform development of measures of children's participation and environment. *Arch Phys Med Rehabil* 92: 765–773.
	Coster W, Bedell G, Law M, et al (2011) Psychometric evaluation of the Participation and Environment Measure for Children and Youth (PEM-CY). *Dev Med Child Neurol* 53: 1030–1037.
	Coster W, Law M, Bedell G, Khetani MA, Cousins M, Teplicky R (2012) Development of the Participation and Environment Measure for Children and Youth (PEM-CY): conceptual basis. *Disabil Rehabil* 34: 238–246.

Acknowledgements

We thank team members Rebecca Braman and Ariel Zwelling for their assistance with the item review of existing measures, the results of which are included in this chapter. We also thank Rebecca Slavin for assistance in retrieving information on measures described in detail in this chapter.

REFERENCES

1. Maulik PK, Darmstadt GL (2007) Childhood disability in low- and middle-income countries: overview of screening, prevention, services, legislation, and epidemiology. *Pediatrics* 120: S1–S55.
2. Brofenbrenner U (1979) *The Ecology of Human Development: Experiments by Nature and Design.* Cambridge, MA: Harvard University Press.
3. Ford DH, Lerner RM (1992) *Developmental Systems Theory: An Integrative Approach.* Thousand Oaks, CA: Sage.
4. Lerner RM (2002) *Concepts and Theories of Human Development.* Mahwah, NJ: Lawrence Erlbaum Associates.
5. Sameroff AJ, Chandler MJ (1975) Reproductive risk and the continuum of caretaking casualty. In: Horowitz FD, Hetherington M, Scarr-Salapatek S, Sigel G, editors. *Review of Child Development Research.* Chicago, IL: University of Chicago Press, pp. 187–244.
6. Sameroff AJ, Fiese BH (2000) Models of development and developmental risk. In: Zeanah CH, editor. *Handbook of Infant Mental Health*, 2nd edition. New York: Guilford Press, pp. 3–19.
7. Thelen E, Smith LB (1994) *A Dynamic Systems Approach to the Development of Cognition and Action.* Cambridge, MA: MIT Press.
8. Bruder MB (2001) Inclusion of infants and toddlers: outcomes and ecology. In: Guralnick MJ, editor. *Early Childhood Inclusion: Focus on Change.* Baltimore, MD: Brookes Publishing, pp. 203–229.

9. Dunst CJ (2001) Participation of young children with disabilities in community learning activities. In: Guralnick MJ, editor. *Early Childhood Inclusion: Focus on Change.* Baltimore, MD: Brookes Publishing, pp. 307–333.

10. Fiese BH, Tomcho TJ, Douglas M, Josephs K, Poltrock S, Baker T (2002) A review of 50 years of research on naturally occurring family routines and rituals: cause for celebration? *J Fam Psychol* 16: 381–390.

11. Hauser-Cram P, Howell A (2003) The development of young children with disabilities and their families: implications for policies and programs. In: Lerner RM, Jacobs F, Wertlieb D, editors. *Handbook of Applied Developmental Science*, Vol. 1. Thousand Oaks, CA: Sage Publications, pp. 259–279.

12. Keogh BK, Bernheimer LP, Gallimore R, Weisner TS (1998) Child and family outcomes over time: a longitudinal perspective on developmental delays. In: Lewis M, Feiring C, editors. *Families, Risk, and Competence.* Mahwah, NJ: Lawrence Erlbaum, pp. 269–287.

13. Rogoff B (2003) *The Cultural Nature of Human Development.* Oxford: Oxford University Press.

14. Weisner TS (2002) Ecocultural understanding of children's developmental pathways. *Hum Dev* 45: 275–281.

15. Baltes PB, Freund AM (1998) Selection, optimization, and compensation as strategies of life management: correction to Freund and Baltes (1998). *Psychol Aging* 14: 700–702.

16. Almqvist L, Granlund M (2005) Participation in school environment of children and youth with disabilities: a person-oriented approach. *Scand J Psychol* 46: 305–314.

17. Law M, Haight M, Milroy B, Willms D, Stewart D, Rosenbaum P (1999) Environmental factors affecting the occupations of children with physical disabilities. *J Occupat Sci* 6: 102–110.

18. Mihaylov SI, Jarvis SN, Colver AF, Beresford B (2004) Identification and description of environmental factors that influence participation of children with cerebral palsy. *Dev Med Child Neurol* 46: 299–304.

19. Rimmer J, Riley B, Wang E, Rauworth A, Jurkowski J (2002) Physical activity participation among persons with disabilities: barriers and facilitators. *Am J Prev Med* 26: 419–425.

20. Coster WJ (1998) Occupation-centered assessment of children. *Am J Occup Ther* 52: 337–344.

21. Law M, Cooper B, Strong S, Stewart D, Rigby P, Letts L (1996) The Person–Environment–Occupation Model: a transactive approach to occupational performance. *Can J Occup Ther* 63: 9–23.

22. Strong S (1998) Meaningful work in supportive environments: experiences with the recovery process. *Am J Occup Ther* 52: 31–38.

23. Cuskelly MM, Hayes A (2004) The evolving nature of intellectual disability: are all things old new again? *Int J Disabil Dev Educ* 511: 117–122.

24. Luckasson R, Brotwick-Duffy S, Buntinx W, et al (2002) *Mental Retardation: Definition, Classification, and Systems of Supports.* Washington, DC: American Association on Mental Retardation.

25. Fougeyrollas P, Noreau I, Bergeron H, Cloutier R, Dion S-A, St-Michel G (1998) Social consequences of long term impairments and disabilities: conceptual approach and assessment of handicap. *Int J Rehabil Res* 21: 127–141.

26. Kramer J, Bowyer P, Kielhofner G (2009) Evidence for practice from the Model of Human Occupation. In: Kielhofner G, editor. *Model of Human Occupation: Theory and Application*, 4th edition. Baltimore, MD: Lippincott and Williams and Wilkins, pp. 466–503.

27. World Health Organization (2001) *International Classification of Functioning, Disability, and Health.* Geneva: WHO.

28. Florian L, Hollenweger J, Simeonsson RJ, et al (2006) Cross-cultural perspectives on the classification of children with disabilities: Part 1. Issues in the classification of children with disabilities. *J Spec Educ* 40: 36–45.

29. Bedell GM, Coster WJ (2008) Measuring participation of school-age children with traumatic brain injuries: considerations and approaches. *J Head Trauma Rehabil* 23: 220–229.

30. Coster WJ, Khetani MA (2008) Measuring participation of children with disabilities: issues and challenges. *Disabil Rehabil* 30: 639–648.

31. Welsh B, Jarvis S, Hammal D, Colver A (2006) How might districts identify local barriers to participation for children with cerebral palsy? *Public Health* 120: 167–175.

32. McManus S, Michelsen I, Parkinson K, et al (2006) Discussion groups with parents of children with cerebral palsy in Europe designed to assist development of a relevant measure of environment. *Child Care Health Dev* 32: 185–192.

33. Bedell GM, Cohn ES, Dumas HM (2004) Exploring parents' use of strategies to promote social participation of school-age children with acquired brain injuries. *Am J Occup Ther* 59: 273–284.

34. Bernheimer LP, Keogh BK (1995) Weaving intervention into the fabric of everyday life: an approach to family assessment. *Top Early Child Spec Educ* 15: 415–433.

35. Law M, Petrenchik T, King G, Hurley P (2007) Perceived environmental barriers to recreational, community, and school participation for children with physical disabilities. *Arch Phys Med Rehabil* 88: 1636–1642.

36. Whiteneck G, Harrison-Felix, CL, Melick D, Brookes CA, Charlifue S, Gerhart KA (2004) Quantifying environmental factors: a measure of physical, attitudinal, service, productivity, and policy barriers. *Arch Phys Med Rehabil* 85: 1324–1335.

37. Bedell G, Khetani MA, Cousins M, Coster WJ, Law M (2011) Parent perspectives to inform development of measures of children's participation and environment. *Arch Phys Med Rehabil* 92: 765–773.

38. McDougall J, DeWit D, King G, Miller L, Killip S (2004) High school-aged youths' attitudes toward their peers with disabilities: the role of school and student interpersonal factors. *Int J Disabil Dev Educ* 51: 287–313.

39. Vignes C, Coley N, Grandjean H, Godeau E, Arnaud C (2008) Measuring children's attitudes towards peers with disabilities: a review of instruments. *Dev Med Child Neurol* 50: 182–189.

40. Verdonschot MML, de Witte LP, Reichrath E, Buntinx WHE, Curfs LMG (2009) Impact of environmental factors on the community participation of persons with an intellectual disability: a systematic review. *J Intellect Disabil Res* 53: 54–64.

41. Harding J, Harding K, Jamieson P, et al (2009) Children with disabilities' perceptions of activity participation and environments: a pilot study. *Can J Occup Ther* 76: 133–144.

42. Khetani MA, Bedell GM, Coster WJ, Law M (2009) Environmental influences on the social participation of children with developmental disabilities: Parent and child perspectives informing measurement development. Poster session presented at the 42nd annual Gatlinburg Conference on Research and Theory in Intellectual and Developmental Disabilities, New Orleans, LA, March.

43. Lollar DJ, Simeonsson RJ (2005) Diagnosis to function: classification for children and youths. *Dev Behav Pediatr* 26: 323–330.

44. Simeonsson RJ, Leonardi M, Lollar D, Bjorck-Akesson E, Hollenweger J, Martinuzzi A (2003) Applying the International Classification of Functioning, Disability, and Health to measure childhood disability. *Disabil Rehabil* 25: 605–610.

45. Law M (2004) Outcome Measures Rating Form. Available at: www.canchild.ca/en/canchildresources/resources/measrate.pdf (accessed 7 May 2012).

46. Forsyth R, Colver A, Alvanides S, Woolley M, Lowe M (2004) Participation of young severely disabled children is influenced

by their intrinsic impairments and environment. *Dev Med Child Neurol* 49: 345–349.

47. Simeonsson R, Carlson D, Huntington G, McMillen JS, Brent JL (2001) Students with disabilities: a national survey of participation in educational activities. *Disabil Rehabil* 23: 49–63.

48. Gray DB, Hollingsworth HH, Stark S, Morgan KA (2008) A subjective measure of environmental facilitators and barriers to participation for people with mobility limitations. *Disabil Rehabil* 30: 434–457.

49. Gray DB, Gould M, Bickenbach JE (2003) Environmental barriers and disability. *J Architect Plan Res* 20: 29–37.

31
ENVIRONMENTAL FACTORS: SUPPORT AND RELATIONSHIPS (E310–E399)

Aline Bogossian, Lucyna M. Lach and Michael Saini

What is the construct?

Within the broad construct of environmental factors, we review measures to assess the extent to which the child/adolescent, family and/or family members experience being supported. The International Classification of Functioning, Disability and Health-Children and Youth Version (ICF-CY)[1] defines the broad category of environmental factors as the 'physical, social and attitudinal environment in which people live and conduct their lives' (p. 189). These environmental factors may act as facilitators or barriers, contributing to, or getting in the way of, the extent to which individuals are able to participate in meaningful activities. The *UN Convention on the Rights of Individuals with Disabilities* identifies that these environmental factors are directly related to the disability creation process,[2] particularly when those environmental factors create barriers for people with disabilities. Among the environmental factors considered in the ICF-CY framework, *support and relationships* are considered key factors for considering the disability creation process. These include the *immediate family (e310; individuals related by birth, marriage or culturally defined as immediate family); extended family (e315; individuals related through family, marriage or culturally defined as extended family); friends (e320); acquaintances, peers, colleagues, neighbours and community members (e325); people in positions of authority (e330); people in subordinate positions (e335); personal care providers and personal assistants (e340); strangers (e345); domesticated animals (e350); health professionals (e355); and other professionals (e360)* (see Table 31.1). Support and relationships are defined as 'the people or animals that provide practical physical or emotional support, nurturing, protection, assistance and relationships to other persons, in their homes, place of work, school or at play or in other aspects of their daily activities' and refer to the 'amount of physical or emotional support' (p. 205)[1] provided to the individual. Each of these supportive relationship factors can have positive or negative influences on the disability creation process, depending on whether these factors are considered facilitators or barriers in supporting children and their families.

In this chapter, we explore a number of measures developed to assess quality, extent and process for supporting children and families. There are a number of measures that have been developed to evaluate the *immediate family environment* and the extent to which the child/adolescent, family and/or family members experience being supported. In the former, 'family' is broadly defined as the 'individuals related by birth, marriage or other relationship recognized by the culture as immediate family, such as spouses, partners, parents, siblings, children, foster parents, adoptive parents and grandparents' (p. 205). Measures evaluating different aspects of the family environment have been included even if they did not evaluate support per se. The rationale for this is that an adaptive, functional family environment is a support and is facilitative, whereas a family environment that indicates clinical distress is problematic and likely to represent a barrier to functioning and health.

Rather than focusing on support at the child level of analysis, we have broadened the analysis of support by also considering measures of how supported the family/family members feel. This represents a slight diversion from the ICF-CY framework in so far as the ICF-CY focuses on the extent to which the individual is supported, not the family or family members. Family support measures are important to the environmental framework because most children and adolescents are raised in a family environment, so consideration of the influence of support for both caregivers[3,4] and the children[5] is essential.

TABLE 31.1
Selected measures described in this overview

Family Adaptability and Cohesion Evaluation Scale (FACES)

Family Inventory of Life Events (FILE)

Family Crisis Oriented Personal Evaluation Scales (F-COPES)

Family Assessment Device (FAD)

Impact-on-Family Scale (IOF)

Family Environment Scale (FES)

Family Impact of Childhood Disability Scale (FICD)

Beach Center Family Quality of Life Scale (FQOL)

Family Support Scale (FSS)

Social Support Scale for Children (SSSC)

Factors to consider when measuring this domain

Clinicians and researchers interested in the evaluation of family environmental factors should first carefully consider the theoretical foundation for selecting the most appropriate measure that best corresponds with the goals and purposes of including family-based measures. Too often, measures of family function are used simply because they exist and because the measures have demonstrated sufficient reliability and validity in previous studies with similar populations. Although these are important considerations, the selection of an appropriate family measure must include a logical connection to the specific aspect of family environment proposed to be evaluated. For example, the practitioner may be interested in screening, in a general way, for difficulties in family function or family distress. Alternatively, the practitioner may be interested in the extent to which an intervention influences the proximity or level of conflict between family members, or how supported the family member feels. Each of these would require a different measure. There are a few ways to go about finding out what aspect of family environment should be evaluated:

1   *Theoretically.* Draw on existing ways of conceptualizing family environment and the quality of relationships among family members.
2   *Inductively.* Reflect on what is clinically relevant to measure (e.g. satisfaction, communication), and then search for measures that evaluate that characteristic of family function or environment. For observational studies, one could ask the question, 'What aspect of family life is of interest?' For intervention studies, one could ask, 'As a result of participating in this intervention, what is it about the family that I think will change?'

3   *Deductively.* Review the conceptual basis of family measures for their proximity to that which is considered clinically relevant. In other words, 'Do the items/subscales come close enough to evaluating what I think is useful and clinically relevant?'

Answering these questions will inevitably be informed by clinical observation as well as existing conceptual models of family function and the constructs embedded in those. Therefore, it is important to consider the various conceptualizations of family.

Family systems theory is a common framework used to evaluate families of children with disabilities because it operates from the position that each member in the family may be differentially impacted by the disability.[2,4] The primary feature of family systems theory is the notion of family as an interactional system that operates within structures (or subsystems). Interactions reflect family concepts such as adaptability, cohesion, boundaries and communication.[6] Viewing the family as an interactional system, family *adaptability* is the degree to which a family is flexible and can regain equilibrium in an environment that challenges core beliefs, values, traditions and rules for behaviours. Family *cohesion* refers to the degree of closeness and connectedness within a family. In 'normative' family function, cohesion is balanced in line with the developmental tasks of the family. *Boundaries* are the relational lines dividing individual family members and family subsystems (e.g. parents, parent–child, spouses) whose quality determine the extent of dependence or growth promotion inherent in a family system.[6] A family's ability to *communicate* in terms of both pragmatic and emotional issues is also considered in family assessment in the context of chronic illness or disability.

Family stress theories have evolved to explain the impact and pile-up of normative and non-normative life events that include acute and unanticipated stressors on the family.[7] Hill's[8] ABCX family crisis model posits that a family experiences differing degrees of stress depending on the stressor event, the family's crisis-meeting resources, and the meaning of the crisis to the family. McCubbin and Patterson[9] advanced the work of Hill[8] within the Double ABCX model. In this model, variables such as (1) the additional life stressors and strains that may influence the course of adaptation; (2) the crisis management resources (psychological, social, intrafamilial) utilized by the family; (3) the evolution of the meanings and definitions ascribed by the family to the event; (4) the coping strategies employed by the family; and (5) the continuum of outcomes shaped by the family efforts[9] are considered.

McCubbin and McCubbin[10] further expanded the Double ABCX model with a process model that delineates a family's course towards adaptation. The Resiliency Model has widely been used in the study of family adaptation in the context of childhood chronic illness or disability[11] and illustrates how a family adapts to stressors, strains and transitions. The model incorporates intervening variables that include family resources, social support, family types and function patterns, situational appraisal, appraisal by the family of the situation, and the family's problem-solving and coping abilities.

The McMaster Model of Family Functioning is a multidimensional model based on systems, roles and communication theory to assess the behaviours that produce relational processes within a family.[12,13] Within this model, the family is viewed as the location where the social, psychological and biological development of its members is maintained and supported[14] through a number of tasks ranging from basic provision of shelter and food to the management of crises such as illness and loss (death, economic loss, etc.).[12] The model describes structural, occupational and transactional properties of families and identifies six dimensions of family function: problem-solving, communication, roles, affective responses, affective involvement and behaviour control.

Similar to the McMaster Model, the Circumplex Model is also a multidimensional model grounded in systems theory. The Circumplex Model is fundamentally focused on the relational system and integrates three dimensions of family function: family cohesion (on a continuum from disengaged to enmeshed), flexibility (from rigid to chaotic) and communication.[15] The concept of cohesion is concerned with how the family system balances togetherness versus separateness and the extent of emotional bonding among family members. Flexibility refers to how the family system balances stability and change and the amount of change in its leadership, role relationships and relationship rules. Communication is considered a facilitating dimension that defines how a family alters levels of cohesion and flexibility.[15]

Overview of recommended measures

An additional source upon which to select the most appropriate measure is the conceptual foundation of the family measures themselves. Table 31.2 lists the measures that will be reviewed in this chapter. Each of the measures is briefly described with more detailed information provided in the summary tables. Some of these are linked to the conceptual family models discussed above, whereas others have their own unique conceptual framework that guides the construction of these measures. For example,

the Family Assessment Device (FAD)[16] measure is consistent with the model of family function developed by the McMaster group. The FAD subscales evaluate the constructs that the authors believe describe how a family functions. On the other hand, family systems theory[17] does not have a corresponding measure. The Family Inventory of Life Events (FILE) and the Family Crisis Oriented Personal Evaluation Scales (F-COPES) correspond to McCubbin and Patterson's[9] model, while the model underlying the Family Enviroment Scale (FES)[18] is inferred from the subscales.

Another important consideration is whether the measure was developed for use with children in general or with children with developmental disabilities. The first five (Family Adaptability and Cohesion Evaluation Scale [FACES], FILE, F-COPES, FAD and FES) are considered generic measures while the Impact-on-Family Scale (IOF) and the Family Impact of Childhood Disability Scale (FICD) are considered disability-related measures. The applicability of generic measures to children with disabilities provides an opportunity to compare the functioning of children with disabilities with that of children without disabilities; however, the relevance of items in a generic measure to children with disabilities is sometimes questionable and rarely are generic measures validated for use with children with disabilities.

FAMILY ADAPTABILITY AND COHESION EVALUATION SCALE

FACES, now in its fourth edition, is a 20-item instrument designed to measure two dimensions of family functioning – family cohesion and family flexibility.[19] FACES IV is designed to place families within the Circumplex Model. The Circumplex Model is designed to measure three key concepts for understanding family functioning. *Cohesion* is defined as the emotional bonding between family members. There are five levels of cohesion ranging on a continuum from disengaged (unbalanced), somewhat connected, connected, very connected or enmeshed (unbalanced). Family *flexibility* refers to the extent to which there is leadership, organization and clear roles and rules within a family. As in the case of measures of cohesion, five levels of flexibility range on a continuum from chaotic (unbalanced), very flexible, flexible, somewhat flexible and rigid (unbalanced). Finally, *communication* refers to the quality of communication skills evidenced within a couple or family system. In the Circumplex Model, communication is viewed as a facilitating dimension used by families to alter their levels of cohesion and flexibility. The Circumplex Model hypothesizes that balanced levels of cohesion and flexibility indicate healthy family functioning whereas unbalanced levels of cohesion

FAMILY ADAPTABILITY AND COHESION EVALUATION SCALE (FACES)

Purpose	FACES is a 42-item instrument designed to measure two dimensions of family functioning: family cohesion and family adaptability. It is plotted on the Circumplex Model of family functioning, which asserts that there are two central dimensions of family behaviour: family cohesion and family flexibility. FACES is intended for use with as many family members as possible to capture the complexity of the family system
Population	The items of the self-report instrument have been developed to be understandable and readable by family members aged 12 years and over
	The instrument can be administered to couples and families in all stages of the family life cycle
Description of domains (subscales)	FACES is composed of six family scales – two balanced and four unbalanced – with seven items each, giving a total of 42 items. The items are based on two dimensions of family functioning: cohesion and flexibility
	The family cohesion dimension refers to the degree to which family members are separated from or connected to their family
	Specific concepts that are used to measure and diagnose family cohesion are emotional bonding, boundaries, coalitions, time, space, friends, decision-making, interests and recreation
	The six levels of family cohesion are as follows: disengaged, somewhat connected, connected, very connected and enmeshed
	The family flexibility dimension refers to the extent to which a family system is flexible and able to change its structures, role relationships and relationship rules in response to situational or developmental stress
	Specific concepts that are used to measure and diagnose family adaptability are as follows: family power (assertiveness, control, discipline), negotiation style, role relationships and relationship rules
	The five levels of family flexibility are the following: chaotic, very flexible, flexible, somewhat flexible and rigid
Administration and test format	FACES-IV contains 42 items. A 10-item Family Communication Scale and 10-item Family Satisfaction Scale accompany the FACES-IV package
	The instrument was developed to provide a self-report measure on an individual basis, in larger groups or for families responding to a mailed survey
	Scoring: FACES is scored by summing all items to obtain a total score, summing all odd items to obtain the cohesion score, and summing even items to obtain the adaptability score. High cohesion scores indicate high enmeshment. High adaptability scores indicate a more chaotic family system
Psychometric properties	*Reliability*
	Internal consistency: alpha reliability on the internal consistency of the six scales range from 0.77 to 0.89
	Validity
	The validity of the balanced cohesion and flexibility and the unbalanced disengaged and chaotic scales are highly supported (range=0.89–0.99 for balanced regions of cohesion and flexibility; range=–0.67 to –0.93 for low extreme of cohesion and high extreme of flexibility). Weakness was noted in the rigid and enmeshed scales (range=–0.11 to –0.31)
How to order	Life Innovations Inc. (www.facesiv.com; cs@facesiv.com)
Key references	Olson D (2011) FACES IV & the Circumplex Model: validation study. *J Marital Fam Ther* 37: 67–80.

Olson DH (1986) Circumplex Model VII: validation studies and FACES III. *Fam Process* 25: 337–351.

Olson DH, Portner J, Lavee Y (1985) *FACES III*. Department of Family Social Science, University of Minnesota, St. Paul, MN, USA.

and flexibility – that is, extreme high or low levels – indicate problematic family functioning.

The 20-item FACES instrument evaluates how family members see their family (perceived) and how family members would like their family to be (ideal). The perceived–ideal discrepancy assesses each family member's satisfaction with the current family system. It is intended for use with all family members to capture the complexity of the family system.

FAMILY INVENTORY OF LIFE EVENTS

The FILE[20] is a self-administered 71-item instrument developed as an index of family stress to measure the cumulative normative and non-normative life events and changes experienced by a family in the preceding year. Items for the FILE have been informed by an integration of research and clinical experiences to represent situational and developmental changes experienced by families in the life course. Seven stages in the family life course have been delineated as (1) couple (no children); (2) preschool; (3) school age; (4) adolescent; (5) launching; (6) empty nest; (7) retirement.

The FILE encompasses nine conceptual domains: intrafamilial strains (17 items), marital strains (four items), pregnancy and childbearing strains (four items), finance and business strains (12 items), work–family transitions and strains (10 items), illness and family care strains (eight items), losses (six items), transitions 'in and out' (five items) and family legal violations (five items). FILE items centre on changes in the family system, resulting in adjustment and adaptation in family interaction patterns. Items are rated as 'yes' or 'no' and scores are summed by the total number of 'yes' responses or a standardized score. The FILE provides an index of vulnerability of the family that has been caused by the cumulative effect of stressful events.

FAMILY CRISIS-ORIENTED PERSONAL EVALUATION SCALES

The F-COPES,[21] derived from the Double ABCX model of family stress, is designed to identify problem-solving behaviours and strategies used by families in response to problems or crises. The instrument operationalizes the coping dimensions of the Double ABCX model and focuses on two levels of interaction: *internal*, the ways in which the family handles difficulties and problems that

arise among members of the family; and *external*, the ways in which the family handles difficulties that arise from the broader social environment but which affect family members.[22] The F-COPES is a 30-item, five-subscale inventory that assesses the domains of acquiring social support (nine items), reframing (redefining stressful events to make them more manageable) (eight items), seeking spiritual support (five items), mobilizing family to acquire and accept help (four items), and passive appraisal (ability to accept problematic issues) (four items).

MCMASTER FAMILY ASSESSMENT DEVICE

The McMaster FAD[16] is a 60-item questionnaire designed to evaluate family function according to the McMaster Model. The FAD operationalizes the six dimensions of family function (problem-solving, communication, roles, affective responses, affective involvement and behaviour control) and includes a seventh subscale, the general functioning dimension, which assesses overall health or pathology in its evaluation of family functioning.[23] Respondents are asked to indicate their agreement or disagreement (on a four-point scale) to a number of statements about families. The FAD may be used with adult and adolescent family members. The FAD has been developed on the responses of a sample of 503 individuals, many of whom were members of families of children and adults in psychiatric hospitals.

IMPACT ON FAMILY SCALE

The IOF[24,25] is designed to measure the perceived reactions of a family member to paediatric illness. The revised and recommended version of the instrument contains 15 items that tap into the social and familial impact of paediatric illness. Respondents are asked to rate their agreement (on a four-point scale) with statements that address perceived reactions of a family member to the quality and quantity of interactions with those inside and outside the immediate family. Examples of these items include 'Nobody understands the burden' and 'Hard to find a reliable person to care for my child'. The balance of the statements addresses the strain experienced by the primary caregiver that is directly linked to the child's illness. These statements include 'Live on a rollercoaster' and 'Live from day to day'. The 15-item instrument may be used as a self-report questionnaire and has been successfully administered by telephone.

FAMILY INVENTORY OF LIFE EVENTS AND CHANGES (FILE)

Purpose	The FILE is a self-administered 71-item instrument developed as an index of family stress to measure the cumulative normative and non-normative life events and changes experienced by a family in the preceding year
	Items for the FILE have been informed by research and clinical experience and represent situational and developmental changes experienced by families in the life course. Seven stages in the family life course have been delineated as (1) couple (no children), (2) preschool, (3) school age, (4) adolescent, (5) launching, (6) empty nest and (7) retirement
	FILE items centre on changes of ample consequence that require adjustment and adaptation in family interaction patterns
Population	One or both adult family members complete the scale to record the events experienced by any or all members of the family unit during the preceding year
Description of domains (subscales)	The FILE encompasses nine conceptual domains: intra-familial strains (including conflict and parenting strains), marital strains, pregnancy and childbearing strains, finance and business strains (including family finances and family business), work/family transitions and strains, illness and family 'care strains' (incorporating illness onset and child care, chronic illness strains and dependency strains), losses, transitions 'in and out' and family legal violations
Administration and test format	The FILE contains a 71-item self-report measure that can be completed separately by each adult member or by the couple
	Scoring: respondents are asked to read statements representing family life events and changes and to answer (yes/no) as to whether a change has occurred during the last 12 months or before the last 12 months. Any item answered with a 'yes' is assigned a score of 1. These scores are summed for each subscale and a total score is assigned. Higher scores represent a higher cumulative (pile-up) of family stress. The FILE provides an index of the vulnerability of the family caused by the cumulative effect of stressful events
Psychometric properties	*Reliability*
	Test–retest reliability (4–5wk) scores range from 0.64 to 0.84 for subscales and 0.80 for the whole scale
	Internal consistency: internal consistency reliability for total scale alphas range from 0.79 to 0.82 and 0.30 to 0.73 for the subscales
	Validity
	Correlations with the Family Environment Scale (FES) range from –0.41 to 0.42 and –0.24 to 0.23 for the total scale score. FES conflict has been positively related to total life changes and FES cohesion has been negatively correlated with total life changes
How to order	Available from David H. Olson, Department of Family Social Services, University of Minnesota, St. Paul, MN, USA
Key references	Corcoran K, Fischer J (2000) *Measures for Clinical Practice: A Sourcebook (Vol. 1)*. New York: The Free Press.
	McCubbin HI, Thompson AI (eds) (1991) *Family Assessment Inventories for Research and Practice*. Madison, WI: University of Wisconsin.

FAMILY ENVIRONMENT SCALE

The FES by Rudolf Moos and Bernice Moos[18,26,27] is a 90-item instrument used to assess the social environment or climate of families from an interactionist framework. The FES is composed of 10 subscales and divided into three sets: social relationships among family members (consisting of subscales on cohesion, expressiveness and conflict); personal growth (independence, achievement orientation, intellectual–cultural orientation, active recreational orientation, moral–religious emphasis); and family systems maintenance (organization and control).

FAMILY CRISIS ORIENTED PERSONAL EVALUATION SCALES (F-COPES)

Purpose	The F-COPES is designed to identify problem-solving and behavioural strategies used by families in response to difficulties or crises. It is based on the Double ABCX model of family stress and considers pile-up, family resources and meanings or perceptions of individual family members
	The measure looks at two levels of interaction:
	(1) Individual to family system: the ways in which a family handles and copes with difficulties and problems between its members
	(2) Family system to social environment: the ways in which a family unit utilizes supports from outside its boundaries
	High scores on the F-COPES indicate adaptive coping behaviours
Population	Designed to be completed by individual members of a whole family who are aged 12y and over or have a reading level of approximately sixth grade
Description of domains (subscales)	The F-COPES is a 30-item self-report instrument that measures five factors related to coping strategies employed by family members:
	Subscales:
	Acquiring social support (nine items) – measures a family's ability to acquire support from friends, neighbours and extended family
	Reframing (eight items) – measures a family's ability to redefine a situation in order to make it more manageable.
	Seeking spiritual support (five items) – measures a family's ability to seek spiritual support
	Mobilizing family to acquire and accept help (four items) – measures a family's ability to actively seek assistance in the community and to accept help from others
	Passive appraisal (four items) – measures a family's problem appraisal strategies
Administration and test format	It generally takes 10–15min to complete the instrument. Individuals rate their agreement or disagreement with each item on a five-point Likert scale (from strongly disagree to strongly agree) on the basis of how well each statement reflects their family
	Scores for each subscale are averaged and range from healthy (1.0) to unhealthy (4.0)
	Scoring: items on the passive appraisal subscale are reverse scored. Scores for subscales are total and derived by summing all item scores
Psychometric properties	*Reliability*
	Internal consistency: Cronbach's alpha for individual subscales range from 0.63 to 0.83. The internal consistency for the tool is $r=0.86$.
	Test–retest reliability: (4-wk) for the five factors ranges from 0.61 to 0.95, and for the total tool it is 0.81.
	Validity
	Construct validity: factor analysis revealed five factors
	Concurrent validity: subscales and items on the F-COPES correlate with several other family measures
How to order	Family Inventories Project, Family Social Science, University of Minnesota, St. Paul, MN, USA
Key reference	McCubbin HI, Thompson AI (eds) (1991) *Family Assessment Inventories for Research and Practice*. Madison, WI: University of Wisconsin.

FAMILY ASSESSMENT DEVICE (FAD)

Purpose	The Family Assessment Device (FAD) is designed to measure and evaluate family functioning using the conceptual framework of the McMaster Model that incorporates structural, occupational and transactional features of families
Population	Designed to be completed by adolescent and adult family members
Description of domains (subscales)	The FAD is a 60-item instrument that measures six dimensions of family functioning. Subscales: Problem solving (six items) – the extent to which a family is able to resolve problems within and outside the family unit while maintaining effective family functioning Communication (seven items) – the quality of the communication in the family (clear and direct or vague and indirect) Roles (nine items) – the extent to which a family has established patterns and role assignments for managing family tasks Affective responsiveness (seven items) – the ability of individual family members to respond to situations with appropriate quality and quantity of emotions Affective involvement (eight items) – measures the degree to which family members are interested and involved in each other's activities Behaviour control (10 items) – the ways in which a family expresses and maintains standards of behaviour for family members General functioning (13 items) – measures the quality of overall family functioning
Administration and test format	Individuals rate their agreement or disagreement with each item on a four-point Likert scale (strongly agree=1, agree=2, disagree=3, strongly disagree=4) on the basis of how well each statement reflects their family Items describing unhealthy functioning are reverse scored. Scores for each subscale are averaged to provide seven scale scores with a possible range from healthy (1.0) to unhealthy (4.0)
Psychometric properties	*Reliability* Internal consistency: Cronbach's alpha for individual subscales range from 0.72 to 0.92. The internal consistency for general functioning subscale ranges from 0.85 to 0.90 Test–retest reliability (1wk): test–retest reliability scores for the total tool range from 0.66 to 0.76 *Validity* Concurrent validity: concurrent validity was assessed by administering the FAD and the FACES II and the Family Unit Inventory Discriminant validity: discriminant validity was assessed by comparing the FAD scores of families rated by a clinician as either healthy or unhealthy on each dimension. Families rated by a clinician as unhealthy had significantly higher family mean FAD scores (poor functioning) Construct validity: factor analysis revealed five factors
How to order	Brown University, Family Research Program, Butler Hospital, Providence, RI, USA
Key references	Epstein NB, Baldwin LM, Bishop DS (1983) The McMaster Family Assessment Device. *J Marital Fam Ther* 9: 171–180. Miller IW, Epstein NB, Bishop DS, Keitner GI (1985) The McMaster Family Assessment Device: reliability and validity. *J Marital Fam Ther* 11: 345–356.

IMPACT-ON-FAMILY SCALE (IOF)

Purpose	The Impact-on-Family Scale (IOF) is designed to measure the perceived reactions of a family member to paediatric illness
Population	To be completed by the caregiver of a child (of any age) with a medical condition. The instrument can be used as a self-report questionnaire or an interviewer-administered form The IOF is available in English and Spanish
Description of domains (subscales)	The IOF questionnaire is a 15-item instrument designed to measure dimensions of the social and familial impact of paediatric illness, which generates a total score Items on the measure reflect parental perceptions of changes in family life and their attributions of those changes to the child's illness. The instrument measures the variability in perceived reactions of a family member to paediatric illness as it relates to perceptions about the quality and quantity of interactions with those inside and outside the immediate household and the strain experienced by the primary caretaker that is directly linked to the demands of the childhood illness
Administration and test format	A 15-item self-administered questionnaire that has been successfully administered by phone Respondents rate their agreement or disagreement on the instrument items based on a four-point Likert-type scale (possible responses range from strongly agree to strongly disagree) Time: it takes approximately 10min to complete the IOF
Psychometric properties	*Reliability* Cronbach's alpha for total impact summary score ranged from 0.54 to values greater than 1.00. Eleven items had a value greater than 1.00 and four other items ranged in value from 0.54 to 0.76
How to order	Email Ruth Stein (ruth.stein@einstein.yu.edu)
Key references	Stein REK, Reissman CK (1980) The development of an Impact-on-Family scale: preliminary findings. *Med Care* 18: 465–472. Stein REK, Jessop DJ (2003) The Impact-On-Family Scale revisited: further psychometric data. *J Dev Behav Paediatr* 24: 9–16.

FAMILY ENVIRONMENT SCALE (FES)

Purpose	The Family Environment Scale (FES) was designed to assess social and environmental characteristics within a family
Population	The FES is a self-report measure that may be completed by any member of the family with a sixth-grade or higher reading level (typically age 11y to adult)
Description of domains (subscales)	The FES is a 90-item instrument designed to assess family members' perceptions of their family functioning with regard to three primary domains, each composed of two or more dimensions. Each of the 10 subscales is composed of nine items. Domains and subscales: *Relationship dimensions* Cohesion (nine items): the degree of help, support and commitment that family members provide for each other Expressiveness (nine items): the degree to which family members are encouraged to act openly and to express their feelings

Description of domains (subscales)	Conflict (nine items): the level of anger, aggression and conflict expressed among family members.
	Personal growth dimensions
	Independence (nine items): the extent to which family members are self-sufficient, assertive and make their own decisions
	Achievement orientation (nine items): the competition and achievement-orientated tendencies of the family
	Intellectual–cultural orientation (nine items): the degree of interest in political, social, intellectual and cultural activities
	Active recreational orientation (nine items): the extent of participation in recreational and social activities
	Moral–religious emphasis (nine items): the degree of moral and/or religious orientation in the family.
	System maintenance dimensions
	Organization (nine items): the importance placed by family members on the organization and structured planning of family activities
	Control (nine items): the degree to which rules and procedures are used to run family life
Administration and test format	The 90-item FES instrument can be used in three different formats:
	Real form (Form R) measures respondents' perceptions of their actual family environment
	Ideal form (Form I) is a reworded version of Form R and aims to measure respondents' perceptions of an ideal family environment
	Expectations form (Form E) asks respondents to indicate their expectations for their family environment following anticipated change
	All forms have a true–false format.
	Administration time: 15–20min
Psychometric properties	Normative data are available on a typical family sample (n=1125), a sample of distressed families (n=500) and subgroups varying in terms of family size and age of parent, single versus two-parent status and family ethnicity
	Reliability
	Internal consistency: estimates for Form R subscales range from 0.61 to 0.78
	Test–retest reliability: test–retest reliability scores for the total tool range from r=0.78 (8wk), r=0.74 (4mo) and r=0.73 (12mo)
	Intercorrelation among subscales: low to moderate ranges with an average value of r=0.25
	Validity
	Evidence of construct validity is presented in the manual through comparative descriptions of homogeneous family structures
How to order	Outsourced online survey and scoring system, paper-and-pencil survey and reproduction licence, or online version with licence to administer the instrument are available
	The FES has been translated into 15 different languages
	See Mind Garden: www.mindgarden.com/forms/contactform.php
Key references	Moos R, Moos B (1994) *Family Environment Scale Manual: Development, Applications, Research*, 3rd edition. Palo Alto, CA: Consulting Psychologist Press.

FAMILY IMPACT OF CHILDHOOD DISABILITY SCALE (FICD)

Purpose	The Family Impact of Child Disability Scale (FICD) is designed to measure parents' positive and negative cognitive appraisals of the impact of their child's disability on family life
Population	The FICD is a self-report measure that may be completed by either or both parents of a child with a disability
Description of domains (subscales)	The FICD is a 20-item scale composed of two subscales: Negative Family Impact (NFI) – 10 items measure parents' negative cognitive appraisals of the impact of the disability on the family Positive Family Impact (PFI) – 10 items measure parents' positive cognitive appraisals of the impact of the disability on the family
Administration and test format	The 20-item scale aims to measure the perception of the impact of child disability on the family. The scale is composed of both positive and negative statements Respondents are asked to indicate the impact of the disability of the family on a four-point Likert-type scale with possible responses ranging from 1 (not at all) to 4 (to a substantial degree) Scoring and interpretation: For research purposes, it is recommended to sum the items in each subscale (PFI and NFI) For clinical purposes, it is recommended to sum the items of each subscale and weigh the balance between the parent report of positive and negative impact The instrument can be administered as a self-report questionnaire or be used as part of a face-to-face or telephone interview
Psychometric properties	*Reliability* Internal consistency: Cronbach's alphas have been reported for the negative subscale (0.86–0.89) and the positive subscale (0.81–0.85) from a random sample of mother and father respondents from studies in Manitoba and Alberta in Canada Test–retest reliability: test–retest reliability scores for the NFI subscale were $r=0.92$ and $r=0.95$ for the PFI subscale, indicating strong stability over a 2-wk interval in a Manitoba sample of parents. Similarly, test–retest reliability scores for the NFI subscale were $r=0.86$ and $r=0.77$ for the PFI subscale, indicating strong stability over a 4-wk interval in an Alberta sample of parents *Validity* Discriminant validity: the PFI and NFI have been found to be weakly related to the construct of overall family functioning Factorial validity: a two-factor solution was supported by confirmatory factor analysis
How to order	For ordering information contact Dr Barry Trute (btrute@ucalgary.ca)
Key references	Trute B, Hiebert-Murphy D (2002) Family adjustment to childhood developmental disability: a measure of parent appraisal of family impacts. *J Paediatr Psychol* 27: 271–280. Trute B, Hiebert-Murphy D, Benzie K, Levine K (2009) *Three Measures for Family-centered Practice in Children's Services: Family Impact of Childhood Disability (FICD), Parenting Morale Index (PMI), and Professional and Parent Alliance Scale (PAPAS).* Calgary, AB: University of Calgary.

FAMILY IMPACT OF CHILDHOOD DISABILITY

The FICD[28,29] is a 20-item instrument design to measure parents' positive and negative cognitive appraisals of the impact of their child's disability on the family.

Respondents are asked to indicate their appraisal of the impact of the disability on the family on a four-point Likert-type scale with possible responses ranging from 1 (not at all) to 4 (to a substantial degree). The questionnaire asks respondents to rate the family consequences of having a child with a disability. Examples of statements include 'It has led to financial costs', 'The experience has made us come to terms with what should be valued in life' and 'There have been extraordinary time demands created in looking after the needs of a child with a disability'. The instrument is scored by summing up the positive appraisal subscale and then the negative appraisal subscale. For clinical purposes it is recommended to weigh the balance between parent report of positive and negative appraisals.

BEACH CENTER FAMILY QUALITY OF LIFE SCALE

The Beach Center Family Quality of Life Scale (FQOL)[30–32] is an instrument designed to measure family quality of life, particularly for families who have children with disabilities. Quality of life is conceptualized as the degree to which a family's needs are met, the extent to which family members enjoy their life together as a family and the extent to which family members have the opportunity to engage in activities that are important to them. The 25-item instrument is composed of five subscales. One member of the family is asked to rate the importance of each item to the quality of life of their overall family. Respondents are also asked to rate their level of satisfaction with each item on the instrument.

The *family interaction* subscale is composed of six items that tap into the things that families do (e.g. spending time together, talking openly with each other, solving problems together, handling life's ups and downs), the quality of their interactions (e.g. showing love and care for each other) and the ways in which members support each other's goals, dreams and priorities. The *parenting* subscale is composed of six items that tap into things that parents do (e.g. helping children with schoolwork and activities, knowing the people in their children's lives). The five items on the *physical/material well-being* subscale include statements about having transportation, getting medical and dental care when needed and feelings of safety in both the home environment and beyond (work, school and community). The *emotional well-being* subscale is composed of four items that ask respondents to rate the importance and satisfaction with having the support they need to relieve stress (e.g. friends, time, outside help). Finally, the *disability-related supports* subscale asks respondents to comment on the importance and their satisfaction with having supports for their child with a disability.

FAMILY SUPPORT SCALE

The Family Support Scale (FSS)[33] is an 18-item instrument (plus two items provided by respondents) to measure the perceived helpfulness of sources of support from kinship relationships, spousal relationships, informal supports, programmes and professional services.

The FSS is administered to parents or caregivers with young children who are asked to evaluate the helpfulness of each source of support on a five-point Likert scale, ranging from 1 (not at all helpful) to 5 (extremely helpful). Responses on the instrument are used by professionals to open up dialogue with parents about their experiences with the various means of support and to help mobilize or strengthen sources of support.

SOCIAL SUPPORT SCALE FOR CHILDREN

The Social Support Scale for Children (SSSC)[34] is a survey of children's perceptions of the social support they receive from their parents, teachers, classmates and close friends. The central construct of 'social support' has been operationalized as the *perceived positive regard from others*, one of the many constructs responsible for one's perception of self-worth.

The four subscales of the SSSC (parent, teacher, close friend and classmate) each contains six pairs of statements designed to measure the child's perceived support. Children are asked to read each pair of statements and to select the one that best describes how they feel. They are then asked to indicate if their selection is 'really true for me' or 'sort of true for me'. The parent subscale surveys the child's perceptions about their relationship with their parents and the extent to which they feel understood, heard and the degree to which the parents care about their feelings and treat them like a person who really matters (e.g. some children have parents who *do not* seem to want to hear about their problems *but* other children have parents who *do* want to listen to their children's problems). The teacher support subscale surveys the child's perceptions of the degree of support he or she receives from his or her teacher. Questions in this subscale tap into the child's experience of his or her teacher as someone who helps him or her and treats him or her fairly and as a person who matters (e.g. some children *do not* have a teacher who helps them to do their very best *but* other children do have a teacher who helps them to do their very best). The classmate subscale surveys children's perceptions about their relationships with school peers. Questions this subscale taps into are the child's perceptions of peers as people who like them, do not make fun of them, listen to what they say and include them in games (e.g. some children have classmates who they can become friends with *but* other children do not have classmates with whom they can become friends). Finally, the close friend subscale asks whether the child has a close friend whom he can rely on for support (e.g. some children have a close friend who really understands

BEACH CENTER FAMILY QUALITY OF LIFE SCALE (FQOL)

Purpose	The Beach Center Family Quality of Life Scale (FQOL) is designed to measure family quality of life in families of children with disabilities
	The FQOL is designed for use as a research tool and should not be used for diagnostic purposes or for assessment to determine eligibility for services
	The FQOL may be used as:
	a pre- and post-test measure;
	an outcome measure for services or supports; or
	a measure of an independent or dependent variable
Population	Families of children with disabilities
Description of domains (subscales)	The FQOL is composed of 25 items across five subscales:
	family interaction (six items);
	parenting (six items);
	emotional well-being (four items);
	physical/material well-being (five items); and
	disability-related support (four items)
Administration and test format	The FQOL scale is a self-report instrument designed to be administered to one member of the family. The scale can be completed in 10min
	Respondents are asked to rate the level of importance of each item on the instrument on a five-point Likert scale, where 1=a little important, 3=important and 5=critically important
	Respondents are also asked to rate their level of satisfaction on each item of the instrument on a five-point Likert scale, where 1=very satisfied, 3=neither satisfied nor dissatisfied and 5=very satisfied
Psychometric properties	*Reliability*
	Internal consistency: Cronbach's alpha on importance ratings across subscales was 0.94 and 0.88 for satisfaction ratings across subscales
	Test–retest reliability: importance and satisfaction responses across all FQOL subscales were significantly correlated ($p=0.01$ or beyond)
	Validity
	Convergent validity with the Family Apgar scale (Smilkstein et al, 1982) and the Family Resource Scale (Dunst and Leet, 1985): each of these measures was significantly correlated with the hypothesized subscales of the FQOL. The Family Apgar was significantly correlated with the satisfaction mean of the FQOL family interaction subscale, $r=0.68$, $p<0.001$
	The Family Resource Scale was significantly correlated with the mean of the five items in the FQOL physical/material well-being subscale: $r=0.60$, $p<0.001$, $n=60$. (Lack of relevant existing measures made it impossible to test convergent validity across all subscales.)
How to order	Information about obtaining permission copies of the Beach Center Family Quality of Life Scale can be obtained from the Beach Center website: wwww.beachcenter.org.
	The Beach Center Family Quality of Life Scale may be ordered via email: beachcenter@ku.edu
Key references	Dunst CJ, Leet HE (1985) *Family Resource Scale*. Morganton, NC: Western Carolina Center.
	Hoffman L, Marquis J, Poston D, Summers JA, Turnbull A (2006) Assessing family outcomes: psychometric evaluation of the Beach Center Family Quality of Life Scale. *J Marriage Fam* 68: 1069–1083.

Key references	Park J, Hoffman L, Marquis J, et al (2003) Toward assessing family outcomes of service delivery: validation of a family quality of life survey. *J Intellect Disabil Res* 47: 367–384.
	Smilkstein G, Ashworth C, Montano D (1982) Validity and reliability of the family APGAR as a test of family function. *J Fam Pract* 15: 303–311.

FAMILY SUPPORT SCALE (FSS)

Purpose	The Family Support Scale (FSS) measures the adequacy of a family's support network and parents' satisfaction with the support they receive with regards to raising young children
Population	Families rearing a young child
Description of domains (subscales)	The FSS consists of 18 items covering an array of sources of support including grandparents, relatives, friends, social groups, medical and allied health professionals and the child's school environment
Administration and test format	Participants are asked to respond on a five-point Likert scale ranging from 'not at all helpful' (1) to extremely helpful (5). Clinicians can use the FSS results to evaluate the areas of a family's support system that need to be reinforced.
Psychometric properties	*Reliability* Internal consistency alpha coefficient=0.77 on the 18-item scale Split-half reliability (using the Spearman–Brown formula)=0.77 Test–retest reliability (1–2y apart) yielded an average correlation of $r=0.42$ (standard deviation=0.15) for the 18 items and $r=0.50$ for the total scale score *Validity* Concurrent predictive validity was tested through correlations of the FSS total helpfulness scores and subscales of the questionnaire on resources and stress[35]: Poor Health/Mood ($r=-0.25$, $p<0.025$), Excessive Time Demands ($r=0.22$, $p<0.025$) and Family Integrity ($r=-0.17$, $p<0.025$)
How to order	The FSS may be purchased by phone, fax or mail from Winterberry Press. Order forms and information are available at www.wbpress.com
Key references	Dunst CJ, Jenkins V, Trivette CM (1984) Family Support Scale: reliability and validity. *J Individ Fam Community Support* 1: 45–52.

SOCIAL SUPPORT SCALE FOR CHILDREN (SSSC)

Purpose	The Social Support Scale for Children is a survey of children's perceptions of the social support they receive and the positive regard they may receive from their parents, teachers, classmates and close friends
Population	Children and youth aged 8–18y may complete the SSSC
Description of domains (subscales)	The SSSC has four subscales (parent, teacher, close friend and classmate), each containing six items and measuring perceived support or regard towards the child The parent subscale surveys the child's perceptions about his or her relationship with his or her parents and the extent to which he or she feels understood, heard and cared for The teacher support subscale surveys the child's perceptions about the degree of support he or she receives from his or her teacher The classmate subscale surveys children's perceptions about their relationships with school peers (e.g. the extent to which they feel liked and included) The close friend subscale asks whether the child has a close friend on whom he or she can rely on for support (e.g. listening to him or her, etc.)

Administration and test format	The scale may be administered individually or in groups. The author recommends reading the items out loud for children below the fourth grade. Children in the fifth grade or above can complete the scale on their own. The scale is introduced to participants as a 'survey'
	The measure assesses the child's perception of social support from his or her parents, teacher, close friend and classmate. The survey requires the participant to select a response from two alternatives that apply to his or her experience (e.g. some children have a teacher who helps them if they are upset and have a problem *but* other children do not have a teacher who helps them if they are upset and have a problem)
	The first statement is on the left-hand side of the page, the second statement is on the right. Participants are asked to make two choices about the two statements. First, they are asked to decide which of the two statements applies most to themselves. Then, based on their selection, they are asked to endorse whether their selected statement is 'sort of' or 'really' true for them
Psychometric properties	The internal consistency reliabilities for the subscales range from 0.72 to 0.88. Additional psychometric properties are available in the manual
How to order	Orders must be mailed to Dr Susan Harter, University of Denver, 2155 S. Race Street, Denver, CO 80208, USA
Key reference	Harter S (1985) *Manual for the Social Support Scale for Children*. Denver, CO: University of Denver.

them *but* other children do not have a close friend who understands them).

Summary

The family system is the social context in which a child develops. This chapter highlights the use of the ICF-CY framework to guide practitioners in the selection of measurement tools to consider aspects of the *immediate family and family functioning*. The evaluation of the family environment can guide efforts to implement services and supports that can ultimately contribute to the well-being of children, adolescents and their families.

Practitioners are encouraged to reflect on the goals and purpose of family evaluation and to consider desired outcomes in their measurement selection process. These decisions should be based on a careful reflection and matching of theoretical frameworks that are most consistent with the goals and purposes of including the family within the evaluation.

Three groupings of measurement tools evaluating different aspects of the support and relationships within the immediate family were proposed: measures that evaluate the *immediate family environment*; measures that evaluate the extent to which the child/adolescent, family and or family members *experiences being supported* within their family environment; and *measures that describe the impact of the disability on the family.*

MEASURES THAT EVALUATE THE IMMEDIATE FAMILY ENVIRONMENT

If the purpose of evaluation is to determine the quality of the *immediate family environment,* such as the strengths and abilities of the family including perceptions of mastery and pride, and coping mechanisms such as acquiring social support, reframing, seeking spiritual support, the F-COPES or the FAD may be a consideration.

Alternatively, if the goal of evaluation is to determine the quality of family interaction patterns such as cohesion, expressiveness, independence, commitment, conflict control and involvement among members, the FACES or the FES may be of greater relevance.

Finally, if practitioners are aiming to determine the context and overall family functioning, including family stress, the FILE could provide a viable option.

MEASURES THAT EVALUATE THE EXTENT TO WHICH AN INDIVIDUAL FEELS SUPPORTED

If the goal of measurement is to determine *the extent to which an individual feels supported* within his or her family environment, the FSS could be a helpful tool. To evaluate a child's perception of the social support and positive regard he or she may receive from family members, teachers and peers, the SSSC can illuminate barriers and facilitators within their environment.

MEASURES THAT DESCRIBE THE IMPACT OF THE
DISABILITY ON THE FAMILY

Families of children with health and functioning difficulties may experience extraordinary challenges. Practitioners interested in measuring *the impact of the disability on the family* may select the IOF to measure the perceived reactions of family members to paediatric illness. The FICD can reveal the positive and negative appraisal of the impact of a child's disability on family life. Finally, researchers interested in quality of life in families of children with disabilities may opt to use the Beach Center FQOL as pre- and post-test measures, an outcome measure for services or supports, or a measure of an independent or dependent variable.

REFERENCES

1. World Health Organization (1992) *International Statistical Classification of Diseases and Related Health Problems, 1989 Revision.* Geneva: WHO.
2. Head LS, Abbeduto L (2007) Recognizing the role of parents in developmental outcomes: A systems approach to evaluating the child with developmental disabilities. *Ment Retard Dev Disabil* 13: 293–301.
3. Benson P (2006) The impact of child symptom severity on depressed mood among parents of children with ASD: the mediating role of stress proliferation. *J Autism Dev Disord* 36: 685–695.
4. Hornby G, Seligman M (1991) Disability and the family: Current status and future developments. *Counsel Psychol Quart* 4: 267–271.
5. Barakat LP, Linney JA (1992) Children with physical handicaps and their mothers: the interrelation of social support, maternal adjustment, and child adjustment. *J Pediatr Psychol* 17: 725–739.
6. Rolland JS (1994) *Families, Illness, and Disability: An Integrative Treatment Model.* New York: Basic Books.
7. Yoav L, McCubbin HI, Olson DH (1987) The effect of stressful life events and transitions on family functioning and well-being. *J Marriage Fam* 49: 857–873.
8. Hill R (1949) *Families Under Stress: Adjustment to the Crises of War Separation and Reunion.* New York: Harper.
9. McCubbin HI, Patterson JM (1983) The family stress process – the Double ABCX Model of Adjustment and Adaptation. *Marriage Fam Rev* 6: 7–37.
10. McCubbin MA, McCubbin HI (1987) Family stress theory and assessment: the Resiliency Model of family stress, adjustment, and adaptation. In: McCubbin HI, Thompson, AI, editors. *Family Assessment Inventories for Research and Practice.* Madison, WI: University of Wisconsin-Madison, pp. 3–32.
11. Patterson JM (2002) Integrating family resilience and family stress theory. *J Marriage Fam* 64: 349–360.
12. Epstein NB, Bishop DS, Levin S (1978) The McMaster Model of Family Functioning. *J Marital Fam Ther* 4: 19–31.
13. Sawin KJ, Harrigan MP, Woog P (1995) *Measures of Family Functioning for Research and Practice.* New York: Springer Publishing Company.
14. Epstein NB, Levin S, Bishop DS (1976) The family as a social unit. *Can Fam Physician* 22: 1411.
15. Olson DH, Gorall DM (2003) Circumplex Model of Marital and Family Systems. In: Walsh F, editor, *Normal Family Processes.* New York: Guilford, pp. 514–547.
16. Epstein NB, Baldwin LM, Bishop DS (1983) The McMaster Family Assessment Device. *J Marital Fam Ther* 9: 171–180.
17. Bertalanffy L (1973) *General System Theory: Foundations, Development, Applications.* New York: George Braziller Inc.
18. Moos RH, Insel PM, Humphrey B (1974) *Family Environment Scale.* Palo Alto, CA: Consulting Psychologists Press.
19. Olson D (2011) FACES IV & the Circumplex Model: Validation Study. *J Marital Fam Ther* 37: 64–80.
20. McCubbin HI, Patterson JM, Wilson LR (1983) FILE – Family Inventory of Life Events. In: McCubbin HI, Thompson AI, editors. *Family Assessment: Resiliency, Coping and Adaptation: Inventory for Research and Practice.* Madison, WI: University of Wisconsin System, pp. 103–178.
21. McCubbin HI, Olson DH, Larsen AS (1991) F-COPES (Family Crisis Oriented Personal Evaluation Scales). In: McCubbin HI, Thompson AI, editors. *Family Assessment Inventories for Research and Practice.* Madison, WI: University of Wisconsin-Madison, pp. 193–207.
22. Theodore J, Tennenbaum DL (1988) *Family Assessment: Rationale, Methods, and Future Direction.* New York: Plenum Press.
23. Miller IW, Bishop DS, Epstein NB, Gabor IK (1985) The McMaster Family Assessment Device: reliability and validity. *J Marital Fam Ther* 11: 345–356.
24. Stein REK, Jessop DJ (2003) The Impact on Family Scale revisited: further psychometric data. *J Dev Behav Pediatr* 24: 9–16.
25. Stein REK, Riessman CK (1980) The development of an Impact-on-Family scale: preliminary findings. *Med Care* 18: 465–472.
26. Moos RH, Moos BS (1986) *Family Environment Scale Manual,* 2nd edition. Palo Alto, CA: Consulting Psychologists Press.
27. Moos RH, Moos BS (1994) *Family Environment Scale Manual,* 3rd edition. Palo Alto, CA: Consulting Psychologists Press.
28. Trute B, Hiebert-Murphy D, Benzies KM, Levine K (2009) *Three Measures for Family-centered Practice in Children's Services: Family Impact of Childhood Disability, Parenting Morale Index, and Professional and Parent Alliance Scale.* Calgary, AB: University of Calgary.
29. Trute B, Hiebert-Murphy D, Levine K (2007) Parental appraisal of the Family Impact of Childhood Developmental Disability: times of sadness and times of joy. *J Intellect Dev Disabil* 32: 1–9.
30. Hoffman L, Marquis J, Poston D, Summers JA, Turnbull A (2006) Assessing family outcomes: psychometric evaluation of the Beach Center Family Quality of Life Scale. *J Marriage Fam* 68: 1069–1083.
31. Park J, Hoffman L, Marquis J, et al (2003) Toward assessing family outcomes of service delivery: validation of a family quality of life survey. *J Intellect Disabil Res* 47: 367–384.
32. Poston D, Turnbull A, Park J, Mannan H, Marquis J, Wang M (2003) Family quality of life: a qualitative inquiry. *Ment Retard* 41: 313–328.
33. Dunst CJ, Jenkins V, Trivette CM (1984) Family Support Scale: reliability and validity. *J Individual Fam Community Support* 1: 45–52.
34. Harter S (1985) *Manual for the Social Support Scale for Children.* Denver, CO: University of Denver.
35. Holroyd J (1974) The questionnaire on resources and stress: an instrument to measure family response to a handicapped member. *J Community Psychol* 2: 92–94.

32
HEALTH AND REHABILITATION SERVICES AND SYSTEMS (E355, E360, E510, E575, E580)

Debbie Feldman and Bonnie Swaine

What is the construct?

Developmental therapists such as physical therapists, occupational therapists, and speech and language pathologists provide rehabilitation services for children and youth with developmental disabilities. Systems designed to deliver these services vary across different contexts (e.g. hospitals, rehabilitation centres, schools, communities), regions (urban, rural), and jurisdictions (provinces or states). Provision of services is dependent on resource availability and allocation, organization of services, legislation and policy. As a result, patients and their families can experience different levels of service provision. This may have an impact on the child's quality of life and functional progress.[1]

Despite the variations in service provision, the Child Care Advocacy Association of Canada outlines principles for developmentally appropriate programming for *all* children (including those with developmental disabilities).[2] The key points include (1) a learning environment in which developmentally appropriate activities are integrated; (2) appropriate adult to child ratios that can engage the children in a range of developmentally appropriate activities; (3) highly qualified and well-trained staff who experience high job satisfaction; (4) public and not-for-profit service delivery that is directed solely to the delivery of the childcare programmes; (5) legislated standards and capacity for monitoring and enforcement; and (6) funding that is stable and adequate to sustain long-term service delivery. In addition, families report that they value well-organized services that are accessible and co-ordinated across a continuum of care.[3] Indeed, there should be early access to rehabilitation services upon confirmation of the child's impairment regardless of the degree of severity, to ensure that timely, comprehensive, well-co-ordinated services are delivered.

To address the issue of access to rehabilitation services, the US Congress passed the Public Law 99-457 in 1986, which mandated the early identification and the organization of comprehensive programmes of early intervention services (including physiotherapy and occupational therapy) of infants and young children with developmental delays.[4,5] Despite mandates for complementarity and coordination of services, there are problems with service delivery.[5-9] Simpson and colleagues[5] report that 69% to 83% (or an estimated 558 000) of infants and young children in the USA with developmental delay do not receive intervention services.

In the early 1990s, Fox and colleagues found that Health Maintenance Organizations (HMOs) in the USA restricted access to a majority of children with special needs who did not meet the established criterion that the child is expected to make significant improvement over a short period of time.[6] These policies impose barriers to care for children with chronic disabilities. In addition, parents of these children do not have the choice to seek providers outside their HMO. Long waiting times and lack of resources may limit access to comprehensive services, especially in community settings.[7] This is consistent with a study that revealed long waiting times for rehabilitation services for children with physical disabilities in the Montreal region in 1999: of 172 children, 6 months after referral, 50% and 36% had not yet received occupational therapy services and physiotherapy services, respectively, at a rehabilitation centre.[9] Grilli et al[8] reported that these delays actually increased within a 5-year span, such that half of the children waited more than 7 and 11 months for physiotherapy and occupational therapy services, respectively. Older children (aged >4y) waited longer for services. They also found that organizational factors (first come, first served, vs organization of services by programme or specific diagnostic category) may also influence service delivery.

Delay in service delivery may have an impact on parent satisfaction, therapist satisfaction[10] and child and

TABLE 32.1
Selected measures described in this overview

Health services and systems: attributes	Measures
Access to care	Service Obstacles Scale (SOS)
Continuity	Continuity of Care Index (COC)
Comprehensiveness	Family Needs Questionnaire (FNQ)
Family-centred care and coordination	Measure of Processes of Care (MPOC-56)
	MPOC-Service Provider (MPOC-SP)
Satisfaction	DISABKIDS
	Client Satisfaction Questionnaire (CSQ)
	Peds-QL Healthcare Satisfaction Generic Module
	Multidimensional Assessment of Parental Satisfaction (MAP)
Maintaining standards of care	Multidimensional Peer Rating of the Clinical Behaviors of Pediatric Therapists (MPR)
	Therapy Intervention Methods Checklist (TIMC)

family function.[1] The current paradigm for high-quality care is a partnership between developmental specialists, the child and his or her parents to promote and enhance the child's health and well-being within his or her environment.[11,12] Measures to describe quality of care of rehabilitation services must take into consideration the notion of partnership and family-centred care. In addition, these measures may also include dimensions of care typically cited in the general medical care literature; services should be accessible, continuous, co-ordinated, integrated, appropriate, comprehensive and of a high standard, and have both a family and community orientation.[13] These attributes closely relate to patient satisfaction, health system equity and effectiveness. They need to be measurable so that healthcare providers and administrators can evaluate levels of service provision and improve them on an ongoing basis.

Specific measures may be developed with a panel of experts, similar to that which has been done for emergency department care in paediatrics[14] and for ambulatory paediatric care.[15] In the case of attention-deficit–hyperactivity disorder, a panel of experts determined outcomes reflecting processes of diagnosis and treatment guidelines, assessing quality of care in terms of adherence to guidelines.[16] Computerized administrative databases such as the Health Plan Employer Data and Information Set HEDIS in the USA can be used to monitor care for children with chronic conditions.[17] Other measures include surveys with mainly open questions to assess parental assessment of care,[18] as well as those with closed questions that require the parent to rank the care received.[19]

Despite the need to evaluate the quality of services and systems for children and youth with developmental disabilities, to date there appear to be only a few measures used to capture structure- and process-related aspects of

service delivery for this important rehabilitation patient group. In this chapter, we present some measures that address the following attributes of service quality: access (and accessibility), continuity, comprehensiveness, family-centred care and coordination, satisfaction and high standards of care. Each of these domains is specifically defined and *general factors to consider when measuring each of these domains* are highlighted. Particular measures are then described and tabulated. We have selected measures that have undergone psychometric testing and either have been used in the paediatric population or can be adapted for use with children and families. We believe that use of these and other similar measures should help ensure that a quality rehabilitation service is delivered to children and youth with developmental disabilities.

Overview of recommended measures

ACCESS TO CARE
According to Mooney,[20] access to care is a question of supply whereas utilization is a function of both supply and demand. Donabedian[21] makes the distinction between *access* and *accessibility*: the latter goes beyond the availability of resources and services; it includes the characteristics of resources that either facilitate or deter use by potential clients. Availability of services supply includes geographic proximity, distribution, number and type of resources. Demand for services is related to cost, knowledge and beliefs, preferences, etc. Data sources relative to access/accessibility include administrative databases that detail service utilization: dates of visits and admissions; and surveys or interviews administered to current and potential clients, clinicians and administrators. In the case of children requiring rehabilitation services, typical measures relating to *access* may include the following:

- time of first concern by parent regarding child's development and date of visit with paediatrician;[22]
- time between visit with paediatrician regarding developmental problem and its confirmation and referral to specialized services: developmental paediatrician, neurologist, physical therapist, occupational therapist or speech and language pathologist;[23]
- time between referral to specialized service and reception of that service, i.e. first appointment with that service;[8,9] and

- time between date of reception of initial rehabilitation consultation and acceptance to a long-term rehabilitation programme.[8,9]

Barriers to care in terms of access and accessibility, such as the Service Obstacles Scale (SOS),[24,25] are described below in further detail. It is important to note that the SOS was developed for use in the brain injury population and their families. However, we believe that it can be easily adapted for children with other conditions, and their families.

SERVICE OBSTACLES SCALE (SOS)	
Purpose	To evaluate individuals' and caregivers' perceptions of brain injury services in the community with regard to quality and accessibility
Population	Patients (all ages) with traumatic brain injury and their families
Description of domains (subscales)	Six-item scale regarding obstacles to receiving brain injury services, knowledge of and availability of resources and satisfaction with the quality of care. There are three main components: satisfaction with treatment resources (four items); finances as an obstacle to receiving services (one item); and transportation as an obstacle to receiving services (one item)
Administration and test format	Administration is brief: it can be completed by interview (face to face or on the telephone) or using a paper-and-pencil response Six items scored from 1 to 7 (1=disagree strongly to 7=strongly agree) Satisfaction subscale is scored by summing the responses to the four items
Psychometric properties	Internal consistency: all items were positively correlated with each other with $p<0.01$ for all values (Spearman's rho). The items regarding satisfaction with the amount of professional help, good brain injury treatment and adequate resources were highly related as indicated by correlations ranging from 0.56 to 0.77. The strength of the correlations among the transportation item, the money item and the remaining items was lower, ranging from 0.29 to 0.48 *Validity* The SOS items were related to Family Needs Questionnaire scale scores (Kreutzer and Marwitz, 1989) with correlations in the expected directions Lower quality of life ratings were associated with reports of more obstacles and less satisfaction with community resources
How to order	In the public domain: www.tbims.org/combi/sos Contact Jeffrey S. Kreutzer (jskreutz@mail2.vcu.edu) for more information
Key references	Kreutzer J (2000) *The Service Obstacles Scale.* The Center for Outcome Measurement in Brain Injury. www.tbims.org/combi/sos Kreutzer J, Marwitz J (1989) *The Family Needs Questionnaire.* Richmond, VA: The National Resource Center for Traumatic Brain Injury. Kolakowsky-Hayner SA, Kreutzer JS, Miner D (2000) Validation of the Service Obstacles Scale for the traumatic brain injury population. *NeuroRehabilitation* 14: 151–158. Marwitz JH, Kreutzer JS (1996) *The Service Obstacles Scale (SOS).* Richmond, VA: Medical College of Virginia Commonwealth University.

CONTINUITY

The definition of continuity is perspective dependent. For patients and their families, it is the perception that providers know what has happened before, that different providers agree on a management plan, and that a provider who knows them will care for them in the future.[26] For providers, it is ensuring that there is sufficient knowledge and information about a patient as well as confidence that their input will be recognized and pursued by other providers. There are three categories of continuity: informational continuity (use of information of past events and personal circumstances to ensure appropriate care); management continuity (consistent and coherent approach to management of the health condition that is responsive to the changing needs of the patient) and relational continuity (ongoing therapeutic relationship between patient and provider[s]). Typical measures of continuity may include the following:

- frequency of treatment and/or follow-up consultations (data source: survey of clients, administrative data);
- seeing the same therapist (data source: interviews with clients, administrative data);
- coherence of approaches between therapists (data source: interviews of clients and therapists) and other clinicians (across the continuum); and
- Continuity of Care Index (COC) first described in 1977 by Bice and Boxerman[27] and used in several paediatrics studies.[28–31] This index is described below.

COMPREHENSIVENESS

Comprehensiveness implies the recognition of the full range of the patient's health needs and arrangement of resources to deal with these needs.[13] Thus, a child who has multiple health needs should be offered all appropriate services throughout the continuum of care. Comprehensiveness can be measured as receipt of all services that are required by the child (comprehensive care). Parents may evaluate this to some degree by articulating their needs with respect to health care. Several authors have proposed methods for evaluating health needs and unmet needs.

Thyen et al[32] and Perrin et al[33] have published studies documenting *unmet needs of children with disabilities and chronic health conditions*. Both groups adapted instruments to document unmet needs in various areas.

Thyen et al[32] developed a questionnaire containing 14 items reflecting four dimensions: medical care; care coordination and communication; education about illness; and social counselling. All questions are answered as follows: yes, yes partly, no but not needed, no but needed. If parents respond that they need a service but do not receive it to any question within one of the four domains, an unmet health need in that domain is recorded.

- Perrin et al[33] developed a list of 23 categories of needs. Parents respond to 'would benefit from…'. There are four subgroups: information needs; counselling needs; specific help needs (e.g. arrangements for school, etc.); and a miscellaneous category. Each of the 23 items is graded dichotomously (yes or no).

CONTINUITY OF CARE INDEX (COC)

Purpose	To describe the consistency of contact between patients and their providers
Population	Has been used in both adult and paediatric populations
Description of index	$$COC = \frac{\sum_{j=1}^{s} n_j^2 - N}{N(N-1)}$$ where N=total number of visits, n_j=number of visits to provider j, and s=number of providers. COC takes on values between 0 and 1. Zero means that a different provider is seen for each visit; 1 means that the same provider is seen at every visit
Data sources	Originally based on administrative physician claims databases. However, it could be used for therapist sessions as well
Key references	Bice TW, Boxerman SB (1977) A quantitative measure of continuity of care. *Med Care* 15: 347–349. Christakis DA, Feudtner C, Pihoker C, Connell FA (2001) Continuity and quality of care for children with diabetes who are covered by Medicaid. *Ambul Pediatr* 1: 99–103.

- The Family Needs Questionnaire,[34–36] a tool assessing family needs was developed for persons with brain injury (although not specifically in a paediatric population). It has been used for spinal cord injuries and may be adapted to other diagnostic groups. This tool is described below.

FAMILY-CENTRED CARE AND COORDINATION

The notion of partnership has brought about a dramatic change to traditional rehabilitation approaches and service delivery for children with disabilities.[11,37,38] This highly valued approach to service delivery is known as family-centred service (FCS), and it is based on the

FAMILY NEEDS QUESTIONNAIRE (FNQ)	
Purpose	To provide information about family members' needs after traumatic brain injury, in terms of perceptions of (1) the importance of needs and (2) the extent to which each need has been met
	The FNQ can be used to develop individualized programmes tailored to a family's needs. It can also provide an indication of intervention effectiveness
Population	Family members of patients with a primary diagnosis of traumatic brain injury; also used in families of patients with a diagnosis of spinal cord injury. There is the possibility of adaptation for other diagnostic categories
Description of domains (subscales)	Forty items representing diverse needs during acute rehabilitation and post discharge. There are six subscales: Health Information / Emotional Support / Instrumental Support / Professional Support / Community Support Network / Involvement with Care
Administration and test format	The FNQ is an auto-administered questionnaire.
	Items are rated as the extent of importance (1=not important, 2=slightly important, 3=important, 4=very important) and the degree to which needs are met (yes, partly, no)
	Scoring: mean importance ratings for each of the 40 items can be calculated. Mean percentage of needs rated as met for the six scales are calculated. Similarly, mean percentage of needs most often rated as not met can be calculated
Psychometric properties	Internal consistency: Spearman–Brown's split-half reliability of 0.75. Cronbach's alphas for individual subscales range from 0.78 to 0.89
	Construct validity: families who perceived the injured person as having more problems will have more unmet needs
How to order	Contact Jenny Marwitz (jhmarwit@vcu.edu)
Key references	Camplair P, Kreutzer JS, Doherty K (1990) Family outcome following adult traumatic brain injury: a critical review. In: Kreutzer J, Wehman P (eds) *Community Integration Following Traumatic Brain Injury*. Baltimore, MD: Paul Brookes, pp. 207–224.
	Kreutzer J, Marwitz J (1989) *The Family Needs Questionnaire*. Richmond, VA: The National Resource Center for Traumatic Brain Injury.
	Kreutzer J, Devany C, Keck S (1994) Family needs following brain injury: a quantitative analysis. *J Head Trauma Rehabil* 9: 104–115.
	Marwitz J (2000) *The Family Needs Questionnaire*. The Center for Outcome Measurement in Brain Injury. www.tbims.org/combi/fnq
	Sander A, Kreutzer J (1999) A holistic approach to family assessment after brain injury. In: Rosenthal M, Griffith E, Kreutzer J, Pentland B (eds) *Rehabilitation of the Adult and Child with Traumatic Brain Injury*, 3rd edn. Philadelphia, PA: F. A. Davis.

acknowledgement of a partnership between children with disabilities, their parents and service providers during the decision-making process concerning the child's rehabilitation services and needs. This approach also recognizes and considers the parents as experts regarding their children's needs. These needs may be associated with the child's functional status as well as with the availability of and satisfaction with rehabilitation services.[39] Coordination of care occurs along a continuum from social to medical settings and can include social models for institutional, residential and in-home long-term care services; medical models that co-ordinate management by various disciplines; and integrated models that bridge the two systems.[40] The integrated model, addressing both social and medical aspects, fits with the goals of paediatric rehabilitation. Further, coordination of care for children with disabilities may comprise elements of parental empowerment, interagency collaboration, a named care co-ordinator and individualized service based on assessment of need.[41]

The Measures of Processes of Care are tools that evaluate parents' (MPOC-56)[19,42] and service providers' (MPOC-SP)[43] perceptions of the family-centeredness of paediatric rehabilitation services. They are the tools that are most commonly used in paediatric rehabilitation services to evaluate processes of care[44] and family centeredness of services,[19] to document parents' perception of the habilitation process[45,46] and to explore relations between processes of care and parenting stress,[47] families' satisfaction[19] and adolescent quality of life.[48] Factors such as children's age, diagnoses and severity, service providers' experience and methods for keeping up to date, settings, team structures, service coordination and information tools used have been reported to influence MPOC and MPOC-SP scores.[10,45,46,49,50,51] Each of the two MPOC tools is described in further detail below.

MEASURE OF PROCESSES OF CARE (MPOC-56)	
Purpose	To assess parents' perceptions of care received from children's rehabilitation treatment centres. It evaluates family-centred behaviours of healthcare providers
Population	Parents whose children range in age from 0y to ≥17y with a variety of neurodevelopmental disabilities or maxillofacial disorders
Description of domains (subscales)	MPOC contains a total of 56 items in five subscales (current work is under way regarding the MPOC-20, a shortened version of the tool): Enabling and Partnership (16 items); Providing General Information (nine items); Providing Specific Information about the Child (five items); Co-ordinated and Comprehensive Care for the Child and Family (17 items); and Respectful and Supportive Care (nine items)
Administration and test format	The questionnaire is auto-administered. For each item, parents respond to a common question: 'To what extent do the people who work with your child…'. A seven-point response scale is used, with three of the options being labelled (7=to a great extent; 4=sometimes; and 1=never). There is also a 'not applicable' category A respondent's data yield five scores, one for each of the factors or scales. There is no total score. A scale score is obtained by computing the average of the items' ratings. Instructions for scoring are included in the manual. Programming statements for use with SPSS-PC+ are available from the first author Time taken: 15–20min for most parents
Psychometric properties	Internal consistency: Cronbach's alphas range from 0.63 to 0.96 Test–retest reliability: intraclass correlation coefficients range from 0.78 to 0.88 *Validity* Positive correlations between MPOC scale scores and a measure of satisfaction; negative correlations between MPOC scale scores and a measure of the stress experienced by parents when dealing with their child's treatment centre

How to order	The manual can be downloaded from www.canchild.ca/Portals/0/measures/1995_MPOC_Manual_MPOC-56_MPOC-20_questionnaires.pdf
Key references	King S, Rosenbaum P, King G (1995) *The Measure of Processes of Care: A Means to Assess Family-centred Behaviours of Health Care Providers*. Hamilton, ON: McMaster University, Neurodevelopmental Clinical Research Unit. King S, Rosenbaum P, King G (1996) Parents' perceptions of care-giving: development and validation of a measure of processes. *Dev Med Child Neurol* 38: 757–772.

MEASURE OF PROCESSES OF CARE – SERVICE PROVIDER (MPOC-SP)

Purpose	To measure, from the service provider's viewpoint, the extent to which the care provided by them is family centred. It can contribute to initiatives of professional development, programme evaluation and research in health service delivery. It can be paired with the Parent Questionnaire (MPOC), and thereby allows users to gain multiple perspectives on service delivery in a clinical setting. It does not measure service provider behaviours, in the objective sense of the word; rather, it measures the service provider's perceptions of his or her behaviours
Population	Paediatric service providers who care for children (and their families) with chronic health or developmental problems
Description of domains (subscales)	This is a discriminative tool that comprises four scales and 27 items: Showing Interpersonal Sensitivity (10 items) – support for families raising a child with a chronic health or developmental problem; Providing General Information (five items) – providing information about the child's condition and services; Communicating Specific Information (three items) – providing information specific to the child's health status, treatment and prognosis; and Treating People Respectfully (nine items) – professionals' treatment of children and families as individuals and equals
Administration and test format	The MPOC-56 is a self-administered questionnaire. Time taken: 10–15min For each item, service providers respond to a common question: 'In the past year, to what extent did you …'. A seven-point response scale is used (7=to a very great extent, 6=to a great extent, 5=to a fairly great extent, 4=to a moderate extent, 3=to a small extent, 2=to a very small extent and 1=not at all). A score of '0' indicates that the item is 'not applicable'. A respondent's data yield four scores, one for each of the factors or scales. There is no total score. Each scale score is obtained by computing the average of the relevant items' ratings
Psychometric properties	Good internal consistency: Cronbach's alphas range from 0.76 to 0.88 Test–retest reliability (5-wk interval): intraclass correlation coefficients range from 0.79 to 0.99 *Validity* Scores discriminate between professionals' ratings of their actual behaviours and what they considered ideal
How to order	Email canchild@mcmaster.ca. Include the title of the measure (i.e. the MPOC-SP) in your message. The MPOC-SP is currently available at no cost
Key references	Woodside J, Rosenbaum P, King S, King G (1998) *The Measure of Processes of Care for Service Providers (MPOC-SP)*. *CanChild* Centre for Childhood Disability Research, McMaster University.

SATISFACTION

Patient satisfaction, defined as an attitude about service or service providers,[52] is an important measure of outcome and of quality of care in the evaluation of healthcare services. It may influence the success of a healthcare organization and has been identified as a factor influencing compliance with medical interventions. Parents who are satisfied with care are more likely to follow medical recommendations for their children.[53] Clinician's interpersonal skills have also been correlated with parental satisfaction.[54] These skills included the clinician's communication to the parent, communication to the child, distress relief and adherence intent. Seeing the same doctor was another important determinant of satisfaction of mothers of children with disabilities.[55,56] Although outcomes of treatment and satisfaction with care are related,[57] Kiser et al[58] found that only 54% of parents were satisfied with their child's psychiatric treatment programme despite the fact that 86% noted improvement in their child's condition.

The American Commission on Accreditation of Rehabilitation Facilities (CARF) recommends that all rehabilitation programmes adopt patient satisfaction as an outcome measure. Thus, there is a need for measures that describe and quantify patient and family satisfaction in the context of paediatric rehabilitation.

Several of these tools are described in more detail below.

DISABKIDS (HEALTHCARE NEEDS AND HEALTHCARE SATISFACTION)

A new battery of tools has been developed by the DISABKIDS group in Europe.[59,60] It is a comprehensive measure that includes structural, process and outcome parameters of care, all from the parent perspective. It contains seven condition-specific modules as well as a DISABKIDS chronic generic module. Domains relevant to services include healthcare needs, the receipt of services, problems with receiving services and satisfaction with quality of care. This comprehensive tool is one to look out for in the future as it is currently undergoing further psychometric testing.

ADAPTATION OF THE GENERIC CLIENT SATISFACTION QUESTIONNAIRE

Although criticized by some as operationalizing patient satisfaction as a unidimensional concept,[61] the Client Satisfaction Questionnaire (CSQ)[62] is a valid and reliable eight-item scale used to assess patient satisfaction with respect to quality of service, type of service, recommending the service, amount of help received, dealing more effectively with problems, satisfaction with

service and returning for the same service. Satisfaction in the CSQ reflects an overall judgement as opposed to the client's perception of the actual behaviours of service providers and the actual events or processes of care that might contribute to satisfaction. The CSQ has good psychometric properties and has been adapted to numerous contexts, including satisfaction with services in paediatrics.[63]

MAINTAINING STANDARDS OF CARE

Having highly qualified and well-trained staff is one of the principles outlined earlier in the chapter. Although there are facility-specific accreditation procedures at the level of the facility, and professional inspections of clinicians by their professional corporation or organization, evaluation by peers may be particularly useful for ensuring a high standard of practice. To maintain a high standard of service delivery (care), it is imperative that rehabilitation interventions practised by therapists are evidence based or reflect best practice.[68] Furthermore, therapists have a wide array of intervention strategies and techniques that they use to maximize results.[69] Measures of these constructs may include the following: Multidimensional Peer Rating of the Clinical Behaviours of Pediatric Therapists (MPR)[70–72] and Therapy Intervention Methods Checklist (TIMC).[69] They can be used to ensure a high quality of care and adherence to practice guidelines (where they exist) or to current best practice. These are both described below in further detail.

Summary

In this chapter, we have presented various tools that may be used to measure different aspects or components of health and rehabilitation service delivery provision to children with disabilities. Although presented individually, some of these tools cut across various structure and process dimensions (e.g. Measures of Processes of Care have elements related to satisfaction as well as family-centred care). We have highlighted those tools that have reported psychometric properties of validity and reliability. Other tools exist that evaluate care in a more global sense (e.g. Parents' Perceptions of Primary Care),[73] which may conceivably be adapted for use with children with special needs. Conversely, other tools developed for groups with specific disabilities may be expanded to other groups with disabilities (e.g. Service Obstacle Scale).[24] Instruments that measure quality and quantity of service provision are crucial for administrators, policy-makers, clinicians and consumers as they provide information that guides ongoing improvement of services to meet the healthcare needs of children with special needs and their families.

PEDS-QL HEALTHCARE SATISFACTION GENERIC MODULE[64,65]

Purpose	To measure satisfaction with healthcare received by a child (and his or her family) at the hospital from the staff
Population	Parents of children and adolescents with or without health problems
Description of domains (subscales)	Six domains (total of 24 items): Information (five items) – describing satisfaction with quantity and timeliness of information provided; Inclusion of Family (four items) – describing satisfaction with attention given to the family; Communication (five items) – describing how well staff communicate; Technical Skills (three items) – describing ability of staff; Emotional Needs (four items) – describing attention to emotional needs; and Overall Satisfaction (three items) regarding overall care, friendliness and helpfulness of staff and the way the child is treated
Administration and test format	Self-administered questionnaire. Each item is scored on a five-point Likert scale (0=never happy to 4=always happy). Scale scores are computed as follows: the mean is computed as the sum of the items divided by the number of items answered. If more than 50% of items are missing, the scale should not be computed. Imputing the mean of the completed items in a scale when 50% or more are completed is the method of choice. The scores are transformed as follows: 0=0 1=25 2=50 3=75 4=100 Higher scores reflect higher satisfaction. To create the Total Scale Score, the mean is computed as the sum of all the items over the number of items answered on all the scales
Psychometric properties	Internal consistency of the haematology/oncology version: Cronbach's alpha=0.96 Content validity of haematology/oncology version: factor analysis revealed four factors – general satisfaction; satisfaction with staff communication and interaction style; satisfaction with information amount and timeliness; and satisfaction with the staff's provision of emotional support for the patient and parent
How to order	Email Christelle Berne (cberne@mapi.fr)
Key reference	Varni JW, Quiggins DJS, Ayala GX (2000) Development of the paediatric hematology/oncology parent satisfaction survey. *Child Health Care* 29: 243–255.

MULTIDIMENSIONAL ASSESSMENT OF PARENTAL SATISFACTION (MAPS)[66,67]

Purpose	To measure satisfaction with providers at the individual level of care
Population	Parents (or primary caregivers) of children with disabilities and chronic illnesses
Description of domains (subscales)	12 items representing five dimensions: developmentally appropriate care (two items); family-centred care (three items); co-ordinated care (four items); technical competence (two items); and interpersonal competence (two items)
Administration and test format	Self-administered, or interviewer administered by telephone. The respondent is asked to identify the person who provides care for the child's condition as well as the person who provides general health care (e.g. care if the child had a cold or influenza). If it is the same person, the items are asked only once with the provider's name as the referent; otherwise, the items are asked twice, with each of the providers indicated separately as referents. Response categories are excellent, very good, good, fair, poor or does not apply. Scoring: to calculate dissatisfaction score, the number of fair or poor responses for each provider should be summed and divided by the total number of responses (excluding items that are not applicable) and multiplied by 10
Psychometric properties	Internal consistency: Cronbach's alpha of 0.87 Discriminant validity: evidence for differential satisfaction ratings for different types of providers and for different individual providers Construct validity: correlations >0.75 with general satisfaction
How to order	The tool is available in Ireys and Perry (1999)
Key references	Ireys HT, Perry JJ (1999) Development and evaluation of a satisfaction scale for parents of children with special health care needs. *Paediatrics* 104: 1182–1191. Liptak GS, Orlando M, Yingling JT, et al (2006) Satisfaction with primary health care received by families of children with developmental disabilities. *J Pediatr Health Care* 20: 245–252.

MULTIDIMENSIONAL PEER RATING OF THE CLINICAL BEHAVIOURS OF PEDIATRIC THERAPISTS (MPR)

Purpose	Originally developed for research on clinical decision-making among paediatric therapists, the MPR also conceptualizes clinical expertise among paediatric rehabilitation clinicians in a multidimensional fashion. It is used to differentiate among therapists with respect to clinical behaviours related to expertise
Population	Paediatric therapists (physiotherapists, occupational therapists and speech and language pathologists) are evaluated by peers. Peers are colleagues in the same or different discipline who meet the following criteria: have experience working with infants/children/youth in a service provision capacity; work directly or indirectly with the target therapist; and have regular opportunities (in their opinion) to observe the clinical decision-making of the target therapists. The peers include individuals who work with the target therapist with the same clients, consult with the target therapist at a clinic or who work with the target therapist in the same school, programme or project. Professionals in different disciplines include social workers, teachers and educational or therapy assistants who work closely with the participants to be able to complete the rating scale

Description of domains (subscales)	A 34-item scale with four subscales:
	    clinical skill (13 items);
	    interpersonal skill (12 items);
	    mentorship (six items); and
	    motivation (three items)

Administration and test format	This is a self-administered tool. Respondents are asked to rate how well the target therapist, for example, 'develops a good rapport with children'. The response is rated on a seven-point scale where 1=not at all and 7=to a very great extent
Psychometric properties	Internal consistency of the scales range from good to excellent (Cronbach's alphas of 0.95, 0.87, 0.89 and 0.71, respectively, for the four subscales) Test–retest reliabilities are good to excellent (intraclass correlation coefficients 0.88, 0.76, 0.76 and 0.91, respectively, for the four scales)
How to order	Email research@tvc.on.ca. See also the website (www.racsn.ca)
Key references	Gilpin M, King G, Currie M, Bartlett D, Willoughby C, Strachan D, Tucker MA, Baxter D (2005) The Multidimensional Peer Rating of the Clinical Behaviours of Paediatric Therapists (MPR). Focus On; 5:Issue 4. London, ON: Research Alliance for Children with Special Needs. King G, Bartlett D, Currie M, et al (2007) Measuring the expertise of paediatric rehabilitation therapists. *Int J Disabil Dev Educ* 55: 5–26.

THERAPY INTERVENTION METHODS CHECKLIST (TIMC)

Purpose	To identify intervention methods used by physiotherapists, occupational therapists, and speech and language practitioners in the school setting. Possible uses include training school-based therapists, providing performance feedback and peer review, and research purposes, e.g. examining methods and improvement on goals
Population	School-based therapists who treat children with special needs

Description of domains (subscales)	Five categories (each includes a list of items plus an 'other' category):
	    cognitive strategies (13 items);
	    teaching/learning techniques (10 items);
	    handling/physical interventions (12 items);
	    environmental/task modifications (four items); and
	    information sharing (five items)

Administration and test format	Evaluators (or observing therapists) who observe treating therapists and complete the checklist to record the types of interventions used
Psychometric properties	Content validity: all items reported at least once in the 36-session testing phase. Test–retest reliability evaluated (over 8-wk time period): physical/handling interventions (r=0.89); cognitive strategies (r=0.75); information sharing (r=0.63); teaching/learning (r=0.54); environmental/task modifications (r=0.21)
How to order	Email research@tvcc.on.ca. See also the website (www.racsn.ca)
Key reference	McDougall J, King G, Malloy-Miller T, Gritzan J, Tucker MA, Evans J (1999) A checklist to determine the methods of intervention using in school-based therapy: development and pilot testing. *Phys Occupat Ther Paediatr* 19: 53–76.

REFERENCES

1. Feldman DE, Swaine B, Gosselin J, Meshefedjian G, Grilli L (2008) Is waiting for rehabilitation services associated with changes in function and quality of life in children with physical disabilities? *Phys Occup Ther Pediatr* 28: 291–304.

2. Childcare Adcocacy Association of Canada. What do we mean by quality child care and developmentally appropriate programming? Available at: www.ccaac.ca/pdf/resources/fact-sheets/quality.pdf (accessed 1 February 2009).

3. L'office des personnes handicapées du Québec (1992) *L'intervention Précoce Auprès de L'enfant Ayant une Déficience et de sa Famille*. Montreal, QC: Bibliothèque nationale du Québec.

4. Campbell SK, Gardner HG, Ramakrishnan V (1995) Correlates of physicians' decisions to refer children with cerebral palsy for physical therapy. *Dev Med Child Neurol* 37: 1062–1074.

5. Simpson GA, Colpe L, Greenspan S (2003) Measuring functional developmental delay in infants and young children: prevalence rates from the NHIS-D. *Paediatr Perinat Epidemiol* 17: 68–80.

6. Fox HB, Wicks LB, Newacheck PW (1993) Health maintenance organizations and children with special health needs. A suitable match? *Am J Dis Child* 147: 546–552.

7. Majnemer A, Shevell MI, Rosenbaum P, Abrahamowicz M (2002) Early rehabilitation service utilization patterns in young children with developmental delays. *Child Care Health Dev* 28: 29–37.

8. Grilli L, Ehrmann FD, Swaine B, Gosselin J, Champagne F, Pineault R (2007) Wait times for pediatric rehabilitation. *Healthcare Policy*. Available at: www.longwoods.com/product.php?productid=18681 (accessed 1 February 2009).

9. Feldman DE, Champagne F, Korner-Bitensky N, Meshefedjian G (2002) Waiting time for rehabilitation services for children with physical disabilities. *Child Care Health Dev* 28: 351–358.

10. Mazer B, Feldman D, Majnemer A, Gosselin J, Kehayia E (2006) Rehabilitation services for children: therapists' perceptions. *Pediatr Rehabil* 9: 340–350.

11. *CanChild*, Centre for Childhood Disability Research (2000) *Children with Disabilities in Ontario: A Profile of Children's Services, Part 1: Children, Families and Services*. Hamilton, ON: McMaster University, CanChild.

12. Law M (2003) Practitioners in pediatric rehabilitation have endorsed the concepts of family-centered service as an approach to the delivery of services to children with disabilities and their families. *Phys Occup Ther Pediatr* 23: 1–3.

13. Starfield B (1998) *Primary Care: Balancing Health Needs, Services, and Technology*. New York: Oxford University Press.

14. Guttmann A, Razzaq A, Lindsay P, Zagorski B, Anderson GM (2006) Development of measures of the quality of emergency department care for children using a structured panel process. *Pediatrics* 118: 114–123.

15. Mangione-Smith R, DeCristofaro AH, Setodji CM, et al (2007) The quality of ambulatory care delivered to children in the United States. *N Engl J Med* 357: 1515–1523.

16. Homer CJ, Horvitz L, Heinrich P, Forbes P, Lesneski C, Phillips J (2004) Improving care for children with attention deficit hyperactivity disorder: assessing the impact of self-assessment and targeted training on practice performance. *Ambul Pediatr* 4: 436–441.

17. Kuhlthau K, Walker DK, Perrin JM, et al (1998) Assessing managed care for children with chronic conditions. *Health Aff (Millwood)* 17: 42–52.

18. Homer CJ, Marino B, Cleary PD, et al (1999) Quality of care at a children's hospital: the parent's perspective. *Arch Pediatr Adolesc Med* 153: 1123–1129.

19. King SM, Rosenbaum PL, King GA (1996) Parents' perceptions of caregiving: development and validation of a measure of processes. *Dev Med Child Neurol* 38: 757–772.

20. Mooney G (1987) What does equity in health mean? *World Health Stat Quart* 40: 296–303.

21. Donabedian A (1973) *Aspects of Medical Care Administration – Specifying Requirements for Health Care*. Cambridge, MA: Harvard University Press.

22. Ehrmann FD, Couture M, Grilli L, Simard MN, Azoulay L, Gosselin J (2005) When and by whom is concern first expressed for children with neuromotor problems? *Arch Pediatr Adolesc Med* 159: 882–886.

23. Shevell MI, Majnemer A, Rosenbaum P, Abrahamowicz M (2001) Profile of referrals for early childhood developmental delay to ambulatory subspecialty clinics. *J Child Neurol* 16: 645–650.

24. Kolakowsky-Hayner SA, Kreutzer JS, Miner KD (2000) Validation of the Service Obstacles Scale for the traumatic brain injury population. *NeuroRehabilitation* 14: 151–158.

25. Kreutzer JS (2000) *The Service Obstacles Scale*. The Center for Outcome Measurement in Brain Injury. Available at: www.tbims.org/combi/sos (accessed 1 February 2009).

26. Haggerty JL, Reid RJ, Freeman GK, Starfield BH, Adair CE, McKendry R (2003) Continuity of care: a multidisciplinary review. *BMJ* 327: 1219–1221.

27. Bice TW, Boxerman SB (1977) A quantitative measure of continuity of care. *Med Care* 15: 347–349.

28. Christakis DA, Kazak AE, Wright JA, Zimmerman FJ, Bassett AL, Connell FA (2004) What factors are associated with achieving high continuity of care? *Fam Med* 36: 55–60.

29. Christakis DA, Wright JA, Zimmerman FJ, Bassett AL, Connell FA (2003) Continuity of care is associated with well-coordinated care. *Ambul Pediatr* 3: 82–86.

30. Christakis DA, Feudtner C, Pihoker C, Connell FA (2001) Continuity and quality of care for children with diabetes who are covered by Medicaid. *Ambul Pediatr* 1: 99–103.

31. Brousseau DC, Meurer JR, Isenberg ML, Kuhn EM, Gorelick MH (2004) Association between infant continuity of care and pediatric emergency department utilization. *Pediatrics* 113: 738–741.

32. Thyen U, Sperner J, Morfeld M, Meyer C, Ravens-Sieberer U (2003) Unmet health care needs and impact on families with children with disabilities in Germany. *Ambul Pediatr* 3: 74–81.

33. Perrin EC, Lewkowicz C, Young MH (2000) Shared vision: concordance among fathers, mothers, and pediatricians about unmet needs of children with chronic health conditions. *Pediatrics* 105: 277–285.

34. Kreutzer JS, Marwitz JH, Kepler K (1992) Traumatic brain injury: family response and outcome. *Arch Phys Med Rehabil* 73: 771–778.

35. Marwitz JH (2000) *The Family Needs Questionnaire*. The Center for Outcome Measurement in Brain Injury. Available at: www.tbims.org/combi/fnq (accessed 1 February 2009).

36. Meade MA, Taylor LA, Kreutzer JS, Marwitz JH, Thomas V (2004) A preliminary study of acute family needs after spinal cord injury: analysis and implications. *Rehabil Psychol* 49: 150–155.

37. King G, Tucker MA, Baldwin P, Lowry K, LaPorta J, Martens L (2002) A life needs model of pediatric service delivery: services to support community participation and quality of life for children and youth with disabilities. *Phys Occup Ther Pediatr* 22: 53–77.

38. Chernoff RG, Ireys HT, DeVet KA, Kim YJ (2002) A randomized, controlled trial of a community-based support program

for families of children with chronic illness: pediatric outcomes. *Arch Pediatr Adolesc Med* 156: 533–539.

39. Law M, Hanna S, King G, et al (2003) Factors affecting family-centred service delivery for children with disabilities. *Child Care Health Dev* 29: 357–366.

40. Mollica RL and Gillespie J (2003) *Care Coordination for People with Chronic Conditions*. Baltimore, MD: Partnership for Solutions, Johns Hopkins University.

41. Appleton PL, Boll V, Everett JM, Kelly AM, Meredith KH, Payne TG (1997) Beyond child development centres: care coordination for children with disabilities. *Child Care Health Dev* 23: 29–40.

42. King S, Rosenbaum P, King G (1995) *The Measure of Processes of Care: A Means to Assess Family-centred Behaviours of Health Care Providers*. Hamilton, ON: McMaster University, Neurodevelopmental Clinical Research Unit.

43. Woodside J, Rosenbaum P, King S, King G (1998) *The Measure of Processes of Care for Service Providers (MPOC-SP)*. Hamilton, ON: CanChild Centre for Childhood Disability Research, McMaster University.

44. Dyke P, Buttigieg P, Blackmore AM, Ghose A (2006) Use of the measure of process of care for families (MPOC-56) and service providers (MPOC-SP) to evaluate family-centred services in a paediatric disability setting. *Child Care Health Dev* 32: 167–176.

45. Bjerre IM, Larsson M, Franzon AM, Nilsson MS, Stromberg G, Westbom LM (2004) Measure of Processes of Care (MPOC) applied to measure parent's perception of the habilitation process in Sweden. *Child Care Health Dev* 30: 123–130.

46. Granat T, Lagander B, Borjesson MC (2002) Parental participation in the habilitation process – evaluation from a user perspective. *Child Care Health Dev* 28: 459–467.

47. O'Neil ME, Palisano RJ, Westcott SL (2001) Relationship of therapists' attitudes, children's motor ability, and parenting stress to mothers' perceptions of therapists' behaviors during early intervention. *Phys Ther* 81: 1412–1424.

48. Mah JK, Tough S, Fung T, Douglas-England K, Verhoef M (2006) Adolescent quality of life and satisfaction with care. *J Adolesc Health* 38: 607.

49. McConachie H, Logan S (2003) Validation of the measure of processes of care for use when there is no Child Development Centre. *Child Care Health Dev* 29: 35–45.

50. Swaine BR, Pless IB, Friedman DS, Montes JL (1999) Using the measure of processes of care with parents of children hospitalized for head injury. *Am J Phys Med Rehabil* 78: 323–329.

51. Stewart D, Law M, Russell D, Hanna S (2004) Evaluating children's rehabilitation services: an application of a programme logic model. *Child Care Health Dev* 30: 453–462.

52. Keith RA (1998) Patient satisfaction and rehabilitation services. *Arch Phys Med Rehabil* 79: 1122–1128.

53. Routh D (1988) *Handbook of Pediatric Psychology*. New York: Guilford Press.

54. Lewis CC, Scott DE, Pantell RH, Wolf MH (1986) Parent satisfaction with children's medical care. Development, field test, and validation of a questionnaire. *Med Care* 24: 209–215.

55. Breslau N, Mortimer EA Jr (1981) Seeing the same doctor: determinants of satisfaction with specialty care for disabled children. *Med Care* 19: 741–758.

56. Corrigan JD, Smith-Knapp K, Granger CV (1998) Outcomes in the first 5 years after traumatic brain injury. *Arch Phys Med Rehabil* 79: 298–305.

57. Kane RL, Maciejewski M, Finch M (1997) The relationship of patient satisfaction with care and clinical outcomes. *Med Care* 35: 714–730.

58. Kiser LJ, Millsap PA, Hickerson S, et al (1996) Results of treatment one year later: child and adolescent partial hospitalization. *J Am Acad Child Adolesc Psychiatry* 35: 81–90.

59. Baars RM, Atherton CI, Koopman HM, Bullinger M, Power M (2005) The European DISABKIDS project: development of seven condition-specific modules to measure health related quality of life in children and adolescents. *Health Qual Life Outcomes* 3: 70.

60. Schmidt S, Thyen U, Chaplin J, Mueller-Godeffroy E, Bullinger M (2008) Healthcare needs and healthcare satisfaction from the perspective of parents of children with chronic conditions: the DISABKIDS approach towards instrument development. *Child Care Health Dev* 34: 355–366.

61. van Campen C, Sixma H, Friele RD, Kerssens JJ, Peters L (1995) Quality of care and patient satisfaction: a review of measuring instruments. *Med Care Res Rev* 52: 109–133.

62. Larsen DL, Attkisson CC, Hargreaves WA, Nguyen TD (1979) Assessment of client/patient satisfaction: development of a general scale. *Eval Program Plann* 2: 197–207.

63. Lawoko S, Soares JJ (2004) Satisfaction with care: a study of parents of children with congenital heart disease and parents of children with other diseases. *Scand J Caring Sci* 18: 90–102.

64. Varni JW, Burwinkle TM, Seid M (2005) The PedsQL as a pediatric patient-reported outcome: reliability and validity of the PedsQL Measurement Model in 25,000 children. *Exp Rev Pharmacoeconomics Outcomes Res* 5: 705–719.

65. Hsieh RL, Huang HY, Lin MI, Wu CW, Lee WC (2009) Quality of life, health satisfaction and family impact on caregivers of children with developmental delays. *Child Care Health Dev* 35: 243–249.

66. Ireys HT, Perry JJ (1999) Development and evaluation of a satisfaction scale for parents of children with special health care needs. *Pediatrics* 104: 1182–1191.

67. Liptak GS, Orlando M, Yingling JT, et al (2006) Satisfaction with primary health care received by families of children with developmental disabilities. *J Pediatr Health Care* 20: 245–252.

68. Majnemer A, Limperopoulos C (2002) Importance of outcome determination in pediatric rehabilitation. *Dev Med Child Neurol* 44: 773–777.

69. McDougall J, King GA, Malloy-Miller T, Gritzan J, Tucker MA, Evans J (1999) A checklist to determine the methods of intervention used in school-based therapy: development and pilot testing. *Phys Occup Ther Pediatr* 19: 53–77.

70. King G, Currie M, Bartlett DJ, et al (2007) The development of expertise in pediatric rehabilitation therapists: changes in approach, self-knowledge, and use of enabling and customizing strategies. *Dev Neurorehabil* 10: 223–240.

71. King G, Bartlett DJ, Currie M, et al (2007) Measuring the expertise of pediatric rehabilitation therapists. *Int J Dis Dev Edu* 55: 5–26.

72. Gilpin M, King G, Currie M, et al (2005) *The Multidimensional Peer Rating of the Clinical Behaviours of Pediatric Therapists (MPR)*. Focus On, vol. 5, issue 4: London, ON: Research Alliance for Children with Special Needs.

73. Seid M, Varni JW, Bermudez LO, et al (2001) Parents' Perceptions of Primary Care: measuring parents' experiences of pediatric primary care quality. *Pediatrics* 108: 264–270.

SECTION VI HOLISTIC VIEW OF HEALTH AND WELL-BEING

33
HEALTH STATUS INSTRUMENTS

Nora Fayed, Anne Klassen and Veronica Schiariti

What is the construct?

In 1948, the World Health Organization (WHO) defined health as 'a state of complete physical, mental, and social well-being and not merely the absence of disease or infirmity'.[1] While this often-quoted definition clarifies that health is much more than not being ill, on its own it fails to offer clarity or consensus about what aspects of a person's life *should* be included in the concept of health. Lack of consensus is problematic because a universal concept of health is needed to describe and to evaluate the needs of children all over the world. Ironically, the original purpose of the 1948 definition was to provide such a definition.

Despite this confusion, the concept of health is viewed internationally as a resource for well-being and positive living.[2,3] The productivity and potential of entire nations is determined at least in part by the health of their children.[3] Furthermore, the efforts of parents, communities and health providers are judged on the basis of improvements to child health. Health status instruments are multidimensional tools that can provide a snapshot of a child's health at any given point in time, but what definition of health do these tools reflect? The answer is that, however implicitly, instruments reflect the developers' ideas of health contextualized to the time, place and purpose for which the instrument was developed. Thus, some historical background to the measurement of health provides a useful starting point to the consideration of health status instruments.

Since the advent of germ theory, health has been expressed using an absence-of-disease approach, which has been found useful in public health contexts. As early as the 1700s, public health proponents were interested in measuring patterns of disease outbreaks and later the effects of clean water and community hygiene practices.[2,4] At that time, health indicators, such as the incidence and prevalence of diseases such as cholera and dysentery, were useful because they showed the proportion of individuals with infirmity in the population. Since the development of antibiotics and vaccination, the incidence and prevalence of infectious disease has declined (at least in the developed world).[4] Health indicators shifted their focus from prevalence and incidence to include symptoms for describing children and adults who were living with disabilities or morbidity as a result of extended illness. Symptom checklists were developed to measure pain or discomfort from the perspective of both the child and parent.[5] As many sources of mortality and morbidity of childhood have become treatable, questionnaires were developed to assess the experience of childhood chronic health conditions or disability and as indicators of health.

More recently, a measurement approach to health has been developed based on child and parent report (otherwise known as patient-reported outcomes [PROs]). PROs are any reports of the status of a patient's condition that come directly from the patient without interpretation by anyone else.[6] PROs measure concepts such as symptoms, satisfaction, health status and health-related quality of life. In order to effectively capture the concept of health through PROs, well-defined, reliable and valid instruments are needed. Such instruments are typically composed of multiple scales that reflect the key aspects of a conceptual framework.

HEALTH AND THE ICF/ICF-CY

Simultaneously with this shift towards using PROs over the last 20 to 30 years came a broadening of the conceptualization of health. In the mid-1970s, Pless and Pinkerton[7] described a non-categorical (i.e. non-diagnosis based) approach to conceptualizing health, which shifted the emphasis of measurement away from diagnosis and onto various psychosocial indicators of health. Non-categorical thinking, combined with an increasing recognition of the importance of the child's daily functioning, has helped to prepare the clinical and research communities for a biopsychosocial concept of health found in the International Classification of Functioning, Disability and Health (ICF) and, more recently, the children and youth version (ICF-CY).[8,9]

The ICF-CY espoused a biopsychosocial approach, which has certain advantages to the measurement of health status. First, it created a definition of health based on the interaction of biopsychosocial factors (*body functions*, *body structures*, *activities and participation*), which occur in a context of the *environment* and *personal factors*.[7,8] The advantage of the ICF-CY definition is the inclusion of the components that constitute functioning, disability and health as opposed to a definition based on what health is not (i.e. the absence of disease). Second, the ICF-CY definition is accompanied by a classification that specifies details about health and health-related components using a standard document. The advantage of the ICF-CY classification is that it serves as a taxonomy that can be applied to describe content from health status instruments (a practice that will also be applied to the measures we review in this chapter). Finally, despite similarities or differences in existing health status instruments, the ICF-CY taxonomy can be used to clarify their content so clinicians and researchers can select instruments that describe and compare the areas of importance to a given time, place and purpose within a biopsychosocial approach to health.

HOW IS PATIENT-REPORTED HEALTH STATUS UNIQUE RELATIVE TO QUALITY OF LIFE?
As questionnaires are developed that include biopsychosocial outcomes of interest to children and their families, there is growing confusion about what distinguishes a health status instrument from other questionnaires that are called quality of life (QOL) instruments or health-related quality of life (HRQOL) tools.[10] Health status includes multidimensional information about health conditions and the ability to perform physically and emotionally in daily life. Ideally, in ICF-CY terms, health status includes the interaction of individual components of body functions, body structures, activities and participation, which occur in a context of environmental and personal factors. Given that these components span the entirety of the experience of life, it is difficult at first glance to see how health status is different from HRQOL or QOL.

Health, HRQOL and QOL include factors pertaining to *biological, psychological* and *social* life. The distinction between health and HRQOL/QOL is in *how* these domains are measured. Chapter 34, on QOL outcomes, specifies that it is the *subjective* element that is common to all QOL outcomes and which makes QOL different from health status. Consistent with the WHO's definition, the primary focus of QOL rests on the 'individual's perception of his or her position in life',[11] with *perception* as the key word. Thus, to measure QOL, the child's or parent's perceptions and values, such as satisfaction, importance or meta-appraisals about biopsychosocial areas of life are the central/intended target of measurement (signal), while the actual presence, absence, severity, intensity or difficulty with the biopsychosocial area of life is secondary or unintended (noise; see Fig. 33.1). Social life, for example, is a component that is relevant to the health of school-aged children and adolescents, and hence is addressed by most health status instruments in some way. The question 'Does your child have difficulty

	Signal (target content)	Noise (extraneous content)
Health Status (Do you have difficulty getting along with other children?)	Actual performance, capacity, severity, frequency, extent of a health domain 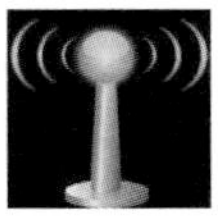	Perceptions i.e., expectations, standards, goals, or concerns about the health domain 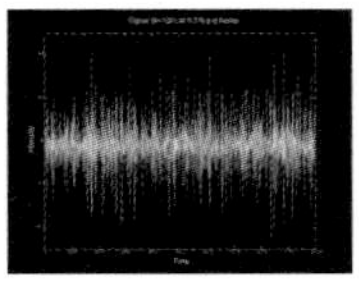
QOL/ HRQOL (Are you satisfied with the way you get along with other children)	Perceptions i.e., expectations, standards, goals, or concerns about the health domain 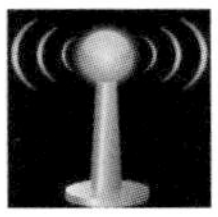	Actual performance, capacity, severity, frequency, extent of a health domain 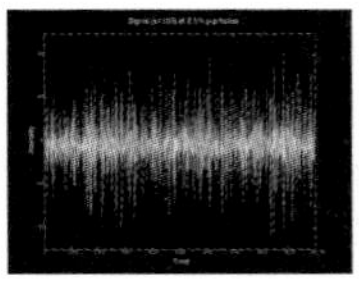

Figure 33.1 Differing emphasis of how health status and quality of life are assessed for the health domain *social interactions*.

TABLE 33.1

Differing emphasis of how health status and quality of life are assessed for the health domain *social interactions*

Standard approach	Health–economics approach
Child Health Questionnaire (CHQ)	Health-Utilities Index III (HUI-III)
Child Health Assessment Questionnaire (CHAQ)	EuroQol 5D-Youth (EQ-5D-Y)
Functional Status II Revised (FS-II R)	
Child Health Illness Profile (CHIP)	

getting along with other children?' represents a health status approach, whereas the question 'Are you satisfied with your child's ability to get along with other children?' reflects a QOL approach.

Thus the concept of health status is distinct from QOL because it seeks to distinguish differences and commonalities in the experience of health for children based on health indicators that are common between children as opposed to individual or personal *perceptions* of those differences and commonalities. Although these distinctions can be made conceptually, deciding on whether an instrument reflects a health status or QOL approach requires some thought on the part of an instrument user. Many health status instruments were developed before these conceptual distinctions were made clear in the literature. This chapter describes considerations in the selection of instruments that are mainly described as health status instruments while recognizing that the reviewed instruments might contain mixed elements of health status and QOL. The chapter is also intended to provide instrument users with basic criteria with which they can appraise instruments of interest for their respective purposes assuming one is interested in measurement using a biopsychosocial definition of health such as that found in the ICF-CY.

We have selected for review in this chapter six popular instruments used to measure health status in children (see Table 33.1). Two of these instruments reflect a health economics perspective while the remaining four instruments reflect a classical or standard approach to testing in PROs. In the next section we describe general factors to consider when choosing a health status instrument.

General factors to consider when measuring this domain

CONTENT VALIDITY AND CONTENT OVERLAP

Content validity is an important measurement property that clinicians and researchers must consider when choosing an instrument.[12] Unfortunately, content validity is commonly overlooked and, once compromised, can lead to a false conclusion that vital outcomes were not affected by an intervention when, in fact, a change occurred. For example, an instrument that focuses on cognitive problems (e.g. attention, planning, mental flexibility) might not detect changes resulting from an educational intervention for a child with a learning disability whereas an instrument focused on school performance detects the improvement based on the child's success in compensating for his or her cognitive issues. Instrument users are often satisfied to choose a so-called 'criterion standard' instrument to assess health status; unaware that content validity is not a property of the instrument itself, but of the fit between an instrument and the purpose for which it is intended.[12] One can only say they expect to achieve content validity if the outcomes that are an issue for the children of interest and the target concept are articulated by the chosen instrument in a comprehensive way.

Often clinicians and researchers are well aware of the aspects of health that they hypothesize are important to the children and families they serve. From the perspective of body functions, these components could include emotional functions, pain, sleep and specific aspects of cognition (e.g. memory and attention). Activities and participation components can vary greatly depending on age and developmental level but typically include play, sports, learning and applying knowledge (e.g. school performance), mobility and self-care. Aspects of the environment that are important to child health, such as social support, the attitudes of others and the availability of educational, social and health services are also often important. All of these health components are articulated in the ICF-CY classification. Thus, the ICF-CY can serve as a standard tool by which clinicians and researchers can define their outcomes of interest, relate them to the classification system and, to ensure content coverage, seek instruments that ask children and families about those specific health outcomes.

Most of the instruments reviewed below were developed prior to the introduction of the ICF-CY. We performed an analysis of the content of each instrument by linking each questionnaire item to the ICF-CY classification[8] in order to understand how the content maps

TABLE 33.2
ICF body functions, activities and participation, and enviroment content assessed according to frequency (number of items). First- and second-level categories appear in bold

ICF category	ICF code	CHQ	CHIP Core section	CHIP Optional section	FS-II R	CHAQ	EQ-5D-Y	HUIIII
Body functions								
Dispositions and intrapersonal functions	b125	1						
Responsivity	b1251				1			
Activity level	b1252				1			
Temperament and personality functions	b126							
Agreeableness	b1261				1			
Psychic stability	b1263		2		1			
Openness to experience	b1264				1			
Energy and drive functions	b130	2			1			
Appetite	b1302							
Sleep functions	b134	1			1			
Onset of sleep	b1341		1					
Maintenance of sleep functions	b1342				1			
Attention functions	b140	1						
Memory functions	b144		1					1
Psychomotor control	b1470	2						
Emotional functions	b152	20	9	1	1		1	1
Appropriateness of emotion	b1521				2			
Thought functions	b160	3						
Expression of spoken language	b16710							
Experience of self and time functions	b180	2						
Experience of self	b1800	1						
Seeing functions	b210							1
Hearing functions	b230							1
Pain	b280	2	1			1	1	1
Pain in head and neck	b28010	1	3					
Activities and participation	d	1		1	1			
Thinking	d163							1
Reading	d166		2					
Writing	d170					1		
Calculating	d172		1					
Solving problems	d175		1					1
General tasks and demands	d2	1						
Carrying out daily routine	d230		1					
Handling crisis	d2402		1					
Managing one's own behaviour	d250	15			1			

TABLE 33.2
Continued

ICF category	ICF code	CHQ	CHIP Core section	CHIP Optional section	FS-II R	CHAQ	EQ-5D-Y	HUIIII
Communication	d3							
Communicating by receiving spoken messages	d310							
Speaking	d330		1					1
Producing non-verbal messages	d335		1					
Communication – producing other specified and unspecified	d349				1			
Conversation	d350	1						
Discussion	d355	1	1					
Discussion with one person	d3550		1					
Changing basic body position	d410					5		
Lying down	d4100	1						
Standing	d4104							
Bending	d4105	1						
Transferring oneself	d420	1						
Lifting and carrying objects	d430	1						
Lifting	d4300							
Fine hand use	d440							
Hand and arm use	d445							
Reaching	d4452		2			1		
Walking	d450	1				2	1	1
Walking short distances	d4500	1	1					
Walking long distances	d4501	2						
Climbing	d4551		1			1		
Running	d4552					1		
Moving around in different locations	d460	3						
Using private motorized transportation	d4701			2				
Driving human-powered transportation (e.g. bicycle)	d4750					1		
Self-care	d5					1	1	
Washing oneself	d510	1				1	1	
Washing body parts	d51000					1		
Washing whole body	d5101					1		
Drying oneself	d5102							
Caring for hair	d5202					1		
Caring for fingernails	d5203					1		
Toileting	d530	1				1		
Dressing	d540	1				3	1	
Taking off clothes	d5401					1		
Eating	d550	1	1		1			
Looking after one's safety	d571			1				
Domestic life	d6							
Acquisition of goods and services	d620					1		

TABLE 33.2
Continued

ICF category	ICF code	CHQ	CHIP Core section	CHIP Optional section	FS-II R	CHAQ	EQ-5D-Y	HUIIII
Doing housework	d640	1				1		
Interpersonal interactions and relationships	d7	4	1					
Complex interpersonal interactions	d720							
Relating with persons in authority	d7400	1	1					
Informal social relationships	d750		3					
Social relationships with friends	d7500	2	2					
Family relationships	d760	5	1					
Family relationships unspecified	d7609		2					
Parent–child relationships	d7600							
Major life areas	d8							
School education	d820	8	3	1				
Maintaining educational programme	d8201	3						
Work and employment other specified and unspecified	d859							
Solitary play	d8800		1					
Recreation and leisure	d920	1	2					
Play	d9200		1					
Sports	d9201	1						
Socializing	d9205	11						
Environment								
Products and technology for personal use in daily living	e115					3		
Products and technology for indoor and outdoor mobility and transportation	e120					4		
Products and technology for communication	e125					1		
Assets	e165			1				
Immediate family	e310			7				
Friends	e320		1					
Health professionals	e355	1						
Attitudes	e4	1	1					
Media services	e5600			1				
Health services, systems and policies	e580	1		7				
Education and training services, systems and policies	e585	1						

CHIP, Child Health Illness Profile; ICF, International Classification of Functioning, Disability and Health; CHQ, Child Health Questionnaire; FS-II R, Functional Status II Revised; CHAQ, Child Health Assessment Questionnaire; EQ-5D-Y, EuroQoL 5D-Youth; HU-III, Health Utilities Index III.

onto the ICF-CY.[13] Table 33.2 provides information about the health domains that are covered by each instrument according to the ICF-CY components of body functions, activity and participation and environment. Table 33.3

shows content that is consistent with personal factors that do not have specific ICF-CY categories, broad health concepts that are conceptually part of the ICF-CY but not specific enough to fit under an ICF-CY component 'not

TABLE 33.3
Life/health/personal factors assessed by the health status questionnaires that are not classified in the ICF according to frequency (number of items)

Life/health/personal factor	Non-ICF category	CHQ	CHIP Core section	CHIP Optional section	FS-II R	CHAQ	EQ-5D-Y	HUIIII
Functioning of family	Not covered	3						
Having fun	Not covered	1	1	2				
Injury	Not covered			9				
Health condition	Not covered	14	3	31		5		
Quality of life	Not covered	1						1
General health	Not defined		1			1	1	
Mental health	Not defined		1					
Physical health	Not defined	2						
Age	Personal factors	1						
Cheating	Personal factors	1	1					
Destroying property	Personal factors		1					
Language	Personal factors			1				
Level of education	Personal factors	1						
Lying	Personal factors	1	1					
Physical abuse	Personal factors			1				
Sex/gender	Personal factors	1						
Solitude	Personal factors	1						
Race	Personal factors			1				
Running away from home	Personal factors	1						
Stealing	Personal factors	2	1					
Things you want from life	Personal factors	1						
Threatening others	Personal factors		1					
Self-perception	Personal factors	1						

CHIP, Child Health Illness Profile; ICF, International Classification of Functioning, Disability and Health; CHQ, Child Health Questionnaire; FS-II R, Functional Status II Revised; CHAQ, Child Health Assessment Questionnaire; EQ-5D-Y, EuroQoL 5D-Youth; HU-III, Health Utilities Index III.

defined', and concepts that are included in the instruments but not covered conceptually by the ICF-CY or using any specific ICF-CY category 'not covered'. These tables are presented so that researchers and clinicians can determine for themselves whether content coverage is present for their intended questions or needs.

Determining content coverage is a relatively simple step that instrument users can perform prior to selecting a tool. Publications are available that have systematically linked existing child self-report instruments to the ICF and the ICF-CY in addition to the instruments that will be reviewed in this chapter.[14–17] Users can refer to such reviews in addition to reviews of psychometric aspects of developed instruments[18–24] prior to deciding on a health status instrument.

EVALUATION VERSUS DESCRIPTION

Evaluative instruments are tools that should be validated as being sensitive to changes that occur as a result of interventions or significant life events. If health status instruments were cameras, ideally they would have quick shutter speed so that they could capture changes to an image between consecutive photographs. When selecting evaluative instruments, one should consider which aspects of a child's health are expected to change following an intervention and determine whether there are questions representing those aspects of health in the instruments. In psychometric terms, this concept is described in Chapter 1 as responsiveness.

Guyatt and colleagues[25] described the issue of responsiveness in clinical research as well as methods for appraising responsiveness. The authors report a variety of statistical approaches (e.g. effect size, standard error of measures [SEM], Guyatt's responsiveness index and receiver operating characteristic [ROC]) that can be used as indicators of responsiveness. Conversely, they caution against over-reliance on statistical indicators to decide on responsiveness because the evaluative power of an instrument must also tap into content vital to represent the construct (in this case health status) for it to be validly measuring what it is intended to measure.[25] These conceptual and psychometric requirements for responsiveness are important because an instrument can show statistical change when it is not measuring the construct of interest, but some separate, although related, concept. For example, a questionnaire measuring physical activity (a body function) could show change for a sports intervention even if participation is actually the construct one wishes to measure.

A useful descriptive instrument should describe the main concerns of a given group of children. Such an instrument can be used to compare the issues that discriminate between groups of children (e.g. children with cerebral palsy show more health status problems related to mobility whereas children with epilepsy have concerns with memory issues). Well-designed descriptive instruments are like cameras set to high resolution, able to capture a snapshot of an individual child or a group of children with accuracy and precision.

Contrary to evaluative instruments, descriptive tools need not focus on the elements of health that are expected to change. Instead, these instruments can probe health areas that are important for a specific group of children. This distinction is important in order to form a basis for comparison between clinical groups of children or to draw attention to the special needs of the children of interest. For example, children with a certain level of severity of cerebral palsy are not likely to show changes in their walking ability, but asking about mobility in these children and non-affected children would show how the issue of mobility affects one group versus the other. Descriptive instruments must have discriminative validity in that they must be able to show quantitatively any differences that exist between groups of children that are expected to be different (e.g. children with cancer in active treatment would be expected to demonstrate more impairments in body functions than children in a remission phase).

In addition to appraising psychometric reports, the onus is on instrument users (i.e. clinicians and researchers) to consider the content of the instrument. Users must determine whether the items contained therein represent health domains that are expected to change following intervention (for evaluation) or items that describe their

population's particular challenges or issues (for description). The ICF-CY content tables (Tables 33.2 and 33.3) presented in this chapter can assist with this task. Additional issues that are unique to childhood will be addressed below.

MEASUREMENT ISSUES UNIQUE TO CHILDHOOD

Child versus parent proxy

Parents and children typically report and emphasize different areas for targeting interventions and often view health differently from each other.[26–28] Whenever possible, children should be surveyed through the use of instruments that have child report questionnaires. Evidence shows that children can reliably report on their experiences from school age.[28] Additionally, school-aged children are the only agents present for the entirety of their daily experience; therefore, in certain ways, they are the most knowledgeable about many aspects of their own daily health experiences. Using appropriately scaled and worded questionnaires, children with various chronic conditions can respond to self-report instruments. A crucial factor for selecting a health-status instrument, therefore, is whether a child self-report version is available with language and a developmentally tailored visual layout.

Negative language

In terms of the content of instruments, it is important to consider how the questions affect children's understanding of themselves.[29–31] Children might be experiencing vulnerable periods, such as an illness or a new diagnosis, when completing self-report questionnaires, and the questions found in an instrument can influence their understanding of themselves.[31] Many self-report health status instruments administered to children were developed for use in a clinical care context. An unanticipated consequence of a clinically orientated approach has often resulted in the development of questionnaires that emphasize problems or negative aspects of life given that the focus of the clinical milieu is to improve upon the areas in which problems occur.

The content of childhood instruments can be considered in terms of negative content and/or negative phrasing or wording of questionnaire items. The items in many questionnaires were developed using negative wording when the same item could easily have been developed using positive or neutral wording. For example, the item 'Do you have difficulty remembering things you learn at school?' could be reworded as 'Are you able to remember things you learn at school?'. Including negative content in instruments can create a psychological burden for respondents,[31] yet also creates an ethical dilemma for those who need to capture the negative as well as positive factors associated with childhood. Including negative content is often necessary to target important concepts such as pain. Regardless, one should be aware of the extent to which negative content is represented in a questionnaire so as to make balanced choices in assessing child health.

Adult valuation of health applied to individual children
Applying a health utilities approach to health status measurement in children gives rise to special issues.[32,33] Instruments that produce health utilities differ from other patient-reported health status instruments by placing a numeric weight based on the health preferences of a general population (a preference score) to the health status of individual children to obtain a single score value for that child's health. In this approach, one needs to consider the original population used to develop the preference scores (usually large numbers of community-based adults) and extrapolate what influences created the weighting or importance placed on any given health domain over another. For example, imagine that the general population was surveyed and walking was determined to be the most important health attribute whereas social support was ranked low. Applying these preference scores to evaluate the health of children with cerebral palsy who have severe mobility restrictions is ethically questionable because the population of children with cerebral palsy might prefer or value very different health attributes than those chosen by the general population.

Development
Although there are studies that have used instruments developed for adults in research with adolescents and preteens, there is very little theoretical foundation for such practice. The use of instruments that were created for adults yet applied to developing groups (e.g. infants or adolescents) remains inappropriate. Health status domains that are universally applicable to all age groups are difficult to isolate and often do not exist. Social life for preschool children focuses on rudimentary social skills with significant others such as siblings or caregivers, whereas the emphasis of social health for adolescents is tied to their peers. Children differ from adults in that their health is not only tied to their environment and context but is also dependent on others (e.g. reliance on parents and communities). Overall, clues about developmental appropriateness should be found by examining the characteristics of the initial group of children with which the developers created and evaluated the content of the instrument, and look for evidence that the children and youth were involved in the development of the items of the measure.

SELECTING HEALTH STATUS INSTRUMENTS
Instruments for assessing health status for research and/ or clinical purposes are diverse and plentiful. Given the breadth of instruments available, the emphasis of this chapter is to provide instrument users with the criteria to select the most appropriate instruments for their intended purposes. As one might expect, no one instrument is likely to represent all the desired characteristics intended by a clinician or researcher. Therefore, we recommend balancing the health status instruments reviewed here with supplementary targets of measurement found in more specific ICF-CY components, as described in other chapters.

As outlined above, elements to consider when selecting a health status instrument include the following: content validity (including overlap of content with the ICF-CY framework); the purpose(s) and properties of the tools (evaluative vs descriptive); general performance in psychometric studies; and issues unique to childhood instruments, such as self-report and the impact of negativity in the wording of items. Users should remain cognizant of these criteria when appraising the reviewed instruments.

The six questionnaires reviewed here span more than one ICF-CY component and represent a concept of health inclusive of the 1948 World Health Organization definition. These six instruments are summarized in tabular format. It should be noted that the complete history of the psychometric properties of many of the instruments reviewed here is extensive and beyond the scope of this chapter. Instead, we have limited our report of reliability and validity to the findings described by the original instrument developers. The content-based criteria proposed above have not been the focus of such reviews, yet are essential to the selection of any one of these instruments over another; hence, we have focused on that information here. Additionally, guidelines for interpreting the psychometric rigour of health status and utility instruments are available and can assist users with the task of sorting through such criteria.

Summary
Health status instruments are complex, owing to their necessarily multidimensional nature and their dependence on the developer's contextual understanding or interpretation of health in a certain time and place. These instruments often have decades of implementation and use, and therefore sorting through the literature and selecting the appropriate questionnaire for a specific purpose can be daunting. We have attempted to delineate the content of some commonly used instruments using the ICF-CY, and provide additional criteria for appraising health status questionnaires that can be used with children. And we

CHILD HEALTH QUESTIONNAIRE (CHQ)	
Development	Developed in the 1990s, the items in the CHQ are based on the WHO's 1948 definition of health, literature review and expert consensus
	Early validation of the instrument occurred among 300 children aged 10–15y from a middle school in north-eastern USA; 54 American children aged 9–16y with attention-deficit–hyperactivity disorder (ADHD); and 20 children aged 10–19y with end-stage renal failure on haemodialysis. Data were collected between 1992 and 1996
ICF-CY components and categories	The CHQ is focused on body functions such as emotions, and activities and participation such as socializing and school, as well as some features relating to personal factors and the environment
Negative content and negative phrasing	Negative content: 33%
	Negative phrasing: 39%
Psychometric properties	Internal consistency (of subscales) reported as Cronbach's alpha >0.7
	Test–retest reliability, assessed by intraclass correlation coefficients, showed 8 of 14 subscales with test–retest reliability above 0.5
	Discriminant validity measured with *F*-statistics: differences between general school group, ADHD group and children with renal failure was significant for all subscales except 'role/social behavioural'
	Responsiveness studies are available for Dutch children with acute asthma, ADHD and children with juvenile arthritis
Author's note	This instrument is detailed and diverse; however, it contains a mixture of health status and QOL items. Users who wish to obtain or partition information about children using health or QOL would not be able to separate these two outcomes by using all of the CHQ's scales
How to order	Short and long versions of parent and child report forms are available in 98-, 87-, 50- and 28-item versions. Child reports are for ages 10–19y and parent/proxy reports are for ages 4–19y. This instrument can be purchased from www.healthact.com/chq.html
Key references	Landgraf JM, Abetz L, Ware JE (1996) Child Health Questionnaire (CHQ): A User's Manual. Boston: The Health Institute, New England Medical.Raata H, Bonselb GJ, Essink-Bota ML, Landgrafc JM, Reinoud JB, Gemke J (2002) Reliability and validity of comprehensive health status measures in children: The Child Health Questionnaire in relation to the Health Utilities Index. J Clin Epidemiol 55: 67–76.
	Raata H, Bonselb GJ, Essink-Bota ML, Landgraf JM, Reinoud JB, Gemke J (2002) Reliability and validity of comprehensive health status measures in children: the Child Health Questionnaire in relation to the Health Utilities Index. *J Clin Epidemiol* 55: 67–76.
	Gorelick MH, Scribano PV, Stevens MW, Schultz TR (2003) Construct validity and responsiveness. Child Health Questionnaire. J Rheumatol 30: 7.
	Rentz AM, Matza LS, Secnik K, Swensen A, Revicki DA (2005) Psychometric validation of the Child Health Questionnaire (CHQ) in a sample of children and adolescents with attention-deficit/hyperactivity disorder. Qual Life Res 14: 719–734.
	Gorelick MH, Scribano PV, Stevens MW, Schultz TR (2003) Construct validity and responsiveness of the Child Health Questionnaire in children with acute asthma. Ann Allergy Asthma Immunol 90: 622–628.
	Selvaag AM, Flato B, Lien G, Sorskaar D, Vinje O, Forre Ø (2003) Measuring health status in early juvenile idiopathic arthritis: determinants and responsiveness of the Child Health Questionnaire. J Rheumatol 30: 1602–1610.

emphasize once again the importance of being clear about the clinical or research question(s) for which any instrument might be used.

Although one often selects instruments to test specific hypotheses about a group of children in a particular situation, every incidence of instrument use is also a test of the conceptual understanding of health reflected in the questionnaire. Using instruments that reflect a biopsychosocial approach as represented by the ICF-CY taps into a broad understanding of health through functioning and disability. Such an approach to measurement considers children's contextual factors (environment and personal) as well as their body functions and structures, activities and participation.

CHILD HEALTH AND ILLNESS PROFILE (CHIP)

Development	Developed originally for adolescents to self-report on their health status. Focus groups with a sample of mothers and fathers, half of whom had children with chronic illness, reported on health issues to create the content of the questionnaire items
	Early versions of the instrument were tested in paediatric outpatient settings in Baltimore with parents of diverse economic backgrounds. Field studies were conducted in four sites in the USA. The developers assert that use of the instrument is intended for research purposes and further validation is required to adapt the instrument to clinical settings
ICF-CY components and categories	The core module of the CHIP focuses on activities and participation with an emphasis on interpersonal aspects such as playing and school performance. Body functions (e.g. emotional functions, experience of self and pain) are included. Environment categories (e.g. attitudes of peers [such as bullying], and social support from parents) are also assessed. The optional modules focus on additional features of the environment, such as health or social services, as well as a checklist of symptoms or diagnoses that can be represented with the International Classification of Diagnoses ICD-10 rather than the ICF-CY
Negative content and negative phrasing	Negative content: 42%
	Negative phrasing: 0%
Psychometric properties	Internal consistency using Cronbach's alpha was 0.79–0.88 for the parent form and 0.70–0.82 for the child form
	Test–retest reliability was reported using intraclass correlation coefficients: 0.63–0.85 for the parent form with the exception of the restricted activity subdomain (0.32); and 0.63–0.76 for the child report form
	Discriminant validity was reported for the adolescent version for the subscales only. A substantial variety in mean group differences was reported, less than half of which was significant, and confidence intervals were reported about the means
	Responsiveness studies are unavailable at this time
Author's note	This instrument has many items, which will reduce its usefulness in clinical settings. An advantage is the breadth of health components that span the body functions, activity and participation, environment and personal factors according to the ICF-CY, and therefore indicating a true biopsychosocial approach to health status measurement
How to order	Self-report, as well as parent-report forms, is available for children aged 6y to adolescence,
	See www.childhealthprofile.org/ for licensing information
Key references	Starfield B, Riley A, Green B, et al (1995) The adolescent child health and illness profile: a population-based measure of health. *Med Care* 33: 553–566.
	Riley AW, Forrest CB, Starfield B, Rebok GW, Robertson JA, Green BF (2004) The parent report form of the CHIP–Child Edition Reliability and Validity. *Med Care* 42(3).
	Riley AW, Forrest CB, Rebok GW, et al (2004) The child report form of the CHIP-Child Edition: reliability and validity. *Med Care* 42: 221–231.

FUNCTIONAL STATUS II REVISED (FS-II R)

Development	Developed conceptually based on Starfield's health framework. Adapted from an earlier version, the authors took 35 items from the Functional Status I and added some items based on literature review
	The FS-II R was validated on a sample of over 700 American children that included children with significant chronic conditions, children with ongoing health conditions seen for regularly scheduled appointments and children seen for routine health care
ICF-CY components and categories	The FS-II R focuses on body functions such as disposition, temperament, energy, sleep, cognition and emotion. General activities, communication and eating from activities and participation are touched upon. No environmental or personal factors are assessed
Negative content and negative phrasing	Negative content: 36%
	Negative phrasing: 0%
Psychometric properties	Internal consistency was measured by Cronbach's alpha and was found to be 0.86–0.87
	Discriminant validity was reported as mean differences without significance testing or confidence intervals of 86.8 (standard deviation [SD]=15.7) for the ill group and 96.1 (SD=8.2) for the well group
	Test–retest reliability was not reported in instrument development studies
	Responsiveness was shown in a study comparing chronically ill children with healthy children
Author's note	This instrument is short, although response errors are likely to occur if the questionnaire is not administered in interview format as the developers intended
How to order	Parent-report forms for children aged 0–16y are administered in interview form. There is no child response form. The 14-item version is common to all age groups and longer age-specific forms are available. To obtain the instrument, contact Ruth Stein, Department of Paediatrics, Albert Einstein College of Medicine/Montefiore Medical Center; Centennial 1, 111 East 210th Street; Bronx, NY 10467, USA
Key references	Stein REK, Jessop DJ (1990) Functional status II(R): a measure of child health status. *Med Care* 28: 1041–1055.
	Drotar D (2004) Health status and quality of life. In: Naar-King S, Ellis DA, Frey MA, editors. *Assessing Children's Well-Being*, 2nd edition. Mahwah, NJ: Lawrence Erlbaum Associates, pp. 1–17.
	Schmidt J, Garratt AM, Fitzpatrick R (year?) Child/parent-assessed population health outcome measures: a structured review. *Child Care Health Dev* 28: 227–237.
	Connolly MA, Johnson JA (1999) Measuring quality of life in paediatric patients. *Pharmacoeconomics* 16: 605–625.

CHILD HEALTH ASSESSMENT QUESTIONNAIRE (CHAQ)

Development	Based on an adaptation of the adult Stanford Health Assessment Questionnaire (HAQ), the CHAQ was developed with at least one 'child-specific' item added to each functional area in an attempt to adapt the measure for use with children with juvenile arthritis. The CHAQ is currently used by the Paediatric Rheumatology International Trials Organization (PRINTO) to collect international health data about children with arthritis
ICF-CY components and categories	The CHAQ focuses on activities such as walking, bicycle riding, washing and dressing. There is no emphasis on participation such as interpersonal aspects of life and there is negligible information about the body functions of pain. The environment is assessed based on needs for assistive devices as opposed to social support or health and social services
Negative content and negative phrasing	Negative content: 3% Negative phrasing: 0%
Psychometric properties	From validation studies: Internal reliability was reported using Spearman's correlation coefficient and was 0.66 for children with juvenile arthritis From use by PRINTO: Discriminant validity was reported as statistically significant mean scores differences. However, there were small differences between the clinical groups and large standard deviations, but no confidence intervals were reported about the mean to establish whether it discriminates between clinical groups Internal consistency was reported using Cronbach's alpha: >0.5 Test–retest reliability was reported using intraclass correlation coefficient: 0.6–0.9 Responsiveness information is available for children with juvenile arthritis in participant countries of the PRINTO trials
Author's note	This questionnaire first asks parents whether an activity is relevant to his or her child based on what is expected for age before assessing the child's level of ability for the activity. Conversely, norms for age are not available. Therefore, one should use caution when applying this instrument to children with delays or chronic conditions Authors not involved in the original development of the CHAQ are attempting to validate its use beyond children with arthritis for children with cerebral palsy
How to order	Parent-report form for all ages of children can be found in the public domain. There is no child-report form available. See www.bspar.org.uk/downloads/registry_forms/CHAQForm.pdf
Key references	Rider LG, Feldman BM, Perez MD, et al (1997) Development of validated disease activity and damage indices for the juvenile idiopathic inflammatory myopathies. I. Physician, parent, and patient global assessments. *Arthritis Rheum* 40: 1976–1983. Ruperto N, Ravelli A, Pistorio A, et al, for the Paediatric Rheumatology International Trials Organisation (PRINTO) (2001) Cross-cultural adaptation and psychometric evaluation of the Childhood Health Assessment Questionnaire (CHAQ) and the Child Health Questionnaire (CHQ) in 32 countries. Review of the general methodology. *Clin Exp Rheumatol* 19(Suppl. 23): S1–S9. Huber AM, Hicks JE, Lachenbruch PA, et al in co-operation with the Juvenile Dermatomyositis Disease Activity Collaborative Study Group (2001) Validation of the Childhood Health Assessment questionnaire in the Juvenile Idiopathic Myopathies. *Journal Rheumatol* 28: 5. Brunner JI, Klein-Gitelman MS, Miller MJ, et al (2005) Minimal clinically important differences of the Childhood Health Assessment Questionnaire. *J Rheumatol* 32: 1.

HEALTH UTILITIES INDEX III (HUI III)

Development	The HUI III evolved from previous versions that were designed to capture the health outcomes of very low birthweight infants. The attributes assessed by HUI III were refined through literature and qualitative work with 84 parent–child pairs. The HUI III was first implemented in the 1990 Statistics Canada Ontario Health Survey and the 1991 Statistics Canada General Social Survey for the general Canadian population
ICF-CY components and categories	The HUI III emphasizes body function attributes such as vision, hearing, cognition and emotion, and activities and participation items such as walking, hand function and communication. Environment domains are assessed directly. There is one quality of life question
Negative content and negative phrasing	Negative content: 12.5% Negative phrasing: 47.5%
Psychometric properties	Test–retest reliability was reported using intraclass correlation coefficient and was found to be 0.77 based on its use in the Canadian General Social Survey Health Questionnaire in 1991 Responsiveness studies are available for children with asthma and Hodgkin's lymphoma
Author's note	As a health utility tool, the instrument can (1) classify the level of health based on norms from the population and (2) provide a final score, where 0 indicates a valuation of death and 1 indicates perfect health for the purpose of health economics or resource allocation decisions When the HUI III classification is interfaced with the preference scoring function (the health preferences are based on adult preferences in Canada) to create a health utilities score value, application of that utility score (e.g. scores less than 0=worse than death) to describe any one particular child has ethical pitfalls
How to order	Parent-report forms for children aged 6–18y; no child-report version. Licence and pricing information can be found at http://healthutilities.com
Key references	Furlong W, Feeny D, Torrance G, Barr R (2008) The Health Utilities Index (HUI®) system undergoing chemotherapy. *J Pediatr Hematol Oncol* 30: 292–297. Horsman J, Furlong W, Feeny D, Torrance G (2003) The Health Utilities Index (HUI®): concepts, measurement properties and applications. *Health Qual Life Outcomes* 1: 54 Furlong WJ, Feeny DH, Torrance GW, Barr RD (2001) The Health Utilities Index (HUI®) system for assessing health-related quality of life in clinical studies. *Ann Med* 33: 375–384. Klaassen RJ, Krahn M, Gaboury I, et al (2010) Evaluating the ability to detect change of health-related quality of life in children with Hodgkin disease. *Cancer* 116: 1608–1614. Juniper EF, Gordon H, Guyatt GH, Feeny DH, Griffith LE, Ferrie PJ (1997) Minimum skills required by children to complete health-related quality of life instruments for asthma: comparison of measurement properties. Eur Respir J 10: 2285–2294. Barr RD, Petrie C, Furlong WJ, Rothney M, Feeny DH (1997) Health-related quality of life during post-induction chemotherapy in children with acute lymphoblastic leukemia in remission: an influence of corticosteroid therapy. Int J Oncol 11: 333–339. Feeny DH, Torrance G, Furlong W (1996) Health utilities index. In: Spilker B, editor. Quality of Life and Pharmacoeconomics in Clinical Trials, 2nd edition. Philadelphia, PA: Lippincott-Raven, pp. 239–252. Furlong W, Boyle M, Torrance GW (1995) Multi-attribute health status classification systems. Health Utilities Index. Pharmacoeconomics 7: 490–502.

EuroQoL Youth (EQ-5D-Y)	
Development	The EQ-5D-Y was adapted from the adult EQ-5D for the purpose of providing children and adolescents with the opportunity to report on their own health. However, the content of the adult version was not created using a developmental approach to child health. The wording was adapted for child self-report using cognitive interviewing with children and adolescents
	The original (adult) EQ-5D contains health components (states) that were described from literature review and formed by expert consensus in the early 1990s within the EuroQoL group
ICF-CY components and categories	Body functions such as emotion and pain are covered. Walking, self-care, washing and dressing are contained in the instrument representing activities. No participation, environment or personal factors were represented by the ICF-CY
Negative content and negative phrasing	Negative content: 47% Negative phrasing: 47%
Psychometric properties	Test–retest reliability using percentage agreement was found to be 69.8–99.7% and using Cohen's kappa was –0.003–0.549 for 8- to 18-year-old children from Italy and Spain for a 7- to 10-day testing interval
	Discriminant validity was reported as a percentage of responses selected for each health state (i.e. mobility, emotions and pain) between chronic and non-chronically affected children. The differences in the proportion of respondents of ill versus well children varied based on the country and were often non-significant for samples composed of at least 200 children
	Responsiveness information was not found for the youth version
Author's note	As with the Health Utilities Index (HUI), this instrument is intended to produce a utilities score, where 0 represents a state of health equivalent to death and 1 represents ideal health. Applying a valuation to any one individual child (as described for the HUI) based on the norms of the majority European population has ethical pitfalls
	EuroQoL developers recommend supplementing the EQ-5D-Y with standard questionnaires to provide information about individuals. Thus, the EQ-5D-Y presents benefit mainly as a crude screen for body function and activities type of health issues that are commonly valued by the adult population at large
How to order	The form is intended for completion by individuals aged 8–18y. Licensing information and agreements can be obtained through www.euroqol.org/home.html
Key references	Williams A (2005) The EuroQol Instrument. In: Kind P, Brooks R, Rabin R, editors. *EQ-5D Concepts and Methods*. Netherlands: Springer.
	Gudex C (2005) The descriptive system of the EuroQol Instrument. In: Kind P, Brooks R, Rabin R, editors. *EQ-5D Concepts and Methods*. Netherlands: Springer, pp. 19–28.
	Wille N, Badia X, Bonsel G, et al (2010) Development of the EQ-5D-Y: a child-friendly version of the EQ-5D. *Qual Life Res*. DOI 10.1007/s11136–010–9648-y.
	Ravens-Sieberer U, Wille N, Badia X, et al (2010) Feasibility, reliability, and validity of the EQ-5D-Y: results from a multinational study. *Qual Life Res* 19: 887–897
	Cieza A, Geyh S, Chatterji S, Kostanjsek N, Ustun B, Stucki G (2005) ICF linking rules: an update based on lessons learned. *J Rehab Med* 37: 212–218.

REFERENCES

1. World Health Organization (2006) *Constitution of the World Health Organization – Basic Documents*, 45th edition, Supplement. Available at: www.who.int/governance/eb/who_constitution_en.pdf (accessed 12 June 2010).

2. Webster C (1993) *Caring for Health: History and Diversity*. Buckingham: The Open University Press.

3. World Health Organization (2010) *Counting Down to 2015 Decade Report with Country Profiles: Taking Stock of Maternal Newborn and Child Survival*. Available at: http://whqlibdoc.who.int/publications/2010/9789241599573_eng.pdf (accessed 17 July 2010).

4. Loudon I (1997) *The Oxford Illustrated History of Western Medicine*. Oxford: Oxford University Press.

5. Wilson IB, Cleary PD (1995) Linking clinical variables with health-related quality of life. *JAMA* 273: 59–65.

6. US Food and Drug Administration (2009) Patient reported outcome measures: use in medical product development to support labeling claims. Available at: www.fda.gov/downloads/Drugs/GuidanceComplianceRegulatoryInformation/Guidances/ucm071975.pdf (accessed 12 June 2010).

7. Pless IB, Pinkerton P (1975) *Chronic Childhood Disorders: Promoting Patterns of Adjustment*. Chicago, IL: Year Book Medical Publishers.

8. World Health Organization (2001) *The International Classification of Functioning Disability and Health*. Geneva: WHO.

9. World Health Organization (2005) *The International Classification of Functioning Disability and Health: Children and Youth*. Geneva: WHO.

10. Bradley C (2001) Importance of differentiating health status from quality of life. *Lancet* 357: 7–8.

11. World Health Organization (1998) *WHOQOL User Manual*. Geneva: WHO.

12. Norman GR, Streiner DL (2008) *Health Measurement Scales: A Practical Guide to their Development and Use*, 4th edition. Oxford: Oxford University Press.

13. Cieza A, Geyh S, Chatterji S, Kostanjsek N, Ustun B, Stucki G (2005) ICF linking rules: an update based on lessons learned. *J Rehab Med* 37: 212–218.

14. Fayed N, Kerr E (2009) Comparing quality of life scales in childhood epilepsy: what's in the measures? *Int J Disabil Community Rehabil* 8: 1–5.

15. Fava L, Muehlan H, Bullinger M (2009) Linking the DISABKIDS modules for health-related quality of life assessment with the International Classification of Functioning, Disability and Health (ICF). *Disabil Rehabil* 31: 1943–1954.

16. Ostensjo S, Bjorbaekmo W, Carlberg EB, Vollestad NK (2006) Assessment of everyday functioning in young children with disabilities: an ICF-based analysis of concepts and content of the Pediatric Evaluation of Disability Inventory (PEDI). *Disabil Rehabil* 28: 489–504.

17. Granlund M, Eriksson L, Ylven R (2004) Utility of International Classification of Functioning, Disability and Health's participation dimension in assigning ICF codes to items from extant rating instruments. *J Rehabil Med* 36: 130–137.

18. Clarke SA, Eiser C (2004) The measurement of health-related quality of life (QOL) in pediatric clinical trials: a systematic review. *Health Qual Life Outcomes* 2: 66–71.

19. Harding L (2001) Children's quality of life assessments: a review of generic and health related quality of life measures completed by children and adolescents. *Clin Psychol Psychotherapy* 8: 79–96.

20. Eiser C, Morse R (2001) A review of measures of quality of life for children with chronic illness. *Arch Disabled Child* 84: 205–211.

21. Ravens-Sieberer U, Erhart M, Wille N (2006) Generic health-related quality-of-life assessment in children and adolescents: methodological considerations. *Pharmacoeconomics* 24: 1199–1220.

22. Solans M, Pane S, Estrada MD, et al (2008) Health-related quality of life measurement in children and adolescents: a systematic review of generic and disease-specific instruments. *Value Health* 11: 742–764.

23. Lidwine B, Mokkink LB, Terwee CB, et al (2010) The COSMIN checklist for assessing the methodological quality of studies on measurement properties of health status measurement instruments: an international Delphi study. *Qual Life Res* 19: 539–549.

24. Schmidt LJ, Garratt AM, Fitzpatrick R (2002) Child/parent-assessed population health outcome measures: a structured review. *Childcare Health Dev* 28: 227–237.

25. Guyatt G, Walter S, Norman G (1987) Measuring change over time: assessing the usefulness of evaluative instruments. *J Chronic Dis* 40: 171–178.

26. Sturgess J, Rodger S, Ozanne A (2002) A review of the use of self-report assessment with young children. *Br J Occup Ther* 65: 108–116.

27. Fayed N, Kerr E (2009) Identifying occupational issues among children with intractable epilepsy: individualized versus norm-referenced approaches. *Can J Occup Ther* 76: 90–97.

28. Riley AW (2004) Evidence that school-age children can self-report on their health. *Ambul Pediatr* 4: 371–376.

29. Schwartz N (1999) How the questions shape the answers. *Am Psychol* 44: 93–105.

30. Heritage J (2002) The limits of questioning: negative interrogatives and hostile question content. *J Pragmatics* 34: 1427–1446.

31. Waters E, Davis E, Ronen G, Rosenbaum P, Livingston M, Saigal S (2009) Quality of life instruments for children and adolescents with neurodisabilities: how to choose the appropriate instrument. *Dev Med Child Neurol* 51: 660–669.

32. Petrou S (2003) Methodological issues for measuring health status of children. *Health Econ* 12: 697–702.

33. Brazier J, Deverill M (1999) A checklist for judging preference-based measures of health related quality of life: learning from psychometrics. *Health Econ* 8: 41–45.

34
QUALITY OF LIFE OUTCOMES

Allan Colver

What is the construct?

Quality of life (QoL) and well-being can be described in broad, multidimensional ways that incorporate objective and subjective accounts of personal feelings, social relationships, local environment, societal values, political institutions, economic conditions and international relations. A Nordic group recommended the classification in Table 34.1 to describe the QoL of an individual;[1] Table 34.2 shows indicators of child well-being reported at a national level in a United Nations International Children's Emergency Fund (UNICEF) report.[2] In practice, such approaches are too wide ranging for meaningful quantitative analysis.

Although such broad definitions are impractical, tighter definitions have been confusing because similar phrases have been used for different concepts. In the early literature on QoL, there was an overlap with terms such as handicap, function and activities of daily living, depending on the authors' philosophies and backgrounds. However, the literature is now clearer and, although a number of definitions of QoL exist, the subjective, self-reported element is now common to all. The World Health Organization (WHO) defines QoL as 'the individual's perception of their position in life in the context of the culture and value systems in which they live, and in relation to their goals, expectations, standards and concerns'.[3] QoL concerns an individual's personal perception of his or her place in the world and society. It is a person's self-reported view, and therefore it is subjective. Most instruments identify a number of crucial dimensions,[4] as shown in Table 34.3.

Because other groups may well continue to use the phrase 'quality of life' for their own purposes, it seems there is now a strong case for calling a person's self-reported, subjective view of his or her life as 'subjective well-being'. However, this article shall not take this argument further and the term 'quality of life' will be used.

There has been a neglect of taking account of children's self-reported subjective views. The United Nations Convention on Rights of the Child Article 12[5] states that 'children's views must be taken into account in all matters concerning them', and the United Nations Convention on Rights of Persons with Disabilities Article 7[6] states that 'disabled children have the right to express their views'. Further, modern sociological thinking regards childhood as a legitimate construct for social analysis, along with categories such as class, sex, ethnicity and disability.[7] Children are seen not as passive objects owned by their parents but rather as social actors in their own right, contributing in various ways to their families and their communities. The new approach is encapsulated by the notion that children should be seen as 'human beings' not 'human becomings'.[8]

Modern QoL instruments should be generated de novo from what young people say, rather than being modified from adult instruments or instruments with items determined by professionals. Such instruments are in accord with the United Nations conventions mentioned earlier because the meaning derives from what the young person says about his or her perception of the world.

QoL cannot be measured directly; rather, its domains are underlying latent variables, the values of which are inferred from a group of questions. All instruments that capture latent variables require their psychometric properties to be carefully evaluated, but this is especially important when the questions ask about subjective, rather than objective, states. Modern psychometric techniques ensure that a latent variable is captured on a unidimensional, arithmetic scale by questions that behave in the same way in different settings and with different children. The KIDSCREEN instrument has recently been developed with these properties and validated across 12 European countries.[9]

TABLE 34.1
Comprehensive description of quality of life proposed by Nordic group[1]

Sphere	Dimension	Example	Objective/subjective
Global	Macro environment	Clean environment	Objective
	Human rights	Political system	Objective
	Policies	Welfare state	Objective
External sphere	Work	Education	Objective
	Economy	Satisfaction with pocket money	Subjective
	Housing	Type of house	Objective
Interpersonal	Family	Family structure	Objective
	Intimate	Satisfaction with close relationships	Subjective
	Extended	Leisure activities with others	Objective
Personal	Physical	Growth and development	Objective
	Mental	Psychological health	Objective
	Spiritual	Fulfilment	Subjective

TABLE 34.2
Overview of child well-being in rich countries[2]

Dimension	Example	Measure
Material well-being	Relative income poverty	Percentage of children living in households with income below 50% of national median
Health and safety	Safety	Deaths from accident and injuries per 100 000 for those aged 0–19y
Educational well-being	School at age 15	Average achievement in reading literacy
Family and peer relationships	Family structure	Percentage of children living in single-parent households
Behaviours and risks	Risk behaviours	Percentage of 15 year olds who smoke
Subjective well-being	School life	Percentage of schoolchildren who 'like school a lot'

IS HEALTH-RELATED QUALITY OF LIFE THE SAME AS QUALITY OF LIFE?

Health-related quality of life (HRQoL) is a concept that has caused confusion because it may be interpreted in many ways. The confusion between HRQoL and QoL appears to stem from the conceptualization of health. Health is defined by WHO as 'a state of complete physical, mental, and social wellbeing and not merely the absence of disease or infirmity'.[10] This definition has been influential in defining HRQoL to include social well-being and emotional/mental well-being as well as physical well-being. QoL and HRQoL are therefore equivalent if this broad view of health is considered.

CONDITION-SPECIFIC PERCEPTION OF HEALTH STATUS, CONDITION AND TREATMENT

How a person views his or her impairment, features of it and its treatment may also be important and may or may not affect his or her QoL. Assessment of such perceptions allows the child's view, or in the case of very young children,[11] the parent's view, to influence areas where health and other services might intervene or improve, such as by dealing with excessive worry about seizures, establishing more sensitive clinical settings or addressing cultural taboos. Such subjective views about impairment are often captured by a condition-specific measure.

Confusingly, instruments to measure this concept are often labelled 'health-related quality of life' or 'condition-specific quality of life'. We suggest instead 'perception of health status, condition and treatment'. Otherwise, there is an implication that perceptions of a health condition are equivalent to subjective well-being and satisfaction with life – an assumption that has been challenged.[12] Perception of health status, condition and treatment is not QoL, but for some children may capture potential condition-specific determinants of QoL.

OTHER CONCEPTS

There are three other concepts that are not QoL but are sometimes mistakenly labelled as HRQoL or incorporated

TABLE 34.3
Dimensions of quality of life

Perception of:

    Emotional well-being

    Social well-being

    Material well-being

    Physical well-being

    Self-esteem

    Self-determination

TABLE 34.4
Characteristics of a quality of life instrument

Original purpose of instrument

Actual focus of instrument

Origin of domains and items

Opportunity for self-report

Clarity of items, using children's own phrases

Potential threat of negative wording to self-esteem

Number of items and time to complete (length)

Psychometric properties

into HRQoL instruments. These concepts are important and are discussed in other chapters. These include the following:

1. Participation, defined by the WHO International Classification of Functioning, Disability and Health (ICF) as 'involvement in life situations'.[13] The ICF, initially developed for adults, was modified for children and young people to include domains that take into account aspects of play, development and dependence on parents.[14]

2. The objective consequences of impairment, such as functional limitation or difficulties with activities of daily living. The ICF[13] defines activity as 'execution of a task or action by an individual'; difficulty in an area is called activity limitation.

3. Economic valuation of a health state. This is used for resource allocation at a systems level rather than as a personalized outcome. For children, there is debate about whether the valuation of the health state should be attributed by the children themselves, their parents or society in general through a reference population. Further, whether the value should be assigned to the level of impairment[15] or to functional health status,[16] or indeed to QoL,[17] is open to debate.

PEOPLE WHO CANNOT SELF-REPORT

People with severe learning disability (the North American term is mental retardation) cannot self-report, but estimating and improving their QoL is no less important. We cannot know their QoL directly so we need to consider how it can best be estimated from objective observations of sounds and facial expressions or the subjective impressions of others such as relatives, friends and professionals.

General factors to consider when measuring this domain

Elizabeth Waters and her co-authors have recently drawn attention to key factors to consider when choosing a QoL instrument.[18] Table 34.4 summarizes these and each is discussed below. These ideas and figures are reproduced with permission.

ORIGINAL PURPOSE OF THE INSTRUMENT

An instrument used to measure QoL may not have been designed for that purpose. For example, in studies of children with cerebral palsy, the Child Health Questionnaire (CHQ)[19] and Lifestyle Assessment Questionnaire[20] have been used to measure QoL but in fact were designed to measure functional health and well-being and impact of disability, respectively. In studies of QoL in childhood epilepsy, the Hague Restrictions in Childhood Epilepsy Scale[21] and Impact of Childhood Illness Scale[22] have been used but were not designed to measure QoL.

ACTUAL FOCUS OF THE INSTRUMENT

An instrument should focus on the personal well-being of an individual and his or her feelings and perceptions about life. However, many instruments designed to be, and which are named as, QoL instruments focus on functioning (what the person can do) rather than well-being. For example, the Pediatric Quality of Life Inventory-CP Module (PedsQL-CP) assesses whether a child has difficulty moving one or both of his or her legs, difficulty using scissors and difficulty brushing his or her teeth.[23] Although functional status and impairment may have an impact on QoL, they are not synonymous with it,[24] and a meta-analysis of adult studies measuring both found them to be distinct concepts.[25] It is not possible to estimate a patient's distress by accumulating his or her range of problems. People with significant health problems can be highly satisfied with some aspects of their lives – the so-called 'disability paradox'.[12] Recent studies of children with cerebral palsy have shown that functioning is only weakly related to domains of QoL.[26]

ORIGIN OF DOMAINS AND ITEMS

Until recently, instruments have measured domains that were decided a priori by professional 'experts' (researchers and clinicians); however, there is an increasing recognition that families and children should be consulted.[27-29] Qualitative research is well suited to this[30] and instrument developers should report in detail the methods they used. Instruments are more likely to have content validity if items are derived from a sample of the population in which the instrument is to be used.[30]

OPPORTUNITY FOR SELF-REPORT

The childhood literature used to suggest that parents may be better able than the child to rate their child's QoL because of their child's cognitive immaturity, limited social experience and continued dependency.[31] However, this view is changing, especially for children aged over 7 years of age for whom test–retest reliability showed acceptable results.[32] New instruments usually have child self-report versions. However, where child or adolescent self-reports cannot be collected owing to age, language ability or cognitive impairment, parent proxy measures are valuable. A systematic review of 14 studies assessing the relationship between parent-proxy and child self-reported QoL demonstrated that the level of agreement depended on the domain.[31] Generally, there was good agreement (correlations >0.5) between parents and children for domains that reflected physical activity, functioning and symptoms, but poorer agreement (correlations <0.30) for domains that reflected social or emotional domains.

THREAT OF NEGATIVE WORDING TO SELF-ESTEEM

Items may threaten self-esteem by making assumptions about an illness. For example, the DISABKIDS-CP[33] includes items such as 'Does it bother you that you have to explain to others what you can and can't do?', 'Is it frustrating to be unable to keep up with other children?' and 'Do people think that you are not as clever as you are?'. Although these items may have sound psychometric properties, there may be ethical objections to including such questions.

NUMBER OF ITEMS AND TIME REQUIRED TO COMPLETE

The number of items and time required to complete a QoL instrument are important considerations, particularly for children. Most agree that completion of a measure should take no longer than 10 to 20 minutes.

PSYCHOMETRIC PROPERTIES

Instruments should demonstrate adequate test–retest reliability, validity and factor structure. If designed to evaluate interventions, they should also demonstrate evidence of sensitivity to change. Factor analysis is important for developing multiconstruct measures because it may reveal patterns of inter-relationships among variables not otherwise apparent, identify redundant domains or items and retain only those items that correlate primarily with a single domain. Cronbach's coefficient α is a useful measure of internal consistency for scales that tap a single domain. Because Cronbach's α is sensitive to the length of the instrument, a long scale may have a high value even where there is heterogeneity. An optimal value of Cronbach's α is a necessary but not sufficient index of reliability, and values over 0.9 are likely to indicate redundancy.[34] Good test–retest reliability confirms that a scale is stable over time and values of the intraclass coefficient should be greater than 0.6. Construct validity assesses an instrument in the absence of a criterion standard and refers to predictions regarding how the instrument should behave based on hypotheses. The process is usually established over a number of studies, tapping into various aspects of the hypothetical construct.

It is helpful in assessing a proposed instrument to locate the status of each key factor on a spectrum. In Figure 34.1 this is done for a number of instruments that might be considered as generic QoL instruments. In Figure 34.2, the same is done for condition-specific instruments for cerebral palsy.

Overview of recommended measures

There are many reviews of available instruments, the most recent being from a Spanish group.[35] Modern reviews try to indicate what an instrument captures as well as the psychometric properties. However, even these reviews usually include instruments that do not capture the concept of QoL used in this chapter.

There are few instruments that have all the desirable features discussed above and summarized in Table 34.4. All the instruments recommended in this chapter (in Table 34.5· and summarized below) have many features on the right side of Figures 34.1 and 34.2. The list includes the instruments thought to have the best features (defined above) and which are available in the English language.

GENERIC QUALITY OF LIFE MEASURES APPLICABLE TO ALL YOUNG PEOPLE, WITH OR WITHOUT IMPAIRMENTS

KIDSCREEN

The KIDSCREEN[36] was developed in a multicultural context and generated items from focus group work with children. There are 52-, 27- and 10-item versions, the last of which generates a global or single factor score.

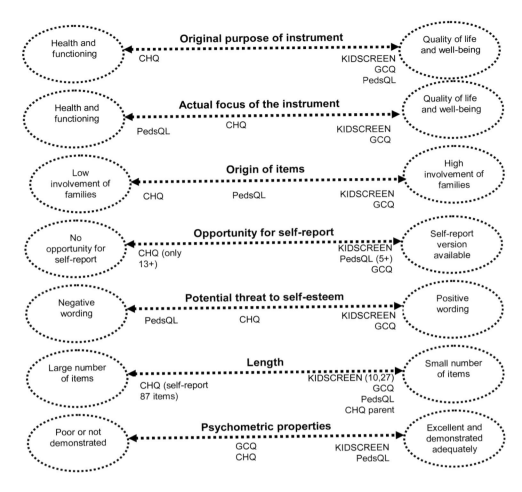

Figure 34.1 Generic quality of life. CHQ, Child Health Questionnaire; GCQ, Generic Children's Quality of Life Measure; PedsQL, Pediatric Quality of Life Inventory.

Normative data are available for 12 European countries, broken down by age and socioeconomic factors. The domains are perception of

- psychological well-being;
- moods and emotions;
- social support and peers;
- relations with parents and home life;
- self-perception;
- autonomy;
- school environment;
- social acceptance and bullying;
- financial resources; and
- physical well-being.

Quality of Life Profile – Adolescent Version

The Quality of Life Profile – Adolescent Version (QOLPAV)[37] instrument captures QoL along the domains of being, belonging and becoming, which were developed

from theoretical and philosophical ideas. Items were then developed from meetings with young people. Conceptually, the instrument is very attractive but some of its predicted associations with constructs such as self-esteem and social belonging were not found. The instrument's subdomains are

- being – physical, psychological and spiritual;
- belonging – physical, social and community; and
- becoming – practical, leisure and growth.

Generic Children's Quality of Life Measure

The Generic Children's Quality of Life Measure (GCQ)[38] was generated from focus-group work with children. The instrument has an attractive and inviting format. Although the questions are the same for each sex, there are separate versions for males and females; the child is invited to see him- or herself as a member of a varied group of males or females. The child answers a question by saying which

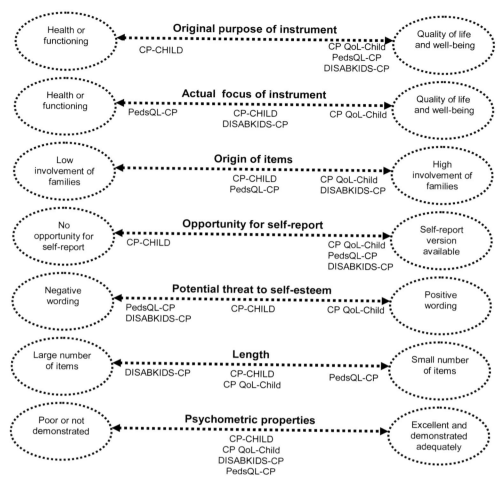

Figure 34.2 Condition specific – cerebral palsy. CP-CHILD, Caregiver Priorites and Child Health Index of Life with Disabilities; CP QoL-Child, Quality of Life Questionnaire for Children with Cerebral Palsy; PedsQL-CP, Pediatric Quality of Life Inventory – Cerebral Palsy; DISABKIDS-CP, DISABKIDS – Cerebral Palsy.

child he or she is most like. Then, in the second section, the participant responds by saying which child he or she would most want to be like. The instrument generates a global or single factor score.

Pediatric Quality of Life Inventory
The Pediatric Quality of Life Inventory (PedsQL)[39] generic scale was generated from work with children with cancer. The domains cover

- physical functioning;
- emotional functioning;
- social functioning; and
- school functioning.

The instrument is short and has excellent psychometric properties. It generates a global or single factor score. Its weakness is that much of it is directed to functioning: what a child can and cannot do and with how much difficulty.

MEASURES TO CAPTURE PERCEPTION OF HEALTH STATUS, CONDITION AND TREATMENT IN CHILDREN AND YOUNG PEOPLE WITH A PARTICULAR CONDITION

Quality of Life Questionnaire for Children with Cerebral Palsy
The Quality of Life Questionnaire for Children with Cerebral Palsy (CP QOL-Child)[40] is a condition-specific instrument for children with cerebral palsy. Its items were developed from focus-group work with children, using the

children's words. It captures some domains of a generic measure, asking children how they feel about their

- social well-being and acceptance;
- functioning;
- participation;
- physical health; and
- emotional well-being.

It also captures some domains of a condition-specific measure, asking children how they feel about their

- special equipment and access to services; and
- pain and feelings about disability.

Health-related Quality of Life in Children with Epilepsy

The Health-related Quality of Life in Children with Epilepsy (CHEQOL)[32] is a condition-specific instrument for children with epilepsy. Its items were developed from focus-group work with children, using the children's words. It captures some concepts of a generic measure

- worries and concerns in daily life;
- interpersonal/social consequences; and
- interpersonal/emotional issues.

It also captures some of a condition-specific measure

- secrecy and concealment of epilepsy;
- quest for normality.

Health-related Quality of Life Instrument for Children with Spina Bifida

The Health-related Quality of Life Instrument for Children with Spina Bifida (HRQL-SB)[41] was developed from in-depth interviews with children and their parents. It has the following 10 domains:

- social;
- emotional;
- intellectual;
- financial;
- medical;
- independence;
- environmental;
- physical functioning;
- recreation; and
- vocational.

Caregiver Priorities and Child Health Index of Life with Disabilities

The Caregiver Priorities and Child Health Index of Life with Disabilities (CP-CHILD)[42] measures caregivers' perspectives on the health status, comfort, well-being, functional abilities and ease of care-giving of children with severe developmental disabilities. It was developed to measure the effectiveness of interventions intended to improve or preserve these outcomes for children with severe disabilities, including non-ambulant children with severe cerebral palsy, and traumatic or other acquired brain injuries. Items were generated from recommendations of parents and caregivers of children with severe cerebral palsy. All questions are answered by a carer. Its domains are

- activities of daily living/personal care;
- positioning, transferring and mobility;
- comfort and emotions;
- communication and social interaction;
- health; and
- overall quality of life.

Quality of Life Measure for Children with Developmental Disabilities

The Quality of Life Measure for Children with Developmental Disabilities[43] was developed from the same framework as the Quality of Life Profile – Adolescent Version described above – namely being, belonging and becoming. Interviews with parents of children with developmental disabilities generated themes and items which were then hung on the structure.

Conclusion

Increasing attention is being paid to QoL as an important outcome to measure in studies of health and illness or disease. Grant-awarding bodies expect assessment of QoL but are usually not specific about what they mean by QoL. This chapter has attempted to clarify the meaning of QoL and related concepts. It has also provided a structure for deciding whether an instrument that purports to measure QoL would actually measure this concept; whether the instrument uses items that are suitable for children; and whether the instrument has strong psychometric properties.

TABLE 34.5
Suggested generic and condition-specific measures

Type (country where developed)	Name	Population	Administration	Internal consistency – Cronbach's alpha	Test–retest ICC	Validity	Sensitivity to change, responsiveness	Cost and how to order (for academic non-commercial studies)	References
Generic (Europe)	**KIDSCREEN**	8–18y	Self-report Carer report	Yes	Not available	Construct validity	Yes	www.kidscreen.de/cms/thekidscreenproject Use of the questionnaires is free	Main article about instrument[9] Cross-cultural analysis and psychometrics[36]
Generic (Canada)	Quality of Life Profile – Adolescent Version (**QOLPAV**)	14–20y	Self-report	>0.7	Not available	Construct validity – convergent	Not available	www.utoronto.ca/qol/profile.htm CA$35 r.renwick@utoronto.ca	Development[37] Validation[44]
Generic (United Kingdom)	Generic Children's Quality of Life Measure (**GCQ**)	6–14y	Self-report	0.7–0.8	Not available	Not available	Not available	Starter pack with manual and 20 questionnaires UK£112 www.hogrefe.co.uk/?/test/show/112/	Development[45] Guide and Manual: www.data-archive.ac.uk/doc/4412/mrdoc/pdf/a4412uab.pdf Normative values[38] A report using the instrument[46]
Generic (United States)	Pediatric Quality of Life Inventory (**PedsQL**)	2–18y	Self-report (5–18y) Carer report (2–18y)	0.8–0.9	Not available	Construct validity – discriminates between those with and without a chronic health condition	Yes	www.pedsql.org/ Non-funded academic: free Funded academic: US$750 per study	Measurement model[47] Main report[39] Psychometrics[48]

Condition (country)	Instrument	Age range	Report type			Validity	Cost	References
Cerebral palsy (Australia)	Cerebral Palsy Quality of Life Questionnaire for Children (**CP QoL-Child**)	4–12y, with cerebral palsy	Self-report (9–12y) Carer report (4–12y)	0.7–0.9	0.7–0.9	Construct validity – both convergent and divergent	Not available	Free. Complete the registration form available in the manual at www.cpqol.org.au/uploads/pdfs/CP_QOL_child_manual_08.pdf	Development of instrument[49] Psychometric properties[40] Manual[50] Paper using the instrument[51]
Epilepsy (Canada)	Health-related Quality of Life in Children with Epilepsy (**CHEQOL**)	6–15y	Self-report Carer report	0.6–0.8	0.3–0.9	Construct validity	Not available	Licensed through McMaster University http://ip.mcmaster.ca/avail_tech/questionnaires.html milo@mcmaster.ca	The model[52] Development and validation[32]
Spina bifida	Health-related Quality of Life for Children with Spina Bifida (**HRQL-SB**)	15–20y	Self-report Carer report	0.9	0.7–0.9	Construct validity – divergent	Not available	Licensed through McMaster University rosenbau@mcmaster.ca	Development[41] Paper using the instrument[53]
Severe physical impairment and learning difficulty (Canada)	Caregiver Priorities and Child Health Index of Life with Disabilities (**CP-CHILD**)	5–12y	Carer report	0.1–0.9	0.8–0.9	Construct validity – convergent and divergent	Not available	Free. Manual and registration at www.sickkids.ca/Research/CPCHILD-Questionaire/CPChild-Questionaire.html	Development of instrument[42] Manual[54]
Developmental disabilities (Canada)	Quality of Life Measure for Children with Developmental Disabilities	3–12y	Carer report	>0.7	>0.7	Construct validity – convergent	Not available	r.renwick@utoronto.ca	Report[43]

ICC, intraclass correlation coefficient.

REFERENCES

1. Berntsson LT, Kohler L (2001) Quality of life among children aged 2–17 years in the five Nordic countries: comparison between 1984 and 1996. *Eur J Pub Health* 11: 437–445.

2. UNICEF (2007) *Child Poverty in Perspective: An Overview of Child Well-being in Rich Countries*. Florence: UNICEF Innocenti Research Centre.

3. The WHOQOL Group (1995) The World Health Organization quality of life assessment (WHOQOL): position paper from the World Health Organization. *Soc Sci Med* 41: 1403–1409.

4. Zekovic B, Renwick R (2003) Quality of life for children and adolescents with developmental disabilities: review of conceptual and methodological issues relevant to public policy. *Disabil Soc* 18: 19–34.

5. United Nations (1989) *Convention on the Rights of the Child*. New York: United Nations.

6. United Nations (2006) *Convention on the Rights of Persons with Disabilities. Resolution 60/232*. New York: United Nations.

7. Prout A, James A (1990) *A New Paradigm for the Sociology of Childhood? Provenance, Promise and Problems*. London: Falmer Press.

8. Qvortrup J (1994) *Childhood Matters: An Introduction*. Aldershot: Avebury.

9. Ravens-Sieberer U, Gosch A, Rajmil L, Erhart M, Bruil J, Duer W, et al (2005) KIDSCREEN-52 quality-of-life measure for children and adolescents. *Exp Rev Pharmacoeconomics Outcomes Res* 5: 353–364.

10. World Health Organization (1948) *Official Records of the World Health Organization*, No. 2, p. 100. Geneva: WHO.

11. McConachie H, Huq S, Munir S, et al (2001) Difficulties for mothers in using an early intervention service for children with cerebral palsy in Bangladesh. *Child Care Health Dev* 27: 1–12.

12. Albrecht GL, Devlieger PJ (1999) The disability paradox: high quality of life against all odds. *Soc Sci Med* 48: 977–988.

13. World Health Organization (2001) *International Classification of Functioning, Disability and Health*. Geneva: WHO.

14. World Health Organization (2007) *World Health Organization Classification of Functioning, Disability and Health. Children and Youth Version*. Geneva: WHO.

15. Feeny D, Furlong W, Torrance GW, et al (2002) Multiattribute and single-attribute utility functions for the Health Utilities Index mark 3 system. *Med Care* 40: 113–128.

16. Rabin R, de Charro F (2001) EQ-5D: a measure of health status from the EuroQoL Group. *Ann Med* 33: 337–343.

17. Dolan P, Kahneman D (2008) Interpretations of utility and their implications for the valuation of health. *Economic J* 118: 215–234.

18. Waters E, Davis E, Ronen GM, Rosenbaum P, Livingston M, Saigal S (2009) Quality of life instruments for children and adolescents with neurodisabilities: how to choose the appropriate instrument. *Dev Med Child Neurol* 51: 660–669.

19. Landgraf J, Abetz L, Ware JE (1999) *Child Health Questionnaire (CHQ): A User's Manual, Second Printing*. Boston, MA: HealthAct.

20. Mackie P, Jessen E, Jarvis S (2002) Creating a measure of impact of childhood disability: statistical methodology. *Public Health* 116: 95–101.

21. Carpay HA, Vermeulen J, Stroink H, et al (1997) Disability due to restrictions in childhood epilepsy. *Dev Med Child Neurol* 39: 521–526.

22. Hoare P, Russell M (1995) The quality of life of children with chronic epilepsy and their families: preliminary findings with a new assessment measure. *Dev Med Child Neurol* 37: 689–696.

23. Varni JW, Burwinkle TM, Berrin SJ, et al (2006) The PedsQL in pediatric cerebral palsy: reliability, validity, and sensitivity of the Generic Core Scales and Cerebral Palsy Module. *Dev Med Child Neurol* 48: 442–449.

24. Hunt SM (1997) The problem of quality of life. *Qual Life Res* 6: 205–212.

25. Smith KW, Avis NE, Assmann SF (1999) Distinguishing between quality of life and health status in quality of life research: a meta-analysis. *Qual Life Res* 8: 447–459.

26. Rosenbaum PL, Livingston MH, Palisano RJ, Galuppi BE, Russell DJ (2007) Quality of life and health-related quality of life of adolescents with cerebral palsy. *Dev Med Child Neurol* 49: 516–521.

27. Ronen GM, Rosenbaum P, Law M, Streiner DL (1999) Health-related quality of life in childhood epilepsy: the results of children's participation in identifying the components. *Dev Med Child Neurol* 41: 554–559.

28. Bjornson KF, McLaughlin FJ (2001) The measurement of health-related quality of life (HRQL) in children with cerebral palsy. *Eur J Neurol* 8: 183–193.

29. Ronen GM, Rosenbaum P, Law M, Streiner DL (2001) Health-related quality of life in childhood disorders: a modified focus group technique to involve children. *Qual Life Res* 10: 71–79.

30. McLaughlin JF, Bjornson KF (1998) Quality of life and developmental disabilities. *Dev Med Child Neurol* 40: 435.

31. Eiser C, Morse R (2001) Can parents rate their child's health-related quality of life? Results of a systematic review. *Qual Life Res* 10: 347–357.

32. Ronen GM, Streiner DL, Rosenbaum P (2003) Health-related quality of life in children with epilepsy: development and validation of self-report and parent proxy measures. *Epilepsia* 44: 598–612.

33. Baars R, Atherton C, Koopman H, Bullinger M, Power M, DISABKIDS group (2005) The European DISABKIDS project: development of seven condition-specific modules to measure health related quality of life in children and adolescents. *Health Qual Life Outcomes* 3: 70.

34. Streiner DL (2003) Being inconsistent about consistency: when coefficient alpha does and doesn't matter. *J Pers Assess* 80: 217–222.

35. Solans M, Pane S, Estrada MD, et al (2008) Health-related quality of life measurement in children and adolescents: a systematic review of generic and disease-specific instruments. *Value Health* 11: 742–764.

36. Ravens-Sieberer U, Gosch A, Rajmil L, et al (2008) The KIDSCREEN-52 quality of life measure for children and adolescents: psychometric results from a cross-cultural survey in 13 European countries. *Value Health* 11: 645–658.

37. Raphael D, Rukholm E, Brown I, Hill-Bailey P, Donato E (1996) The Quality of Life Profile – Adolescent Version: background, description, and initial validation. *J Adolesc Health* 19: 366–375.

38. Collier J, MacKinlay D, Phillips D (2000) Norm values for the Generic Children's Quality of Life Measure (GCQ) from a large school-based sample. *Qual Life Res* 9: 617–623.

39. Varni JW, Burwinkle TM (2005) The PedsQL 4.0 generic score scales as a pediatric PRO instrument: experiences with over 18,000 children and their parents. *PRO Newsletter* 35(Fall): 1–4.

40. Waters E, Davis E, Mackinnon A, et al (2007) Psychometric properties of the Quality of Life Questionnaire for Children with Cerebral Palsy. *Dev Med Child Neurol* 49: 49–55.

41. Parkin PC, Kirpalani HM, Rosenbaum PL, et al (1997) Development of a health-related quality of life instrument for use in children with spina bifida. *Qual Life Res* 6: 123–132.

42. Narayanan UG, Fehlings D, Weir S, Knights S, Kiran S, Campbell K (2006) Initial development and validation of

the Caregiver Priorities and Child Health Index of Life with Disabilities (CPCHILD). *Dev Med Child Neurol* 48: 804–812.

43. Renwick R, Schormans A (2004) *Final Research Report. Quality of Life for Children with Long Term Disabilities. Instrument Development and Validation*. Toronto, ON: University of Toronto.

44. Bradford R, Rutherford DL, John A (2002) Quality of life in young people: ratings and factor structure of the Quality of Life Profile – Adolescent Version. *J Adolesc* 25: 261–274.

45. Collier J, MacKinlay D (1997) Developing a generic child quality of life measure. *Health Psychol Update* 28: 12–16.

46. Jirojanakul P, Skevington SM, Hudson J (2003) Predicting young children's quality of life. *Soc Sci Med* 57: 1277–1288.

47. Varni JW, Seid M, Rode CA (1999) The PedsQL™: measurement model for the Pediatric Quality of Life Inventory. *Med Care* 37: 126–139.

48. Varni JW, Seid M, Kurtin PS (2001) PedsQL 4.0: reliability and validity of the Pediatric Quality of Life Inventory version 4.0 generic core scales in healthy and patient populations. *Med Care* 39: 800–812.

49. Waters E, Maher E, Salmon L, Reddihough D, Boyd R (2005) Development of a condition-specific measure of quality of life for children with cerebral palsy; empirical thematic data reported by parents and children. *Child Care Health Dev* 31: 127–135.

50. Waters E, Davis E, Boyd R, et al (2006) *Manual: Cerebral Palsy Quality of Life Questionnaire for Children (CP QOL-Child)*. Melbourne: Deakin University.

51. Davis E, Shelly A, Waters E, et al (2009) Quality of life of adolescents with cerebral palsy: perspectives of adolescents and parents. *Dev Med Child Neurol* 51: 193–199.

52. Lach LM, Ronen GM, Rosenbaum PL, et al (2006) Health-related quality of life in youth with epilepsy: theoretical model for clinicians and researchers. Part I: the role of epilepsy and co-morbidity. *Qual Life Res* 15: 1161–1171.

53. Kirpalani HM, Parkin PC, Willan AR, et al (2000) Quality of life in spina bifida: importance of parental hope. *Arch Dis Child* 83: 293–297.

54. Narayanan U, Weir S, Fehlings D (2007) *CPCHILD: Manual and Interpretation Guide*. Toronto, ON: Hospital for Sick Children.

INDEX OF TESTS

SUBJECT INDEX

Notes: Page numbers in *italics* indicates material in figures or tables. *vs.* indicates a differential diagnosis or comparison.

DATE DUE FOR RETURN

0 4 JAN 2016

2 7 JAN 2016

3 0 APR 2016

WEN

TG

Renewals
www.liverpool.gov.uk/libraries
0151 233 3000